The Evidence for Cardiothoracic Surgery

Edited by

Tom Treasure

Ian Hunt

Bruce Keogh

Domenico Pagano

Publisher

tfm Publishing Limited
Castle Hill Barns
Harley
Shrewsbury
SY5 6LX
UK

Tel: +44 (0)1952 510061
Fax: +44 (0)1952 510192
E-mail: nikki@tfmpublishing.com
Web site: www.tfmpublishing.com

Design and layout: Nikki Bramhill
Cartoon on front cover: Barry Foley

First Edition © 2005

ISBN 1 903378 20 6

Neither the authors, the editors nor the publisher can accept responsibility for any injury or damage to persons or property occasioned through the implementation of any ideas or use of any product described herein. Neither can they accept any responsibility for errors, omissions or misrepresentations, howsoever caused.

Whilst every care is taken by the authors, the editors and the publisher to ensure that all information and data in this book are as accurate as possible at the time of going to press, it is recommended that readers seek independent verification of advice on drug or other product usage, surgical techniques and clinical processes prior to their use.

The authors, editors and publisher gratefully acknowledge the permission granted to reproduce the copyright material where applicable in this book. Every effort has been made to trace copyright holders and to obtain their permission for the use of copyright material. The publisher apologizes for any errors or omissions and would be grateful if notified of any corrections that should be incorporated in future reprints or editions of this book.

Printed by Gutenberg Press Ltd., Gudja Road, Tarxien, PLA 19, Malta.

Tel: +356 21897037; Fax: +356 21800069.

Contents

Contributors

Ani C Anyanwu MD MSc FRCS, Specialist Registrar, Cardiothoracic Surgery, Harefield Hospital, Harefield, Middlesex, UK.

Nick G Bellenger BSc MD MRCP, Specialist Registrar, Cardiology, Wessex Cardiothoracic Centre, Southampton, UK.

Robert S Bonser FRCP FRCS FESC, Consultant Cardiothoracic Surgeon, Queen Elizabeth Hospital, University Hospital Birmingham NHS Trust, Birmingham, UK.

Robert J Cerfolio MD FACS, Associate Professor of Cardiothoracic Surgery, University of Alabama, Birmingham, Alabama, USA.

Aman S Coonar BSc MD MRCP FRCS, Specialist Registrar, Cardiothoracic Surgery, Guy's and St. Thomas' Hospitals, London, UK.

David Crossman MD FRCP FESC FACC, Professor of Cardiology, Northern General Hospital, Sheffield, UK.

Nicholas P Curzen PhD FRCP, Consultant Interventional Cardiologist, Wessex Cardiothoracic Centre, Southampton, UK.

Richard C Daly MD, Consultant in Cardiac Surgery & Director of Cardiac and Pulmonary Transplantation, Mayo Clinic, Rochester, MN, USA.

Brian M Fabri MD FRCS (Ed), Consultant Cardiac Surgeon, The Cardiothoracic Centre, Liverpool, UK.

S William Fountain FRCS, Consultant Thoracic Surgeon, Harefield Hospital, Harefield, Middlesex, UK.

P Jeremy George MD FRCP, Consultant Thoracic Physician, Middlesex Hospital, London, UK.

Martin J Goddard FRCS FRCPath, Consultant Histopathologist, Papworth Hospital, Cambridge, UK.

Jennifer Hill MSc PhD, Research Fellow, National Collaborating Centre for Acute Care, The Royal College of Surgeons of England, London, UK.

Ian Hunt BSc (Hons) MRCS, Specialist Registrar, Cardiothoracic Surgery, St Thomas' Hospital, London, UK & Research Fellow, National Collaborating Centre for Acute Care, The Royal College of Surgeons of England, London, UK.

Parag Jaiswal MRCS, Senior House Officer, Cardiothoracic Surgery, Guy's and St. Thomas' Hospitals, London, UK.

WR Eric Jamieson MD, Professor of Surgery, St. Paul's Hospital, Vancouver, Canada & Department of Surgery, University of British Columbia, Vancouver, Canada.

Bruce Keogh KBE BSc MD FRCS FESC FETCS, Professor of Cardiac Surgery, University College London, London, UK.

Gregory YH Lip MD FRCP, Professor of Cardiovascular Medicine, Haemostasis, Thrombosis and Vascular Biology Unit, University Department of Medicine, City Hospital, Birmingham, UK.

Frank M McCaughan MRCP, Specialist Registrar, Thoracic Medicine, Middlesex Hospital, London, UK.

Shafi Mussa MA MRCS, Specialist Registrar, Cardiothoracic Surgery, John Radcliffe Hospital, Oxford, UK.

Domenico Pagano MD (Naples) MD (Birmingham) FRCS (Eng-C-Th) FETCS FESC, Consultant Cardiothoracic Surgeon, Queen Elizabeth Hospital, University Hospital Birmingham NHS Trust, Birmingham, UK.

Kiran CR Patel MA PhD MRCP, Specialist Registrar, Cardiology, Queen Elizabeth Hospital, University Hospital Birmingham NHS Trust, Birmingham, UK.

John R Pepper MA MChir FRCS, Professor of Cardiothoracic Surgery, Royal Brompton Hospital and The National Heart & Lung Institute, London, UK.

David R Ramsdale MD FRCP, Consultant Cardiologist, The Cardiothoracic Centre, Liverpool, UK.

Aaron M Ranasinghe MRCS, Specialist Registrar, Cardiothoracic Surgery, Queen Elizabeth Hospital, University Hospital Birmingham NHS Trust, Birmingham, UK.

Stephan Schueler MD FRCS, Professor and Consultant in Cardiothoracic Surgery and Transplantation, Freeman Hospital, Newcastle upon Tyne & Honorary Lecturer, University of Newcastle upon Tyne, Newcastle upon Tyne, UK.

Artyom Sedrakyan MD ScC, Honorary Lecturer and Research Scholar, The Royal College of Surgeons of England and The London School of Hygiene and Tropical Medicine, London, UK.

Paul J Sheridan MB ChB MRCP PhD, Specialist Registrar, Cardiology, Northern General Hospital, Sheffield, UK.

Simon Swift MB BS BSc MRCS, Specialist Registrar, Thoracic Surgery, Harefield Hospital, Harefield, Middlesex, UK.

David P Taggart MD (Hons) PhD FRCS, Professor of Cardiovascular Surgery, University of Oxford (*from Oct 2004*) and Consultant Cardiothoracic Surgeon, John Radcliffe Hospital, Oxford, UK.

Carol Tan MB ChB MRCS(Eng), Specialist Registrar, Thoracic Surgery, Guy's and St Thomas' Hospitals, London, UK.

Kiat T Tan MRCP, Research Fellow, Cardiovascular Medicine, Haemostasis, Thrombosis and Vascular Biology Unit, University Department of Medicine, City Hospital, Birmingham, UK.

Louise Thomas BA MA, Research Associate, National Collaborating Centre for Acute Care, The Royal College of Surgeons of England, London, UK.

Tom Treasure MD MS FRCS, Professor of Cardiothoracic Surgery, Guy's and St Thomas' Hospitals, London, UK.

David Waller MB BS FRCS (C/Th) FCCP, Consultant Thoracic Surgeon, Glenfield Hospital, Leicester, UK.

Francis C Wells MA MS FRCS, Consultant Cardiothoracic Surgeon, Papworth Hospital, Cambridge, UK.

Donald C Whitaker FRCS (Ed), Specialist Registrar, Cardiothoracic Surgery, Guy's and St. Thomas' Hospitals, London, UK.

Joseph Zacharias FRCS (CTh), Consultant Cardiothoracic Surgeon, Blackpool Victoria Hospital, Blackpool, UK.

Foreword

The phrase "evidence-based medicine" was coined in the early 1990s and, love it or hate it, it has entered the language of Health Services Research. Health care providers in caring societies want to find the best value for their pounds, euros and dollars. It makes sense to spend money where it will get the best health gains and to stop spending it where there is less health gain, no net benefit, or where the benefits can be gained more cheaply, more safely or with less inconvenience.

We asked our writers to look systematically at the literature and review selected topics. In some instances where practice has developed recently (for example lung volume reduction surgery, video-assisted thoracic surgery and adjuvant chemotherapy) we knew there were randomised controlled trials (RCTs). Some of the big topics such as surgery for lung cancer and heart valve surgery were already well developed before it was considered appropriate to do randomised trials and there, the evidence is from case series. Our ideal (not always achievable) was to come as close as possible to a series of systematic reviews. For that purpose the literature is searched formally and thoroughly according to search protocols. Evidence tables are created and only then does writing start. The emphasis is on the evidence with relatively less on opinion. It is in marked contrast to the old approach to a review where the article is dominated by opinion and is written from a breadth and depth of knowledge and experience. The literature is consulted to confirm the details and finally cited for further reading. But in many areas of surgery, however thorough the search, there are no RCTs. Then we rely heavily on the authoritative voice of experts and masters.

We are grateful to all our writers for taking on the huge task we set them and hope they will be proud to be part of a book which attempts to set out "The Evidence for Cardiothoracic Surgery".

The Editors

Tom Treasure MD MS FRCS

Tom Treasure is Professor of Cardiothoracic Surgery at Guy's and St Thomas' Hospitals. Previously, he was at the Middlesex and University College Hospitals from 1982 to 1990 and then at St George's Hospital, all in London, England. For twenty years he did a wide range of adult heart and chest surgery, including cardiac transplantation, and had a special interest in aortic surgery. In 2001, he was invited to join the Thoracic Unit at Guy's Hospital. Professor Treasure is an experienced editor, and has held several editorial positions, currently at the *BMJ*, and previously *The Lancet* (until 2003), *Heart* and the *World Journal of Surgery*.

Bruce Keogh KBE BSc MD FRCS FESC FETCS

Bruce Keogh is Professor of Cardiac Surgery at University College London. Prior to this he has held posts as a Consultant Cardiothoracic Surgeon at the University Hospital Birmingham and as a British Heart Foundation Senior Lecturer and Consultant Surgeon at the Royal Postgraduate Medical School, Hammersmith Hospital in London. He spent his childhood in Zimbabwe, but undertook his medical and surgical training in the UK. He is Secretary General of the European Association for Cardio-Thoracic Surgery.

Domenico Pagano MD (Naples) MD (Birmingham) FRCS (Eng-C-Th) FETCS FESC

Domenico Pagano is a Consultant Cardiothoracic Surgeon at the Queen Elizabeth Hospital in Birmingham. He undertook undergraduate medical studies at the University of Naples (II Faculty) and surgical training in the UK.

Ian Hunt BSc (Hons) MRCS

Ian Hunt is currently working as a Specialist Registrar in Cardiothoracic Surgery at St Thomas' Hospital. He qualified from University College London Medical School and completed his basic surgical training at the Hammersmith Hospital in London before spending a year as a general surgical registrar in New Zealand. He has recently worked as a systematic reviewer, developing guidelines for the National Collaborating Centre for Acute Care.

Acknowledgement

The editors would like to thank Clare Jenkin for her support and help in progressing this book.

Introduction

Applying evidence-based medicine to cardiothoracic surgery

Jennifer Hill MSc PhD, Research Fellow [1]
Ian Hunt BSc (Hons) MRCS, Specialist Registrar, Cardiothoracic Surgery [2] & Research Fellow [1]

1 National Collaborating Centre for Acute Care, London, UK
2 St Thomas' Hospital, London, UK

What is evidence-based medicine?

In evidence-based medicine, individual patient care is based on the best evidence currently available, used in conjunction with the expertise of clinicians and patient preferences.

The best evidence is provided by studies that are well-conducted, and relevant to the issue of interest.

Why use evidence-based medicine?

Analysis of the body of research evidence available enables informed judgements to be made about the most suitable management strategy for an individual patient. In order to do this the clinician needs to keep up-to-date with the best practice in a particular area. This is a time-consuming activity that can be difficult for a busy clinician to fit into their working week. The amount of literature published and the fast pace of research in many areas leads to rapid changes in best practice, as new studies reveal better patient management strategies than were previously used. However, selective reading of the literature is likely to reveal only part of the story, as single results may not be representative of the wider body of literature and better-designed studies may have been conducted but published elsewhere.

Fortunately, it is becoming easier to practise evidence-based medicine. The reasons for this include:-

- The development of computer-based databases of references and reference searching software. These have made feasible the task of comprehensively searching the millions of articles published (see under "Useful sources of evidence").
- The availability of software designed to help reviewers manage and sort large numbers of references. References with abstracts can usually be imported directly from electronic databases.
- The development of rigorous methods for undertaking systematic reviews. This has provided guidance and standardisation of methods for people undertaking evidence-based review work.
- Additionally, there are an increasing number of dedicated journals and books that specialise in

the dissemination of evidence-based reviews in medicine. They provide valuable resources for those looking for the best available evidence.

Useful sources of evidence

- Cochrane Central Register of Controlled Trials (CENTRAL).
- MEDLINE - (USA) 3900 journals.
- EMBASE - (Europe) 4000 journals.
- CINAHL - nursing and allied health literature.
- SIGLE - grey literature: research reports, thesis, conference proceedings, technical reports.
- Hand searching, particularly relevant journals, conference proceedings, etc.

How do you practise evidence-based medicine?

A systematic review of literature is based on a thorough literature search and critical appraisal of studies. Before starting the literature search however, it is essential that a well-defined question has been formed that is specific to the problem that you are trying to solve.

For example, to find out whether lobectomy is a more effective treatment than wedge resection for lung cancer, a detailed question should be formulated as the starting point for the investigation. The question must specify the patient group of interest (eg. stage I non-small cell lung cancer patients who are candidates for surgery), the intervention to be examined (eg. lobectomy), an alternative with which to compare this intervention (eg. wedge resection), and the outcome with which to judge the intervention (eg. survival at two years).

When the question is formulated, a search strategy must be designed that will find the references to help answer the question. There is a balance between sensitivity and specificity of the search. An overly selective search will miss some useful papers, but an overly inclusive search will provide too large a number of papers to sift through. Searches should be conducted using comprehensive databases such as MEDLINE and EMBASE. It is valuable to search on both of these databases as MEDLINE contains mostly North American journals, whereas EMBASE has more European titles. Other specialist databases may be available depending on the topic of interest, and hand searching of specific journals may be useful.

Titles and abstracts are sifted for relevance when the search is complete. This can be a time-consuming process, but having a specific question formed prior to the search helps the reviewer tailor the search criteria for finding references and aids selection of the papers of interest.

Once a set of papers have been identified which look like they will be useful, the next important step is to assess the validity of each study along with the size of the effect and the usefulness or applicability to clinical practice. To assess whether the study is valid, the methodology is closely examined to check, for example, whether patients were randomly assigned to receive a specific treatment, that this randomisation was concealed from the clinicians and the patients and whether a control group was included in the study. Studies of therapies that use this methodology are called randomised controlled trials (RCTs).

In evidence-based medicine a "hierarchy of evidence" has been developed. It classifies the type of literature based on its perceived power of the method as an evidence provider (see Table 1) [1]. The highest level of evidence is the RCT design, which is classified using Table 1 as "level-I" evidence. However, in the field of surgery, studies of this design are rare due to the obvious difficulties of blinding either the patients or clinicians to the intervention type. When there is no level-I evidence available, one then looks for the next best level of evidence available according to the hierarchy. In addition, levels of evidence are then tied as "grades of evidence or recommendations". Table 2 shows an example of a grading system for recommendations used previously by NICE [2].

Surgical outcomes are affected not only by the surgical technique chosen but the presence of significant co-morbidities, prognostic factors and

Table 1. Levels of evidence.

Level	Type of evidence
Ia	Evidence obtained from systematic review of meta-analysis of randomised controlled trials
Ib	Evidence obtained from at least one randomised controlled trial
IIa	Evidence obtained from at least one well-designed controlled study without randomisation
IIb	Evidence obtained from at least one other type of well-designed quasi-experimental study
III	Evidence obtained from well-designed non-experimental descriptive studies, such as comparative studies, correlation studies and case studies
IV	Evidence obtained from expert committee reports or opinions and/or clinical experience of respected authorities

Table 2. Grades of evidence.

Grade of evidence	Evidence
A	At least one randomised controlled trial as part of a body of literature of overall good quality and consistency addressing the specific recommendation (evidence levels Ia and Ib)
B	Well-conducted clinical studies but no randomised clinical trials on the topic of recommendation (evidence levels IIa, IIb, III)
C	Expert committee reports or opinions and/or clinical experience of respected authorities. This grading indicates that directly applicable clinical studies or good quality are absent (evidence level IV)

other aspects of patient selection. For example, if studying the outcomes of two groups of patients, one of which had coronary artery bypass grafting (CABG) and the other medical therapy, it would be important to check whether possible confounding factors had been taken into account (eg. severity of illness, age and comorbidities such as history of stroke). These factors should be approximately the same in the two groups of studies or else there is the possibility that differences in the outcomes of the groups may be due to these factors rather than the intervention itself.

Even if full "blinding" of all investigators involved in the study is not possible, as used in drug trials, randomisation of patients into treatment and control groups using methods of allocation concealment will help to counter potential confounding factors. In addition, follow-up should be of adequate length after surgery to measure all relevant outcomes and ideally carried out by clinicians not involved in the early parts of the trial and "blind" to the group allocation. Patients who dropped out of the study should be detailed so that it is clear whether these were random occurrences or systematic in some way. In practice, much of the surgical evidence does consist of case-control studies and their systematic reviews, case-series or evidence from expert opinion and clinical experience of expert bodies (eg. committee reports).

All types of study should also be assessed using rigorous methods of critical appraisal in order to produce a quality systematic review. This involves careful examination of the methods for possible ways that the study could be biased. If it appears from the methodology that there is a high probability the results are biased in one direction or the other, it may well be wise to discard this paper from the review.

In this manner the past literature can be summarised and compared logically and conclusions about best practice made. When putting the findings into practice, the evidence should be combined with the patients' own preferences and the expertise of the clinician.

In this book, the authors have conducted this rigorous procedure, providing an up-to-date guide of the best evidence available in each of the areas of cardiothoracic surgery that follow.

References

1. Eccles M, Mason J. How to develop cost-conscious guidelines. *Health Technol Assess* 2001; 5(16).
2. National Institute for Clinical Excellence. Information for National Collaborating Centres and Guideline Development Groups. National Institute for Clinical Excellence, London, 2001.

Chapter 1

A brief history of evidence

Tom Treasure MD MS FRCS

Professor of Cardiothoracic Surgery

Guy's and St Thomas' Hospitals, London, UK

The phrase "evidence-based medicine" appeared for the first time on a keyword search of PubMed in 1992 when there were two citations using this phrase. Over the next three years there were 6, 12 and 77 citations, reaching over a 1000 in 1998 and over 2000 in 2001 (Figure 1). It peaked in 2001 and there was a small drop in 2003 almost like an epidemic, that had peaked and was probably now declining. Phrases come and go, in and out of fashion; authors want to be published and use words that are of their time. If the vogue term at the end of the twentieth century was "evidence-based medicine", it would be interesting to ask on what basis did our predecessors in surgery justify what they offered to patients, if it was not on the available evidence?

An occasional look at history gives us insight and a better perspective about what we do now. The surgeons of 100 and 200 years ago had human attributes identical to our own; as a species we have not evolved, but there are at least two differences in how doctors see themselves. One is that we have a very different repertoire of scientific knowledge. We are likely to believe that it is a more complete knowledge - that we have biological science just about right now. The other is the context of health care and society's expectation within which we work as surgeons.

> *For hundreds ... of years two forms of serious chronic disease dominated medical practice ... One, consumption thinned and shrank the body; the other, dropsy, bloated and dulled it* [1].

Dropsy or, as we would now call it, oedema, was a familiar condition. Samuel Johnson wrote to his friend Boswell in 1784:-

> *A dropsy gains ground upon me; my legs and thighs are very much swollen with water, which I should be content if I could keep it there, but I am afraid it will soon be higher* [1].

Physicians of the time had a unifying concept that dropsy was a failure of the body's ability to handle water and keep it in its rightful compartment. In dropsy, water from the blood moved into the "cellular texture" rather than forming urine. How much better we understand oedema now - but in fact, we have an understanding based on present beliefs which serves us as well as theirs served them. It might be a mistake to regard it as complete, finished and immutable. I heard a scientific physician explaining an illness recently as due to "mitochondrial stress". That sounds good but what does it mean? What will doctors 100 years from now make of that explanation? I have no

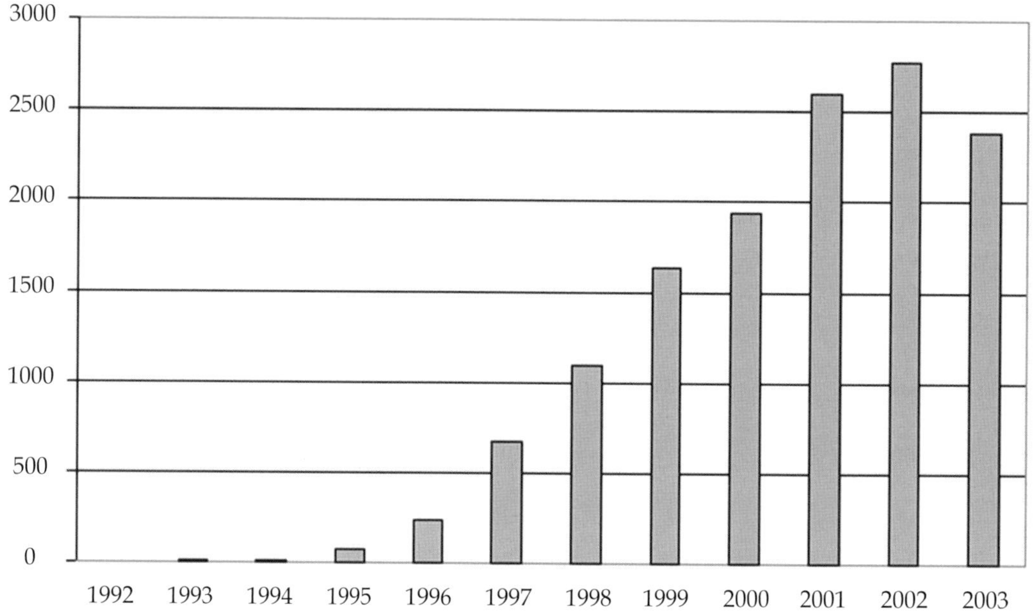

Figure 1. Years 1992 to 2003 with the number of citations found on the keyword search for "evidence-based medicine".

idea but it helps to remember that many of our present beliefs and practices are very different from those of even a few years ago.

We believe that whenever we treat patients, suggest a diagnostic test, or recommend anything from an operation to change in lifestyle we should have good reason to believe it to be effective and beneficial. From our present perspective, 50 to 100 years ago, health care was delivered patchily and unevenly, much less of it was effective, and was based on an image of a kindly doctor treating the sick who were glad of whatever help could be offered. Now we have some really effective treatments, operations and health care strategies. Much of what we do in medicine is effective, but a lot of it is probably not. Whether you look at it from the point of view of the civil purse (that is government expense) or big business in private health care insurance, there is no sense in spending money on ineffective treatments while we do not have enough to spend on what is of proven worth. Individual doctors cannot read everything and cannot possibly synthesise what they do read, in order to be sure of what is proven to be effective and what probably is not. Being confident that what we do is proven to be effective, and if there are choices, that the most effective of treatments are available, is the kernel of what is understood by evidence-based medicine in current parlance. In this chapter I will look at the types of evidence cardiothoracic surgeons have relied upon and briefly analyse them from a historical perspective.

By applying what is known to be effective we can prevent or minimise the seven ubiquitous health care problems [2]:-

1. Errors and mistakes.
2. Poor quality of care.
3. Waste.
4. Unknowing variations in policy and practice.
5. Poor patient experience.
6. Over enthusiastic adoption of interventions of low value.
7. Failure to get new evidence into practice.

Medical knowledge on which we base our decisions about health care can be considered under three headings:-

- Knowledge from research = evidence.
- Knowledge from databases = statistics.
- Knowledge from experience = mistakes.

It is under heading six and seven that we look to research evidence. To the current way of thinking, scientifically rigorous randomised trials provide the best (Levels Ia and Ib) evidence [3] that:-

- a treatment is effective;
- if there is a placebo arm, that treatment is better than doing nothing; and
- which of two or more possible treatments should be used.

Only with evidence from trials can we make Grade A recommendations. Does that mean that in the absence of a trial a treatment cannot be recommended? In surgery that would leave us with very little to offer. From the coining of the phrase "evidence-based medicine" which seems to have been about 1992 judging from PubMed, one might jump to the conclusion that medical and surgical practice was based simply on the beliefs and inherited wisdom of its practitioners before that date - and with no evidence. If we looked at medical practice throughout the world and throughout the history of man, it would be seen that the practice of medicine has been based on belief systems and the authority of respected practitioners far more often than on what we would now regard as evidence; scientific plausibility, objective evaluation, and the scrutiny of outsiders are perhaps unwelcome late comers to medical practice [4]. What we call western scientific medicine has existed only in the last two centuries, and some would narrow it down to the last 50 years [5]. In this chapter I will look at what surgeons have relied upon as the evidence on which to base the practice of surgery of the chest.

Who obtains the evidence and how is it passed on?

Historically, it is doctors themselves who suggest ideas for treating disease. They try out their treatments, draw some conclusions as to efficacy, and they report to their colleagues in journals (Figure 2). My first contention is that evidence usually follows innovation, rather than leads to it. Dissemination may depend on evidence and quite rightly so, but historically, the publication burst follows rather than precedes the first attempts on patients. It might be different in the future but the concept that basic science research leads and lights the way as in the nice phrases "molecules to man" and "bench to bedside" remains hypothetical [5].

As an area of practice becomes sufficiently large and productive to justify it, a journal is started up. The *Journal of Thoracic Surgery* was first published in 1931. To give some historical context, operations such as empyema drainage, lobectomy for bronchiectasis, thoracoplasty to collapse tuberculous cavities, were all in use at the time the journal was first published; operations for persistent ductus arteriosus and coarctation were not performed until the 1940s. In 1959 the journal changed its name to the *Journal of Thoracic and Cardiovascular Surgery* (JTCVS), reflecting the changing practice from thoracic to cardiothoracic surgery. This was about ten years after the first successful series of mitral valvotomies and about five years after the first use of cardiopulmonary bypass.

It is also interesting to reflect on why cardiac surgery in London started at general hospitals (Guy's and The Middlesex) and at chest hospitals (Brompton and Harefield) rather than at the Heart Hospital. It was because the surgeons doing thoracic surgery turned their hands to the duct, coarctation and the mitral valve. The Heart Hospital had no surgeons until heart surgery was established as a practice [6]. The specialty of cardiac surgery followed an evolving practice - it could not lead it.

I have looked at the contents of the JTCVS for the month of May at the end of each decade from 1940 to 2000 to discover what chest surgeons have wanted to present to each other as evidence to guide practice. It is far from a scientific analysis; I have not formally tested the sample against Gallivan's rule [7]. Whether this simple sampling technique is valid or not for the JTCVS (it would still fail to take account of the other journals setting up such as the *Annals of Thoracic Surgery* in 1965 and the *European Journal of Cardiothoracic Surgery* in 1987), it will serve well enough for the purpose of illustration.

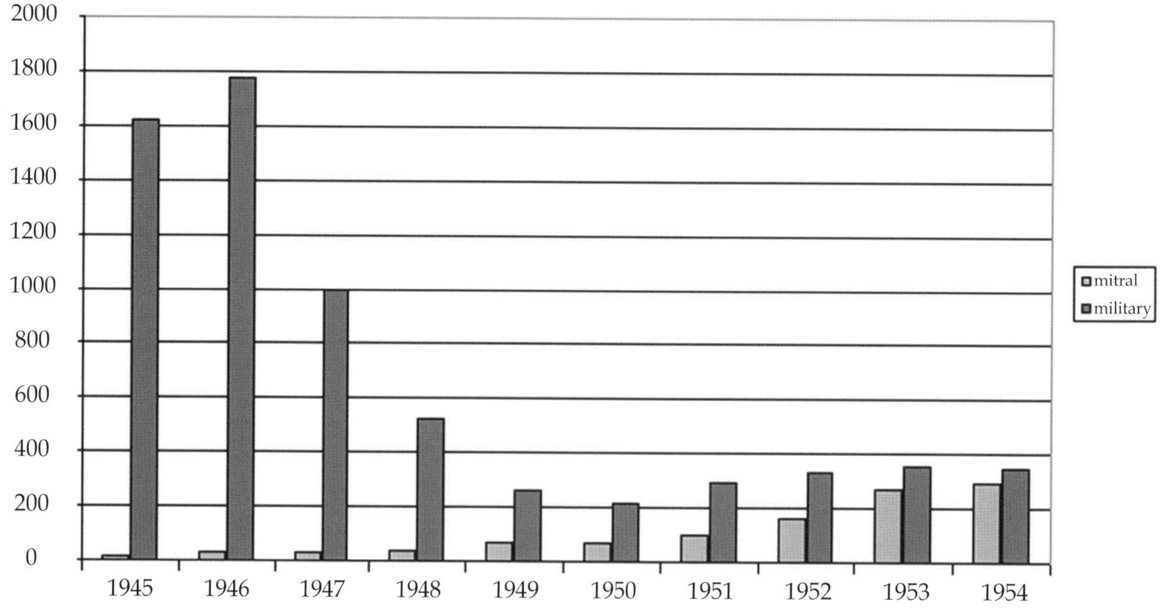

Figure 2. **Research publications do not precede but follow innovation. In pale grey are the number of citations in Index Medicus for 'mitral' covering all aspects of the mitral valve for the ten years spanning the introduction of mitral valvotomy into practice [1]. Conveniently close in Index Medicus is "military medicine". As the war came to an end the very large number of publications under that subject heading rapidly diminished. It provides some sort of comparison or reference point; not every subject is remorselessly increasing.**

In May 1940, five of the eight papers published were descriptions of operative technique. There were 1-3 authors per paper with an average of two. In the same month for 1950 the journal was dominated by clinical series and case reports (I have quite arbitrarily made the distinction at fewer than five cases being case reports). Retrospective reports of clinical series filled about half of the May edition for the next three decades. The rest of the journal is divided between laboratory and clinical science. The number of authors per paper has risen decade by decade to a median of six (IQR 5-7) in May 2000 when there were more than ten authors on some papers. This reflects collaboration with basic scientists and other medical disciplines [3]. I will look at these and some other sources of justification for the work we do and the practices we teach; the word "evidence" may not be regarded as applicable to all but that is to see the world only through contemporary eyes.

Quick fixes, beliefs and revelations: fractures, blood letting and homeopathy

Many aspects of surgery are based on mechanistic solutions to the body's problems: immobilising a fracture, draining an abscess, cutting for a bladder stone. For these the evidence of efficacy was that it worked. More difficult to understand is the very widespread and longstanding practice of blood letting [4], a practice which depended on authority. There was a renaissance debate (1522) about whether it should be performed on the same side as the source of the illness (as taught by Hippocrates and Galen) or on the opposite side which had become the practice due to a mistranslation. We still have a practice of medicine based almost completely on the vision and authority of a single man, Samuel Hahnemann (1755-1833). Concerned by the frequent deleterious effects of medicines (put simply he believed that doctors were systematically poisoning people with treatments such as arsenic), he formulated his own principles of treatment. He taught two laws: his first law of similars (let like be cured by like) and his second law of infinitesimals (the smaller the dose the more efficacious the medicine). Homeopathy is widely practised [8] and patronized by the British Royal Family.

Case reports

One of the best known quotes in cardiac surgical folklore is from Paget [9] who in 1896 wrote:-

Surgery of the heart has probably reached the limits set by Nature to all surgery: no new method, and no new discovery can overcome the natural difficulties that attend a wound of the heart.

The book has one after another elegantly written and meticulously described case reports, of wounds, empyema, lung hernias, tubercular phthisis and so on.

On hernia of the lung (pp5-6) he describes three cases:-

1. A child aged 13 fell from a height coming down on a sharp piece of wood ...
2. A man, while drunk, received a penetrating wound below the nipple, but was too drunk to heed it ...
3. A young soldier in the American war was shot in the left side of the chest ...

And then writes:-

From these cases ... we draw a good clinical picture of hernia of the lung after injury.

There is a long and still thriving tradition of presenting and writing up cases which persists in grand rounds, mortality and morbidity meetings, and most medical journals. They are popular and as a means of enlivening and giving a concrete example in teaching, they are valuable. They rely on a senior figure of knowledge and authority drawing illustrative points from the case. Note that Paget chooses three to illustrate what he wants to teach. He is in reality using a much wider experience of chest surgery than these three cases as evidence on which to base his teaching, but does not need to set it all out; the cases are there to make his teaching alive and to illustrate its applicability in the tangible and real world of injured people and working surgeons.

By present standards case reports are suspect as a form of "evidence" on which to base any practice or predict the likely outcome. When N=1 what credibility can they have in an era when we are looking for statistical power in larger and larger trials, and then performing meta-analyses on accumulated trials? However, to return to the three types of medical knowledge on which we base the delivery of health care [2]:-

- Knowledge from research = evidence.
- Knowledge from databases = statistics.
- Knowledge from experience = mistakes.

If we document a case where there was a single mistake, that might provide sufficient evidence to change practice. For example, if the wrong drug was given (because of easily confused names), in the wrong site (intrathecal rather than intravenous), or at ten times the dose (because we store 1:1000 ampoules and 1:10,000 ampoules in the same cupboard), it only requires one case to provide the evidence on which to change practice. No one inserts a UK plug in the wrong way because there is only one way it will fit. The *BMJ*, the British bastion of evidence-based medicine, publishes reports of single cases as a *Lesson of the Week*. Case reports are very poor evidence on which to base a conclusion "in future always do this" but may be sufficient evidence on which to say "never do that again".

Case series

Writing in 1956 Brock's physician colleague, Maurice Campbell, gave his opinion on the importance of studying case series [10]. Campbell wrote:-

I should like to give one message, ... the importance of following up groups of patients:

we sometimes think of this as an uninteresting form of research, but now that we have to take decisions about when to advise operation for these patients we realise the urgent need of accurate knowledge of the natural history and prognosis, and this is often incomplete even for common conditions.

Retrospective case series (defined as more than five cases), constitute over 30% of all the publications in our sample and if reports of five and fewer cases are included, more than half of the publications are in this format. They are therefore arguably the biggest evidence base for cardiothoracic surgical practice. What form of "evidence" do they provide? I will try to demonstrate how they have served well as evidence and where they are now failing us.

If we know the natural history of a disease, and a series of cases are operated on and a much better clinical course ensues, this has been regarded as evidence on which to base a change in practice. The "breakthroughs" in medicine have relied upon this. The natural course of mitral stenosis was very well known from the Victorian era and was well summarized by Lauder Brunton when in 1902 he wrote in the *Lancet* suggesting it might be surgically relieved [11]. Over 20 years later in 1925, Souttar performed the operation of transatrial mitral valvotomy, with success, very much as Brunton had proposed [12]. Mitral stenosis remained familiar but the received wisdom of the time was that this was a condition that surgery could not improve. The myocardium was the main problem and the single success of Souttar was not evidence enough to contradict that belief. In 1948, Bailey and Harken (each after a run of failures) wrote up single survivors [13]. These were single case reports. But between 1948 and 1950 Brock operated on nine cases with seven survivors (the ninth case, the seventh survivor is in a foot note). Instead of going to press with a single report Brock stayed his pen and waited until he had sufficient cases to constitute evidence for change [14] and by 1952 when he wrote up his first 100 cases with 13 deaths the evidence was widely accepted [15]. Brock and mitral valvotomy is just one example of how early in the introduction of a new drug or a new technique the difference between the known natural history for a condition (and remember Campbell's argument above about the importance of case histories [10]) and what is observed with the innovation, appears so striking that this is accepted as evidence.

The reverse is the case where the disease has a variable course, where there is heterogeneity of cases in different series, where the problems are multifactorial, or where the degree of benefit is marginal. Thoracic cancer management in clinically difficult situations has bleak outcomes though patients are desperate for help; giving the opinion "case hopeless" [16] is not one that is always or readily accepted by patients or referring physicians. I will give two illustrations from surgical case series in the 21st century. Superior sulcus lung cancer (or Pancoast tumour) managed by surgery after induction chemotherapy was studied in 111 patients of whom 83 had operations. These were various combinations of lobectomy, pneumonectomy, with or without chest wall resection, and some were just opened and closed. Of them, 53 had further postoperative chemotherapy. This was a multicentre study and 76 surgeons provided cases making an average of one case per surgeon [17]. Survival is reported for eligible patients with complete resections.

Malignant mesothelioma is a disease on the increase due to asbestos exposure in the 1950s to 1970s [18]. Claims for good results by surgery are not only in the prestigious thoracic surgical journals [19] but on web pages [20]. The absence of control groups and the complete failure to make any realistic attempt to analyse how these results might be better than less damaging treatments or indeed, no treatment at all, is out of step with other efforts to ensure that we have evidence for what cardiothoracic surgeons do. However, case series are the commonest form of evidence in the world's most prestigious cardiothoracic surgical journal.

Framing of disease

There are crucial caveats. When we say the "disease" are we all talking about the same condition? There must be an agreed definition of the diagnosis and the stage of the patients. Prior to mitral valvotomy being taken up in practice little attention was paid to making a clear distinction between mitral stenosis and regurgitation, but if the operation for mitral stenosis which Brock had carried out with such success was performed on patients with mixed mitral valve disease, aortic and mitral valve disease, or pure mitral regurgitation, the results were very different.

The first concept to understand is how we categorise diseases. It is very dependent on the view taken of disease at a given time by doctors and society. This is a construct extensively studied by social historians of medicine who use the term "framing" a disease [21]. A simple example familiar to thoracic surgeons is the apparent change in name from consumption to tuberculosis. In an era before microbes were recognised, before Pasteur (1822-1896) and before Koch (1843-1910) who identified the tubercle bacillus, there was a disease called pulmonary consumption characterised by weight loss, the body's tissues wasting away or being consumed [1] which if associated with lung disease was called pulmonary consumption. Once the tubercle bacillus was discovered it became clear that many of these cases were caused by this organism - but not all wasting disease associated with lung pathology is caused by the tubercle bacillus. The diagnosis of tuberculosis is not equivalent to consumption. Once discovered "TB" was used as the diagnosis for any illness in which the organism is deemed to be the cause, whether or not there is weight loss and whether or not the lungs are involved. The diagnostic "frames" are different or at least the frame has shifted. Consumption is framed by a clinical description, and TB by a bacteriological finding. Some of the cases of consumption were caused by lung cancer but to reclassify the cases according to our present frame is not helpful. Pulmonary consumption was (and should remain) whatever was within that diagnostic frame.

There is a tendency for doctors to think we are becoming more scientific and precise in diagnosis. That is not necessarily the case. Lung cancer is an instance in which we have become less precise. The diagnostic frame is defined by histological proof and once we have proven that the tumour is malignant, we then divide cases into small cell and non-small cell cancers. We used to always specify the type (squamous, adenocarcinoma, large cell anaplastic), but now "non-small cell lung cancer" (NSCLC) is an operational diagnostic "frame" which includes a range of much more subtle histological types which for the present are subsumed in NSCLC to distinguish them as a group from small cell lung cancer. Why? Because chemotherapy rather than surgery is the preferred first-line treatment for these. So the "frame" for lung cancers is determined by treatment options. So we have seen examples of disease being framed by its clinical picture, its causative organism, and now by treatment options. All are equally valid. Consumption has not been replaced by TB. We need to understand this concept particularly in diseases where the frame seems to be shifting.

Firsts and breakthroughs

What is often called history by surgeons is the charting of firsts and landmarks [22], and recording the deeds of famous men. Viewed from now these are clear. We can look behind us and find the footprints leading to where we are now - the only logical place to be and the men of vision pointed the way. This is what a professional historian calls "Whig history". The problem is that it just isn't like that. In our own time there is a breaking medical story every week, but very few change the world and enter into the repertoire of standard care [23]. Similarly, if we go back to the now known landmarks and read the papers around them in the journal in which they first appeared, most of them lead nowhere. And yet the editor accepted and published them all and rarely flagged that one as the paper that will change the world. Look up clitoridectomy in the *Lancet*, the *BMJ* and other eminent journals for the 1860s to learn about a then reputable operation for various ills including epilepsy - which it does not relieve.

Basic science and animal laboratories

Our JTCVS sample is not a reliable indicator for the prevalence of laboratory evidence; it has taken more of its share of laboratory work in recent years than the other more clinically based journals while most basic scientists do not publish in the surgical literature. However, the concept that we set up a hypothesis, test it in the animal laboratory, and then take it into practice is in my view fundamentally flawed. This is a continuum variously known by slogans such as "bench to bedside" or "molecules to man" or more obscurely as translational research. It has not been the usual sequence of events in cardiothoracic surgery.

Although all departments in those days had an animal laboratory programme, surgeons did not necessarily find the animal laboratory very helpful in the early days to the extent that Belsey, a pioneer in the use of profound hypothermia and circulatory arrest, wrote:-

> *... experimental animals appear to be more vulnerable to hypothermia than humans and little information of practical value has emerged from this source* [24].

Probably more commonly surgeons "had a go" in the operating theatre first (or early in the process) and went back to the laboratory to resolve the problems they identified. Cardioplegia to protect the myocardium is an example of successful use of this approach. The limiting factor in operating on the heart has been the durability of the heart muscle. We can replace the valves and redirect macroscopic blood flow through the chambers and coronaries, but all was lost too frequently because the ventricle would not contract. Teaming up as a surgeon and basic science duo, Braimbridge and Hearse [25] completed a series of animal laboratory studies exploring the concentrations of potassium and magnesium that would best conserve the myocardial energy substrates so that when cardiac surgery was complete the heart would take over from the bypass machine. It would make an interesting historical study to tease out more about the relative roles of animal laboratory experimentation versus clinical science in the acquisition of evidence in cardiothoracic surgery.

Clinical science

The greatest advances in cardiac surgery were made from the 1950s to the 1980s. This matches an era of great activity in clinical science [5]. The clinical scientist used the human being as the experimental subject and was at times castigated for it [26]. The studies were not of the outcomes of treatment, they were not clinical trials, but the exploration of physiological and pathophysiological mechanisms in both patients and healthy subjects. This form of research continues and features strongly in the sample of publications from the JTCVS. In cardiac surgical research it is usually patients undergoing surgery or intensive care where we take the opportunity to measure flows, pressures, inflammatory mediators, humoral agents - in fact, anything at all. The questions have not always been well framed, the hypotheses often ill-defined, and the effort often driven by a need to get a publication. Someone knows someone in a laboratory who can measure something new.

I will give two examples, one from early in this era and one late, which provided evidence on which practice was changed.

In the early days of cardiac surgery the maintenance of arterial pressure was paramount. Brock began to emphasise the importance of flow and was one of the first to actively dilate the periphery, to monitor the peripheral temperature as an indication that he was achieving the objective - to make the cold peripheries warm - and he led a change in how we thought about the circulation [27].

In the 1980s, we and others were working to reduce the damaging effect of cardiopulmonary bypass on the brain. There was an area of debate about whether a filter placed in the arterial line of the bypass was beneficial by filtering out bubbles or particles, or detrimental by creating a stimulus for platelet aggregation. Wilf Pugsley devised and ran a study in which patients undergoing surgery were randomised into two groups of 50, one half to have an arterial line filter, the other not to have one. The benefit in terms of outcome was shown by better performance on neuropsychological testing in the filtered group and the mechanism was confirmed by a dramatic reduction in high frequency signals over the middle cerebral artery [28]. On a show of hands at the next meeting of the Society of Cardiothoracic Surgeons of Great Britain and Ireland (SCTS), it was agreed that there was sufficient evidence to persuade the majority who did not use filters to change.

Note that in these examples we research both the mechanism and its outcome and those two together provide evidence we trust. In Western medicine we prefer to have both a plausible mechanism and objective evidence of outcome. If we cannot have both the more important is evidence that the treatment is beneficial; if a treatment is unequivocally effective we can use it while remaining uncertain about exactly how it does the good. My continuing disbelief in homeopathy is that it offers neither.

Randomised controlled trials, statistical claims, and meta-analyses

Where they are applicable randomised controlled trials (RCTs) are regarded as the best evidence on which to base practice. The essential features are that the patients must be allocated to the two or more treatment groups (or arms) by a process that ensures there is no bias; randomisation is the usual way but minimisation has advantages [29]. The patient must not know or be able to discern whether the treatment is active or not in order to exclude the placebo effect which is remarkably strong. Those measuring the outcomes must not know either because a biased judgement is remarkably pervasive. Unbiased allocation is possible in surgery, but requires patient and surgeon to forego the right to choose. Blinding is often impossible.

Because of the high prestige of RCTs there is a tendency to call any study with a comparison group a controlled trial, whereas in fact it may be a clinical study of a mechanism (with a control group) rather than a trial of outcome [3]. True trials of outcome are extremely difficult to set up in surgery but the need for trials is of paramount importance. Series of untreated patients directly comparable to the ones in the operated series do not exist now. Historical controls against which early results of surgery might be compared in the 1950s [10] are not valid now. One of the first formal RCTs was in the management of TB with streptomycin [30] and a notorious one was the management of heart attack at home or coronary care [31]. Archie Cochrane after whom the Cochrane Collaboration is named (the shrine of evidence-based medicine if you like), claimed in his autobiography to have mischievously reversed the headings on the results to give his colleagues time to appreciate that there was a difference - in fact, the RCT showed that staying at home was safer. Has that trial ever been repeated? It is also interesting to reflect that the development of cardiac defibrillation and thrombolysis mandated admission to hospital. However, further development of defibrillators and paramedic delivery of thrombolysis might turn that back again. Who knows?

There have been relatively few RCTs in cardiothoracic surgery but those in coronary artery surgery are the largest by far and the best known. At the time it seemed obvious to some that:-

- if people with narrowed arteries died of heart attacks and,
- vascular grafts provided a mechanism to bypass the narrowings, then
- a policy of grafting those discovered to have a narrowing would save lives.

This did not turn out to be the case [32]. Insertion of "some" people in premise 1 and "selected patients at high risk" in premise 3 would have made the hypothesis correct but in fact, the evidence for saving life was slim [33]. Unfortunately, surgeons have not wanted to or have been unable to put patients into randomised trials and have been criticised for it [34]. Case series are still the commonest form of clinical evidence. Surgeons still make claims for benefits based on these series which are so fundamentally flawed that they cannot stand up to scrutiny. When subjected to randomised trial some of our favourite beliefs crumble. The Starr Edwards valve was long ago considered old-fashioned but a review of case histories showed that there were bigger differences attributable to confounders than valve type [35]. We did a randomised trial showing that his caged ball valve was as good at relieving the left ventricle and no worse as regards thromboembolism as the bileaflet valve favoured in the market place [36], but it is unlikely to change beliefs. Arthroscopic surgery of the knee [37] when compared with placebo had no benefit, and laparoscopic removal of the gall bladder [38] had no advantage over open surgery in a randomised trial. Practice continued driven by other considerations. These include the most venal economics of the market place but now "patient choice" is a justification for many unproven practices, conventional and alternative.

Before leaving this matter it is worth reflecting on patient choice. Long before there was a "scientific" evidence base for medicine as we understand it, medicine was a profession, and the clientele had to be served, their wishes subject to whimsy and fashion. For those who think that patient preference is new I quote from an American novel first published in 1911 which recounts the miserable relationship of Ethan Frome and his hypochondriac wife [39]:-

Ethan was aware that, in regard to the important question of surgical intervention, the female opinion of the neighbourhood was divided, some glorying in the prestige conferred by operations while others shunned them as indelicate. Ethan, from motives of economy, had always been glad that Zeena was of the latter faction.

Surgeons and audit

A well known plea for collection and publication of outcome data for comparative audit was made by a Bristol surgeon, Hey Groves, in 1908 [40], but hospitals such as the Rotunda, the Dublin obstetric hospital, and St Thomas' Hospital in London, published detailed annual reports of cases and outcome in 1900. Cardiac surgery was built on counting; the UK cardiac register was published from the 1970s allowing surgeons to see how they were doing compared with their peers [41]. It is now highly politicized.

Surgeons were introduced to statistical analysis

In the beginning of our attempts to claim differences in our experiments and benefits from our treatments, surgeons had to be taught to understand the question "Is it significant?" In a small study there may be an apparent big difference. For instance, an event rate of 80% is much bigger than 20%, but if the groups are only five each the 95% confidence limits are 28% to 99% for 4/5 and 0.5% to 72% for 1/5. To claim a difference which is not significant statistically is called a type I or alpha error. This mistake is not made now. Surgeons have been well taught in that regard. The situation in which this still occurs is for example, if a surgeon claims his operation is "safe" because there have been no deaths in his first ten patients. The 95% confidence limits around 0/10 are 0-31%.

Much more commonly now, rather than lay claim to evidence we do not have, we fail to find the evidence we should because the studies are too small. This is called a type II or beta error; the study is "underpowered" to refute the hypothesis is another way of saying it. A good historical example of this is in studies of prevention of deep vein thrombosis and pulmonary embolism in surgical patients [42]. It seemed that every surgical unit in the 1960s and 1970s was running a little study on this problem and not showing benefit - but not because nothing worked but because they could not show the difference in these small studies. Eventually, a study in over 4,000 patients published in the *Lancet* in 1975 [43] showed a reduction in fatal pulmonary embolism from 0.7% to 0.1%. This is a very big difference but a very small absolute number of events. When the event rate is in single figures, trials of 100 or 1000s are required to have any prospect of showing a difference. From statistics such as this come concepts such as "number needed to treat" to save a life. About 150 patients have to be treated with subcutaneous heparin to save one life if these results are generally applicable.

Meta-analysis

Where there are adequate quality RCTs but individually without sufficient power to give an answer, results can be pooled [44]. This was done for the question of prophylaxis of pulmonary embolism [45].

Consensus

The formal process of finding consensus is a further source of support or justification for what we do. The first use of this in the UK was to explore the applicability of coronary artery surgery in wider practice and contributed its dissemination from the few centres doing reasonably large numbers at the time [46]. The approach has become formalised into smaller expert panels informed by more formally presented "evidence" [47,48]. The process is known generically as a nominal group technique and a particular form, the RAND appropriateness method (RAM), has been used to good effect, again in coronary artery surgery [49].

And so interestingly, we come full circle to the use of experts' advice to determine what we do. When Paget considered heart surgery as "reaching the limits set by nature to all surgery" he was giving a consensus view based on the evidence at the time. The essential feature of creating contemporary guidelines for practice is that available evidence is formally gathered, a process transformed by the use of computer searches and data management, and presented to "experts". They have the power and indeed exercise it, setting the hard won evidence from trials to one side in favour of a synthesis based on their own perception of what should be recommended. It is a social process which is only partly based on science and perhaps the emphasis is shifting away from the scientific model [5]. Caring for our fellow men has more to it than just numerical evidence. It is a caring profession and in it we have to mould science, care, and an internal and external view of surgery as a profession: it comprises caring, counting and accountability [50].

References

1. Peitzman Steven J. From Bright's disease to end-stage renal failure. In: *Framing Disease: studies in cultural history.* Rosenberg CE, Golden J, Eds. Rutgers University Press, New Brunswick, New Jersey, 1992: pp 3-19.
2. Gray, Muir. Presentation to the National Programme for Information Technology (NPfIT). 15-1-2004. Personal Communication.
3. Anyanwu A, Treasure T. Surgical research revisited: clinical trials in the cardiothoracic surgical literature. *Eur J Cardiothorac Surg* (in press) 2004.
4. Porter R. *The Greatest Benefit to Mankind. A medical history of humanity from antiquity to the present.* HarperCollins, London, 1997.
5. Le Fanu J. *The Rise and Fall of Modern Medicine.* Little Brown, London, 1999.
6. Treasure T. Cardiac Surgery. In: *British Cardiology in the 20th Century.* Silverman ME, *et al*, Eds. Springer, London Berlin Heidelberg, 2000: pp192-213.
7. Gallivan S. Gallivan's rule: the size of sample required is that when addition of further cases in not making any difference to the conclusion. This rule must be applied with discretion and in the spirit intended. Professor Steve Gallivan is the Director of the Clinical Operational Research Unit, UCL. 2004. Personal Communication
8. Coulter HL. *Homeopathic Science and Modern Medicine.* North Atlantic Books, Berkley, California, 1980.
9. Paget S. *The Surgery of the Chest.* John Wright and Co, Bristol, 1896.
10. Campbell M. Acyanotic congenital heart disease. Guy's Hospital Gazette 1956; 70: 246-56.
11. Brunton L. Preliminary note on the possibility of treating mitral stenosis by surgical methods. *The Lancet* 1902; i: 352.
12. Souttar HS. The surgical treatment of mitral stenosis. *BMJ* 1925; ii: 603-7.
13. Treasure T, Hollman A. The surgery of mitral stenosis 1898-1948: why did it take 50 years to establish mitral valvotomy? *Ann R Coll Surg Engl* 1995; 77: 145-51.
14. Baker C, Brock RC, Campbell M. Valvulotomy for mitral stenosis. Report of six successful cases. *BMJ* 1950; i: 1283-93.
15. Baker C, Brock RC, Campbell M, Wood P. Valvotomy for mitral stenosis. A further report, on 100 cases. *BMJ* 1952; i: 1043-55.
16. Sullivan D. In his book *Navvyman* Sullivan reprints a letter dated 20/9/22 about the death of a young doctor from septicaemia including the fatal words "case hopeless". Coracle, London, 1983.
17. Rusch VW, Giroux DJ, Kraut MJ, Crowley J, Hazuka M, Johnson D, *et al.* Induction chemoradiation and surgical resection for non-small cell lung carcinomas of the superior sulcus: Initial results of Southwest Oncology Group Trial 9416 (Intergroup Trial 0160). *J Thorac Cardiovasc Surg* 2001; 121: 472-83.
18. Treasure T, Waller D, Swift S, Peto J. Radical surgery for mesothelioma. *BMJ* 2004; 328: 237-8.
19. Sugarbaker DJ, Flores RM, Jaklitsch MT, Richards WG, Strauss GM, Corson JM, *et al.* Resection margins, extrapleural nodal status, and cell type determine postoperative long-term survival in trimodality therapy of malignant pleural mesothelioma: results in 183 patients. *J Thorac Cardiovasc Surg* 1999; 117: 54-63.
20. Sugarbaker DJ, Norberto JJ, Bueno R. Current therapy for mesothelioma. http://moffitt.usf.edu/pubs/ccj/v4n4/article4.html 2002.
21. Rosenberg CE, Golden J, Eds. *Framing Disease: studies in cultural history.* Rutgers University Press, New Brunswick, New Jersey, 1992.
22. Westaby S. *Landmarks in Cardiac Surgery.* Isis Medical Media Ltd, Oxford, UK, 1997.
23. Treasure T. Recent advances. Cardiac surgery. *BMJ* 1997; 315: 104-7.
24. Belsey RH, Dowlatshahi K, Keen G, Skinner DB. Profound hypothermia in cardiac surgery. *J Thorac Cardiovasc Surg* 1968; 56: 497-509.
25. Braimbridge MV, Hearse DJ, Stewart DA. Myocardial preservation during cardiac arrest. *Proc R Soc Med* 1976; 69: 197-9.

26. Papworth M. *Human Guinea Pigs.* Pelican, London, 1969.
27. Ross BA, Brock L, Aynsley-Green A. Observations on central and peripheral temperatures in the understanding and management of shock. *Br J Surg* 1969; 56: 877-82.
28. Pugsley W, Klinger L, Paschalis C, Treasure T, Harrison M, Newman S. The impact of microemboli during cardiopulmonary bypass on neuropsychological functioning. *Stroke* 1994; 25: 1393-9.
29. Treasure T, MacRae KD. Minimisation: the platinum standard for trials?. Randomisation doesn't guarantee similarity of groups; minimisation does. *BMJ* 1998; 317: 362-3.
30. Medical Research Council. Streptomycin treatement of pulmonary tuberculosis: a report of the streptomycin in tuberculosis trials committee. *BMJ* 1948; ii: 769-82.
31. Mather HG, Morgan DC, Pearson NG, Read KL, Shaw DB, Steed GR, *et al.* Myocardial infarction: a comparison between home and hospital care for patients. *BMJ* 1976; 1: 925-9.
32. Myocardial infarction and mortality in the coronary artery surgery study (CASS) randomized trial. *N Engl J Med* 1984; 310: 750-8.
33. Hampton JR. Coronary artery bypass grafting for the reduction of mortality: an analysis of the trials. *Br Med J (Clin Res Ed)* 1984; 289: 1166-70.
34. Horton R. Surgical research or comic opera: questions, but few answers. *Lancet* 1996; 347: 984-5.
35. Treasure T. Which heart valves should we use? *Lancet* 1990; 336: 1115-7.
36. Murday AJ, Hochstitzky A, Mansfield J, Miles J, Taylor B, Whitley E, *et al.* A prospective controlled trial of St. Jude versus Starr Edwards aortic and mitral valve prostheses. *Ann Thorac Surg* 2003; 76: 66-73.
37. Moseley JB, O'Malley K, Petersen NJ, Menke TJ, Brody BA, Kuykendall DH, *et al.* A controlled trial of arthroscopic surgery for osteoarthritis of the knee. *N Engl J Med* 2002; 347: 81-8.
38. Majeed AW, Troy G, Nicholl JP, Smythe A, Reed MW, Stoddard CJ, *et al.* Randomised, prospective, single-blind comparison of laparoscopic versus small-incision cholecystectomy. *Lancet* 1996; 347: 989-94.
39. Wharton E. Ethan Frome (first published 1911). Oxford University Press, Oxford,1996.
40. Hey Groves EW. A plea for a uniform registration of operation results. *BMJ* 1908 (ii): 1008-9.
41. English TA, Bailey AR, Dark JF, Williams WG. The UK cardiac surgical register, 1977-82. *Br Med J (Clin Res Ed)* 1984; 289: 1205-8.
42. Treasure T, Griffin S. Postoperative thromboembolic disease: a tantaliizing enigma. In: *Current Surgical Practice* (Volume 5). Hadfield J, Hobsley M, Treasure T, Eds. Edward Arnold, London,1990: pp38-51.
43. Prevention of fatal postoperative pulmonary embolism by low doses of heparin. An international multicentre trial. *Lancet* 1975; 2: 45-51.
44. Collins R, Peto R, GR, Parish S. Large scale randomised evidence: trials and overviews. In: *Non-random Reflections on Health Services Research.* Maynard A, Chalmers I, Eds. BMJ, London,1997: pp197-230.
45. Collins R, Scrimgeour A, Yusuf S, Peto R. Reduction in fatal pulmonary embolism and venous thrombosis by perioperative administration of subcutaneous heparin. Overview of results of randomized trials in general, orthopedic, and urologic surgery. *N Engl J Med* 1988; 318: 1162-73.
46. Stocking B. First consensus development conference in United Kingdom: on coronary artery bypass grafting. I. Views of audience, panel, and speakers. *Br Med J (Clin Res Ed)* 1985; 291: 713-6.
47. Jones J, Hunter D. Consensus methods for medical and health services research. *BMJ* 1995; 311: 376-80.
48. Lomas J, Anderson G, Enkin M, Vayda E, Roberts R, MacKinnon B. The role of evidence in the consensus process. Results from a Canadian consensus exercise. *JAMA* 1988; 259: 3001-5.
49. Hemingway H, Crook AM, Feder G, Banerjee S, Dawson JR, Magee P, *et al.* Underuse of coronary revascularization procedures in patients considered appropriate candidates for revascularization. *N Engl J Med* 2001; 344: 645-54.
50. Treasure T. Caring, counting and accountability. *Progress in Pediatric Cardiology* 2003; 18: 85-8.

Chapter 2

Screening for lung cancer: the current evidence

Ian Hunt BSc (Hons) MRCS, Specialist Registrar

Cardiothoracic Surgery [1] & Research Fellow [2]

1 St Thomas' Hospital, London, UK and
2 National Collaborating Centre for Acute Care,
The Royal College of Surgeons of England, London, UK

Introduction

Lung cancer continues to claim 29,000 lives a year in the UK, and though new cases are falling in certain groups, approximately 40,000 people are diagnosed annually [1]. The majority will have advanced disease at presentation making a cure unlikely. However, in those diagnosed with early stage disease, a cure - usually surgical resection - is achievable. Survival rates for lung cancer are very poor. In England, for patients diagnosed between 1993 and 1995 and followed-up to 2000, 21% with lung cancer were alive one year after diagnosis and only 5.5% were alive after five years [2]. These figures are around 5% lower than the European average and 7-10% lower than in the USA.

The criteria for appraising whether to screen for a disease are well established (Table 1).

There are many studies that suggest lung cancer discovered incidentally is associated with better survival than cancer detected because of symptoms [3]. But despite its obvious disease burden and that early intervention is likely to improve outcome, there is still

Table 1. Criteria for a disease to be deemed appropriate for screening.

- The illness in question must clearly impose a sufficient disease burden
- The screening test must provide benefit to individuals who have the disease so that early effective intervention in the natural course of the disease would likely improve outcome
- Such a test must be accurate with few false-positive results that cause anxiety or lead to further, more invasive investigations
- It must be acceptable to the patient and not dangerous
- The programme should be cost-effective

no public health strategy for the early detection of lung cancer.

Much of the early evidence against lung cancer screening came from several large randomised screening trials (RCTs) completed during the 1970s. These studies appeared to show no clear reduction in mortality in a population screened with chest radiography compared to the control. However, recent critical discussion and analysis of these early studies along with the development of other potential screening tools, such as low-dose Computerised Tomography (LDCT), has re-kindled interest in lung cancer screening [4].

Methodology

A systematic review of the current literature on lung cancer screening was completed with a search of databases including the Cochrane Library, MEDLINE and EMBASE between 1966 to 2002. In total, 41 publications were identified, of which three were recent systematic reviews (Manser *et al* 1999, Cochrane review [updated 2003]; Detterbeck *et al* 2001, ch.4 *Diagnosis and treatment of Lung Cancer,* and Bach *et al* 2003, ACCP review). A further five non-systematic reviews were also identified. In total, eight clinical trials were found, six of which were prospective randomised controlled studies. The remaining papers were a mixture of observational and population-based publications with only 12 studies having appropriate methodology.

Methods to evaluate lung cancer screening

Screening programmes have focused on the evaluation of asymptomatic individuals believed to be at high risk for lung cancer. In assessing such programmes several research methods can be applied which include randomised controlled trials, population-based studies of screening and observational studies.

Evidence-based medical practice places the RCT at the top of a hierarchy of study designs (see *Applying evidence-based medicine to cardiothoracic surgery* in the Introduction to the book). Typically, individuals are subjected to different intensities of screening. For example, in the Mayo Lung Project, individuals were randomised to receive regular scheduled screening with 4-monthly chest x-rays and sputum cytology (intervention arm) or routinue care, which was an annual chest x-ray (CXR) and sputum cytology (control arm). By convention, when examining the efficacy of a medical intervention in screening, the outcome measure is usually disease-specific mortality. The other outcome measures, such as fatality and survival, are felt to be open to screening biases. The issue of "improved outcome" as measured by the early-randomised screening trials has provoked intense debate and further analysis of these studies.

An alternative to the RCT is the population-based study whereby the impact of a broadly implemented screening programme is assessed through changes in disease-specific mortality rates within the population. In Japan, supported by the Japanese Ministry of Health and Welfare, population-based research groups have published results on lung cancer screening. Japan has a long tradition of cancer screening and has established several population-based cancer registries having set up the Japanese Association of Cancer Registries in 1992.

A third approach is screening in selected cohorts, whereby the efficacy of the screening test is inferred from the frequency of detecting early stage cancers. Such observational studies are regarded less highly according to the EBM hierarchy of evidence as they are felt to be open to certain biases.

Sputum cytology and chest X-ray screening studies

Screening for lung cancer began in the 1960s with several observational studies and one early study, the North London Lung Cancer study [5], a cluster randomised controlled trial. Commenced in 1960, it randomised (based on industrial firms) around 55,000 London male smokers over the age of 40 years to a study group receiving a CXR every six months for three years or to a control group who had a CXR at the beginning and end of the study only. Though the study showed additional cases detected in the study group, with more resections, there was no difference in lung cancer mortality.

The Erfurt County Study [6] compared a biannual CXR study group with a control group receiving a CXR every 1-2 years. Like the North London study, randomisation was group-based (place of residence in this case) and not randomisation of individual patients. As before, there was an increased incidence of lung cancer in the screened patients but no reduction in mortality.

With doubts remaining on the benefits of screening as well as improvements in CXR and sputum cytology techniques, the National Cancer Institute through the mid 1970s and early 1980s, funded the Co-operative Early Lung Cancer group, who sponsored three large RCTs (see Table 2). These trials were powered to detect a 50% reduction in mortality in the intervention arm. Along with one European RCT, the Czech Study, a total of 38,000 patients were entered into the four big RCTs. The Mayo Lung Project [7,8] has been viewed as the most "definitive" trial to date.

The Mayo Lung Project recruited 10,933 male smokers over 45 years of age who underwent a prevalence screen for lung cancer with a combination of CXR and sputum cytology. Subjects with negative and satisfactory prevalence screens were then randomised to either a screened group who had 4-monthly CXR and sputum cytology for six years or a control group who were advised to have an annual CXR and sputum cytology. The screened group had lung cancer detected more often, with more localised tumours and therefore more likely to be resectable. But, there were no differences in lung cancer-specific mortality between the groups; in fact, mortality was slightly higher in the screened patients. A further analysis as part of an extended follow-up 15 years after study completion, still showed no difference in lung cancer mortality between the screened and control groups [9].

The other NCI-funded trials, the Memorial Sloan Kettering [10] and Johns Hopkins Lung Project [11] were primarily designed to assess the incremental impact of sputum cytology in a CXR-screened cohort. No mortality reduction was detected between the randomised groups or even any differences in the number of cancers detected. The fourth RCT, was conducted in the former Czechoslovakia [12]. Following a prevalence screen, the trial randomly assigned male smokers between 40 and 65 years of age to either a CXR and sputum cytology every six months for three years (screened group) or CXR and sputum cytology once every three years (control group). Like the Mayo study, more cancers were detected in the screened group, a higher number had early stage disease and survival was greater. However, it also showed a non-statistically significant increase in mortality in the screened group.

As well as the RCTs mentioned, "lesser" studies that would constitute level II evidence, such as non-randomised controlled, uncontrolled and observational studies, have attempted to evaluate the role of CXR and/or sputum cytology as screening tools. Several early non-randomised uncontrolled trials including the South London Lung Cancer study [13] and the Veterans Administration trial [14], found little evidence supporting the hypothesis that CXR screening would be associated with a mortality benefit. This was despite often showing improved survival, staging, and resectability in the screened patients.

In Japan, where an annual screening programme for lung cancer has been carried out widely since 1987, there is still insufficient evidence to confirm its efficacy in reducing mortality. In attempting to assess this screening programme, a retrospective case-control study was conducted [15]. It claimed a 46% reduction in mortality since screening began.

Assessing the evidence

In reviewing the large randomised screening trials, all recruited males, over the age of 45 who were currently smoking. All used prevalence screening as an initial evaluation designed to eliminate subjects with detectable lung cancers at the time of entry into the study. Furthermore, all the studies were really assessing more intense screening versus less intense screening, as all involved a CXR at regular intervals in the control group. Study compliance ranged from 65% to 94% in the screened groups. Two of the studies specifically addressed the addition of sputum cytology to chest radiography as a screening tool.

The results of the RCTs are shown in Table 2 and from the evidence presented, there appears to be no significant reduction in mortality in a population screened by intensive CXR compared with less intensive screening. However, despite these studies being extremely large, they still only had a 50% power to detect a 20% reduction in lung cancer mortality. Furthermore, there was considerable contamination of the control groups in the RCTs. For example, in the Mayo Lung Project, 55% of patients in the control group had a CXR in the last year of the study. In addition, the rate of adherence to trial protocol was just 75% in the screened group and 50% in the control. Similar criticisms of contamination have been made regarding the Czech study, as after three years both control and study group underwent an identical CXR protocol.

Despite criticism of certain aspects of the methodology of the RCTs reviewed, the number of cases of lung cancer detected was higher in the screened patients in four out of six RCTs reporting this data (see Table 2). In the two studies that had included sputum cytology in addition to annual CXR, a slightly higher incidence of lung cancer was seen in the control groups. Apart from one of these CXR and sputum cytology studies, all the CXR screening trials reported that the lung cancers occurring in the screened group were more likely to be curatively resected and that 5-year survival was higher.

Overall, the RCTs consistently demonstrated a higher incidence, a higher rate of resection and better survival in the screened group. But, despite these improvements, the mortality due to lung cancer of the entire study population was consistently the same in the screened and the control groups. Much of the subsequent discussion in the literature has attempted to explain this apparent disparity in the conclusions drawn from the RCTs.

When examining the efficacy of a medical intervention in screening, it is conventional for disease-specific mortality as opposed to other measures such as fatality or survival, to be the outcome measure. Mortality is equal to the product of incidence and fatality. Therefore, although fatality, and therefore, survival was improved in the Mayo Lung Project, the increased incidence of lung cancer in the screened group, meant there was no reduction in lung cancer mortality from screening. In fact, both the Mayo and Czech studies showed higher lung cancer mortality in the screened group compared to the controlled groups.

Different explanations have been proposed to explain the increased incidence of lung cancer in the screened groups and the role of biases that are inherent to such screening trials have been hotly debated. One explanation is that it is a result of an imbalance of covariates of risk for lung cancer that was not controlled in the process of randomisation. In large screening trials of these sorts, even quite small heterogeneities in the control and screening arms can greatly outweigh any effect that the screening programmes itself may have [16].

A further explanation is that screening for lung cancer detects "biologically unimportant" tumours as well as those that are significant. Such tumours have such an indolent pattern of growth that they will never become clinically significant before the patient dies of other causes. The comorbidity of smoking-related disease in this population provides some intuitive evidence that such a screening bias exists. This **overdiagnosis bias** in screening trials would explain the increased incidence of lung cancer in the screened group and better survival of patients with a diagnosed lung cancer, but that overall disease-specific mortality in the population will be unaffected.

There is currently no consensus on whether such a class of indolent lung cancer truly exists. Proponents of such an explanation use autopsy data [17], data derived from lung volume reduction surgery studies [18] and series documenting doubling times in the growth of lung cancer [19]. Further support for the existence of indolent "screened-detected" lung tumours can be drawn from experiences with other organ sites, most notably breast and prostate. However, the natural history of lung cancer, albeit lesions presenting symptomatically is one of rapid death, even in early stage disease and so the high fatality rate of lung cancer is offered as a reason that such lesions do not exist [16].

Table 2. Randomised controlled trials of lung cancer screening with CXR +/- sputum cytology.

Study *Recruitment dates*	**Sample**	**Method**	**Study arms**		**Lung cancer detection rate in pop.** *Per 1000 patients/year*		**% Resectable of patients with lung cancer**		**% 5-yr survival of patients with lung cancer**		**Lung cancer mortality in pop.** *Per 1000 patients/year*		**Benefit** *reduction in lung cancer mortality*	**Level of evidence**
			Control (C)	**Intervention (I)**	**C**	**I**	**C**	**I**	**C**	**I**	**C**	**I**		
North London Study [5] 1960-1964	55034	Cluster RCT	CXR entry & exit of study	6-monthly CXR	0.38	0.44	29	44	6	15	0.8	0.7	No benefit	Ib
Erfurt County Study [6] 1972-1977	104880	Cluster RCT	18-monthly CXR	6-monthly CXR	0.65	0.95	19	28	8	14	0.8	0.6	No benefit	Ib
Johns Hopkins Study [11] 1973-1978	10384	RCT	Annual CXR	Annual CXR & 4-monthly sputum	5.5	4.8	44	47	20	20	4.6	3.6	No benefit	Ib
Mayo Lung Project [7,8] 1971-1976	9211	RCT	Advised annual CXR & sputum	4-monthly CXR & sputum	3.5	4.5	32	46	15	33	3.0	3.2	No benefit	Ib
Mem Sloan Kettering [10] 1974-1978	10040	RCT	Annual CXR	Annual CXR & sputum	3.8	3.7	51	53	33	37	2.7	2.7	No benefit	Ib
Czech Study [12] 1976-1982	6364	RCT	CXR yrs 4,5,6	6-monthly CXR yrs 1,2,3 & Annual CXR 4,5,6	2.0	3.9	16	25	0	26	1.5	1.7	No benefit	Ib

Case survival refers to the time from diagnosis to death and is calculated using only participants who were diagnosed with lung cancer, whereas mortality is calculated for all participants in the study: those who were diagnosed with lung cancer as well as those who were not. In the recent extended follow-up of the Mayo Lung Project [9], lung cancer survival was significantly different in the two arms. Examining all lung cancers, the median survival was higher in the intervention arm (1.3yrs vs. 0.9yrs). Such a finding is consistent with the previous findings of a higher survival in the screened group from the original Mayo Lung and Czech studies. However, in the absence of a mortality benefit, an improvement in case survival for the screened group is commonly ascribed to biases inherent in this type of screening study. As well as overdiagnosis bias previously discussed, other biases inherent to the type of studies reviewed are recognised and include lead-time bias and length bias.

Lead-time bias occurs because the asymptomatic diagnoses within the screening group as a result of intervention, will occur at an earlier point in time than the corresponding symptomatic diagnoses in the control group. It is responsible for an apparent increase in incidence and case survival as screened-detected cases of lung cancer are diagnosed earlier, and therefore live longer from time of diagnosis, even if death is ultimately not delayed as compared to a unscreened population. In the Mayo study, an adjustment for lead-time did not eliminate the longer case survival in the screened arm, suggesting another screening bias is responsible.

Length bias occurs because screening reveals a different set of tumours to those diagnosed as a result of symptoms. Assuming a spectrum of cancer aggressiveness, the more indolent cancers have a prolonged pre-clinical phase and are more likely to be detected by screening before becoming symptomatic. Therefore, cases detected at screening tend to be less aggressive and progress more slowly than those that are not detected at screening and ultimately manifest clinically (interval cases). As extended follow-up of the Mayo Lung project subjects, was more than 13 years on average, and therefore probably long enough for the slow growing cancers to manifest themselves clinically, length bias is an unlikely explanation for the longer case survival.

Conclusions

Evaluating the evidence from CXR and/or sputum cytology screening studies and interpreting such results remains unclear. Whereas overdiagnosis may easily explain an increased incidence of lung cancer unscreened patients without a reduction in mortality, this explanation is not without its critics. A clear conclusion is also hampered by the lack of a no-screening control arm, thus no determination of true efficacy can be made [20]. Therefore, routinue screening for lung cancer with CXR or sputum cytology in asymptomatic persons is not recommended. No organisation currently recommends routinue screening of either the general population or smokers.

Future studies

Currently ongoing is the NCI-sponsored Prostate, Lung, Colorectal and Ovarian Cancer screening (PLCO) study. This large-scale RCT based in ten American centres and involving 155,000 men and women over 55 years of age, is designed to further determine the role of CXR screening in a low-risk population. It commenced in 1994, and it involves a 14-year follow-up of participants. Results are not yet available [21]. In addition, further large-scale trials are planned or currently recruiting, including the National Lung Screening Trial (NLST), which compares screening with spiral CT (low radiation-dose computed tomography or LDCT) every three years or screening with CXR annually [22].

Low-dose computed tomography screening studies

It appears that if surgery for lung cancer is to be effective, detection of early stage disease is essential. A major limitation of screening may result from the limited sensitivity for the detection of early stage cancer of the screening tests used. This suggests that improvements in detection may substantially alter the effectiveness of screening for lung cancer. Not surprisingly, there has been considerable interest in the use of low-dose spiral computed tomography (LDCT) as a screening test. LDCT is a technique that allows a low-resolution image of the entire thorax to be

Table 3. Baseline results of observational LDCT screening studies.

Study (Date of publication)	Country	Sample	Abnormal lesions detected		Malignant lesions detected		% stage I tumours detected	Average size of cancer (mm)	Level of evidence
			N	%	N	%			
Henschke *et al* [24] 1999	USA	1000	233	23	27	2.7	81	10	IIb
Sone *et al* [25] 1998	Japan	5483	676	12	22	0.4	100	17	III
Sobue *et al* [27] 2002	Japan	1611	186	11.5	14	0.87	77	-	III
Swenson *et al* [28] 2002	USA	1520	782	51	22	1.4	59	-	IIb

obtained in a single breath-hold with low radiation exposure. Currently, LDCT has only been evaluated in observational studies, although several prospective RCTs of spiral CT in lung cancer screening are awaited [22].

Much of the experience of lung cancer screening with CT comes from Japan, which since 1993 has run public-funded CT screening programmes. A recent retrospective report compared the two screening strategies performed in Japan from 1975 to 1993 (CXR and sputum cytology) and the same strategy plus LDCT carried out between 1993 to 1998 [23]. A higher number of stage IA tumours were detected (42% to 81%) and the 5-year survival improved (48% to 82%) in the later years when spiral CT was included in the screened cohort. Such evidence suggests that screening with spiral CT can increase the ability to diagnose early stage lung cancer, but clearly as a non-randomised retrospective comparison, offers only weak support for a mortality benefit as it is open to biases.

One of the most publicised CT screening studies is the Early Lung Cancer Action Project (ELCAP), a single-arm cohort study that reported the baseline prevalence results of 1000 high-risk subjects [24]. The ELCAP design has subsequently been included in other non-randomised studies (see Table 3). In the study, 1000 asymptomatic smokers aged 60-years or over who were fit for surgery, underwent yearly LDCT and CXR. Non-calcified lung nodules were detected in 233 participants (23%) as compared with 68 (7%) patients by CXR. The ELCAP protocol then recommended further high-resolution CT follow-up. By following the protocol, just 28 patients underwent a biopsy, with 27 nodules proving to be malignant. Among these 27 malignant nodules, 20 nodules (74%) were not found on standard CXR; in contrast, no malignant nodules were detected by CXR that were not also seen on CT scanning. Twenty-three of the 27 malignant nodules (85%) proved to be stage I disease and the majority were resectable (26 of 27, 97%). Although LDCT generates more false positives, the ELCAP design for dealing with suspicious lesions has limited the use of invasive tissue diagnosis.

A prevalence screen conducted in Japan [25] reported that a single-spiral CT scan in 5483 persons detected lung cancer in 0.48%. In comparison, screening with CXR and sputum cytology performed in the same region previously, detected a lung cancer rate of just 0.03-0.05%. Many of the lesions were too small to have been found by conventional CXR. In this study, sensitvity and specificity of spiral-CT were calculated to be

95%. However, it had a weak positive predictive value and was criticized for the number of unnecessary and invasive investigations it engendered [26].

Assessing the evidence

LDCT can detect smaller nodules than CXR, with CT typically detecting a peripheral tumour with a mean size of 12mm as compared to CXR, detecting tumours averaging 30mm [29]. In Table 3 the results of LDCT screening studies are presented. Few patients in the studies reported, who underwent surgical biopsy, turned out not to have cancer (average 8%).

Clearly, based on prevalence screening and observational studies so far conducted, LDCT is capable of detecting early stage lung cancer. However, whether LDCT screening will be associated with a reduction in lung cancer mortality has been enthusiastically debated. Advocates for LDCT screening cite the consistently higher detection rates of early stage disease in observational studies. Critics however, have argued that the findings in these studies may reflect the impact of biases and not a true effect.

One study examined whether detection of small lesions leads to an actual reduction in lung cancer mortality. In over 500 persons screened with CT, no correlation between the size of T1N0M0 tumours and survival was found, with 3cm cancers having the same outcome as 1cm cancers [30].

Another criticism is that LDCT may be detecting malignant pulmonary nodules that are "indolent" in their behaviour and treating them will not increase the person's life expectancy. This concept of overdiagnosis first met in the debate on screening with CXR and/or sputum cytology, remains an area of much discussion, particularly on whether such a thing as an "indolent" lung cancer exists.

Evidence that LDCT is detecting atypical lung cancer has been suggested from ELCAP, in that the number of cancers detected in the annual follow-up LDCT is far less than that detected during the initial scan, even though the size of the nodules detected are similar. If all the lesions grew at similar rates, as would be expected with malignant tumours, there should be consistence in the rates of detection. However, ELCAP found significant differences in rate of detection despite the fact that the size of the lesions detected at the initial scan varied little from those detected at later scans. This has been interpreted as a proportion of cancers detected during the initial CT as behaving in an indolent manner.

A further issue is the high numbers of false positive results that CT screening appears to generate with subsequent need for further invasive investigation. For example, in the ELCAP study, 23% of participants were noted to have at least one non-calcified nodule, and only around 3% had diagnosed lung cancer. However, by following a protocol such as ELCAP to deal with suspicious lesions, the number of invasive tests were limited to those with highly suspicious lesions (3%) of which almost all, were histologically lung cancer.

Little has been published on the cost-effectiveness of CT as a mass screening tool. The cost however, is expected to be high, as screening would involve a large "high-risk" population combined with a high rate of findings that necessitate follow-up serial CT scanning, if unnecessary invasive procedures are to be kept to a minimum [31].

Conclusions

The ELCAP trial highlighted the numbers of resectable and curable stage I lung cancers that LDCT could detect among high-risk individuals. Furthermore, it set out a protocol for follow-up and further scanning to deal with the high positive findings. However, currently no RCT has been conducted and therefore no organisations are recommending the use of LDCT to screen for the presence of lung cancer.

Future studies

Currently, the NCI is conducting the National Lung Screening Trial (NLST), an RCT with the primary objective of determining whether screening with spiral CT, as compared with CXR, reduces lung cancer mortality among high-risk individuals. The trial, which aims to enrol 50,000 participants throughout the USA, will be completed in 2009.

Recommendations	Evidence level
◆ Routine screening for lung cancer with CXR and/or sputum cytology in individuals without symptoms or a history of cancer is not recommended.	Ib/A
◆ Routine screening for lung cancer with single or serial LDCT in individuals without symptoms or a history of cancer is not recommended.	IIb/III/B

References

1. Office for National Statistics 2001b. Mortality statistics cause. Review of the Registrar General on deaths by cause, sex and age, in England and Wales. Office for National Statistics, London, 2000: 27.
2. Office for National Statistics 2001a. Cancer survival, England 1993-2000. Office for National Statistics, London.
3. Early Lung cancer detection. Summary and conclusions. *Am Rev Respir Dis* 1984; 130: 565-570.
4. Shimizu N, Ando A, Teramoto S, *et al.* Outcome of patients with lung cancer detected via mass screening as compared to those presenting with symptoms. *J Surg Oncol* 1992; 50: 7-11.
5. Brett GZ. The value of lung cancer detection by six-monthly chest radiographs. *Thorax* 1968; 23: 414-20.
6. Wilde J. A 10-year follow-up of semi annual screening for early detection of lung cancer in the Erfurt County, GDR. *Eur Respir J* 1989; 2: 656-62.
7. Fontana RS, Sanderson DR, Taylor WF, *et al.* Early lung cancer detection: results of the initial (prevalence) radiologic and cytologic screening in the Mayo Clinic study. *Am Rev Respir Dis* 1984; 130: 561-5.
8. Fontana RS, Sanderson DR, Woolner LB, *et al.* Lung cancer screening: the Mayo program. *J Occup Med* 1986; 28: 746-50.
9. Marcus PM. Lung Cancer Screening: an update. *J Clin Oncol* 2001; 19: 83s-86s.
10. Melamed MR, Flehinger BJ, Zaman MB, *et al.* Screening for early lung cancer: results of the Memorial-Sloan Kettering study in New York. *Chest* 1984; 86: 44-53.
11. Frost JK, Ball WC, Levin ML, *et al.* Early lung cancer detection: results of the intial (prevalence) radiologic and cytologic screening in the Johns Hopkins study. *Am Rev Respir Dis* 1984; 130: 549-54.
12. Kubik A, Polak J. Lung cancer detection: results of a randomized prospective study in Czechoslovakia. *Cancer* 1986; 57: 2427-37.
13. Nash FA, Morgan JM, Tomkins JG, *et al.* South London Lung Cancer Study. *BMJ* 1968; 2: 715-21.
14. Lilienfield A, Archer PG, Burnett CH, *et al.* An evaluation of radiologic and cytologic screening for the early detection of lung cancer: a co-operative pilot study of the American cancer Society and the Veterans Administration. *Cancer Res* 1966; 2083-121.
15. Okamoto N, Suzuki T, Hesegawa H, *et al.* Evaluation of a clinical based screening program for lung cancer with a case control design in Kanagawa, Japan. *Lung Cancer* 1999; 25: 77-85.
16. Strauss GM, Gleason RE, Sugarbaker DJ, *et al.* Screening for lung cancer. Another look; a different view. *Chest* 1997; 111: 754-68.
17. McFarlane MJ, Feinstein AR, Wells CK, *et al.* Clinical features of lung cancers discovered at a postmortem "surprise". *Chest* 1986; 90: 520-523.
18. Geedales D, Davies M, Koyanna H, *et al.* Effect of lung volume reduction surgery in patients with severe emphysema. *N Engl J Med* 2000; 343: 239-45.
19. Meyer J. Growth rate versus prognosis in resected primary bronchiogenic carcinomas. *Cancer* 1973; 31: 1468-72.
20. Prorok PC, Chamberlain J, Day NE *et al.* UICC workshop on the evaluation of screening programmes for cancer. *Int J Cancer* 1984; 34: 1-4.
21. Gohagan JK, Prorok PC, Hayes RB, *et al.* The Prostate, Lung, Colorectal, and Ovarian Cancer Screening Trial of the National Cancer Institute: history, organisation, and status. *Control Clin Trial* 2000; 21(6 suppl): 251S-272S.
22. The National Lung Screening Trial. www.nci.nih.gov/nlst.
23. Kakinuma R, Ohmatsu H, Kaneko M, *et al.* Detection failures in spiral CT screening for lung cancer: analysis of CT findings. *Radiology* 1999; 212: 61-66.
24. Henschke CI, McCauley DI, Yankelevitz, *et al.* Early Lung Cancer Action Project: overall design and findings from baseline screening. *Lancet* 1999; 354: 99-105.
25. Sone S, Takashima S, Li F, *et al.* Mass screening for lung cancer with mobile spiral computed tomography scanner. *Lancet* 1998; 351: 1242-1245.
26. Dalrymple-Hay MJR. Screening for lung cancer. *J R Soc Med* 2001; 94: 2-5.
27. Sobue T, Moriyama N, Kaneko M, *et al.* Screening for lung cancer with low-dose helical computed tomography: anti-lung cancer association project. *J Clin Oncol* 2002; 20: 911-920.
28. Swenson SJ, Jett JR, Sloan JA, *et al.* Screening for lung cancer with low-dose spiral computed tomography. *Am J Respir Crit Care Med* 2002; 165: 153-159.
29. Kaneko M, Eguchi K, Ohmatsu H, *et al.* Peripheral lung cancer: screening and detection with low-dose spiral CT versus radiography. *Radiology* 1996; 201: 798-802.

30. Patz EF Jr, Rossi S, Harpole DH Jr, *et al.* Correlation of tumour size and survival in patients with stage 1A non-small cell lung cancer. *Chest* 2000; 117: 1568-71.
31. Marshall D, Simpson KN, Earle CC, *et al.* Economic decision analysis model of screening for lung cancer. *Eur J Cancer* 2001; 37: 1759-67.

Future reading

1. Manser RL, Irving LB, Stone C, *et al.* Screening for lung cancer. In: *The Cochrane Library*, issue 1, 2004.
2. Detterbeck FC, Rivera MP. Clinical presentation and diagnosis Ch. 4. In: *Diagnosis and treatment of lung cancer: An evidence-based guide for the practising clinician.* WB Saunders, New York, 2001.
3. Bach PB. Screening for Lung Cancer: A review of the current Literature. *Chest* 2003; 123 (supplement): 72S-82S.

Chapter 3

Classification and staging of lung cancer

Ian Hunt BSc (Hons) MRCS, Specialist Registrar, Cardiothoracic Surgery [1] & Research Fellow [2]

Louise Thomas BA MA, Research Associate [2]

1 St Thomas' Hospital, London, UK and
2 National Collaborating Centre for Acute Care,
The Royal College of Surgeons of England, London, UK

Introduction

The basis of staging in the surgical management of lung cancer is that the likelihood of surviving (usually counted at five years) is dependent on the extent of cancer spread. In the case of lung cancer, operation is for cure, not local control, as it might be in many cases of breast and bowel cancer. If the cancer has spread outside the field of resection (that is, into the mediastinal nodes or beyond or remote metastatic disease), then surgery is usually futile adding neither to length nor quality of life. This was formalised into the TNM classification, a system of classifying the anatomical extent of the tumour based on the primary tumour (T), regional lymph node involvement (N) and distant metastases (M). This was first proposed by Denoix in 1946 [1]. In 1973, the American Joint Committee on Cancer (AJCC) proposed a scheme for lung cancer based on this TNM system. The system was revised in 1986 [2] and most recently in 1997, being published on behalf of the AJCC and the Union Internationale Contre le Cancer (UICC) [3]. In addition, at the same time, a classification of regional lymph node stations according to anatomic landmarks into 14 mediastinal, hilar (N2) and intrapulmonary (N1) lymph node stations was published [4] (Figure 2. Regional lymph node map. Chapter 4). This allowed consistent lymph node mapping when staging patients, particularly during mediastinoscopy.

Methodology

Following a broad search of the literature, the current classification systems for small cell lung cancer (SCLC) and non-small cell lung cancer (NSCLC) are presented. In addition, a systematic review of the current literature on lung cancer staging for NSCLC was conducted using the Cochrane library, MEDLINE and EMBASE from 1966 to 2003. Studies identified were appraised for their methodology. In total, 45 publications were identified, of which four were recent systematic reviews [5,6,7,8]. A further two recent substantive non-systematic reviews [9,10], were also identified and one previous meta-analysis [11]. This chapter focuses on current staging strategies in evaluating mediastinal involvement; we begin with a brief overview of classification.

Staging for small cell lung cancer

Small cell lung cancer (SCLC) accounts for approximately 20-25% of lung tumours and because of its tendency to undergo early and widespread dissemination, is staged differently from NSCLC. The simple staging system introduced by the Veterans Administration Lung Cancer Study Group (VALG) of "limited" and "extensive" disease is generally applied in clinical practice and has proven adequate for most clinical situations [12]. In addition, the revised TNM system [3] has limited use in SCLC, except in those patients undergoing surgical resection [13].

The VALG system (Table 1) is sufficient for management decisions regarding the use of local radiotherapy, and carries prognostic information independent of whether chemotherapy is used or not. Patients with tumour confined to the chest are described as having limited disease (LD) and are eligible for treatment with thoracic radiotherapy. These patients represent about 30% of small cell cases. Patients with systemic metastasis are described as having extensive disease (ED) and are commonly treated with systemic chemotherapy. These patients account for 70% of SCLC.

A small proportion of patients with limited stage disease will have long-term survival, although this is very rare for patients presenting with extensive disease. In this group, surgery as part of a multi-modality approach may be considered. These are the patients who according to the revised TNM system, can be classified as having stage I, II, or resectable stage IIIa disease. Extensive disease SCLC is equivalent to stage IIIb and IV.

Performance status and biochemical variables are at least as important as the LD/ED distinction in terms of prognosis and should be taken into account when treatment management decisions are being made [14].

TNM staging for non-small cell lung cancer

In the TNM classification system for NSCLC (Table 2), T represents the size, location and extent of the primary tumour, with progression of T-stage denoting a larger tumour that invades extraparenchymal tissue. N denotes the extent of regional lymph node involvement and logically, the increasing numbers represent the advancement of disease from parenchymal lymph nodes to mediastinal lymph nodes and more remote spread into the neck. In designating regional lymph node stations according to anatomic landmarks, Mountain and Dressler [4] have allowed for consistent, reproducible lymph node mapping that is compatible with the international staging system for lung cancer (Figure 2. Regional lymph node map. Chapter 4). M represents presence of blood-borne metastasis.

Table 1. Staging of small cell lung cancer.

Limited	Defined according to the possibility of encompassing all detectable tumour within a "tolerable" radiotherapy port Disease confined to one hemithorax - ipsilateral hilar lymph nodes - ipsilateral and contralateral supraclavicular lymph nodes - ipsilateral and contralateral mediastinal lymph nodes - with or without ipsilateral pleural effusions independent of cytology
Extensive	Defined as disease at sites beyond the definition of limited disease - metastatic lesions in contralateral lung - distant metastatic involvement (such as brain, bone, liver or adrenals)

Table 2. The TNM Staging Classification System.

Primary Tumour (T)

Tx	Primary tumour cannot be assessed, or tumour proven by the presence of malignant cells in sputum or bronchial washings but not visualised by imaging or bronchoscopy.
T0	No evidence of primary tumour.
Tis	Carcinoma *in situ.*
T1	Tumour <3cm in greatest dimension, surrounded by lung or visceral pleura, without bronchoscopic evidence of invasion more proximal than the lobar bronchus.
T2	Tumour with any of the following features of size or extent: >3cm in greatest dimension; involves main bronchus >2cm distal to the carina; invades the visceral pleura; associated with atelectasis or obstructive pneumonitis that extends to the hilar region but does not involve the entire lung.
T3	Tumour of any size that directly invades the following: chest wall (including superior sulcus tumours); diaphragm; mediastinal pleura; parietal pericardium; or tumour in the main bronchus <2cm distal to the carina but without involvement of the carina; or associated atelectasis or obstructive pneumonitis of the entire lung.
T4	Tumour of any size that involves any of the following: mediastinum; heart; great vessels; trachea; oesophagus; vertebral body; carina; or tumour with a malignant pleural or pericardial effusion, or with satellite tumour nodule(s) within the ipsilateral primary tumour lobe of the lung.

Regional lymph nodes (N)

Nx	Regional lymph nodes cannot be assessed.
N0	No regional lymph node metastases.
N1	Metastases to ipsilateral peribronchial and/or ipsilateral hilar lymph nodes and intrapulmonary nodes involved by direct extension of primary tumour.
N2	Metastases to ipsilateral mediastinal and/or subcarinal lymph nodes.
N3	Metastases to contralateral mediastinal, contralateral hilar, ipsilateral or contralateral saclene or supraclavicular lymph nodes.

Distant metastases (M)

Mx	Presence of distant metastases cannot be assessed.
M0	No distant metastases.
M1	Distant metastases present.

Stage grouping TNM subsets

Stage	**TNM subset**
0	Carcinoma *in situ*
IA	T1N0M0
IB	T2N0M0
IIA	T1N1M0
IIB	T2N1M0; T3N0M0
IIIA	T3N1M0; T1N2M0; T2N2M0; T3N2M0
IIIB	T4N0M0; T4N1M0; T4N2M0; T1N3M0; T2N3M0; T3N3M0; T4N3M0
IV	Any T Any N M1

Table 3. Stage grouping of lung cancer and current 5-yr survival [3]. ***Reproduced with permission from Mountain [3] and the American College of Chest Physicians.***

Stage	TMN Subset	5-yr survival cTNM	5-yr survival pTNM
0	Carcinoma *in situ*		
IA	T1N0M0	61	67
IB	T2N0M0	38	57
IIA	T1N1M0	34	55
IIB	T2N1M0 T3N0M0	24 22	39 38
IIIA	T1-3N2M0 T3N1M0	13 9	23 25
IIIB	T4N0-3M0 T1-4N3M0	7 3	
IV	Any T any N M1	1	

cTNM = clinical stage TNM; pTNM = pathological stage

Various combinations of TNM descriptors are grouped together resulting in different categories or stages [15] (Table 3). The stages define and influence patient therapeutic decisions as having prognostic implications. In the most recent revision [3], stage I disease was sub-divided into stage IA and IB which reflect the significantly better five years survival outcome compared to stage IB disease (67% vs. 57% respectively). For the same reason, stage II disease was also divided; T1N1M0 was reclassified as stage IIA while T2N1M0 and T3N0M0 were redefined as stage IIB. Stage IIIA, now includes T1-3N2M0 and T3N1M0 while stage IIIB includes T4 and N3 TNM subsets.

Despite the more recent stage revision, issues still arise in classifying lung cancer according to a TNM system and the way TNM descriptors are grouped. One example currently debated relates to the presence of a malignant pleural effusion in NSCLC. This is currently considered a T4 (stage IIIB) lesion and therefore, has an apparently more favourable prognosis than patients with M1 (stage IV) disease. However, it has been demonstrated by Naruke *et al* [16] that the survival of patients with stage IIIB disease who have malignant effusions is considerably worse than those with stage IIIB disease who do not have malignant effusions. Thus, stage IIIB disease in the presence of malignant effusion has a similar prognosis to patients with stage IV disease. More data analysis and further refining of stage groupings is ongoing, with a revision now planned in 2009 [17].

Staging procedures for SCLC

The extent of clinical staging necessary depends on the clinical situation of the patient. In SCLC, the staging procedures used depend on whether a local modality is considered as part of the treatment and whether the patient is part of a clinical trial [18,19]. The recommended staging procedures include chest x-ray, CT chest, blood screen and histological (biopsy) or cytological (pleural aspiration) confirmation of small cell lung cancer. Additional investigations will depend on presence of specific symptoms, such as CT scan of the brain in the presence of neurological abnormalities. Extensive disease can be excluded by bone scan, ultrasound or CT of the abdomen, bone marrow aspiration and/or brain CT.

Staging procedures for NSCLC

The focus of the current literature on lung cancer staging is on invasive and non-invasive methods of staging NSCLC. Clinically, disease involving the mediastinum, as reflected by the N status, often determines the appropriateness of the patient for surgical resection. Patients with stage IA, IB, IIA and IIB NSCLC generally benefit from surgical resection with intention to cure. Patients with stage IIIA disease may be candidates for surgery as part of combination therapy with neoadjuvant chemotherapy and/or radiotherapy. Patients with stage IIIB and IV NSCLC rarely meet the criteria for surgery.

Non-invasive staging of the mediastinum

CT scan of the chest

As the most widely available and commonly used non-invasive method of evaluating the mediastinum, since the early 1990s many studies have compared clinical staging by CT scanning with the reference or "gold standard" of mediastinoscopy or surgery. Based on a meta-analysis of 42 studies conduced in 1990, the most widely accepted criterion for malignant involvement of lymph nodes is a short-axis diameter of >1cm on a transverse CT scan [11]. However, amongst the numerous studies on the use of CT as a diagnostic or staging tool, various criteria are used in the assessment of individual nodal stations.

Despite this heterogeneity, several recent systematic reviews have evaluated CT for staging the mediastinum. The Health Technology Report (HTA) for Scotland [8] reported on 17 studies that considered the diagnostic accuracy of CT at determining malignancy and likely operability as compared to histologically proven NSCLC (surgery or biopsy). The weighted average sensitivity was 0.65, and specificity 0.72.

A recent systematic review by Toloza *et al* [5], as a background to the American College of Chest Physicians (ACCP) guidelines, evaluated 20 studies (n=3438) that used standard CT scanning for staging the mediastinum. The pooled sensitivity of CT scanning was 0.57 (95% CI, 0.49-0.66), and the pooled specificity was 0.82 (95% CI 0.77-0.86). Marked heterogeneity in the sensitivity and specificity of the individual studies was noted. The overall Predictive Positive Value was 0.56 (range, 0.26-0.84) and Negative Predictive Value was 0.83 (range, 0.63-0.93). The overall prevalence of mediastinal disease among the patients was 28% (range, 18-50%).

In assessing the evidence, regardless of the criterion used by many of the studies, CT scan findings in isolation could not be taken as clear evidence of malignant nodal involvement. Detterbeck *et al* [7] in systematically reviewing 22 studies that report on reliability of CT against surgical confirmation, included assessment of the false-negative (FN) and false-positive (FP) rates. The average FP rate for CT detected lymph nodes was 45% (range, 18-72%) and the average FN rate was 13% (range, 3-26%).

CT scanning clearly plays an important role in the evaluation of patients with lung cancer. However, considering the limitations of its sensitivity and specificity, it would be inadvisable to rely only on a CT scan to assess presence of malignancy in mediastinal lymph nodes.

PET scan of the mediastinum

Positron Emission Tomography (PET) scans provide an insight into the biochemical processes of regions suspicious of cancer. Fluoro 18-2-deoxy-D-glucose (FDG), a glucose analogue labelled with positron emitting fluorine, is generally used in the evaluation of lung cancer patients. This radioactive tracer introduced into the patient is metabolised at a faster rate by any tumour cells, compared to surrounding non-malignant cells, with areas of high activity detected by a scanner. PET scanning is thus a metabolic imaging technique based on the function of a tissue rather than on its anatomy. Because of limitations with CT scans, in the last few years interest in the use of FDG-PET scanning to stage the mediastinum in lung cancer has grown.

As a background to the ACCP guidelines published in 2003, Toloza *et al* [5] systematically reviewed 18 studies that evaluated mediastinal staging by FDG-PET (n=1166). Inclusion criteria included >20 patients, and histological or cytological confirmation of mediastinal lymph nodes or extrathoracic sites, as well as the primary tumour. Overall, sensitivity was 0.84 (95% CI, 0.78-0.89) and overall specificity was 0.89 (95% CI, 0.8-0.93). The overall PPV and NPV were 0.79 (range, 0.40-1.00) and 0.93 (range, 0.75-1.00) respectively. The overall prevalence of mediastinal disease among the patients was 32% (range, 5-56%).

Based on this, and similar systematic reviews [7,8] FDG-PET scanning appears to have a higher sensitivity and specificity for the assessment of mediastinal lymph nodes than does CT scanning. In addition, in the systematic review by Detterbeck [7], including many of the studies reviewed by Toloza, the average FN and FP rate was 7% and 16% respectively. However, despite the apparent improvement over CT scanning, PET is not without limitations. Firstly, PET is not an anatomic scan but a functional test; therefore, there is often poor anatomic localization, with difficulties reported on differentiating hilar from mediastinal nodes. Difficulties can also arise in differentiating nodal metastases from primary centrally located tumours, so adding to the FN rate. In addition, though the average reported FP rate of 16% might be acceptable, there was significant variability in range reported by Detterbeck (0-52%) reflecting geographical variation and the varying incidence of granulomatous inflammatory disease. Inflammatory foci including infection are frequently positive, though usually weakly. Finally, the cost and availability of PET scanners in the UK remain a real issue.

PET scanning is a fairly reliable method of staging the mediastinum but with limitations. A negative PET scan of the mediastinum prior to surgical resection may reduce the need for mediastinoscopy before proceeding, but at present a positive PET should not negate further evaluation or the possibility of resection.

The limitations of PET may be overcome with improved technology and in particular, the increasing use of combination PET and CT imaging. The combination of the two imaging tests may achieve greater staging accuracy than either test alone. Future studies should include the evaluation of a combination of CT and PET scanning in prospective clinical trials. Furthermore, the ongoing development of fusion scanners that combine CT and PET warrants clinical trials and may provide an optimal method for non-invasive clinical staging.

MRI scan of the chest

MRI offers an alternative to CT scanning as an anatomic assessment of mediastinal involvement. It appears to offer little above CT scanning in assessing tumour size, chest wall and local mediastinal invasion (T-stage assessment) [7]. But few reports have assessed MRI in the detection of mediastinal lymph nodes. One cohort study [20] of 170 patients, comparing MRI versus CT in detecting N2,3 disease obtained a sensitivity of 48% versus 52%, and a specificity of 79% versus 79%. However, later work has suggested that use of contrast enhancement (with gadolinium) may improve the accuracy of MRI in assessing mediastinal lymph nodes [21]. Further studies using the latest MR imaging with enhancement are awaited.

The value of MRI in terms of its greater contrast resolution and its multiplanar capabilities is in the context of superior sulcus or Pancoast tumours. In this regard, many authors have advocated its use in assessing invasion of the root of the neck, including the brachial plexus, vertebral bodies and blood vessels. However, in reviewing the literature on the staging of superior sulcus tumours little evidence was found.

Mediastinal staging by endoscopic ultrasound

Endoscopic ultrasound (EUS) was originally developed for the local staging of gastrointestinal cancers, but it also provides excellent access to the posterior mediastinum through the oesophageal wall. Through such an approach access to the subcarinal, aortopulmonary and posterior mediastinal lymph nodes is possible. Toloza *et al*[5] recently systematically reviewed five eligible studies (n=163) using lymph node size and heterogeneity to assess likely malignancy. The pooled sensitivity of EUS was 0.78 (95% CI, 0.61-0.89) and pooled specificity was 0.71 (95% CI, 0.56-0.82). The overall PPV was 75% (range, 38-100%) and the overall NPV was 79% (range, 57-89%), with an overall prevalence of mediastinal involvement of 50% (range, 25-76%).

Though invasive, it is possible to perform needle aspiration (EUS-NA) of abnormal subcarinal and aortopulmonary window lymph nodes with a very low risk of bleeding or infection. The overall sensitivity and specificity reported by Toloza *et al* [6] of five studies (n=215) was 0.88 (95% CI, 0.82-0.93) and 0.91 (95% CI, 0.77-0.97). The overall PPV was 98% (range, 96-100%) and NPV was 77% (range, 23-79%), with an overall prevalence of 69% (range, 63-79%). These findings reflect the patient population tested, who generally had radiological evidence of enlarged mediastinal lymph nodes in sites accessible to EUS-NA as reflected by the high prevalence. Currently, this technique is offered in a few specialised centres in the UK only.

Invasive staging of NSCLC

Transbronchial (Wang) needle biopsy

A flexible fibreoptic bronchoscopy allows visualisation of the tracheo-bronchial tree down to the sub-segmental braches, while sampling techniques accumulate cytohistological information. Transbronchial needle aspiration (TBNA) was developed in the 1980s by Wang and Terry [22]. It is generally regarded as a safe procedure, being most frequently used to assess subcarinal lymph nodes, as well as paratracheal lymph nodes and occasionally, aortopulmonary window nodes. The recent ACCP systematic review of 12 studies (n=910) demonstrated an overall sensitivity of 0.76 (95% CI, 0.72-0.79) and a specificity of 0.96 (95% CI, 0.91-1.00). The average NPV was 71%, but with a range of 36-100%, and the average prevalence was 70% [6]. As noted, in the accompanying guideline [23], the sensitivity tended to be higher in studies that had a high prevalence N2,3 disease and therefore, one assumes significantly enlarged mediastinal nodes. Furthermore, with a NPV of 71%, a high FN rate makes any test less useful as a staging tool. Recently, TBNA has been used with ultrasound guidance. Endobronchial Ultrasound (EBUS), was initially developed to assess the depth of endobronchial invasion, but is likely to have a role in the assessment of mediastinal and hilar metastases [24].

Transthoracic needle aspiration

A percutaneous or transthoracic needle aspiration (TTNA) under CT guidance allows access to most regions of the mediastinum and as well as lesions in the lung parenchyma. TTNA of mediastinal lymph nodes often involves traversing the lung, but despite this it is regarded as a safe procedure [25]. However, the rate of pnuemothoraces requiring chest drain insertion is estimated at around 10% post-TTNA [7]. Toloza *et al* [6] systematically reviewed five studies that assessed TTNA for staging the mediastinum (n=215) and found an overall sensitivity of 0.91 (95% CI, 0.74-0.97). The NPV overall was 78% (range, 42-100%), with an average prevalence of 83% (range, 63-93%). As with TBNA, prevalence was high, reflecting the fact that most of the patients had significantly enlarged mediastinal lymph nodes. The overall FN rate was 22%, but varied widely. Immediate cytological interpretation by the pathologist present, and further biopsy if the quality of the sample is unsatisfactory, may reduce the FN rate [26]. As with TBNA, this modality may be more appropriate as a diagnostic tool rather than to stage the mediastinum.

Mediastinoscopy

Surgical staging of the mediastinum by mediastinoscopy has been the historical "gold standard" for evaluating mediastinal lymph nodes. The most common technique is cervical mediastinoscopy [27], which gives access to the pre-tracheal (station 1 and 3) and paratracheal (station 2 and 4) lymph nodes, as well as lymph nodes between the left and right main bronchus (anterior subcarinal nodes, station 7). Areas which are more difficult or impossible to access include the posterior subcarinal nodes (station 7), inferior mediastinal nodes (stations 8,9) and in particular, aortopulmonary and subaortic nodes (station 5,6) (see Figure 2. Regional lymph node map. Chapter 4). Alternatively, an anterior mediastinotomy [28] via the second or third intercostal space on the left side allows exploration of the aortopulmonary window, and is useful particularly in patients with tumours of the left lung. A modified technique, an extended cervical mediastinoscopy [29] has also been described for assessing this region.

Mediastinoscopy, as with any surgical procedure has potential risks. It requires general anaesthesia, but can be performed as an outpatient procedure [30]. In most experienced centres complications are minimal. In a series of eight of the largest studies (n=8007) reported since 1985 [7], the non-weighted mortality was 0.07% and morbidity was under 2%. The most common complication was significant bleeding requiring tamponade or thoracotomy (0.6%), pneumothorax (0.3%) and recurrent laryngeal nerve injury (0.3%). Emergency thoracotomy for treatment of an operative injury was reported as 0.12%. In the context of SVC obstruction it is felt to be a safe procedure in experienced hands [31].

The ACCP systematic review of mediastinal staging by standard cervical mediastinoscopy included 14 studies (n=5867) [6]. The pooled sensitivity was 0.81 (95% CI, 0.76-0.85). The overall NPV was 91% (range, 58-97%) with a prevalence of 37% (range, 21-54%). This gives an average false negative (FN) rate of roughly 10%. However, in at least four of the studies reviewed, the FN rate was affected by detection of positive nodes at surgery that were inaccessible by conventional mediastinoscopy. In addition, the FN rate is likely to be affected by the diligence with which nodes are sampled at mediastinoscopy [7].

The specificity and PPV for mediastinoscopy was reported as 1.0 and 100% respectively. These values cannot really be assessed, as patients with positive lymph nodes were not then subject to any further procedures. However, several commentators have suggested that the FP rate is likely to be low [23].

The indications for mediastinoscopy remain an area of much debate and reflect the evidence presented in this chapter on the accuracy of mediastinal staging by less or non-invasive methods, in particular CT and PET. The indications of mediastinoscopy include mediastinal lymph nodes larger than 1cm in the shortest axis detected with a chest CT scan; tumour histology of adeno or large cell lung cancer with detectable mediastinal lymph nodes of any size; clinical T4 tumours; clinical T3 tumours with central location and; the potential entry into neoadjuvant therapy protocols [32].

The issue of routine mediastinoscopy for patients with a CT negative for mediastinal nodal disease, remains controversial [33,34]. Proponents of routine mediastinoscopy cite its low complication rate, the higher rate of thoracotomies that lead to curative resection, and the average FN rate of 13% (range, 3-26%) with CT (see earlier). Proponents of selective mediastinoscopy cite the high rate of negative mediastinoscopy examinations, and the ability to completely resect patients with unsuspected N2 disease (assuming appropriate mediastinal lymph node dissection at the time of resection). The developing role of PET in this debate may tip the balance toward an increasingly non-invasive approach to mediastinal staging [35], though its exact role in replacing or complementing invasive surgical staging is still undefined.

Left anterior mediastinotomy or extended cervical mediastinoscopy

These techniques are generally applied in the context of tumours in the left upper lobe and are used to assess lymph node stations 5 and 6, which are not accessible by standard mediastinoscopy. Typically, in the presence of enlarged lymph nodes in the aortic-pulmonary window on CT, cervical mediastinoscopy precedes anterior mediastinotomy or extended cervical mediastinoscopy, even in the absence of obvious lymphadenopthy in the paratracheal stations [36]. If mediastinoscopy is negative, left anterior mediastinotomy should be done. Alternatively, the surgeon may proceed directly to surgical resection of the primary tumour and all enlarged lymph nodes in station 5 and 6 [37].

In the Toloza *et al* [6] review of the current literature, only two papers had evaluated anterior mediastinotomy in isolation (n=84) and in combination with cervical mediastinoscopy (n=71). The overall sensitivity for detecting mediastinal disease in patients with left upper lobe tumours was 87%, higher than the sensitivity of each procedure in isolation. In assessing extended cervical mediastinoscopy the same review identified two non-randomised studies (n=206) that assessed standard mediastinoscopy alone, or combined with extended mediastinoscopy in patients with left upper lobe tumours and/or CT positive mediastinal lymph nodes in station 5 and 6. As with anterior mediastinotomy, the combined approach had a higher sensitivity (69% and 81%) than the procedures in isolation.

Thoracoscopy

Video-assisted thoracoscopy (VATS) is increasingly used in the diagnosis and management of the indeterminate pulmonary nodule [38]. In the context of staging, VATS has been used to assess for locally invasive pleural disease, unsuspected pleural effusion or mediastinal infiltration. With respect to mediastinal lymph node staging, the role of VATS is similar to that of anterior mediastinotomy and extended cervical mediastinoscopy, as an aid to standard mediastinoscopy in assessing stations 5 and 6. In addition, subcarinal lymph nodes (station 7) paraoesophageal (station 8) and pulmonary ligament nodes (station 9) are accessible to VATS. As few studies were identified and those that were involved small numbers of patients, the role of VATS in mediastinal staging requires further evaluation, but is likely to be complementary to mediastinoscopy in selected patients.

Recommendations - Non-invasive staging of the mediastinum	**Evidence level**
No single imaging method alone was conclusive in evaluating potential mediastinal involvement in apparently operable lung cancer and routine clinical conditions. However, based on available evidence the following recommendations are appropriate:-	
• To perform a CT scan as part of a staging assessment in patients with known or suspected NSCLC.	IIa/B
• In the presence of enlarged mediastinal lymph nodes on CT, further assessment of the mediastinum is required prior to surgical resection of the primary tumour.	IIa/B
• Where available, patients who are surgical candidates should undergo a PET scan to further evaluate the mediastinum.	IIa/B
• MRI as an additional staging modality should be performed only in patients with NSCLC involving the superior sulcus.	IIb/B
• In the presence of abnormal imaging that suggests mediastinal involvement, patients with NSCLC should not be denied assessment for potentially curative surgery without tissue confirmation wherever possible.	IIb/B
Recommendations - Invasive staging of NSCLC	
A tissue diagnosis is extremely helpful. The most appropriate method depends on the size and extent of mediastinal lymph node involvement. Based on the available evidence, the recommendations for invasive staging of the mediastinum are:-	
• In patients with NSCLC who have radiological evidence of significantly enlarged mediastinal lymph nodes, the aim is to provide confirmation of the diagnosis through histological or cytological means. In such patients this can be achieved through TTNA or where available, EUS-NA (high sensitivity and low morbidity). TBNA offers an alternative, if mediastinal disease is appropriately located (lower sensitivity). Mediastinoscopy is a further alternative but remains the most invasive method.	IIb/B
• In patients with NSCLC who have enlarged but discrete mediastinal lymph nodes on CT, mediastinoscopy is the invasive method of choice. Alternatively, TTNA, TBNA and EUS-NA can be used but generally result in less thorough mediastinal staging.	IIa/B
• In patients with NSCLC who have normal mediastinal nodes on CT (high FN rate of CT) and invasive staging is recommended, mediastinoscopy is the method of choice.	IIa/B
• In patients with Left Upper Lobe primary NSCLC, who have either enlarged discrete or normal mediastinal lymph nodes, additional to mediastinoscopy, an anterior mediastinotomy, extended mediastinoscopy or thoracoscopy should be performed to assess specifically the aortopulmonary station.	III/B

References

1. Denoix PF. Enquete permanent das les centers anticanceras. *Bull Inst Nat Hyg* 1946; 1: 70-75.
2. Mountain CF. A new international staging system for lung cancer. *Chest* 1986; 89(suppl): 225S-233S.
3. Mountain CF. Revision in the international system for staging lung cancer. *Chest* 1997; 111: 1710-1717.
4. Mountain CF, Dressler CM. Regional lymph node classification for lung cancer staging. *Chest* 1997; 11: 1718-1723.
5. Toloza EM, Harploe L, McCrory DC. Non-invasive staging of Non-small Cell Lung Cancer. *Chest* 2003; 123: 137S-146S.
6. Toloza EM, Harploe L, Detterbeck FC, McCrory DC. Invasive staging of Non-small Cell Lung Cancer: a review of the current evidence. *Chest* 2003; 123: 157S-166S.
7. Detterbeck FC, Jones DR, Parker Jr, LR. Intrathoracic staging. In: *Diagnosis and Treatment of lung cancer: an evidence-based guide for the practicing clinician.* Detterbeck FC, Rivera MP, Socinski MA, Rosenman JG, Eds. WB Saunders, Philadelphia, 2001: 73-93.
8. Bradbury I, Bonell E, Boynton J, *et al.* Positron emission tomography (PET) imaging in cancer management (Health Technology Assessment Report 2.) Glasgow: Health Technology Board for Scotland 2002.
9. Spiro SG, Porter JC. Lung Cancer - Where are we today? Current advances in staging and nonsurgical treatment. *Am J Respir Crit Care Med* 2002; 166: 1166-1196.
10. Passlick B. Initial surgical staging of lung cancer. *Lung Cancer* 2003; 42: S21-25.
11. Dales RE, Stark RM, Raman S. Computed tomography to stage lung cancer: approaching a controversy using meta-analysis. *Am Rev Respir Dis* 1990; 141: 1096-1101.
12. Zelen M. Keynote address on biostatistics and data retrieval. *Cancer Chemother Rep* Part. 3. 1973; 4: 31-42.
13. Shields TW, Karrer K (Eds). In: *Surgery for Small-Cell Lung cancer.* Ch.7, 2nd ed. Blackwell Scientific Publications, Cambridge, Massachusetts, 1998: 115-134.
14. Rawson NS, Peto J. An overview of prognostic factors in small cell lung cancer. A report from the Subcommittee for the Management of Lung Cancer of the United Kingdom Coordinating Committee on Cancer Research. *Br J Cancer* 1990 Apr; 61(4): 597-604. Erratum in: *Br J Cancer* 1990; Sep; 62(3): 550.
15. Deslauriers J, Gregoire MD. Clinical and Surgical staging of Non-Small cell lung cancer. *Chest* 2000; 117; 4: 96S-103S.
16. Naruke T, Tsuchiya R, Kondo H, *et al.* Implications of staging in lung cancer. *Chest* 1997; 112: 242S-248S.
17. Watanabe Y. TNM classification for Lung cancer. *Ann Thorac Cardiovasc Surg* 2003; 9; 6: 343-350.
18. Stahel RA, Ginsberg R, Havemann K, *et al.* Staging and prognostic factors in small cell lung cancer: a consensus report. *Lung Cancer* 1989; 5: 119-126.
19. Shepherd FA, Ginsberg RJ, Haddad R, *et al.* Importance of clinical staging in limited small-cell lung cancer: a valuable system to separate prognostic subgroups. *J Clin Oncol* 1993; 11: 1592-1597.
20. Webb WR, Gatsonis C, Zerhouni EA, *et al.* CT and MR imaging in staging non-small cell bronchogenic carcinoma: report of the Radiologic Diagnostic Oncology Group. *Radiology* 1991; 178: 705-713.
21. Crisci R, Di Cesare E, Lupattelli L, *et al.* MR study of N2 disease in lung cancer: contrast-enhanced method using gadolinium-DTPA. *Eur J Cardiothorac Surg* 1997; 11: 214-217.
22. Wang KP, Terry PB. Transbronchial needle aspiration in the diagnosis and staging of bronchogenic carcinoma. *Am Rev Respir Dis* 1983; 127: 344-347.
23. Detterbeck FC, Decamp MM, Kohman LJ, Silvestri GA. Invasive Staging. The Guidelines. *Chest* 2003; 123: 167S-173S.
24. Shannon JJ, Bude RO, Oren JB, *et al.* Endobronchial ultrasound-guided needle aspiration of mediastinal adenopathy. *Am J Respir Crit Care Med* 1996; 153: 1424-1430.
25. Westcott JL. Percutaneous transthoracic needle biopsy. *Radiology* 1988; 169: 593-601.
26. Padhani AR, Scott WW Jr; Cheema M, Kearney D, Erozan YS. The value of immediate cytologic evaluation for needle aspiration lung biopsy. *Invest Radiol* 1997; 32(8): 453-8.
27. Carlens EL. Mediastinoscopy: a method for inspection and tissue biopsy in the superior mediastinum. *Dis Chest* 1959; 36: 343-52.
28. McNeil TM, Chamberlain J. Diagnostic anterior mediastinotomy. *Ann Thorac Surg* 1966; 2: 532-9.
29. Ginsberg RJ, Rice TW, Goldberg M, *et al.* Extended cervical mediastinoscopy: a single staging procedure for bronchiogenic carcinoma of the left upper lobe. *Thorac Cardiovasc Surg* 1987; 94: 673-678.
30. Cybulsky IJ, Bennett WF. Mediastinoscopy as a routine outpatient procedure. *Ann Thorac Surg* 1994; 58: 176-8.
31. Jahangiri M, Goldstraw P. The Role of Mediastinoscopy in Superior Vena Caval Obstruction. *Ann Thorac Surg* 1995; 59(2): 453-455.
32. Toker A, Bayrak Y, Tanju S, *et al.* Invasive staging of superior mediastinum in non-small cell lung cancer patients with specific indications. *ICVTS* 2003; Vol. 2 (4): 472-476.
33. Daly BD Jr, Faling LJ, Pugatch RD, *et al.* Computed tomography. An effective technique for mediastinal staging in lung cancer. *J Thorac Cardiovasc Surg* 1984 Oct; 88(4): 486-94.
34. Luke WP, Pearson FG, Todd TR, *et al.* Prospective evaluation of mediastinoscopy for assessment of carcinoma of the lung. *J Thorac Cardiovasc Surg* 1986; 91(1): 53-6.
35. Kernstine KH, Mclaughlin KA, Menda Y, *et al.* Can FDG-PET reduce the need for mediastinoscopy in potentially resectable non-small cell lung cancer? *Ann Thorac Surg* 2002 Feb; 73(2): 394-401.
36. Pearson FG, Cooper JD, Deslauriers J, *et al* (Eds). *Thoracic Surgery*, Ch.7. Churchill Livingstone, 1995: 813-836.
37. Patterson GA, Piazza D, Pearson FG, *et al.* Significance of metastatic disease in subaortic lymph nodes. *Ann Thorac Surg* 1987 Feb; 43(2): 155-9.

38. Landreneau RJ, Hazelrigg SR, Mack MJ, *et al.* Thoracoscopic mediastinal lymph node sampling: a useful approach to mediastinal lymph node stations inaccessible to cervical mediastinoscopy. *J Thorac Cardiovasc Surg* 1993; 106: 554-58.

Further Reading

1. Detterbeck FC, Jones DR, Parker Jr, LR. Intrathoracic staging. In: *Diagnosis and Treatment of lung cancer: an evidence-based guide for the practicing clinician.* Detterbeck FC, Rivera MP, Socinski MA, Rosenman JG, Eds. WB Saunders, Philadelphia, 2001: 73-93.
2. Spiro SG, Porter JC. Lung Cancer - Where are we today? Current advances in staging and nonsurgical treatment. *Am J Respir Crit Care Med* 2002; 166: 1166-1196.
3. Passlick B. Initial surgical staging of lung cancer. *Lung Cancer* 2003; 42: S21-25.

Chapter 4

Curative intent surgery for lung cancer

S William Fountain FRCS

Consultant Thoracic Surgeon

Harefield Hospital, Harefield, Middlesex, UK

Introduction

When Evarts A Graham (Figure 1) performed the first dissectional pneumonectomy for bronchial carcinoma in 1933 [1] the only evidence he had that it was good treatment was the anecdotal experience of a few surgeons who had performed similar resections. His next 19 patients succumbed before he had another survivor [2] and yet he persevered with an operation which has now become a standard procedure in lung cancer surgery. In terms of the US Agency for Health Care Policy and Research (AHCPR) grading [3] there is still virtually no positive grade A evidence for the procedures commonly performed in the treatment of lung cancer. The data on which modern surgery is based comes from a large number of well constructed observational studies performed over the last 30 years, which show such consistency that their results cannot reasonably be doubted.

Early studies showed what could be done by skilled surgeons but lack of proper staging meant that long-term outcomes were poor [4]. More recent work [5] enables analysis which is sufficiently sophisticated to allow for the development of a reliable staging system, for non-small cell lung cancer (NSCLC) at least [6] (Figure 2 and Table 1 [TNM classification, see Table 2, Chapter 3]). The validity of Mountain's work is confirmed, in practical terms, by large single centre studies in the UK [7,8] and elsewhere.

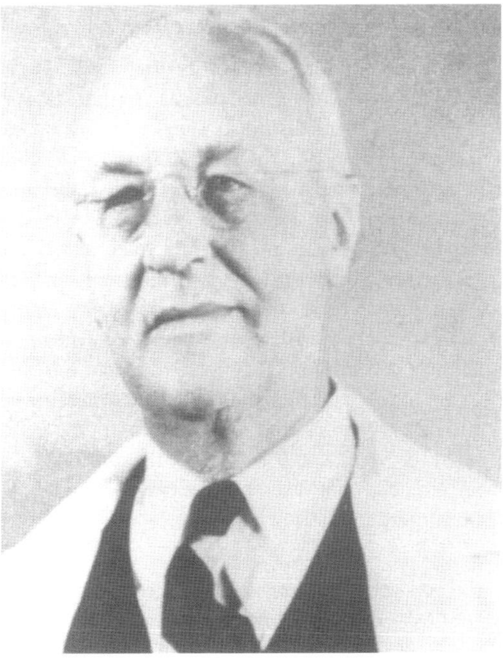

Figure 1. Evarts A Graham (1883-1957).

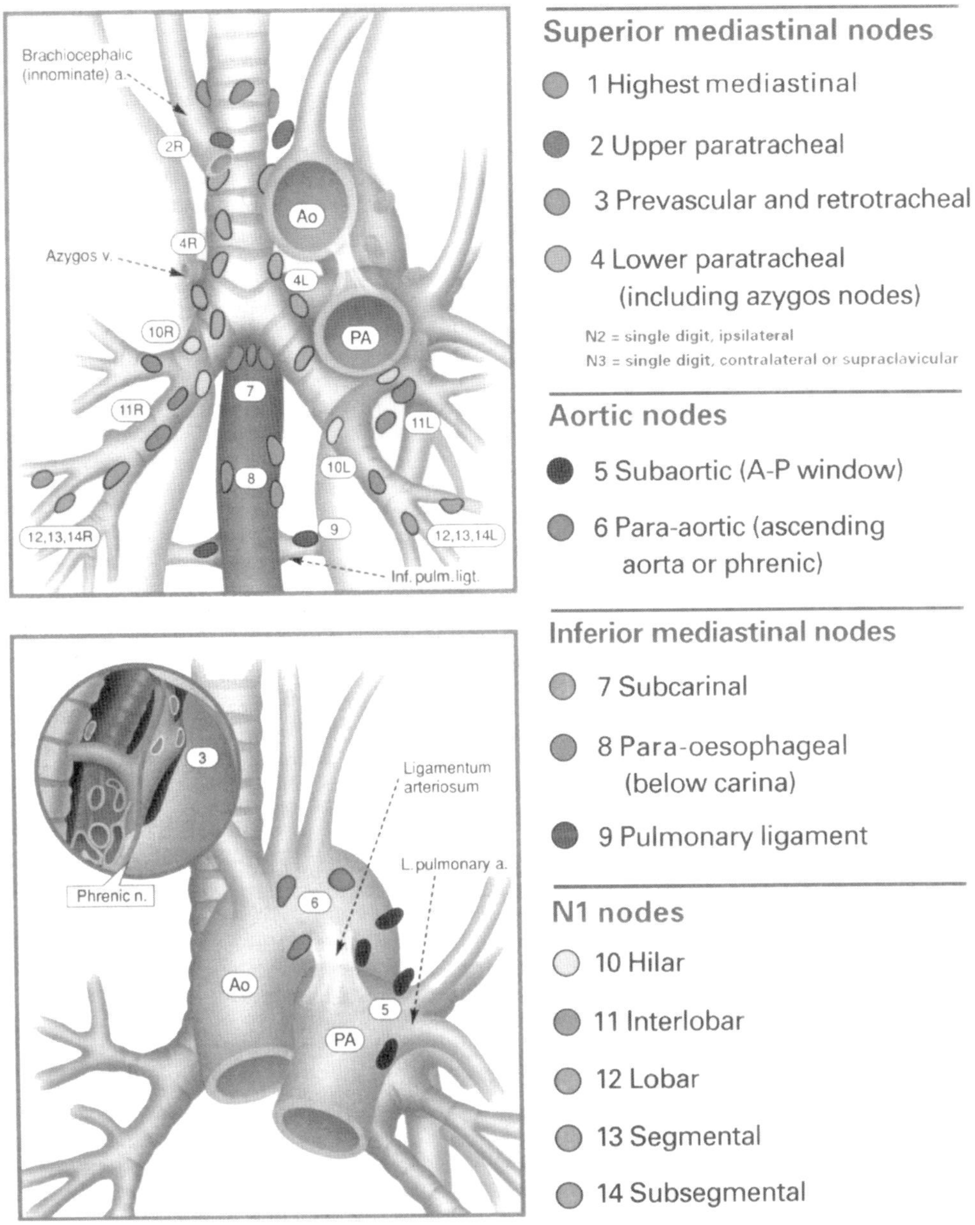

Figure 2. **Regional lymph node map.** *Reproduced with permission from Mountain and Dresler [6] and the American College of Chest Physicians.*

Table 1. **Lymph node map definitions.** ***Reproduced with permission from Mountain and Dresler [6] and the American College of Chest Physicians.***

Nodal station	Anatomic landmarks
N2 nodes - All N2 nodes lie within the mediastinal pleural envelope	
1 Highest mediastinal nodes	Nodes lying above a horizontal line at the upper rim of the bracheocephalic (left innominate) vein where it ascends to the left, crossing in front of the trachea at its midline.
2 Upper paratracheal nodes	Nodes lying above a horizontal line drawn tangential to the upper margin of the aortic arch and below the inferior boundary of No. 1 nodes.
3 Prevascular and retrotracheal nodes	Prevascular and retrotracheal nodes may be designated 3A and 3P; midline nodes are considered to be ipsilateral.
4 Lower paratracheal nodes	The lower paratracheal nodes on the right lie to the right of the midline of the trachea between a horizontal line drawn tangential to the upper margin of the aortic arch and a line extending across the right main bronchus at the upper margin of the upper lobe bronchus, and contained within the mediastinal pleural envelope; the lower paratracheal nodes on the left lie to the left of the midline of the trachea between a horizontal line drawn tangential to the upper margin of the aortic arch and a line extending across the left main bronchus at the level of the upper margin of the left upper lobe bronchus, medial to the ligamentum arteriosum and contained within the mediastinal pleural envelope. Researchers may wish to designate the lower paratracheal nodes as No. 4s (superior) and No. 4i (inferior) subsets for study purposes; the No. 4s nodes may be defined by a horizontal line extending across the trachea and drawn tangential to the cephalic border of the azygos vein; the No. 4i nodes may be defined by the lower boundary of No. 4s and the lower boundary of No. 4, as described above.
5 Subaortic (aorto-pulmonary window)	Subaortic nodes are lateral to the ligamentum arteriosum or the aorta or left pulmonary artery and proximal to the first branch of the left pulmonary artery and lie within the mediastinal pleural envelope.
6 Para-aortic nodes (ascending aorta or phrenic)	Nodes lying anterior and lateral to the ascending aorta and the aortic arch or the innominate artery, beneath a line tangential to the upper margin of the aortic arch.
7 Subcarinal nodes	Nodes lying caudal to the carina of the trachea, but not associated with the lower lobe bronchi or arteries within the lung.
8 Paraesophageal nodes (below carina)	Nodes lying adjacent to the wall of the esophagus and to the right or left of the midline, excluding subcarinal nodes.
9 Pulmonary ligament nodes	Nodes lying within the pulmonary ligament, including those in the posterior wall and lower part of the inferior pulmonary vein.
N1 nodes - All N1 nodes lie distal to the mediastinal pleural reflection and within the visceral pleura	
10 Hilar nodes	The proximal lobar nodes, distal to the mediastinal pleural reflection and the nodes adjacent to the bronchus intermedius on the right; radiographically, the hilar shadow may be created by enlargement of both hilar and interlobar nodes.
11 Interlobar nodes	Nodes lying between the lobar bronchi.
12 Lobar nodes	Nodes adjacent to the distal lobar bronchi.
13 Segmental nodes	Nodes adjacent to the segmental bronchi.
14 Subsegmental nodes	Nodes around the subsegmental bronchi.

The place of surgery in lung cancer

In terms of absolute fact, surgery is the only established method of cure for lung cancer. It is only possible however, in a relatively small proportion of patients with the disease. The UK has one of the lowest resection rates in the civilised world at 13%, well below that in the United States [9] and most of Europe [10] where it is generally 25-30%. While the denominator for population-based studies is not always the same, it is accepted that the low UK rate is real. Better access to surgery may be part of the solution [11] and the National Cancer Plan and other initiatives are designed to address this [12,13]. Selection criteria vary little from country to country and UK long-term survival rates compare well with others (Table 2). While short-term results may to some extent reflect technical competence, long-term survival depends on appropriate case selection, which in turn depends on accurate pre-operative staging.

Staging

The international staging system for NSCLC [6] is the basis for all surgical treatment modalities and the success of novel methods must be measured against this yardstick.

From the data available it is clear that the principal influence on long-term prognosis and therefore cure is tumour stage. For patients with NSCLC who are fit for surgery, lung resection is the best form of treatment for stage I and stage II disease. At the other extreme, surgery with curative intent has no place in the management of stage IV disease.

The position of patients with stage III disease is uncertain, particularly with respect to the prognostic significance of lymph node spread. Most of the recent and current clinical research being undertaken in the area of surgery for lung cancer is aimed at improving cure rates in this group.

Pre-operative assessment

Clinical (c) staging is the estimate of stage based on pre-operative investigations. Pathological (p) staging is that derived from histological examination of the resected specimen. In some groups there is a significant difference in long-term survival between the two [5] implying that (c) staging underestimates the extent of disease. As more sensitive staging modalities are developed, this difference should diminish.

Imaging

Plain radiology and Computed Tomography (CT) scans have been established as the baseline imaging techniques for many years [14]. Magnetic Resonance Imaging (MRI) has some applications but radioactive isotope scanning has a low positive yield in NSCLC and is not widely used. Positron Emission Tomography (PET) scanning promises much [15] but is not foolproof and cannot yet replace mediastinoscopy for assessment of superior mediastinal nodes [16].

Invasive staging

Bronchoscopy may contribute information about both cell type and tumour (T) stage for central lesions. Percutaneous biopsy may be necessary to obtain a histological diagnosis. At present, mediastinoscopy remains the gold standard for assessing bulky superior mediastinal nodes.

Surgical procedures

Lobectomy

Anatomical lobectomy has been the most commonly performed procedure for lung cancer for over 50 years and little has changed in terms of technique in that time. There is no evidence to show that if complete macroscopic tumour clearance can be achieved by lobectomy, better results will follow a more radical procedure.

Pneumonectomy

As indicated above, pneumonectomy has been performed for lung cancer for 70 years. Despite advances in case selection and pre- and

Table 2. **Long-term results of surgery.**

		5-year survival (%)		
Study	**No of patients**	**Stage I**	**Stage II**	**Stage IIIa**
Mountain *et al*	5319	51	32	17
Al Kattan *et al*	207	59	30	16
Kadri and Dussek	479	55	35	16

postoperative care however, it remains a procedure with a stubbornly high operative mortality. Respiratory and cardiac complications are the commonest causes [17] but age, probably as a surrogate for accumulative comorbidity is also a factor, particularly for right-sided resections [18].

Other procedures

Anatomical segmental resection and more recently, unanatomical wedge resection has been described but neither deals as well as the more radical procedures with intrapulmonary lymphatic permeation and node spread and so local recurrence rates are higher. Segmental resection has no advantage over wedge resection in terms of local treatment and has largely been abandoned for the treatment of lung cancer. Wedge resection for small, peripheral tumours in patients with poor pulmonary reserve or other significant comorbidity is therefore probably the treatment of choice for these groups [19]. This procedure is also well adapted to the application of video-assisted thoracic surgical (VATS) techniques. The use of wedge resection for blood-borne metastatic disease to the lung is also well established [20].

VATS lobectomy and pneumonectomy have also been validated as techniques with results as good as, but in most respects, no better than standard open operations [21,22].

Extended resection

Radical procedures for locally advanced disease are associated with good results so long as the extent of disease is confined to T stage. When advanced N (nodal) disease is also involved, prognosis is dictated by this aspect of the disease and the higher morbidity and mortality of extended resection may not be justified by long-term results. Bronchoplastic lobar resection involving a sleeve, usually of bronchus but occasionally of pulmonary artery is a good combination of both radical and conservative surgery [23]. Sleeve pneumonectomy is a highly specialised procedure with few applications and acceptable results in only a few series [24]. Chest wall resection for T3 tumours invading parietal pleura is well established and attended by good long-term survival [25]. The place of resection in the special situation of patients with superior sulcus tumours causing Pancoast's syndrome is less clear. Initial reports that pre-operative radiotherapy was able to downstage such tumours [26] have not been borne out by general experience, but there are some fairly small, single centre studies employing radical resection [27]. Interpretation of results in the area of extended resection is sometimes made difficult by the inclusion of different methods of adjuvant therapy during the course of an individual study.

Results

Short-term

Currently, information from recent studies [5,7,8] and from the UK thoracic surgical Register, which has been collecting mortality data from all UK centres for over 20 years [28], shows that mortality following lobectomy and pneumonectomy respectively, are 3% and 7%. These figures have changed little during the Register's existence, but the ratio of lobectomy to pneumonectomy has changed from 2:1 to 4:1 in recent years. This probably reflects the risk profile of patients at presentation. Unfortunately, no information of predictive value is available on morbidity, and virtually no data of any kind exists concerning quality of life after surgery.

Long-term

Table 2 shows the long-term results which can be expected following standard surgery for stage I and II disease.

The position of patients with stage III disease is much less clear. Within this group, T and N status each separately influence prognosis and the influence of N status varies between (c) and (p) stage. In stage IIIA, many studies have shown that 5-year survival following resection for disease with a pN2 component is around 15% [5,7,8], whereas with cN2 disease, survival for more than three years is unusual [29]. In stage IIIB there is evidence of good long-term survival in T4 N0 disease however radical the resection, but nodal disease is again associated with poor prognosis [30].

Adjuvant therapy

Attempts to alter these outcomes have concentrated on two areas: radical lymphadenectomy and adjuvant therapy. In retrospective observational studies, radical lymphadenectomy has been shown to give good results [31] but a prospective randomised controlled trial (RCT) comparing it with systematic dissection for staging purposes only showed no survival advantage [32].

The situation with adjuvant therapy is much more complex because of the different modalities, timing and agents available (Figure 3). Pre-operative radiotherapy has not been shown to improve resectability or long-term survival and it is currently believed that postoperative radiotherapy in addition to surgery has no beneficial effect [33].

An initial meta-analysis of adjuvant chemotherapy showed a small survival benefit [34] but this has not been confirmed by a more recent multicentre RCT [35].

The value of neoadjuvant chemotherapy is not proven, but it is widely used in contemporary practice. A large number of studies have been conducted to evaluate neoadjuvant chemotherapy but many are single centre observational studies [36]. RCTs have been performed [29,37] but their study designs have been criticised and others have shown no benefit [38]. Although most studies showing value employ platinum-based drugs, there is little consistency about the total drug regimens and it is likely that these

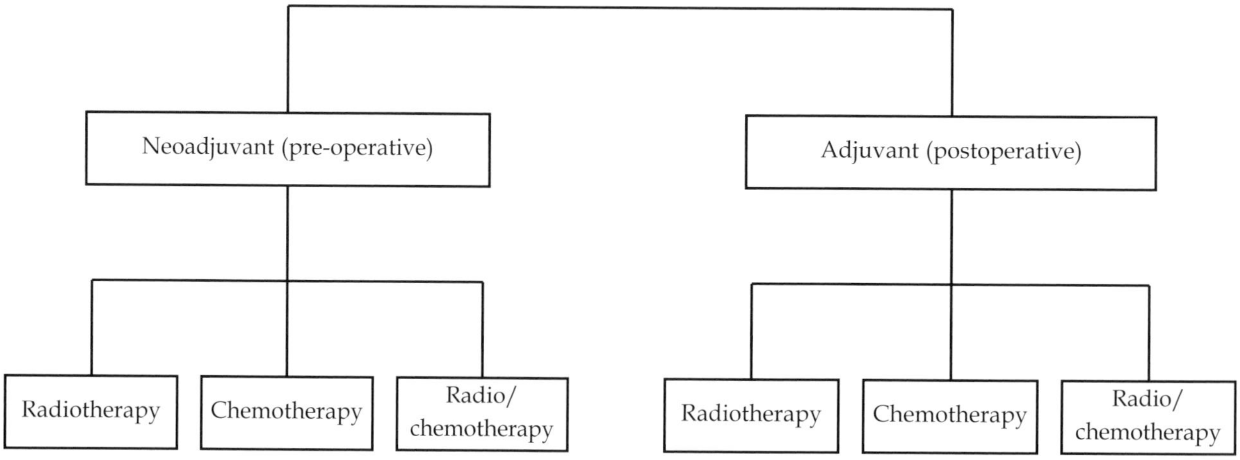

Figure 3. **Adjuvant therapy.**

regimes will be overtaken by the use of more modern agents. It is also generally accepted that the response rate of NSCLC to induction chemotherapy is relatively low. A multicentre RCT on the effects of neoadjuvant chemotherapy on early stage NSCLC - MRC LU22 - is currently underway and may resolve some of these issues [39]. Despite the lack of irrefutable evidence that neoadjuvant chemotherapy works, it is common practice for it to be given to patients with stage III tumours in an attempt to downstage their disease and adjuvant therapy is recommended by some [40]. Individual small studies show benefit from combining neoadjuvant chemotherapy with radiotherapy, but again the response rate is low [41]. Not surprisingly, these treatments cause increased morbidity but no studies measure quality of life, which is particularly important to the majority of patients who do not respond to the treatment.

Small Cell Lung Cancer (SCLC)

A trial conducted by the Medical Research Council in the 1970s [42] indicated that there was virtually no place for surgical treatment of this aggressive form of lung cancer, which is almost always systemic at presentation. Nevertheless, a few studies have shown that in the very small proportion of patients who present with early stage, peripheral tumours, surgical results compare favourably with those of chemotherapy [43]. Although the TNM staging system strictly applies only to NSCLC it can be seen by applying the same criteria to SCLC that surgical treatment is appropriate for patients with the equivalent of stage I disease, who have a 5-year survival of 44%. For stage II it is 20% and for stage IIIA, 4%. Because of the high chance of subclinical metastatic disease in SCLC it is normal practice to carry out extensive pre-operative scanning and to give postoperative chemotherapy, although the evidence for the value of this treatment is equivocal [44].

Conclusions

Surgery is the treatment of choice for patients with stage I and II NSCLC but accurate pre-operative staging is essential for good results. Patients with stage III disease may benefit from a combination of surgery and adjuvant therapy but the evidence in this area is currently equivocal. Surgery is also indicated for patients with stage I SCLC.

Recommendations	Evidence level
◆ Surgery is the best form of treatment for patients with stage I and stage II NSCLC.	II/A
◆ Accurate pre-operative staging is essential to achieve good long-term results.	I/B
◆ Adjuvant therapy may improve long-term survival for patients with stage III NSCLC but current studies show conflicting results.	I/A

References

1. Graham EA, Singer JJ. Successful removal of an entire lung for carcinoma of the bronchus. *JAMA* 1933; 101: 1371-4.
2. Naef AP. The mid-century revolution in thoracic and cardiovascular surgery: Part 1. *Interactive Cardiovascular and Thoracic Surgery* 2003; 2: 219-26.
3. Agency for Health Care Policy and Research. Acute pain management, operative or medical procedures and trauma. Clinical Practice Guideline 92-0032. Rockvilee, Marland, USA: Agency for Health Care Policy and Research Publications, 1992.
4. Smith RA. The importance of mediastinal lymph node invasion by pulmonary carcinoma in selection of patients for resection. *Ann Thorac Surg* 1978; 25: 5-11.
5. Mountain CF. Revisions in the International System for Staging Lung Cancer. *Chest* 1997; 111: 1710-7.
6. Mountain CF, Dresler CM. Regional lymph node classification for lung cancer staging. *Chest* 1997; 111: 1718-23.
7. Kadri MA, Dussek JE. Survival and prognosis following resection of primary non-small cell bronchogenic carcinoma. *Eur J Cardiothorac Surg* 1991; 5: 132-6.
8. al Kattan K, Sepsas E, Townsend ER, Fountain SW. Factors affecting long-term survival following resection for lung cancer. *Thorax* 1996; 51: 1266-9.
9. Humphrey EW, Smart CR, Winchester DP, Steele GD, Jr., Yarbro JW, Chu KC, *et al.* National survey of the pattern of care for carcinoma of the lung. *J Thorac Cardiovasc Surg* 1990; 100: 837-43.
10. Janssen-Heijnen ML, Gatta G, Forman D, Capocaccia R, Coebergh JW. Variation in survival of patients with lung cancer in Europe, 1985-1989. *Eur J Cancer* 1998; 34: 2191-6.
11. Laroche C, Wells F, Coulden R, Stewart S, Goddard M, Lowry E, *et al.* Improving surgical resection rate in lung cancer. *Thorax* 1998; 53: 445-9.
12. DoH. Expert Advisory Group on Cancer. http://www.chi.nhs.uk/cancer/ch1/07.shtml 1995.
13. Treasure T, Dussek J, Eraut D, Muers M, Rudd R, Fountain W, Morgan A, and Vaughan R. The Critical Under-Provision of Thoracic Surgery in the UK. Report of a joint Working Group of The British Thoracic Society and The Society of Cardiothoracic Surgeons of Great Britain and Ireland. 2002. British Thoracic Society and the Society of Cardiothoracic Surgeons of Great Britain and Ireland.
14. BTS guidelines: guidelines on the selection of patients with lung cancer for surgery. *Thorax* 2001; 56: 89-108.
15. Lowe VJ, Naunheim KS. Positron emission tomography in lung cancer. *Ann Thorac Surg* 1998; 65: 1821-9.
16. Gonzalez-Stawinski GV, Lemaire A, Merchant F, O'Halloran E, Coleman RE, Harpole DH, *et al.* A comparative analysis of positron emission tomography and mediastinoscopy in staging non-small cell lung cancer. *J Thorac Cardiovasc Surg* 2003; 126: 1900-5.
17. Patel RL, Townsend ER, Fountain SW. Elective pneumonectomy: factors associated with morbidity and operative mortality. *Ann Thorac Surg* 1992; 54: 84-8.
18. Au J, el Oakley R, Cameron EW. Pneumonectomy for bronchogenic carcinoma in the elderly. *Eur J Cardiothorac Surg* 1994; 8: 247-50.
19. Ginsberg RJ, Rubinstein LV. Randomized trial of lobectomy versus limited resection for T1 N0 non-small cell lung cancer. Lung Cancer Study Group. *Ann Thorac Surg* 1995; 60: 615-22.
20. Pastorino U, Boyse M, Friedel G, *et al.* Long-term results of lung metastasectomy: prognostic analysis based on 5206 cases. *J Thorac Cardiovasc Surg* 1997; 113: 37-49
21. Walker WS. Video-assisted thoracic surgery (VATS) lobectomy: the Edinburgh experience. *Semin Thorac Cardiovasc Surg* 1998; 10: 291-9.
22. Roviaro GC, Varoli F, Rebuffat C, Sonnino D, Vergani C, Maciocco M, *et al.* Videothoracoscopic operative staging for lung cancer. *Int Surg* 1996; 81: 252-4.
23. Vogt-Moykopf I, Fritz T, Meyer G, Bulzerbruck H, Daskos G. Bronchoplastic and angioplastic operation in bronchial carcinoma: long-term results of a retrospective analysis from 1973 to 1983. *Int Surg* 1986; 71: 211-20.
24. Mathisen DJ, Grillo HC. Carinal resection for bronchogenic carcinoma. *J Thorac Cardiovasc Surg* 1991; 102: 16-22.
25. Trastek VF, Pairolero PC, Piehler JM, Weiland LH, O'Brien PC, Payne WS, *et al.* En bloc (non-chest wall) resection for bronchogenic carcinoma with parietal fixation. Factors affecting survival. *J Thorac Cardiovasc Surg* 1984; 87: 352-8.
26. Paulson DL. Carcinomas in the superior pulmonary sulcus. *J Thorac Cardiovasc Surg* 1975; 70: 1095-104.
27. Dartevelle PG, Chapelier AR, Macchiarini P, Lenot B, Cerrina J, Ladurie FL *et al.* Anterior transcervical-thoracic approach for radical resection of lung tumors invading the thoracic inlet. *J Thorac Cardiovasc Surg* 1993; 105: 1025-34.
28. Society of Cardiothoracic Surgeons. http://www.scts.org/file/thoracicregister1999-00.xls. 2002.
29. Rosell R, Gomez-Codina J, Camps C, Maestre J, Padille J, Canto A, *et al.* A randomized trial comparing preoperative chemotherapy plus surgery with surgery alone in patients with non-small-cell lung cancer. *N Engl J Med* 1994; 330: 153-8.
30. DeMeester TR, Albertucci M, Dawson PJ, Montner SM. Management of tumor adherent to the vertebral column. *J Thorac Cardiovasc Surg* 1989; 97: 373-8.
31. Naruke T, Goya T, Tsuchiya R, Suemasu K. The importance of surgery to non-small cell carcinoma of lung with mediastinal lymph node metastasis. *Ann Thorac Surg* 1988; 46: 603-10.
32. Izbicki JR, Thetter O, Habekost M, Karg O, Passlick B, Kubuschok B, *et al.* Radical systematic mediastinal lymphadenectomy in non-small cell lung cancer: a randomized controlled trial. *Br J Surg* 1994; 81: 229-35.
33. Postoperative radiotherapy in non-small-cell lung cancer: systematic review and meta-analysis of individual patient data from nine randomised controlled trials. PORT Meta-analysis Trialists Group. *Lancet* 1998; 352: 257-63.

34. NSCLC Collaborative Group. Chemotherapy in non-small cell lung cancer: a meta-analysis using updated data on individual patients from 52 randomised clinical trials. Non-small Cell Lung Cancer Collaborative Group. *BMJ* 1995; 311: 899-909.
35. Fairlamb DJ, Gower N, Milroy R, *et al.* The Big Lung Trial. *Proc Am Soc Clin Oncol* 2003; 22:639
36. Martini N, Kris MG, Flehinger BJ, Gralla RJ, Bains MS, Burt ME, *et al.* Preoperative chemotherapy for stage IIIa (N2) lung cancer: the Sloan-Kettering experience with 136 patients. *Ann Thorac Surg* 1993; 55: 1365-73.
37. Roth JA, Fossella F, Komaki R, Ryan MB, Putnam JB, Jr., Lee JS, *et al.* A randomized trial comparing perioperative chemotherapy and surgery with surgery alone in resectable stage IIIA non-small-cell lung cancer. *J Natl Cancer Inst* 1994; 86: 673-80.
38. Scagliotti GV, Fossati R, Torri V, Crino L, Giaccone G, Silvano G, *et al.* Randomized study of adjuvant chemotherapy for completely resected stage I, II, or IIIA non-small-cell Lung cancer. *J Natl Cancer Inst* 2003; 95: 1453-61.
39. Preoperative Chemotherapy in Resectable NSCLC. Medical Research Council 1998.
40. Blum RH Adjuvant chemotherapy for lung cancer: a new standard of care. *N Engl J Med* 2004; 350: 404-5
41. Machtay M, Lee JH, Stevenson JP, Shrager JB, Algazy KM, Treat J, *et al.* Two commonly used neoadjuvant chemoradiotherapy regimens for locally advanced stage III non-small cell lung carcinoma: long-term results and associations with pathologic response. *J Thorac Cardiovasc Surg* 2004; 127: 108-13.
42. Fox W, Scadding JG. Medical Research Council comparative trial of surgery and radiotherapy for primary treatment of small-celled or oat-celled carcinoma of bronchus. Ten-year follow-up. *Lancet* 1973; 2: 63-5.
43. Shields TW, Higgins GA, Jr., Matthews MJ, Keehn RJ. Surgical resection in the management of small cell carcinoma of the lung. *J Thorac Cardiovasc Surg* 1982; 84: 481-8.
44. Shepherd FA, Ginsberg RJ, Patterson GA, Evans WK, Feld R. A prospective study of adjuvant surgical resection after chemotherapy for limited small cell lung cancer. A University of Toronto Lung Oncology Group study. *J Thorac Cardiovasc Surg* 1989; 97: 177-86.

Chapter 5

Lobectomy for lung cancer by video-assisted thoracic surgery (VATS)

Artyom Sedrakyan MD ScC
Honorary Lecturer and Research Scholar [1]
Tom Treasure MD MS FRCS
Professor of Cardiothoracic Surgery [2]

1 The Royal College of Surgeons of England and The London School of Hygiene and Tropical Medicine, London, UK
2 Guy's and St. Thomas' Hospitals, London, UK

Introduction

The technical developments in television cameras and the ability to display a brilliantly lit and magnified view of the inside of the chest on large television screens opened the way to video-assisted thoracic surgery [1,2]. Thoracoscopy by direct vision (in our experience it was an uncomfortable operation, often performed crouching and peering through an inadequate instrument) has been possible for many years as summarised by Wakabayashi [3], but in the discussion of that paper at the American Association of Thoracic Surgery in Washington DC in 1991, Lewis announced his group's addition of a video camera to thoracoscopy. There soon followed a series of papers on video-assisted thoracic surgery for lung biopsy [4], wedge excision [5,6] and, in Lewis's first 100 patients, a variety of other indications [2]. The rapid spread of laparoscopic procedures in abdominal surgery had resulted in a series of surgical disasters [7], particularly with technical errors involving the gall bladder. Promptly, a joint committee of the American Association for Thoracic Surgery and the Society of Thoracic Surgeons issued a joint statement on appropriate training [8]. The newly developed term of video-assisted thoracic surgery (VATS) was rapidly popularised and the development and manufacture of a range of stapling and cutting devices for operating through ports of a centimetre or less in diameter followed. It seemed evident that if patients could be managed with "keyhole" surgery rather than thoracotomy, there would be advantages in reduced pain and shorter hospital stays. Now, lung biopsies for parenchymal lung disease or excision biopsies of solitary lesions at the lung edge can be readily performed for diagnostic purposes. Virtually all operations for pneumothorax can be performed by VATS and clinical experience is that it makes inspection and biopsy of the pleura easier. At the more challenging end of the spectrum is lobectomy for lung cancer by VATS, an operation which Lewis published in 1995 [9]. In this chapter we explore the evidence for VATS lobectomy.

We have performed a systematic review of randomised clinical trials to determine if VATS is associated with better clinical outcomes as compared to thoracotomy for lobectomy.

Methodology

Systematic review

Only randomised clinical trials (RCTs) comparing VATS to conventional surgery were included. The following inclusion criteria were applied:-

- Random allocation of patients.
- Enrolment of only general thoracic surgery patients.
- No concurrent use of another experimental medication or device.

Randomised trials were identified by searching the MEDLINE, EMBASE and Cochrane Controlled Trials Register from 1980 to 2003. Only studies in humans were considered and no language restrictions were applied. We used MeSH terms "thoracic surgery", "video-assisted" "thoracoscopy", and various combinations of text words that might be related to this specific procedure. A standard RCT filter designed by the Cochrane Collaboration for identifying RCTs was used for MEDLINE and EMBASE (adapted from the Scottish Intercollegiate Guideline Network SIGN (http://www.sign.ac.uk/methodology/filters.html)). In addition, we searched the reference lists of randomised trials and reviews to look for additional studies.

Search of the databases identified 142 unique abstracts. Independent review of these abstracts identified 12 unique studies of VATS meeting all inclusion criteria of which three were for lobectomy (Tables 1 and 2). For each trial, abstracted data included the number of patients randomised and the frequency of the events in the VATS and control groups. Further outcomes such as surgery time, pain measurement/medication, any major complications, length of hospital stay (LOS) and costs were collected for the two groups under comparison. Finally, information on age and gender were collected. Meta-analysis was not attempted because as will be seen these three RCTs had very different objectives and reported very different outcomes.

The methodological quality of included studies was evaluated using modified Jadad criteria [10] which were based on the following:-

- "Randomised" study description.
- Description of randomisation procedure.
- Allocation concealment.
- Dropouts and intention to treat analysis.

Blinding was not applicable in this setting.

The trials

There were three reported trials (Tables 1 and 2) of VATS lobectomy versus conventional lobectomy enrolling 196 patients [11-13]. The average age of patients in these studies was 64 years and 48% were females. None of the studies reported information on method of randomisation and analysis was not based on intention to treat methodology in two studies [11,12].

The first reported RCT in 1995 was a collaboration between three USA centres in Cleveland, Dallas and Pittsburgh. The control group had a muscle-sparing thoracotomy (MST: neither serratus anterior nor latissimus dorsi were divided) and the VATS group had a 6-8cm access thoracotomy (without rib spreading). In 52/61 patients, staging mediastinoscopy was performed with similar proportions in each arm of the trial (MST 28/30, VATS 24/25) to ensure as far as possible that these were stage I disease (T1/2N0M0). It is not clear whether randomisation was before or after this procedure, but a determined attempt was made to sample lymph nodes for operative staging. Three patients who turned out to have benign disease were excluded and three intended VATS cases were converted to thoracotomy and excluded.

We will use the phrase "periprocedural indices" to summarize such measures as operative time, blood loss, air leak, conversion rate, drain days and length of stay as we discuss the evidence and present a summary of evidence and recommendations.

The operative time was about 2.7 hours for thoracotomy and averaged 14 minutes longer for

Table 1. Characteristics of the randomised trials of VATS and conventional strategy.

Study	Randomisation	Description of randomisation	Allocation concealment	Intention to treat	Age (mean)	% Female	% Malignant
Lobectomy							
Sugi *et al* 2000	'Randomised'	Not described	Not reported	No	65	43	100
Craig *et al* 2001	'Randomised'	Not described	Concealed	Yes	63	46	87
Kirby *et al* 1995	'Randomised'	Not described	Concealed	No	60	57	100

Table 2. Outcomes reported in the randomised trials of VATS and conventional strategy.

Study	Surgical group comparison	N of people	Recurrence/ Failure	Surgery time (min)	Length of stay (days)	Pain/ medication use	Other complications	Costs
Sugi *et al* 2000	VATS lobectomy	48	Not reported	Not reported	Not reported	Not reported	No survival difference between the groups	
	Thoracotomy	52	Not reported	Not reported	Not reported	Not reported		
Craig *et al* 2001	VATS lobectomy	22	Not reported	141 ± 39	8.6 ± 3.0	Not reported	2/22	Not reported
	Thoracotomy	19	Not reported	121 ± 31	7.9 ± 3.2	Not reported	4/19	Not reported
Kirby *et al* 1995	VATS lobectomy	25	Not reported	161 ± 61	7.1 ± 5.5	Disabling pain 1/25	Mostly air leaks 6/25†	Not reported
	Thoracotomy	30	Not reported	175 ± 93	8.3 ± 5.7	Disabling pain 2/30	Mostly air leaks 19/30	Not reported

Values are reported as means ± standard deviations or median (range) for surgery time, length of stay and pain/medication use, unless specified otherwise.

† Difference is statistically significant ($p<0.05$).

VATS, but the differences were not significant. With standard deviations of 1.5 hours and one hour respectively, these were unlikely to reach significance unless part of a much larger study for reasons of statistical power. Blood loss was uniformly small (rarely more than 250ml). Chest tube drainage and hospital stay were both shorter by a day for VATS but at 5-6 days chest drainage and hospital stays averaging 7-8 days, both were conservatively long (in our view) and are witness to an appropriate caution in the study of a radically different approach to a major operation. We can conclude that in a non-blinded study, VATS compared favourably with conventional surgery in a study ten years old at the time this chapter went to press.

We should remark while summarizing this trial that an "intention to treat" analysis would have been preferred and should always be conducted when a new technique is under evaluation. Exclusions, failures and conversions are necessary, but need to be known in evaluating a technique and the techniques should be analyzed in the groups they were assigned initially.

If a comparison is being made with a very well established technique it is important of course that the very earliest part of the learning curve has been overcome for fair comparison to be made. An early trial of laparoscopic versus open surgery for cholecystectomy [14] was robustly criticized because other surgeons believed that they were still in their learning curve [15,16].

Sugi *et al* [11] reported a series of 100 cases of lobectomy randomised to VATS (48) or thoractotomy (52). Lung cancer was staged IA pre-operatively and in only eight were positive nodes found. Their focus was on survival. After three and five years, they found no difference. The survival for VATS versus open surgery was 90% vs 93% and 90% vs 85% at these two time points. We can conclude that it would be hard to sustain an argument that VATS compromises the oncological quality of the surgery in stage IA disease given these results, provided they can be replicated by others in larger series and cohort studies.

Craig *et al* [13] hypothesised that VATS being less traumatic would induce a less acute phase response which might prove beneficial in terms of preservation of immune function. In 41 patients randomised to VATS (22) or thoracotomy (19) they measured C-reactive protein, interleukin 6 (IL-6), tumour necrosis factor (TNF), P-selectin and an index of oxygen free radical activity. There were impressive differences with open surgery creating significant changes in these markers of the inflammatory response, which were significantly less for VATS. The use of surrogate markers to look for benefit makes it possible to reach significant differences to report in a study which is far too small (and hence, underpowered) to show differences in clinically important periprocedural indices. This and similar studies report far too early to be able to make any claims about cancer cure and survival. This is common in contemporary surgical research [17]. The advantages in terms of getting a publishable result are clear but we are left uncertain as to how to interpret differences in C-reactive protein, P-selectin and reactive oxygen species in deciding whether to adopt VATS as our surgical practice for lobectomy.

Conclusions

It seems clear that with practice and experience lobectomy can be performed safely and with very satisfactory periprocedural indices. The George Washington group [18] have reported on 179 selected cases of stage I lung cancer with one death and excellent periprocedural indices, including operative times averaging 75 minutes. Five-year survival was 85%. Walker from Edinburgh, UK, has reported on 158 patients with one in-hospital death [19]. Operative time was a median of 130 minutes and blood loss was very small. However, at six days the median length of stay does not indicate that the advantages of avoiding thoracotomy are yielding much faster recovery. In summary, with increasing experience cohort studies report shorter operating time, fewer conversions from VATS to conventional thoracotomy [18,19] and satisfactory long-term results, particularly in stage IA patients (T1N0M0). On the basis of their results Walker believes that VATS lobectomy should become the procedure of choice [19], but it has not as far as can be judged from registry reports.

We used the data from the UK Register of the Society of Thoracic Surgeons of Great Britain and Ireland (2000-2002) to determine the use of VATS procedures in all participating centers. Taking pneumothorax surgery for which VATS is well established as a reference point, there were 2,606 procedures performed in 40 units; 57% of these procedures were performed by VATS leaving 41% of patients having a thoracotomy for pneumothorax. From unit to unit, the use of VATS for pneumothorax surgery ranged from 0% to 100%. For minor resections such as excision biopsy of peripheral lesions, data are available for 2,691 procedures performed in 39 centers; 56% were done by VATS. Variation in VATS usage was not related to surgical volumes of the units. To return to lobectomy, during this same time frame there were 3,879 lobectomies performed in 40 hospitals. VATS lobectomy was reported in only 123 cases, that is only 3%. Only six units did any VATS lobectomy with two hospitals accounting for over 60% of the cases. The variation in use of medical procedures may well be related to uncertainty about the best strategy for particular patients and particular conditions [20,21]. However, variation cannot be fully explained by diversity of the populations, prevalence of the disease in question, or health characteristics of the populations [22,23]. There is evidence that the willingness of the physician/surgeon to provide a procedure, rather than the appropriateness of the procedure to the disease and the patient, explains a substantial variation in practice [20,21,24].

VATS may have higher costs as far as the equipment and consumables are concerned [25] and the more complex the procedure the more these costs are likely to be. The trade-off is shorter time in hospital and of course, if there is a clinical benefit in terms of pain reduction, better mobility and early recovery, these must be offset as advantages worth paying for. Quality of life evaluation, patient satisfaction assessments and cost-effectiveness analyses are warranted in this setting.

Those who have adopted VATS for pleural disease, lung biopsy and pneumothorax surgery appreciate considerable advantages. There seems little doubt that the advantages of a much better view, both well lit and magnified, allow better surgery with less tissue injury to the patient. Units where VATS expertise is well developed would be loath to subject an otherwise fit young patient to thoracotomy for pneumothorax. Similarly, we would want the advantages of VATS for an old frail patient with any condition, including pneumothorax, excision of peripheral lesions or haemothorax. VATS lobectomy is technically a much greater challenge and uptake has been strikingly less where we have been able to obtain registry data. It is probable that VATS lobectomy can be performed with similar periprocedural indices [11], reduction in biochemical measures of insult [13] and equivalent survival data at three and five years [12] as has been shown in RCTs. At present, the evidence of advantage does not seem strong enough to persuade most surgeons to change their practice, nor for us to recommend that they should.

Recommendations	**Evidence level**
◆ Periprocedural indices after VATS lobectomy such as operative time, blood loss, air leak and length of stay are not substantially different from those after open thoracotomy.	Ib/A
◆ VATS has advantages in terms of pain and mobility.	IV/C
◆ VATS lobectomy in selected cases is associated with survival figures comparable with open surgery.	Ib/A

References

1. Lewis RJ, Caccavale RJ, Sisler GE. Imaged thoracoscopic surgery: a new thoracic technique for resection of mediastinal cysts. *Ann Thorac Surg* 1992; 53: 318-20.
2. Lewis RJ, Caccavale RJ, Sisler GE, Mackenzie JW. One hundred consecutive patients undergoing video-assisted thoracic operations. *Ann Thorac Surg* 1992; 54: 421-6.
3. Wakabayashi A. Expanded applications of diagnostic and therapeutic thoracoscopy. *J Thorac Cardiovasc Surg* 1991; 102: 721-3.
4. Mack MJ, Aronoff RJ, Acuff TE, Douthit MB, Bowman RT, Ryan WH. Present role of thoracoscopy in the diagnosis and treatment of diseases of the chest. *Ann Thorac Surg* 1992; 54: 403-8.
5. Miller DL, Allen MS, Trastek VF, Deschamps C, Pairolero PC. Videothoracoscopic wedge excision of the lung. *Ann Thorac Surg* 1992; 54: 410-3.
6. Landreneau RJ, Hazelrigg SR, Ferson PF, Johnson JA, Nawarawong W, Boley TM, *et al.* Thoracoscopic resection of 85 pulmonary lesions. *Ann Thorac Surg* 1992; 54: 415-9.
7. Scurr JH. Medico-legal aspects of laparsocopy. In: *Laparoscopic Surgery.* Hobsley M, Treasure T, Northover J, Eds. Arnold, London, 1998: 309-14.
8. McKneally MF, Lewis RJ, Anderson RJ, Fosburg RG, Gay WA, Jr., Jones RH, *et al.* Statement of the AATS/STS Joint Committee on Thoracoscopy and Video-Assisted Thoracic Surgery. *J Thorac Cardiovasc Surg* 1992; 104: 1.
9. Lewis RJ. Simultaneously stapled lobectomy: a safe technique for video-assisted thoracic surgery. *J Thorac Cardiovasc Surg* 1995; 109: 619-25.
10. Jadad AR, Moore RA, Carroll D, Jenkinson C, Reynolds DJ, Gavaghan DJ, *et al.* Assessing the quality of reports of randomized clinical trials: is blinding necessary? *Control Clin Trials* 1996; 17: 1-12.
11. Kirby TJ, Mack MJ, Landreneau RJ, Rice TW. Lobectomy - video-assisted thoracic surgery versus muscle-sparing thoracotomy. A randomized trial. *J Thorac Cardiovasc Surg* 1995; 109: 997-1001.
12. Sugi K, Kaneda Y, Esato K. Video-assisted thoracoscopic lobectomy achieves a satisfactory long-term prognosis in patients with clinical stage IA lung cancer. *World J Surg* 2000; 24: 27-30.
13. Craig SR, Leaver HA, Yap PL, Pugh GC, Walker WS. Acute phase responses following minimal access and conventional thoracic surgery. *Eur J Cardiothorac Surg* 2001; 20: 455-63.
14. Majeed AW, Troy G, Nicholl JP, Smythe A, Reed MW, Stoddard CJ, *et al.* Randomised, prospective, single-blind comparison of laparoscopic versus small-incision cholecystectomy. *Lancet* 1996; 347: 989-94.
15. Rhodes M, Gompertz H, Armstrong K, Lennard T, Rees B. Randomised trial of laparoscopic versus small-incision cholecystectomy. *Lancet* 1996; 347: 1621-2.
16. Wellwood J. Randomised trial of laparoscopic versus small-incision cholecystectomy. *Lancet* 1996; 347: 1622-3.
17. Anyanwu AC, Treasure T. Surgical research revisited: clinical trials in the cardiothoracic surgical literature. *Eur J Cardiothorac Surg* 2004; 25: 299-303.
18. Gharagozloo F, Tempesta B, Margolis M, Alexander EP. Video-assisted thoracic surgery lobectomy for stage I lung cancer. *Ann Thorac Surg* 2003; 76: 1009-14.
19. Walker WS, Codispoti M, Soon SY, Stamenkovic S, Carnochan F, Pugh G. Long-term outcomes following VATS lobectomy for non-small cell bronchogenic carcinoma. *Eur J Cardiothorac Surg* 2003; 23: 397-402.
20. Detsky AS. Regional variation in medical care. *N Engl J Med* 1995; 333: 589-90.
21. Wennberg JE. Understanding geographic variations in health care delivery. *N Engl J Med* 1999; 340: 52-3.
22. Pilote L, Califf RM, Sapp S, Miller DP, Mark DB, Weaver WD, *et al.* Regional variation across the United States in the management of acute myocardial infarction. GUSTO-1 Investigators. Global Utilization of Streptokinase and Tissue Plasminogen Activator for Occluded Coronary Arteries. *N Engl J Med* 1995; 333: 565-72.
23. Guadagnoli E, Hauptman PJ, Ayanian JZ, Pashos CL, McNeil BJ, Cleary PD. Variation in the use of cardiac procedures after acute myocardial infarction. *N Engl J Med* 1995; 333: 573-8.
24. Laycock WS, Siewers AE, Birkmeyer CM, Wennberg DE, Birkmeyer JD. Variation in the use of laparoscopic cholecystectomy for elderly patients with acute cholecystitis. *Arch Surg* 2000; 135: 457-62.
25. Hazelrigg SR, Nunchuck SK, Landreneau RJ, Mack MJ, Naunheim KS, Seifert PE, *et al.* Cost analysis for thoracoscopy: thoracoscopic wedge resection. *Ann Thorac Surg* 1993; 56: 633-5.

Chapter 6

Multimodality treatment in non-small cell lung cancer surgery

Artyom Sedrakyan MD ScC
Honorary Lecturer and Research Scholar [3]
Ian Hunt BSc (Hons) MRCS, Specialist Registrar,
Cardiothoracic Surgery [1] & Research Fellow [2]
Jennifer Hill MSc PhD, Research Fellow [2]

1 St Thomas' Hospital, London, UK
2 National Collaborating Centre for Acute Care, London, UK
3 The Royal College of Surgeons of England and
The London School of Hygiene and Tropical Medicine, London, UK

Introduction

Over 3,000 operations in the United Kingdom and 70,000 similar procedures in the United States are performed for early stage lung cancer annually [1,2] (Figure 1) and most of these procedures are performed for early stage non-small cell lung cancer (NSCLC). Despite the curative intent of surgery, 5-year survival in patients with early stage (localised) disease still varies between 50-70% [3], with much of the subsequent mortality associated with disseminated recurrence.

As the predominant pattern of recurrence following curative resection of non-small cell lung cancer is systemic, and chemotherapy is effective in disseminated lung cancer, chemotherapy is likely to be useful in controlling distant metastatic disease before or after resection [3]. If the treatment is aimed to control local disease, radiotherapy is considered suitable as it may help to improve the control of macroscopic intrathoracic disease [3]. Finally, for more advanced disease, a combination of chemotherapy and radiotherapy may also potentially be beneficial as chemotherapy may enhance the effect of radiotherapy.

In this chapter we review the current evidence for surgical resection combined with chemotherapy and/or radiotherapy in the treatment of NSCLC. Various combinations and orders of treatment are included:-

- Pre-operative radiotherapy.
- Pre-operative chemotherapy.
- Postoperative chemotherapy.
- Postoperative radiotherapy.
- Postoperative chemotherapy + radiotherapy.

Methodology

The systematic review performed by Detterbeck *et al* 2001 [3] was determined to be of high quality and included studies up to April 2000. New randomised controlled trials (RCTs) and systematic reviews were identified by searching MEDLINE, EMBASE and the Cochrane Controlled Trials Register from 2000 to 2003. Standard filters identifying RCTs were used for MEDLINE and EMBASE. These RCT search filters are available at the Scottish Intercollegiate Guideline (SIGN) Network website:-

http://www.sign.ac.uk/methodology/filters.html

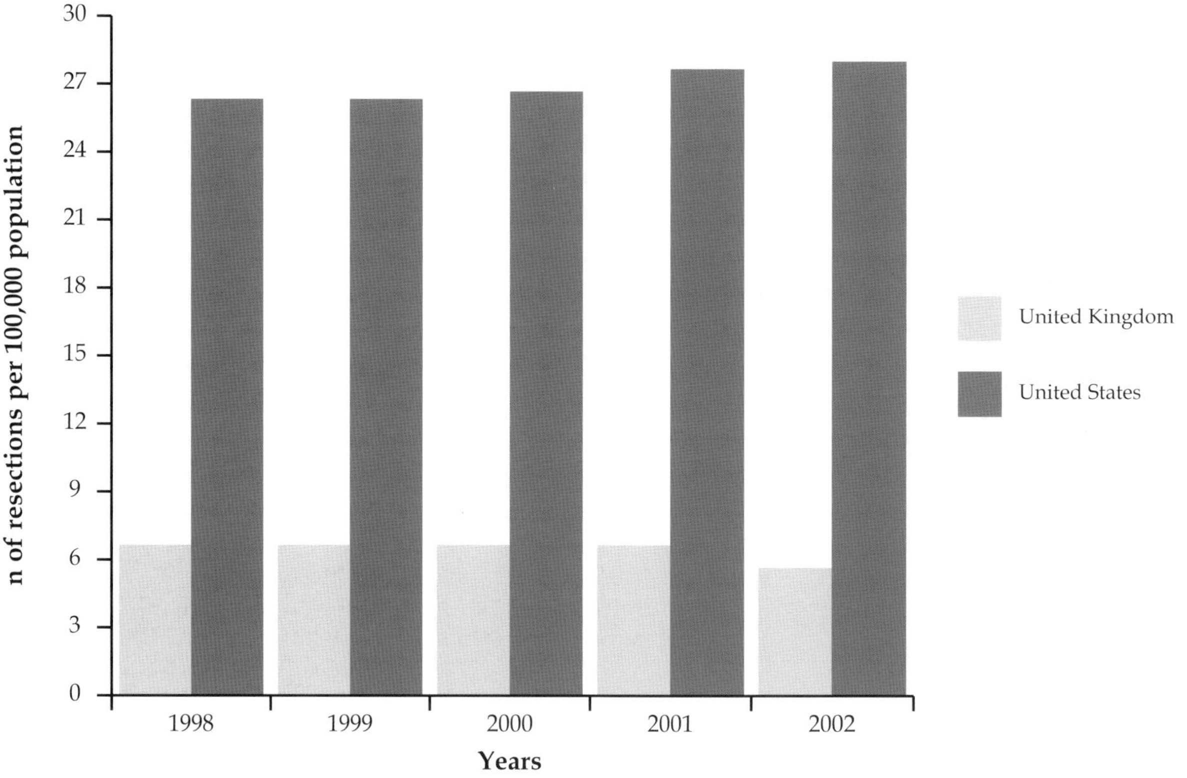

Figure 1. **Rates of lung resections per 100,000 population in the United Kingdom and United States.**

Topics not covered within Detterbeck *et al* 2001 were searched for in MEDLINE and EMBASE from 1990 onwards.

Meta-analyses were performed whenever it was appropriate. We abstracted the estimates of risk from the original reports and calculated the logarithm of the hazard ratio (HR) and its standard error [4]. RevMan 4.2 (available from the Cochrane Collaboration) was used to combine the HR estimates from the trials.

Assessing the evidence

Pre-operative radiotherapy

Four decades ago, pre-operative radiotherapy was regarded as a treatment of choice as it was thought to be useful in controlling the residual disease and dissemination of tumour cells at the time of resection [3,5]. There were two randomised trials [6,7] conducted in the 1960s. Both studies [6,7] reported no advantage for pre-operative radiotherapy as compared to surgery alone. Five-year survival after randomisation was 2% higher in the surgery alone arm in one study [6] that randomised 568 patients and, 2-year survival was over 10% higher in the surgery alone arm in the second [7] study, which randomised 339 patients.

We found another pilot study published in 1984 that had randomised 33 early stage cancer patients (T1-2, N0, M0). Although it reported a 5-year survival benefit associated with pre-operative short-course radiotherapy as compared to surgery alone (58% vs 43%) [8], the results were not statistically significant and the study was too small to reach reliable estimates of standard error.

The trials of pre-operative radiotherapy also reported that the rate of recurrence was likely to be similar in the pre-operative radiotherapy and surgery alone arms (55% vs. 52%) [3]. Thus, pre-operative radiotherapy did not seem to be useful in controlling local macroscopic disease as compared to surgical resection alone.

However, there were major limitations in the trials of pre-operative radiotherapy that need to be considered when interpreting the results. The dose of radiotherapy used in these studies ranged from 30 Gy to 60 Gy with over 50% receiving less than 50 Gy. In addition, radiotherapy equipment was based on Colbalt (Co^{60}), the standard of the time but now increasingly obsolete and is likely to be more toxic (particularly in the long-term) than linear accelerators (LINACs) that are the current standard of care. Approximately 30% of patients in the radiotherapy and surgery series had T4 disease and approximately 15% of patients had nodal involvement (N2, N3). Thus, many patients included in the two large trials were likely to have stage IIIb disease while the pilot study enrolled stage I-II patients. The rate of complete surgical resection was approximately 66%. Finally, the two large studies included 10% to 15% of patients with small cell lung cancer.

No other randomised trials of pre-operative radiotherapy have been published since and this is likely to reflect the increasing popularity of pre-operative chemotherapy in treating NSCLC.

Conclusions

There is limited information about the outcome, selection, design and the quality of the trials assessing pre-operative radiotherapy for NSCLC. Based on the RCTs reviewed, there is no evidence that patients would benefit from pre-operative radiotherapy and therefore, its use is not recommended.

Pre-operative chemotherapy

The rationale for pre-operative therapy (rather than postoperative) is that blood supply to the tumour might be compromised after major resection and, therefore in theory, tumour cells might be more sensitive to chemotherapy in the pre-operative period [5].

The evidence regarding the survival benefits associated with pre-operative chemotherapy was outlined in the 2002 Cancer Care Ontario Guidelines [9]. The pooled estimate from two well known trials [10,11] has shown a statistically significant and substantial reduction in mortality (OR 0.18, 95% CI 0.06-0.51). There was one more RCT [12] not included in the meta-analyses. This study was not included as there was routine use of radiotherapy in the arm randomised to surgery alone. However, the study still found a tendency toward reduced mortality associated with pre-operative chemotherapy. Our search identified one more study published in 2002 that has shown a reduction of mortality associated with pre-operative chemotherapy in stage IIIA patients [13]. The latter trial has also shown a tendency toward survival benefit in early stage cancer patients. It should be noted that in-hospital surgical mortality from resection following chemotherapy was similar to that after surgery alone with the rates of complications reported to be similar in both groups [3]. Thus, most of the survival benefit seems to occur after surgical resection of the cancer and there was no trade-off between increased peri-operative risk of death and later survival.

Radiological response rate after chemotherapy was over 65% in these trials [3]. Radiological response rate is based on disappearance (complete response) or over 50% reduction of tumour size (partial response). Histological complete response was also substantial and it was observed in 47% of patients [3].

Most patients enrolled in the trials of pre-operative chemotherapy were stage IIIA patients with limited number of early stage patients. These early stage patients are the subject of a Medical Research Council LU22 study that aims to enrol 450-1,000 patients (225-500 per treatment arm) within five years into a trial of surgery with and without pre-operative chemotherapy in patients with operable NSCLC.

Despite the evidence of substantial benefits associated with pre-operative chemotherapy there are some limitations to be considered:-

- There is substantial heterogeneity in stage IIIA patient selection in these trials.

- Different chemotherapy regimens and doses were used in the trials.
- The toxicity data were not well reported although the trials uniformly stated that the therapy is well tolerated. Most common toxicities and side effects were neutropenia, nausea, vomiting, diarrhoea, oesophagitis, hypomagnesemia and alopecia.

Conclusions

Most studies of pre-operative chemotherapy included stage IIIA patients with histologically proven N2, N3 involvement. There is evidence of a mortality benefit associated with pre-operative chemotherapy in stage IIIA patients as compared to surgery alone. Thus, pre-operative chemotherapy may be recommended in stage IIIA NSCLC patients, ideally enrolled into a clinical trial. However, there is little evidence to recommend the use of pre-operative chemotherapy in stage I-II patients.

Postoperative radiotherapy

Postoperative radiotherapy has been examined with the hypothesis that cure rates should be improved by reducing local recurrence. A Cochrane meta-analysis produced by the Postoperative Radiotherapy (PORT) meta-analysis trialists group [14] updated in 2002, includes the results from nine studies and 2128 patients. In these trials radiotherapy after surgery was compared to surgery alone. There was a 21% higher risk of death found with PORT and overall survival was reduced from 55% to 48% at two years. Although the most detrimental effect was evident for stage I-II patients, there was still no advantage of PORT found even for stage III patients. The Cancer Care Ontario Practice Guidelines reported by Logan *et al* [15] provided an update to the PORT meta-analysis. Two additional RCTs were found [16,17] that had not been incorporated into the original PORT-Cochrane review. Our literature search uncovered one more RCT [18]. This study included 104 stage I patients.

Local recurrence rates were reduced in the postoperative radiotherapy group according to the PORT meta-analysis [14]. There were 195 recurrences in the radiotherapy arm and 276 recurrences in the surgery alone arm (approximately 8% difference and 40% reduction).

As a major criticism of the Cochrane review, seven out of nine studies included in the meta-analysis used Co^{60} based radiation sources rather than linear accelerators (LINACs). We updated the meta-analysis and stratified the RCTs into two major subgroups (according to Co^{60} use or LINAC). We found that radiotherapy was associated with higher mortality compared to surgery when the Co^{60} radiation method was used (RR 1.22, 95% CI 1.09-1.35) (Figure 2). However, in the studies where the LINAC method was used, the adjuvant radiation therapy tended to be associated with lower mortality compared to surgery alone (RR 0.86, 95% CI 0.73-1.01).

Conclusions

The results of previous meta-analyses and our update should be treated with some caution. Modern techniques seem to show a tendency toward a beneficial effect of postoperative radiotherapy. The evidence is also conflicting regarding the importance of stage (I-II or IIIA-B) in predicting the benefits or demerits of the therapy. Therefore, currently there is no strong evidence for the use of postoperative radiotherapy.

Postoperative chemotherapy

The strongest evidence regarding the usefulness of postoperative chemotherapy came from the Non-Small Cell Lung Cancer Collaborative Group (NCLCCG) that has published the first systematic review in this area [19]. There were 12 studies included in the meta-analysis. These trials enrolled mostly early stage I-II patients as compared to mostly stage IIIa enrolled in the trials of pre-operative chemotherapy. The review found only a tendency toward mortality reduction after postoperative chemotherapy with cisplatin as compared to surgery alone (RR 0.87, 95% CI 0.74-1.02, p=0.08). Similarly, chemotherapy with Uracil + Tefagur (UFT) also tended to be associated

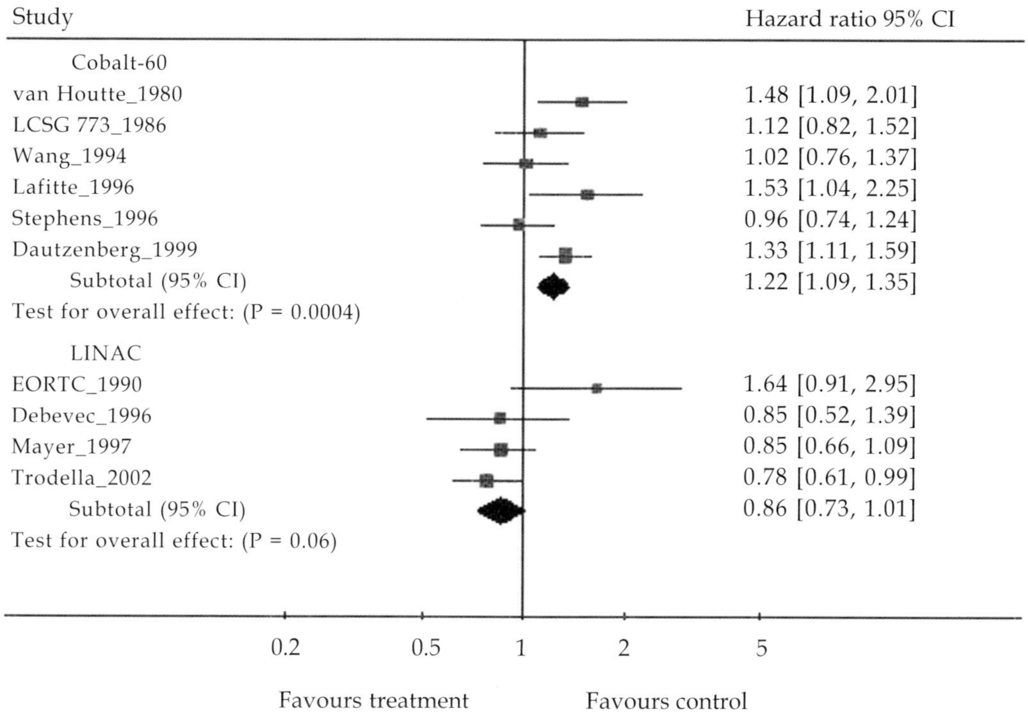

Figure 2. Survival in the trials of postoperative radiotherapy in the subgroups with Co^{60} based radiation sources and linear accelerators (LINACs).

with survival benefit in the treatment of early stage lung cancer (RR 0.89, 95% CI 0.73-0.08, p=0.31).

Based on the evidence from the meta-analysis, postoperative chemotherapy was not recommended after complete resection of early stage (I-II) lung cancer [15]. These decisions were mostly guided by statistical insignificance of the pooled estimate of the hazard ratio, relatively small overall benefit of chemotherapy (55% vs 50% by five years) found in these trials and toxicity concerns associated with chemotherapy.

The major shortcomings of the trials included in the NCLCCG review were the outdated chemotherapy regimens and dosages, which probably affected the compliance and efficacy. Detterbeck *et al* [3] also reported that in the past the rates of complete resections were much lower than in current practice. There was also heterogeneity in the selection of early stage cancer patients.

In light of these limitations, we attempted to update current evidence and found three new studies published after 2000. Two of them [20,21] randomised in total 968 patients into a postoperative cisplatin-based regimen and 965 patients into a control arm. One last study [22] randomised 109 patients into Uracil + Ftorafur (UFT) arm and 110 patients into the control arm (surgery alone).

We have combined the estimates from the two cisplatin studies with studies included in the NCLCCG report. The RR has changed from 0.87 (95% CI 0.74-1.02, p=0.08) to 0.85 (95% CI 0.77-0.94) (Figure 3) and the estimates become highly statistically significant (p=0.001).

We also combined the estimate from the new UFT study with those included in the NCLCCG report and found that the RR estimate did not change (HR 0.89, 95% CI 0.73-1.08). Although the results of several other trials of cisplatin and UFT are expected, relative

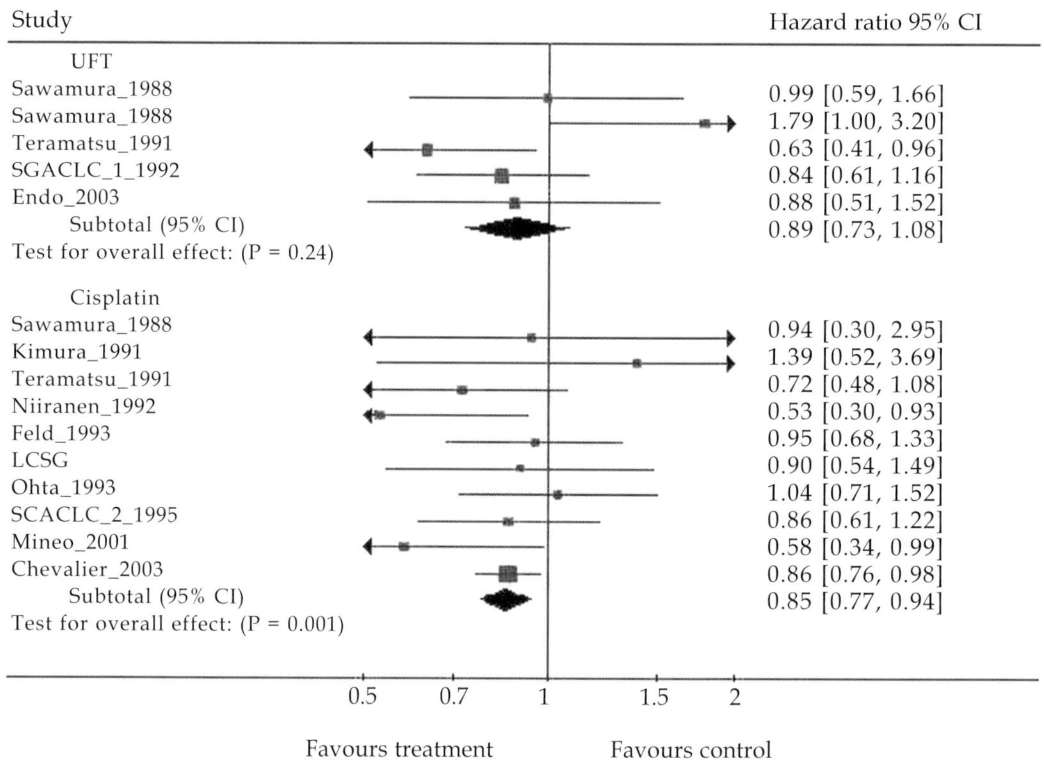

Figure 3. Survival in the trials of Cisplatin and Uracil + Ftorafur (UFT) based postoperative chemotherapy groups.

risk estimates favouring postoperative chemotherapy are less likely to change substantially.

Conclusions

Surgery in stage I and stage II patients carries a high probability of cure (5-year survival is 70% for stage IA, 55% for stage IB). However, it leaves a large number of patients who will die within five years of recurrent disease that is sub-clinical at the time of surgery. There is new evidence that postoperative chemotherapy might be associated with reduced mortality as compared to surgery alone in resected stage I-II NSCLC. The fact that there is a 'small' improvement in survival is common to many oncological strategies and toxicity concerns might be insufficient to refute this therapeutic strategy as modern chemotherapy regimens are less toxic and well tolerated.

Postoperative chemotherapy + radiotherapy

Postoperative chemotherapy + radiotherapy is currently used in clinical trials enrolling the patients with stage II and IIIA NSCLC. It is proposed that the addition of chemotherapy to the radiotherapy regimen will "radiosensitise" patients and shorten the duration of the therapy.

The NCLCCG performed a meta-analysis that was published in 1995 [23] and provided the best evidence for clinical efficacy of postoperative chemotherapy + radiotherapy as compared to postoperative radiotherapy alone. Interestingly, there were no trials that compared the postoperative chemotherapy + radiotherapy with chemotherapy alone. The meta-analysis combined the data from seven trials, six of which used a cisplatin-based regimen. The overall hazard ratio of 0.98 (p=0.76) was reported in this review. However, in the six trials of cisplatin-based chemotherapy + radiotherapy, there was a 6% lower risk of death (HR 0.94, 95% CI 0.79-1.11).

We found one more study [24] published in 2000 that randomised 488 patients into postoperative chemotherapy + radiotherapy and postoperative radiotherapy arms. There was a tendency toward a 7% reduction in mortality observed in the combination arm (HR 0.93, 95% CI 0.74-1.18). Combining this new evidence with the NCLCCG report yielded an estimate of a 6% reduction (HR 0.94, 95% CI 0.82-1.07) in the risk of mortality which was still not statistically significant (p=0.35).

Conclusions

The evidence is inconclusive and patient eligibility into the trials of postoperative chemotherapy + radiotherapy is not well addressed. There is a tendency toward a 6% reduction in mortality associated with chemotherapy + radiotherapy as compared to radiotherapy alone. This evidence is in line with benefits associated with chemotherapy reported in the studies of pre-operative and postoperative chemotherapy. The use of postoperative chemotherapy + radiotherapy cannot therefore be recommended.

Recommendations	Evidence level
◆ Patients with stage IIIa NSCLC who are suitable for resection should be considered for preoperative chemotherapy.	I/A
◆ There is evidence of a survival benefit associated with postoperative chemotherapy in patients with stage I-IIIa disease and it might be considered for selected patients after weighing the risk of toxicity and patient preferences.	I/A
◆ There is inconclusive evidence regarding the use of preoperative radiotherapy, postoperative radiotherapy and postoperative chemotherapy + radiotherapy. However, modern radiotherapy techniques may be associated with survival benefit. Future studies should elucidate if modern radiotherapy regimens can improve survival in surgical patients and if combined chemotherapy + radiotherapy can be superior to either strategy alone. Furthermore, eligibility of the patients for these therapies should be defined.	I/A & I/B

References

1. Agency for Health Care Research and Quality HCCaUP. http://hcup.ahrq.gov/HCUPNet.asp. 2001.
2. Goldstraw P. The expansion of consultant provision for thoracic surgery in the UK. http://www.scts.org 2003.
3. Detterbeck FC, Rivera MP, Socinski MA, Rosenman JG. *Diagnosis and treatment of lung cancer: an evidence-based guide for the practicing clinician.* WB Saunders, Philadelphia, 2001.
4. Parmar MK, Torri V, Stewart L. Extracting summary statistics to perform meta-analyses of the published literature for survival endpoints. *Stat Med* 1998;17(24): 2815-34.
5. Einhorn LH. Neoadjuvant and adjuvant trials in non-small cell lung cancer. Ann Thorac Surg 1998; 65: 208-11.
6. Warram J. Preoperative irradiation of cancer of the lung: final report of a therapeutic trial. A collaborative study. *Cancer* 1975; 36(3): 914-25.
7. Shields TW, Higgins GA, Lawton R, Heilbrunn A, Keehn RJ. Preoperative X-ray therapy as an adjuvant in the treatment of bronchogenic carcinoma. *J Thorac Cardiovasc Surg* 1970; 59(1): 49-59.
8. Kazem I, Jongerius CM, Lacquet LK, Kramer G, Huygen PL. Evaluation of short-course preoperative irradiation in the treatment of resectable bronchus carcinoma: long-term analysis of a randomized pilot-study. *Int J Radiat Oncol Biol Phys* 1984; 10(7): 981-5.
9. Initiative CCOG. Use of Preoperative chemotherapy with or without postoperative radiotherapy in technically resectable stage IIa non-small-cell lung cancer. Practice guideline report No 7-4 2002.
10. Roth JA, Atkison EN, Fossella F, *et al.* Long-term follow up of patients enrolled in a randomized trial comparing perioperative chemotherapy and surgery with surgery alone in resectable stage IIIa non-small-cell lung cancer. *Lung Cancer* 1998; 21(1): 1-6.
11. Rosell R, Gomez-Codina J, Camps C, *et al.* A radomized trial comparing preoperative chemotherapy plus surgery with surgery alone in patients with non-small-cell lung cancer. *N Engl J Med* 1994; 330(3): 153-8.
12. Pass HI, Pogrebniak HW, Steinberg SM, Mulshine J, Minna J. Randomized trial of neoadjuvant therapy for lung cancer: interim analysis. *Ann Thorac Surg* 1992; 53(6): 992-8.
13. Depierre A, Milleron B, Moro-Sibilot D, *et al.* Preoperative chemotherapy followed by surgery compared with primary surgery in resectable stage I (except T1N0), II, and IIIa non-small-cell lung cancer. *J Clin Oncol* 2002; 20(1): 247-53.
14. "PORT" Meta-analysis Trialist Group. Postoperative radiotherapy for non-small-cell lung cancer (Cochrane Review). In: The Cochrane Library, Issue 2, 2003. Oxford. 2002.
15. Logan DM, Lochrin CA, Darling G, Eady A, Newman TE, Evans WK. Adjuvant radiotherapy and chemotherapy for stage II or IIIA non-small-cell lung cancer after complete resection. Provincial Lung Cancer Disease Site Group. *Cancer Prev Control* 1997; 1(5): 366-78.
16. Mayer R, Smolle-Juettner FM, Szolar D, Stuecklschweiger GF, Quehenberger F, Friehs G. Postoperative radiotherapy in radically resected non-small-cell lung cancer. *Chest* 1997; 112: 954-9.
17. Feng QF, Wang M, Wang LJ, YZ Y, Zhang YJ, Zhang DW. A study of postoperative radiotherapy in patients with non-small-cell lung cancer: a randomized trial. *Int J Radiat Oncol Biol Phys* 2000; 47: 925-9.
18. Trodella L, Granone P, Valente S, *et al.* Adjuvant radiotherapy in non-small cell lung cancer with pathological stage I: definitive results of a phase III randomized trial. *Radiotherapy & Oncology* 2002; 62: 11-19.
19. Non-small Cell Lung Cancer Collaborative Group. Chemotherapy for non-small cell lung cancer (Cochrane Review). In: The Cochrane Library, Issue 2, 2003. Oxford. 2000(2): CD002139.
20. Mineo TC, Ambrogi V, Corsaro V, Roselli M. Postoperative adjuvant therapy for stage IB non-small-cell lung cancer. *Eur J Cardiothorac Surg* 2001; 20(2): 378-84.
21. Le Chevalier T. Results of the randomized international adjuvant lung cancer trial (IALT): cisplatin-based chemotherapy vs no cisplatin therapy in 1867 patients with resected non-small cell lung cancer. Meeting of the American Society of Clinical Oncology, Abstract. June 2003.
22. Endo C, Saito Y, Iwanami H, *et al.* A randomized trial of postoperative UFT therapy in p stage I, II non-small cell lung cancer: North-east Japan Study Group for Lung Cancer Surgery. *Lung Cancer* 2003; 40(2): 181-6.
23. Chemotherapy in non-small cell lung cancer: a meta-analysis using updated data on individual patients from 52 randomised clinical trials. Non-small Cell Lung Cancer Collaborative Group. *BMJ* 1995; 311(7010): 899-909.
24. Keller SM, Adak S, Wagner H, *et al.* A randomized trial of postoperative adjuvant therapy in patients with completely resected stage II or IIIa non-small-cell lung cancer. *N Engl J Med* 2000; 343(17): 1217-22.

Chapter 7

Endobronchial therapies

Frank M McCaughan MRCP
Specialist Registrar, Thoracic Medicine
P Jeremy George MD FRCP
Consultant Thoracic Physician

Middlesex Hospital, London, UK

Introduction

Bronchoscopy was first performed by Gustav Killian at the University of Freiburg in 1897. The first case report refers to a therapeutic indication in which foreign bodies were removed from the tracheobronchial tree using a rigid bronchoscope. Rigid bronchoscopy rapidly became a standard procedure worldwide, but was superseded in the late 1960s with the advent of fibreoptic bronchoscopy. More recently, there has been a resurgence of interest as its interventional capabilities are rediscovered and used to treat growing numbers of patients with lung cancer. The main clinical indications include palliation in patients with advanced malignant disease, treatment with curative intent in patients with early disease who are unfit for surgery, and treatment of pre-invasive lesions that have the potential to progress to lung cancer.

Although endobronchial therapies are now widely used, the evidence base is particularly sparse. Relatively few randomised controlled trials have been undertaken and, in most instances, the best level of evidence is based on recommendations made from large retrospective case series.

There are two reasons for this relative paucity of evidence. Firstly, many patients are at risk of asphyxia when referred for treatment and there is often no alternative to endobronchial therapy. A trial in which intervention is withheld would clearly be unethical. Secondly, patients referred for endobronchial treatment are frequently receiving other treatments, such as chemotherapy and external radiotherapy, and it is extremely difficult to adjust for the effects of such treatments when evaluating their responses to endobronchial treatment.

Methodology

A systematic review of the current literature was completed by searching Medline between 1966 and 2003 using the following terms: laser therapy, photodynamic therapy, brachytherapy, cryotherapy, electrocautery, stents, in the context of "LUNG" and "LUNG NEOPLASMS". There are no meta-analyses, Cochrane reviews or randomised controlled trials comparing interventional bronchoscopic techniques with the best available alternative practice. There are two relevant systematic reviews: one on the treatment of early stage lung cancer [1] and one on the role of photodynamic therapy in the management of early and advanced lung cancer [2]. Two text books provided additional references and background information [3,4].

Palliation of advanced lung cancer: principles of treatment

There is a tendency for patients with lung cancer to present late when there is no prospect of cure. Over 33,000 patients die in the UK from lung cancer each year [5]. Approximately a third of these will develop potentially fatal complications associated with localised intrathoracic disease, such as haemoptysis, pulmonary sepsis and asphyxia, and a proportion derive undoubted benefit from endobronchial palliation with an improved quality and, possibly, duration of life. There is therefore, potentially a very great demand for appropriate endobronchial palliative interventions.

It should be appreciated that the success of treatment depends on appropriate patient selection. Patients with localised airway obstruction and viable distal lung tissue are likely to benefit from treatment, whereas patients with extensive tumours invading and destroying peripheral lung tissue cannot benefit. In addition, tumours obstructing a central airway are likely to compromise breathing more than tumours obstructing a more peripheral airway. As a consequence, treatment for central airway obstruction is likely to lead to correspondingly greater benefit. In the absence of randomised controlled clinical trials, it is difficult to compare different treatments, as outcomes may reflect differences in patient selection rather than differences in the efficacy of treatment.

There are several techniques for debulking endobronchial tumours. These include laser resection, cryotherapy, photodynamic therapy (PDT), electrocautery and mechanical debulking, using rigid forceps. Although these treatments usually provide rapid relief, the duration of palliation may be relatively brief and is limited by the rate at which tumour grows back to re-obstruct the airway. More durable palliation, however, may be obtained with endobronchial radiotherapy (brachytherapy) and the use of endoluminal stents, and these techniques may be regarded as being complementary to tumour debulking.

Endobronchial laser resection

Laser resection via a bronchoscope is used for direct thermal ablation of intraluminal tumours. The Neodymium yttrium-aluminium garnet (Nd YAG) laser is the most popular device, and has been used in the palliation of advanced lung cancer, endobronchial metastases and in the management of benign endobronchial tumours [3,4]. The thermal action of the Nd YAG laser is illustrated in Figure 1.

Safety is of obvious importance in view of the often severely compromised respiratory state of patients at the time of referral. Potential risks include tracheobronchial wall perforation, haemorrhage, airway burning, together with postoperative complications such as infection, respiratory failure and delayed airway obstruction by exudate. Treatment may be given using either a flexible bronchoscope under local anaesthesia with sedation or via a rigid bronchoscope under general anaesthesia. The laser beam is transmitted via an optical fibre inserted into the biopsy channel of a flexible bronchoscope or into the treatment port of the rigid bronchoscope. One retrospective study compared outcomes in patients treated under local and general anaesthesia and concluded that rigid bronchoscopy under general anaesthesia provided a more controlled environment enabling treatment to be conducted more efficiently and in greater safety [6].

Palliation is the most common indication for laser therapy. A number of case series have been reported and the majority have evaluated treatment by making subjective assessments of the patient's airway and symptoms before and after treatment. The largest published series has reported retrospectively on 2915 treatments in 2069 patients [7]; part of this cohort has been published in a peer-reviewed journal article [8]. Tumour site, rather than cell type, was the most important factor determining the outcome of therapy. Initial treatment was judged to have been successful in 97% with tracheal obstruction, and in 95% and 92% respectively, with right and left main bronchial obstruction. Treatment for tumours causing more peripheral obstruction was judged to be less successful (62% and 66% for obstruction of the left upper lobe bronchus and the apical segmental bronchus of the right lower lobe respectively). The

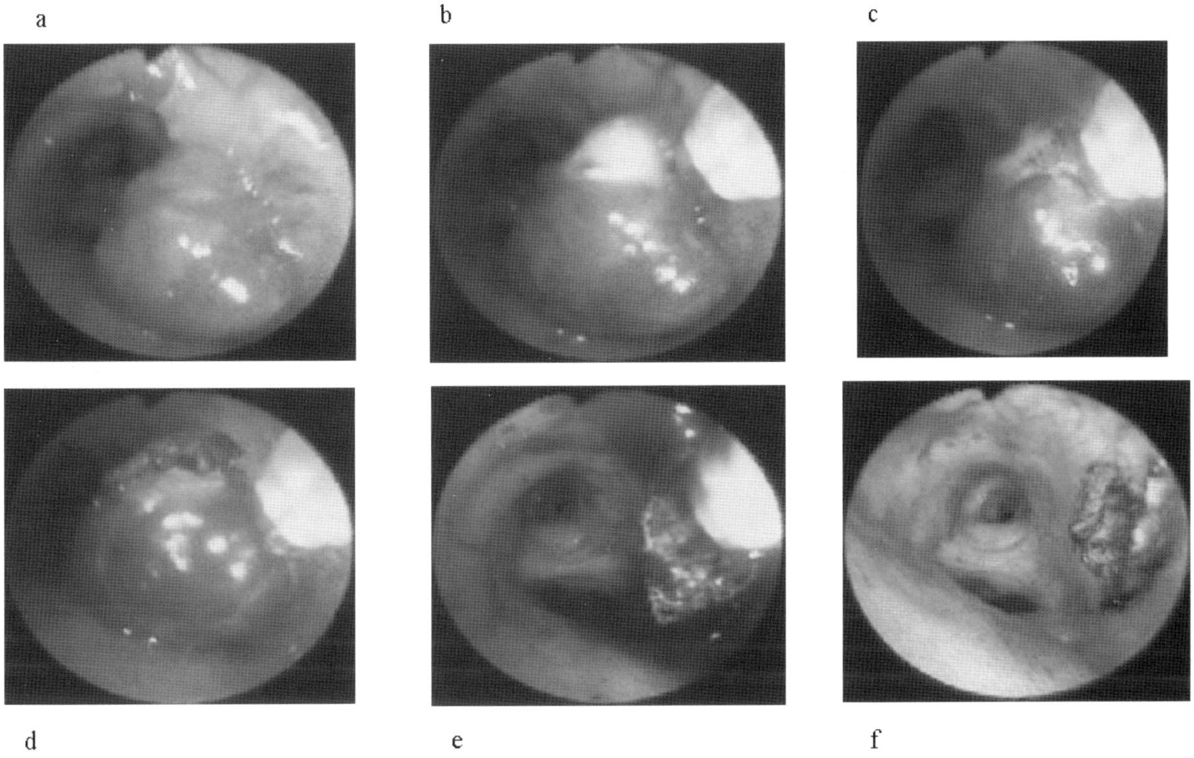

Figure 1. An illustration of the thermal properties of the YAG laser employed to resect a vascular carcinoid tumour. a) The tumour can be seen arising from the anterior wall of the left main bronchus. b) and c) The YAG laser beam is directed via an optical fibre at the pedicle of the tumour and leads to superficial blanching as the tumour blood vessels constrict. d) The tumour changes colour as its blood supply is compromised by continued laser treatment, allowing it to be removed relatively bloodlessly (e and f).

two main complications were haemorrhage (1.2%) and respiratory failure (0.9%) [8].

Smaller studies have been published in which formal symptom scores and indices of performance status and lung function have been used to evaluate treatment, and further support the importance of tumour site in determining the success of treatment [9,10]. In patients with central airway obstruction who are at imminent risk of asphyxia, the particular advantage of laser treatment is that it provides an immediate improvement in airway diameter, allowing more definitive treatments to be given electively and in greater safety [9,10]. Treatment for more peripheral obstruction of a main bronchus produces less dramatic improvement, but has been shown to lead to matched improvements in scores of ventilation and perfusion (see Figure 2) in association with improved symptom scores, and indices of lung function and performance [11].

Complication rates of between 1% and 33% are reported following Nd-YAG laser treatment, but an experienced operator should achieve a mortality rate of less than 2% in this sick group of patients [4]. The largest published series quotes a complication risk per patient of 3.7% and a mortality risk per patient of 0.7% [8].

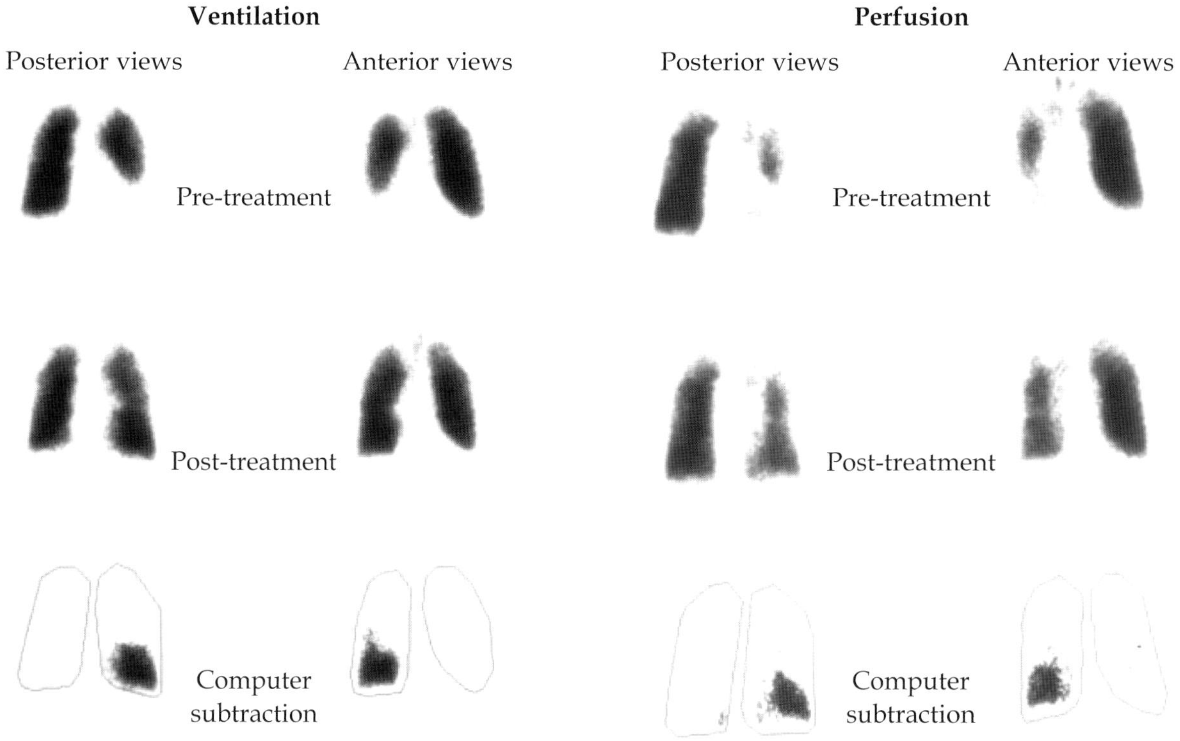

Figure 2. **Changes in ventilation (left figure) and perfusion (right figure) are shown for a patient with a tumour obstructing the right intermediate bronchus before and after laser treatment. The areas of change are highlighted by performing a computer subtraction in which the pre-treatment image is subtracted from the post-treatment image. When this is done, areas of improved ventilation can be seen to be matched topographically with areas of improved perfusion.** *Reproduced with permission from the BMJ Publishing Group. George et al. Thorax 1990; 45: 248-253.*

Cryotherapy

The aim of cryotherapy is to provoke intracellular freezing rapidly in the target tissue. The combination of freezing and then slow thawing causes cell death as a delayed response. Toilet bronchoscopy is required after an interval of 1-2 weeks to remove necrotic slough and assess any need for further therapy. The delayed treatment effect means that the technique is unlikely to be appropriate for patients with imminent central airway obstruction, where there is an urgent need to rescue the airway. There is no reported risk of tracheobronchial perforation. The technique can be performed using either a flexible or rigid bronchoscope.

There is one large prospective study which evaluated the response to therapy in 153 patients with symptomatic obstructing inoperable lung cancers [12]. One hundred and thirty-three patients had dyspnoea, 120 had a cough and 55 had haemoptysis. Both rigid and flexible bronchoscopy was used. The results showed an overall subjective improvement in 72%. Dyspnoea improved in 64%, cough in 68% and haemoptysis in 93%. There was a significant mean improvement in FEV1, but this was a modest 110mls. Only 11 patients had complications including bleeding and respiratory failure, but there were no deaths.

A much larger case series from the same group (n=600) reported a subjective improvement in 78% of patients after cryotherapy [13]. However, no physiological parameters were reported. Others have reported success with cryotherapy, for example a further series of 22 patients in which cryotherapy was delivered solely via the flexible bronchoscope has also been published [14]. Again, no physiological data were included, but dyspnoea improved in 12 of 17 patients who were suitable for assessment. Those patients not suitable included three who had luminal occlusion due to extrinsic compression. One patient died prior to reassessment and in another, treatment was unsuccessful. There was one serious complication - cardiorespiratory arrest - although the patient survived to discharge with a patent airway; two other patients developed bronchospasm.

There is therefore, evidence to suggest that cryotherapy provides effective relief from airway obstruction with an acceptable risk. However, multiple bronchoscopies are required for each treatment schedule and there is less efficacy data available than for laser resection.

The complication risk per patient is approximately 7% and cryotherapy associated deaths are unusual - there were none in the largest prospective series [12].

Photodynamic therapy (PDT)

Photodynamic therapy (PDT) enables tumour to be destroyed with some selectivity while preserving the structural integrity of surrounding tissues. This is achieved by administering a non-toxic photosensitising dye, which becomes highly cytotoxic when exposed to light at a wavelength corresponding to one of its absorption peaks. The toxic effect is mediated via the production of singlet oxygen, which migrates less than 0.02μm after its formation, thereby limiting its effects to the region where it is formed. The mechanisms of action of PDT are non-thermal and include cell death through direct toxicity on cell membranes and mitochondria, apoptosis of tumour cells, and damage to tumour microvasculature with vessel constriction.

The compound, Photofrin ™, has now been approved for use in the UK. An intravenous dose is administered and, after 48 hours, laser light of 630nm is delivered to the tumour via an optical fibre passed through the working channel of a bronchoscope. Its therapeutic effect extends to a depth of up to 0.5cm. Potential complications include local inflammation, swelling and bleeding. A second bronchoscopy is indicated at 48-72 hours to ensure adequate bronchial toilet. In addition, the compound is retained by the skin so that patients are at risk of sunburn for the next 4-6 weeks even in normal daylight.

There is an increasing global experience in using PDT for palliation. Only patients with intraluminal or mural tumours are suitable. If the cause of airway narrowing or obstruction is extrinsic, then PDT is not appropriate. Careful patient selection with fibreoptic bronchoscopy and / or thoracic CT scanning is therefore necessary prior to planning PDT.

In a recent overview of PDT for symptomatic patients with inoperable lung cancer (predominantly non-small cell lung cancer) (NSCLC), 12 papers describing 636 patients were reviewed [2]. Although the majority were treated with Photofrin, other photosensitising agents were also used. Treatment was judged to have been successful with almost all patients reporting a symptomatic benefit. The most important factor in determining post-treatment survival was pre-treatment tumour stage [15].

Two randomised controlled studies have been published which compare YAG laser resection with PDT in advanced lung cancer [16,17]. Although the number of patients in these studies is small, both treatment modalities appear to be equally effective. The response to treatment appears to be more rapid with the YAG laser but is more durable with PDT.

The complication rate per patient is high with the incidence of photosensitivity between 5% and 28%. Respiratory complications are also reported infrequently - haemoptysis, infection and dyspnoea. The mortality rate per patient based on figures from the systematic review is 0.3% [2].

Electrocautery

Electrocautery is synonymous with diathermy and involves the heating and coagulation of tumour using an electric current. High frequency oscillating current is delivered using a small endoscopic probe with immediate effects. In addition to tumour debulking, it is used to stop superficial haemorrhage from vascular tumours. Treatment can be administered via a flexible or rigid bronchoscope.

The published experience with this technique is considerably less than for laser resection. The available data consists of retrospective case series, the largest of which reported on 56 patients [18]. The success rate using mainly flexible bronchoscopy was high - 39/56 or 70%. Treatment failures only occurred in those with extraluminal tumour, emphasising the importance of patient selection [15]. Other smaller case series using electrocautery report comparable levels of success.

It is generally well tolerated with significant haemorrhage being the only frequently reported complication with a rate per patient of 2.5% [19].

Mechanical debulking with forceps

This technique is often used in conjunction with other debulking strategies. The rigid forceps are more effective than forceps used with the flexible bronchoscope because they enable larger volumes of tumour to be removed with each "bite". One study has been published in which tumour debulking was achieved solely with rigid biopsy forceps in a consecutive series of 56 patients [20]. Fifty-one (91%) were judged to have an improved airway and this was associated with an improvement in symptoms. However, measurements of lung function were not given and it is therefore difficult to draw comparisons with other treatment modalities.

Nineteen potentially serious complications were reported, representing a risk per patient of 34%.

Brachytherapy

Brachytherapy (BT) is synonymous with endobronchial radiotherapy and involves the local application of radiotherapy from within the airway. The dose of radiation falls off steeply with distance from the source, with the result that relatively high doses of radiation are delivered to the tumour and peribronchial tissues, but negligible doses to the surrounding normal lung parenchyma. It has been advocated as a sole treatment for early lung cancer and for inoperable lung cancer, and as a salvage treatment for patients who have already received full courses of external radiotherapy (ext RT). It is generally a well-tolerated procedure with the major reported complication being haemoptysis, though it is not known whether this is related primarily to treatment or disease progression.

A number of techniques for delivering endobronchial radiotherapy have been developed. The most sophisticated involve the use of high activity Iridium-192 sources which are loaded by remote control into afterloading catheters, which have been positioned bronchoscopically within the airways. Treatment can be completed within 10-15 minutes under sedation to deliver doses of up to 15Gy in a single fraction at 1cm radius from the source. Treatment has the advantages of being simple and easy to administer and can be offered on a day-case basis.

There is only one randomised controlled trial comparing Ext RT and BT as a primary palliative treatment [21]. Ninety-nine patients were randomised to receive Ext RT or BT. The main endpoints were symptom relief, the acute and late side effects of treatment and the effect of treatment on patients' functional status and quality of life. The results of treatment were similar, though ext RT achieved more durable palliation and was associated with a modest gain in median survival (287 vs. 250 days). Ext RT therefore, appears to be the treatment of choice for first-line palliation.

A further prospective randomised controlled trial from a different group has compared Ext RT alone with Ext RT and BT [22]. Ninety-five patients with previously untreated endobronchial NSCLC affecting the proximal airways (stages I-IIIB, and WHO-performance status of 0-3) were recruited. A significantly higher rate of lung re-expansion was observed in the dual treatment arm (57%) compared to Ext RT only (35%) and this was associated with a significant increase in lung function. Dyspnoea scores were also superior in this group but this advantage was confined to the first three months and was only apparent in patients with proximal obstruction of a main bronchus. No difference was noted in the incidence of massive haemoptysis (13% vs. 15%).

In a separate prospective study of 19 patients undergoing BT alone for obstructing NSCLC, improved scores of ventilation and perfusion were demonstrated in association with improved symptoms, spirometry and airway calibre assessed by follow-up bronchoscopy [23]. A proportion of these patients had already received other treatments before BT, testifying to its value as a salvage treatment.

Table 1. **Major retrospective case series: experience with endobronchial stenting.**

Series	Patients	Stents	Main stent type used	Malignant	Benign	Complication rate
Wood *et al* [23]	143	309	Silicone (Hood)	96 (67%)	47 (33%)	131 (42%)
Dumon *et al* [24]	1,058	1,574	Silicone (Dumon)	698 (66%)	360 (34%)	21.5%
Cavaliere *et al* [25]	306	308	Silicone (Dumon)	100%	N/A	Not given

Stenting

Stents may be used to treat airway obstruction due to both benign and malignant conditions. The principal types are silicone rubber stents and expandable metal stents, which are either covered or uncovered. Although a detailed discussion is beyond the scope of this chapter, it should be appreciated that these stents are intended for different clinical situations.

The easiest stents to place within the airway are uncovered expandable metal stents. They can be compressed and loaded into narrow delivery catheters and then released under radiographic control. Their expansile properties then dilate the strictured airway. They do not interfere with ventilation and so they can be deployed within the peripheral airways. Their important disadvantage is that they cannot prevent the encroachment of intraluminal tumour through their metal lattice and so they can only be used in patients with airways that are compressed by extrabronchial tumour.

Expandable metal stents with polyurethane covers have been designed which prevent encroachment by intraluminal tumour. However, they are liable to interfere with ventilation and can only be used in the proximal airways. Neither covered nor uncovered stents can be removed after placement and so they are not generally recommended for use in patients with benign strictures who have relatively long life expectancies.

Silicone rubber stents are more difficult to place within the airway, but they can be removed after placement. They are therefore, more appropriate for conditions requiring temporary stenting. Their important limitations are that they may interfere with mucociliary clearance and ventilation. They can therefore, only be used within the proximal airways.

Stents tend to be used as part of a multimodality approach and are extremely difficult to evaluate in randomised controlled studies. Recommendations for their use must therefore be based on reported case series. In general, they are used when more conventional options, such as surgery and ext RT, are not possible.

To design the ideal stent one would incorporate technical properties reducing the risk of:-

- stent migration;
- growth of granulation tissue;
- penetration by infiltrating tumour;
- bronchial wall perforation;
- secretion retention; and
- stent distortion.

The results from three large retrospective series (all using mainly silicone stents) have now been published and are summarised in Table 1 [8,24,25]. In these trials, well over 90% of stent placements were regarded as being successful, but objective measurements of lung function and symptom scores are not given. However,

Dineen *et al* [26] summarised a number of very small case series which have illustrated an improvement in lung function as a result of stenting.

Wood *et al* have recently reported their experience in stenting in great detail [23]. Although the immediate results were very impressive with 95% of patients palliated, there was a relatively high complication rate (42%). The most common complications were partial stent blockage by retained secretions (27%) or granulation tissue (9%), stent migration (5%) and bronchial wall perforation (1%). Many patients (41%) in this series required further endobronchial intervention and all patients required long-term specialist follow-up.

Curative treatment for central early lung cancer

Central early lung cancers may be defined as superficial invasive carcinomas involving the proximal airways, which have not invaded bronchial cartilage nor metastasised, and whose upper and lower margins are visible bronchoscopically. The majority are squamous cell carcinoma.

The main management decision lies between surgical resection and endobronchial treatment. Surgery has the advantages of clearing tumour with greater reliability and excluding N1 and N2 disease, whereas endobronchial treatment is associated with less operative risk and conserves lung tissue.

Photodynamic therapy (PDT)

PDT is not currently licensed for early stage lung cancers in the UK but is licensed in the USA, Japan and some European countries. The ACCP has recently reviewed the published literature on PDT and other endobronchial treatments [1]. In addition there has been a recent systematic review [2].

In an overview of the Japanese literature involving PDT in 145 patients [1], a long-term complete response was obtained in 75% of 154 lesions treated. The size of the lesion was found to have a bearing on the outcome, such that a complete response was seen in 95% of lesions whose greatest dimension was less than 1cm, but in only 46% of lesions greater than 2cms. Treatment success was also dependent on the lower margin of the tumour being visualised. However, it should be appreciated that 99 of these lesions were carcinoma *in situ* (CIS) rather than invasive lung cancer. Review of the Mayo Clinic PDT data, which do not include CIS lesions, reveals a long-term complete response in 38 of 58 (66%) patients [27].

These results raise the question as to whether PDT should be used to treat early stage lung cancers in patients who are eligible for surgery. This question has been addressed in a study of 21 patients who were offered PDT as an alternative to surgical resection [28]. Bronchoscopy was carried out at 3-6 monthly intervals after PDT and a further treatment was administered if there was an incomplete response. If there was no response to the first treatment, or an incomplete response to the second, then the patient received surgery. Overall, surgery was successfully avoided in nine patients (43%). However, three patients, who later required surgery, were found to have previously undetected N1 disease. Nodal disease is beyond the therapeutic range of PDT and this study therefore underlines the inherent limitations of this type of treatment.

A further limitation of PDT is its inability to eradicate tumour invading beyond bronchial cartilage. However, it may now be possible to assess invasion more precisely with endobronchial ultrasound and thereby improve patient selection. Miyazu *et al* used endobronchial ultrasound to assess 16 early stage cancers and three CIS lesions [30]. Nine were found to be entirely intra-cartilaginous and were managed with PDT; all of these patients exhibited a complete response with a median follow-up of 32 months. The remaining nine patients with extra-cartilaginous spread were managed with other treatments; six of these patients received surgery and it was subsequently possible to confirm the accuracy of endobronchial ultrasound histologically.

Laser resection

This has not been widely studied. There has been one published series of 17 patients by Cavaliere *et al* [8]. Although the early outcome results were excellent

(100% complete remission), no follow-up data has been published and so no conclusions can be drawn. Other groups have used laser therapy in this way but long-term comparative data are not available.

Brachytherapy

There are no randomised controlled trials addressing this but two case series have been published. In the first paper, 34 patients with early-stage non-small cell bronchial carcinoma were recruited [31]. All patients were medically inoperable and external radiotherapy was contraindicated. The treatment protocol was six sessions of 5Gy over six weeks. In half of the patients the treatment catheter positioning was a CT-guided procedure. Local disease recurrence occurred in five patients (15%). With a median follow-up of two years, the survival rate was 78%. There was no significant brachytherapy-related morbidity.

In another smaller series, 15 patients with early lung cancer were treated with 7Gy per week over 3-5 weeks [32]. The results showed 25% local recurrence at one year, and 1-year disease-free survival figures of 70%. There were more significant complications - one patient with no evidence of local recurrence died from massive haemoptysis 12 months after treatment. Two further patients had severe treatment-related mucosal necrosis, one of whom died from a related haemoptysis. Both of these patients were treated with 7Gy for five weeks raising the possibility of dose-related morbidity.

Cryotherapy

There is only one relevant paper which is a case series of 35 patients collected in a number of French institutions [33]. The duration of enrolment, 12 years one month, attests to the difficulty in finding these patients. Twenty-seven patients had carcinoma *in situ*, and the remaining eight had early lung cancer. Local recurrence at the site of cryotherapy occurred in only three patients at one year but seven further patients developed late local recurrences. During follow-up five other patients developed an incidental lung carcinoma at a distant site and only 20 of 35 patients survived two years. The results of this study are difficult to interpret as the distinction between CIS and early invasive lung cancer is not made clear when assessing the outcomes.

Electrocautery

Electrocautery is gaining favour as an alternative to PDT in patients with early lung cancer. Much of the published work in this field comes from one group. In a prospective study of 13 patients (15 lesions) with early lung cancer, who were treated with electrocautery (30W) and followed for a median of 21 months, ten patients (12 lesions) exhibited a complete response and the remaining three did not respond [34]. Two of these proceeded to resection and the other to Ext RT.

The management of pre-invasive bronchial epithelial lesions

It is widely believed that pre-invasive bronchial epithelial lesions, such as severe dysplasia and carcinoma *in situ*, have the potential to progress to squamous cell carcinoma. Auerbach first raised the possible clinical relevance of these lesions in his classical post-mortem studies in which he demonstrated that CIS was prevalent in the airways of heavy smokers and that its distribution corresponded with that seen in squamous cell carcinoma [35]. Until recently, the management of these lesions was of academic interest as they could not be detected bronchoscopically. However, with the recent development of fluorescence bronchoscopy, these lesions can now be detected with greater reliability and this raises the important question as to how they should be managed.

In view of their undoubted malignant potential, some groups have advocated prompt treatment [36,37,38]. However, careful review of the Auerbach data suggests that the majority are unlikely to progress to malignancy. His systematic post-mortem studies demonstrated CIS in 75% of heavy smokers [35]. As only 10-20% of heavy smokers actually develop clinically significant lung cancers and as CIS is only implicated in the development of squamous cell carcinoma, it could be argued that the majority will not progress to clinically significant cancers [41]. There are no randomised controlled trials comparing intervention with surveillance in the management of pre-invasive lesions.

Treatments for pre-invasive lesions vary but have included surgical resection and endobronchial therapies [2,33,39] such as photodynamic therapy, brachytherapy, electrocautery, cryotherapy, and laser coagulation. Surgery undoubtedly provides an effective method of eradicating these lesions but carries an appreciable risk, which is difficult to justify when there is no certainty that some or all will progress. Moreover, patients harbouring pre-invasive lesions are known to be at risk of developing other cancers at remote sites within their lungs, with the result that prior lung resection may render them unfit for curative treatment when they eventually develop an invasive tumour.

Endobronchial treatments have the advantage of conserving lung tissue and have been used more extensively. Although it is claimed that these treatments are successful in up to 80% cases, it has been difficult to assess the value of intervention when the natural history of pre-invasive lesions remains unclear. Moreover, the detection and treatment of pre-invasive lesions on a large scale will inevitably be time-consuming and costly, particularly if they are as prevalent as suggested by Auerbach's studies, and it is difficult to justify without objective evidence of clinical benefit.

At the Middlesex Hospital, we have been undertaking surveillance of patients with pre-invasive lesions. Preliminary findings from this long-term study are now in press [40] and suggest that approximately one in six high-grade lesions progress to invasive squamous cell carcinoma, while a similar proportion regress either to normal or to a lesser grade. The remaining high-grade lesions have persisted for up to four years. We have also found that patients harbouring pre-invasive lesions are at high risk of developing incidental cancers at remote sites within their lungs, in keeping with a "field change" effect. The advantage of maintaining surveillance in these patients is that it has ensured that treatment is targeted to the most appropriate site while also facilitating the prompt detection and treatment of new carcinomas.

Recommendations - Management of advanced lung cancer	**Evidence level**
Laser resection, photodynamic therapy, electrocautery, cryotherapy, brachytherapy, stenting and debulking with forceps are regarded as appropriate treatments.	
◆ Laser resection, PDT.	IIa/B
◆ Cryotherapy and diathermy.	IIb/B
◆ Debulking with forceps.	III/B
◆ PDT and cryotherapy are not recommended for patients with severe obstruction of their central airways who are at risk of asphyxia and who require immediate relief.	IV/C
◆ Brachytherapy is an appropriate endobronchial treatment for patients with advanced lung cancer.	IIa/B
◆ Stenting is an appropriate endobronchial treatment for patients with advanced lung cancer.	IIb/B
Recommendations - Management of early lung cancer	
◆ PDT should be regarded as a treatment option for early superficial squamous cell carcinomas in patients who are not surgical candidates.	IIa/B
◆ Brachytherapy, cryotherapy and electrocautery may be alternatives to PDT for treating early superficial squamous cell carcinomas in patients who are not surgical candidates, but more experience is needed.	IIb/B
◆ PDT is a promising alternative to surgery in patients with early superficial squamous cell carcinomas who are fit for surgery but more experience is needed. No recommendation can be made at present.	
◆ No recommendation can be made on the use of laser therapy to treat early superficial lung cancer.	
Recommendations - Management of pre-invasion lesions	
◆ No recommendation can currently be made on the management of pre-invasive bronchial epithelial lesions. More information on the natural history of these lesions is required.	

References

1. Mathur PN, Edell E, Sutedja T, Vergnon J-M. Treatment of Early Stage Lung Cancer. *Chest* 2003; 123: 176S-180S.
2. Moghissi K, Dixon K. Is bronchoscopic photodynamic therapy a therapeutic option in lung cancer? *Eur Resp J* 2003; 3: 535-541.
3. Bolliger CT, Mathur PN, Eds. Interventional Bronchoscopy. *Progress Resp Res* 2001; 30. Karger, Basel, 2001.
4. Hetzel MR, Ed. *Minimally invasive techniques in thoracic medicine and surgery.* Chapman and Hall, London, 1995.
5. Cancer research UK. Cancerstats. Mortality-UK. Feb 2004. www.cancerresearchuk.org/aboutcancer/statistics/statsmisc/pdfs/cancerstats_ mortality.pdf. Accessed 25 April 2004.
6. George PJ, Garrett CP, Nixon C, *et al.* Laser treatment for tracheobronchial tumours: local or general anaesthesia? *Thorax* 1987; 42 : 656-60.
7. Cavaliere S, Dumon J-F. Laser Bronchoscopy. In: Interventional Bronchoscopy. Bollinger CT, Mathur PN, Eds. *Progress Resp Res* 2000; 30: 108-119.
8. Cavaliere S, Venuta F, Foccoli P, *et al.* Endoscopic treatment of malignant airway obstructions in 2008 patients. *Chest* 1996; 110: 1536-42.

9. George PJM, Garrett CPO, Hetzel MR. Role of the neodymium YAG laser in the management of tracheal tumours. *Thorax* 1987; 42: 440-444.
10. George PJM. Assessment of the response to laser resection. In: *Minimally invasive techniques in thoracic medicine and surgery.* Hetzel MR, Ed. Chapman and Hall, London, 1995.
11. George PJ, Clarke G, Tolfree S, *et al.* Changes in regional ventilation and perfusion of the lung after endoscopic laser treatment. *Thorax* 1990; 45: 248-53.
12. Maiwand MO. The role of cryosurgery in palliation of tracheo-bronchial carcinoma. *Eur J of Cardiothorac Surg* 1999; 15: 764-768.
13. Maiwand MO, Homasson J-P. Cryotherapy for tracheobronchial disorders. *Clin Chest Med* 1995; 16: 427-443.
14. Mathur PN, Wolf KM, Busk MF, *et al.* Fiberoptic bronchoscopic cryotherapy in the management of tracheobronchial obstruction. *Chest* 1996; 110: 718-23.
15 McCaughan JS, Williams TE. Photodynamic therapy for endobronchial malignant disease: a prospective 14-year study. *J Thor Cardiothoracic Surg* 1997; 114: 940-7.
16. Moghissi K, Dixon K, Parsons RJ. Controlled trial of NdYAG laser versus photodynamic therapy for advanced malignant bronchial obstruction. *Lasers Med Sci* 1993; 8: 269-273.
17. Diaz-Jiminez, JP, Martinez-Ballarin JE, Llunell A, *et al.* Efficacy and safety of photodynamic therapy versus Nd-YAG laser resection in NSCLC with airway obstruction. *Eur Respir J* 1999; 14: 800-805.
18. Sutedja G, van Boxem T, Schramel F, *et al.* Endobronchial electrocautery is an excellent alternative for Nd:YAG laser to treat airway tumors. *J Bronchology* 1997; 4: 101-105.
19. Homasson JP. Endobronchial electrocautery. *Semin Respir Crit Care Med* 1997; 18: 535-43.
20. Mathisen DJ, Grillo HC. Endoscopic relief of malignant airway obstruction. *Ann Thoracic Surg* 1989; 48: 469-475.
21. Stout R, Barber P, Burt P, *et al.* Clinical and quality of life outcomes in the first United Kingdom randomized trial of endobronchial brachytherapy (intraluminal radiotherapy) vs. external beam radiotherapy in the palliative treatment of inoperable non-small cell lung cancer. *Radiotherapy & Oncology* 2000; 56: 323-7.
22. Langendijk H, de Jong J, Tjwa M, *et al.* External irradiation versus external irradiation plus endobronchial brachytherapy in inoperable non-small cell lung cancer: a prospective randomized study. *Radiotherapy & Oncology* 2001; 58: 257-68.
23. Goldman J. Physiological effect of endobronchial radiotherapy in patients with major airway occlusion by carcinoma. *Thorax* 1993; 48(2): 110-4.
24. Wood DE, Yun-Hen Liu Y-H, Vallieres E, *et al.* Airway Stenting for Malignant and Benign Tracheobronchial Stenosis. *Ann Thorac Surg* 2003; 76: 167-74.
25. Dumon J-F, Cavaliere S, Diaz-Jimenez JP, *et al.* Seven-year experience with the Dumon prosthesis. *J Bronchol* 1996; 3: 6-10.
26. Dineen KM, Jantz MA, Silvestri GA. Tracheobronchial Stents. *J Bronchology* 2002; 9: 127-137.
27. Edell E, Cortese DA. Bronchoscopic phototherapy with hematoporphyrin derivative for treatment of localized bronchogenic carcinoma: a 5-year experience. *Mayo Clin Proc* 1987; 62: 8-14.
28. Cortese DA, Edell ES, Kinsey JH. Photodynamic therapy for early stage squamous cell carcinoma of the lung. *Mayo Clin Proc* 1997; 72: 595-602.
30. Miyazu Y, Miyazuma T, Kurimoto N, *et al.* Endobronchial Ultrasonography in the assessment of Centrally Located Early-Stage Lung Cancer before Photodynamic Therapy. *Am J Respir Crit Care Med* 2001; 165: 832-37.
31. Marsiglia H, Baldeyrou P, Lartigau E, *et al.* High-Dose Brachytherapy as sole modality for early stage lung cancer. *Int J Radiat Oncol Biol Phys* 2000; 47: 665-72.
32. Perol M, Caliandro R, Pommier P, *et al.* Curative irradiation of limited endobronchial carcinomas with high-dose rate brachytherapy. Results of a pilot study. *Chest* 1997; 111: 1417-1423.
33. Deygas N, Froudarakis M, Ozenne G, *et al.* Cryotherapy in early superficial bronchogenic carcinoma. *Chest* 2001; 120: 26-31.
34. van Boxem TJ, Venmans BJ, Schramel FM, *et al.* Radiographically occult lung cancer treated with fibreoptic bronchoscopic electrocautery: a pilot study of a simple and inexpensive technique. *Eur Respir J* 1998; 11: 169-72.
35. Auerbach O, Stout AP, Hammond EC, *et al.* Changes in bronchial epithelium in relation to cigarette smoking and in relation to lung cancer. *N Engl J Med* 1961; 265: 253-267.
36. Bota S, Auliac JB, Paris C, *et al.* Follow-up of bronchial precancerous lesions and carcinoma *in situ* using fluorescence endoscopy. *Am J Respir Crit Care Med* 2001; 164: 1688-93.
37. Thurer RJ. Cryotherapy in early lung cancer. *Chest* 2001; 120: 3-5.
38. Venmans BJ, van Boxem TJ, Smit EF, *et al.* Outcome of bronchial carcinoma *in situ. Chest* 2000 117: 1572-6.
39. Lorchel F, Spaeth D, Scheid P, *et al.* High dose rate brachytherapy: a potentially curative treatment for small invasive T1N0 endobronchial carcinoma and carcinoma *in situ. Rev Mal Respir* 2003; 20: 515-20.
40. Banerjee, AK, Rabbitts PH, George PJ. Pre-invasive bronchial lesions: surveillance or intervention? *Chest* 2004; 125: 95S-96S.
41. Banerjee A, Rabbitts PH, George PJ. Lung cancer 3: fluorescence bronchoscopy: clinical dilemmas and research opportunities. *Thorax* 2003; 58: 266-271.

Chapter 8

The solitary pulmonary nodule

Francis C Wells MA MS FRCS
Consultant Cardiothoracic Surgeon
Martin J Goddard FRCS FRCPath
Consultant Histopathologist

PAPWORTH HOSPITAL, CAMBRIDGE, UK

Introduction

The use of the term "solitary pulmonary nodule" to describe an indeterminate, distinct lesion within the pulmonary parenchyma, has been in common usage for many years. Attempts to define the management of this clinical conundrum continue to generate a significant amount of literature. By implication this entity is a radiological finding. A solitary pulmonary nodule may be defined as a lesion measuring up to 3cm in maximum diameter, confined within aerated pulmonary parenchyma, without distinctive radiological features of malignancy.

The reasons for increasing interest in this entity are as follows. Lung cancer remains the most common cancer cause of death resulting in 28% of all cancer deaths in the USA and the UK [1]. Complete surgical resection remains the only likely cure for lung cancer, and the potential for "cure" depends upon complete resection. A cancer that presents as a solitary lesion within the lung measuring less than 3cm in diameter, without nodal metastases, represents stage I lung cancer (T1 N0 M0), and is likely to yield a 5-year survival of ~80% [2]. In other words, complete surgical resection at this stage of the disease, providing that there has not been prior dissemination, will likely result in cure for the patient [3]. The conundrum is how to achieve this without subjecting many people to unnecessary surgery, if the lesion is benign.

Over-investigation and treatment of patients wastes precious resources and money that could be spent on improving the management of others. All intervention carries some risk of complications [4]. Hence, the appropriate use of resources to give the most accurate management plan is the goal of evidence-based management of the solitary pulmonary nodule.

In addition to the appropriate desire to optimise the management of this condition on cost-effectiveness and quality care grounds, there is renewed interest in screening programmes for the earliest detection of lung cancer. Earlier attempts in the 1970s had been discredited. In 1999, an editorial by Smith [5] outlined the flaws in the previous trials and underscored the need for current evaluation of CT-based screening protocols in high-risk patients.

It is axiomatic that the earliest detection of this disease will lead to the best hope of cure. As screening programmes develop, the finding of the solitary undiagnosed pulmonary nodule is becoming a frequent event. Hence, effective management strategies are more important than ever before. The two main questions raised by the increased radiological screening for lung cancer are, who is responsible for the follow-up of indeterminate nodules and how should such lesions be managed?

The magnitude of the problem was demonstrated by the results of the Early Lung Cancer Action Project [6]. One thousand symptom-free volunteers, 60 years of age or older with at least ten pack-years of smoking history, were enrolled in this study. Patients with previous cancer and patients regarded as unfit to undergo a surgical resection, should an operable lung cancer be discovered, were excluded. On the initial chest radiograph 68 patients were found to have a pulmonary nodule, which proved to be malignant in seven individuals. In addition, baseline low-dose CT scans demonstrated 233 non-calcified pulmonary nodules, which in 27 individuals ultimately proved malignant. Hence, in both groups approximately 90% of lesions discovered ultimately proved to be benign. This expensive process throws up a significant work-load cost and legal implications. The management of these lesions will therefore depend upon the nature of the nodule, the state of the patient and the approach of the physician or surgeon responsible for the patient [7].

General approach

Many patients in whom a solitary nodule is discovered, will have a pre-existing chest radiograph. The presence of a long-term, pre-existing nodule, with no demonstrable change in size is very reassuring for both patient and clinician. In this circumstance, in the absence of any other features of malignancy, it is sensible to continue to watch with interval chest radiographs. Whether CT scanning is indicated at this stage will be dependent upon other findings. Simple tests such as sputum cytology and the general state of the patient, will add important additional information with regard to the likelihood of malignancy. One of the most important factors in the management of this condition is the reassurance of the patient. The obvious pre-existence of the nodule without identifiable change is usually enough to allay the fears of the patient.

The next question, having decided to wait and watch a nodule, is how long may be regarded as a safe period? Quaterman and colleagues [8] retrospectively studied the effect of delay in surgical intervention on survival for patients with early stage non-small cell lung cancer. Lung tumours of approximately 1cm in diameter contain approximately 10^8 cells, which approximates to 30 cell doubling times [9]. Tumour biology studies have revealed that doubling times for squamous cell carcinomas and adenocarcinomas are approximately 88 and 161 days respectively. Thus, even tumours that are barely visible on a chest radiograph may have been present for up to seven years. Detection by spiral CT at ~0.5cm translates into a saving of only three doubling times or 10% of the tumour's life span. Not only does this suggest that a short extended period of observation of the indeterminate nodule that is eventually demonstrated to be malignant of perhaps little consequence, but that there has already been considerable opportunity for dissemination. This fact explains why <100% of patients survive for five years even at the earliest clinical presentation. This observation also raises the interesting question of why as many as 80% of patients with stage IA non-small cell lung cancer do survive five years.

The study of Quaterman and colleagues revealed no difference in survivorship of patients with early stage NSCLC, who underwent resection either within 90 days of first detection or after 90 days. This paper allows very limited deductions, but points the way for more planned prospective analyses.

However, a watching brief for lesions measuring ≤1cm in diameter with interval spiral CT scanning at approximately three months, would seem to be an acceptable protocol. Further evidence in support of this approach is the fact that increasing tumour size up to 3cm in diameter has no apparent impact on survival rate [10,11].

The site within a lobe of an indeterminate nodule is also important in the decision-making process. If the lesion is centrally placed within the lung, resection is much more likely to involve a lobar resection. Lobectomy for an ultimately benign lesion is a much more egregious intervention than a wedge resection of a peripheral lesion.

Whilst other factors in the patient's history, such as smoking, industrial or environmental exposure may heighten suspicion, the anxiety level of the patient may in the end determine the attitude towards early resection.

The attitude of the patient's surgeon or physician will also have bearing on the management protocol. To wait and watch will need a surgeon who is prepared to take the time to give a very clear explanation of the decisions taken and to take on board the anxieties of the patient. This modus operandi will also require meticulous follow-up plans.

From the contrary point of view, does the resection of a benign nodule represent a failure in management? Theoretically, the answer to this question is yes, but there are also potential benefits from this action. The alleviation of anxiety for some patients cannot be underestimated. In addition, there is an undoubted saving to be made from abbreviating the monitoring period and eliminating repeated CT and PET scans. As a rough guide, no more than 10% of resections should be benign. Reversed logic would suggest that if the positivity for malignancy rate is close to 100%, it is likely that some cancers are being missed.

Diagnostic tools for evaluation of lung nodules

Table 1 lists the diagnostic tools available for the assessment of newly discovered lung lesions.

Chest radiograph

Solitary pulmonary nodules are often incidental findings on chest radiographs. The discovery of a nodule should lead to a clinical assessment. Important risk factors for malignancy are a smoking history, previous malignancy and age >35 [12].

CT scan

High resolution CT scanning allows a more detailed non-invasive assessment of the nodule. Repeat scanning and careful volumetric analysis allows any changes in size of the nodule to be monitored. There are a number of radiological characteristics that can be assessed that are of value in determining the likelihood of malignancy and can be used to inform the clinician in planning the patient's management.

Calcification

Calcification within a nodule is most commonly seen in benign lesions [13,14]. Granulomatous lesions may show diffuse, solid or central calcification [15], whilst hamartomas are typically described as having a popcorn-like calcification [16]. However, 6-14% of malignancies show calcification often amorphous or stippled [17,18]. CT has been shown to be more sensitive than plain film radiography in detecting the presence of calcification and has been used to undertake quantitative assessment of the calcification.

Table 1. Diagnostic tools for evaluation of lung cancer.

X-ray or CT scan
Sputum cytology
Bronchoscopy (including direct biopsy, needle biopsy and brushings and washings for cytology)
Percutaneous fine needle aspiration or biopsy
PET scan
Excision biopsy [?]
- Video-assisted
- Thoracotomy

Edge characteristics

A spiculated margin with fine linear strands radiating outward from the nodule has a high positive predictive value with quoted figures of 88-94% [12,19]. The appearance is due to the radial extension of tumour cells along interlobular septa or lymphatics [17]. Conversely, smooth borders are not a reliable indicator of a benign lesion and are seen in up to 23% of malignant lesions, many of which are subsequently shown to be metastases [20,21].

Internal characteristics

The size of the nodule is also an indicator of likely diagnosis. The majority of nodules >2cm are malignant, whereas for those <2cm, the incidence of malignancy is about 50% [22]. Non-calcified nodules <1cm are malignant in 8-36% depending on the published series [20,23]. Cavitation is commonly associated with malignancy, but may also be seen in inflammatory and infectious conditions. In this setting, the wall thickness can further aid in discriminating benign from malignant nodules. A wall thickness >15mm is associated with malignancy in 84% of cases, whilst those with a wall thickness <5mm are benign in 95% of cases [24,25]. Nodules displaying fat are most likely benign, most usually hamartomas.

Enhancement

The blood supply and metabolism of malignant nodules differ from those of benign ones. Nodules are scanned before and after the application of contrast material. An enhancement of <15 Hounsfield units (HU) is strongly predictive of benignity, but the technique has a relative poor positive predictive value (68%), because of false positives being associated with central necrosis [26]. Maximum attenuation rates of 20-60 HU are reliable predictors of malignancy [27-29]. The technique however, lacks a standard protocol and is affected by scanning time, scan intervals and contrast injection rates. Comparison between different studies is therefore difficult.

Rates of growth

Neoplastic lesions grow and this can be expressed as the time taken to double their volume (doubling time). CT studies have confirmed doubling times for lung cancers of 20 to 400 days [30]. This range of doubling times, has led to the practice of equating 2-year stability with benignity. However, a doubling in volume equates to a 1.25 times increase in linear dimension, which may be difficult to detect in small lesions [31,32]. Conversely, an increase in size over a short period of time in an indeterminate lesion is more likely to reflect a malignant lesion. It has been argued that adding a time delay to potentially curative surgical treatment could adversely affect outcome. However, one study with a time delay of 48 days did not show any deleterious impact on outcome [33].

Positron Emission Tomography (PET)

Positron emission tomography (PET) using 18-fluorodeoxyglucose (18-FDG) has been used widely for tumour imaging. The FDG is taken up by cells for glycolysis, but cannot be utilised and accumulates. Increased activity is seen in highly metabolic cells particularly within tumours and areas of inflammation. A meta-analysis of 40 studies published in 2001 showed a sensitivity of 96.8% and specificity of 77.8% for detecting malignancy. For benign nodules the technique has a sensitivity of 96% and a specificity of 88% [34].

The technique is limited because it only has a spatial resolution of 8mm and hence, imaging of solitary pulmonary nodules less than 1cm in diameter is unreliable. False negative results may be seen in carcinoids and broncho-alveolar carcinomas, whilst false positives are seen in infectious or inflammatory lesions. In patients with a solitary pulmonary nodule with a low likelihood of malignancy (<20%) then the finding of a negative PET scan reduces the likelihood of malignancy to <1% [34]. In highly suspicious lesions, then a negative PET scan still leaves a significant risk of malignancy and adds little to the decision-making process.

Magnetic Resonance Imaging (MRI)

MRI has a limited role in the evaluation of the solitary pulmonary nodule. It allows for better anatomic evaluation of the lung apices and chest wall, but the imaging from CT is usually adequate for most nodules. MRI has been reported to help in distinguishing between benign lesions and those requiring further investigation, either malignant or with active infection, by comparing the relative enhancement ratios and slope of enhancement [35].

Pathology

The only way to establish a definitive diagnosis is to obtain a sample for pathological examination. Other than an excision biopsy, all other biopsy techniques may potentially give false negative results due to sampling errors.

Relative non-invasive techniques can be by bronchoscopy with biopsy or washings and by a percutaneous needle biopsy depending on the site of the nodule. Routine sputum cytology is little used because of the low diagnostic yield [36].

Bronchoscopy

Bronchoscopy has a variable sensitivity in detecting malignancy in a solitary pulmonary nodule depending on the size of the nodule and its proximity to the bronchial tree. Larger nodules (2-3cm diameter) are more likely to be diagnosed with a sensitivity of 40-60%, but for nodules 1.5cm diameter, the sensitivity falls to just 10% [37]. The diagnostic yield is improved when there is a "bronchus sign" on the CT scan, such that a fourth order bronchus or higher can be seen within or directly leading to the nodule. In one study, the diagnostic yield was 59% with a positive bronchus sign against 18% without [38]. The diagnostic yield can be increased by the use of endobronchial needle aspiration. This is particularly beneficial when sampling submucosal or peribronchial disease. In one study, this led to an increase in positive diagnoses from 76% to 96% [39]. Diagnostic yield is further enhanced through the use of fluoroscopy and multiple sampling methods [40].

Transthoracic needle biopsy

Percutaneous needle biopsy is useful in determining the nature of the solitary pulmonary nodule. Using CT imaging a cutting biopsy needle is directed into the nodule. The sensitivity for malignancy ranges from 64% to 100% [41,42], depending on the series. A meta-analysis of 48 studies showed that given a 50% probability of malignancy prior to needle biopsy, then the post-test probabilities of malignancy upon receiving the results would be malignant, 99%, suspicious, 94%, and non-specific benign, 7% [43]. Needle biopsy is relatively contraindicated in patients with a previous pneumonectomy, severe emphysema or a bleeding diathesis. Pneumothorax is the most common complication following the procedure and occurs in approximately 24.5% of cases [43]. The use of enhanced imaging techniques has meant that smaller lesions are now detected. However, high diagnostic yields can still be achieved in nodules <1cm in diameter [44], although results are less good in subpleural lesions and those <0.8cm.

Surgery

Nearly all solitary pulmonary nodules are resectable. With the use of radiological investigations and needle biopsy techniques, the majority of patients should have a tissue diagnosis before being considered for surgery. Some patients will have a radiologically suspicious lesion, but needle biopsy techniques will have failed to produce a diagnostic sample. The use of video-assisted thoracoscopy (VATS) has been widely used for the diagnosis of solitary pulmonary nodules. Depending on the criteria used for referral for an excision biopsy, 50-75% of the nodules have proven benign [45,46]. The specimen may be sent for frozen section so that conversion to a thoracotomy and lobectomy can be performed. This should only be undertaken if the patient has been subjected to the usual pre-operative staging.

A suggested diagnostic algorithim for the investgation of SPN is given in Figure 1.

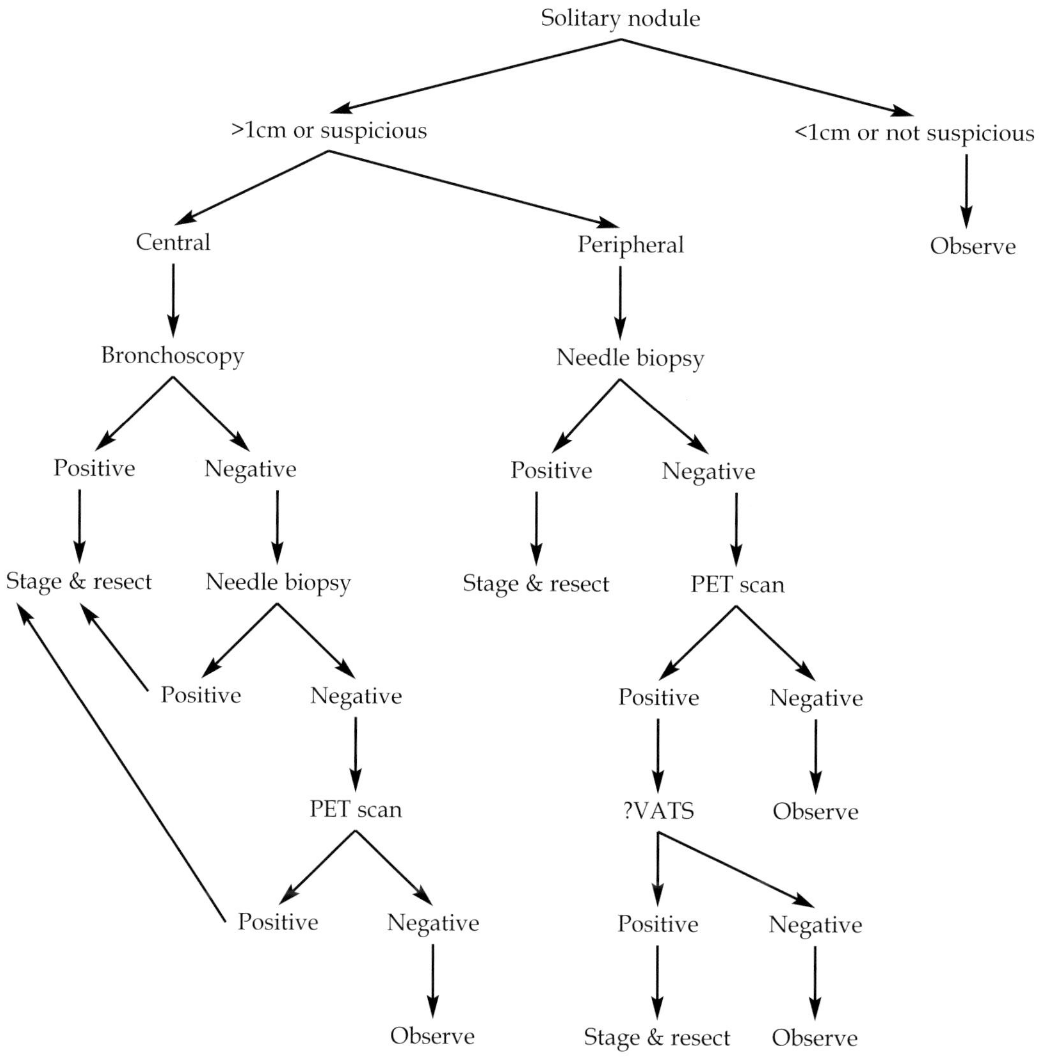

Figure 1. **Flow diagram to show the diagnostic pathway for a solitary pulmonary nodule.**

Recommendations	**Evidence level**
◆ Patients with a solitary pulmonary nodule should have a CT scan to characterise the nodule. Assessment of size, calcification, edge and internal characteristics can be useful in identifying nodules that are more likely to be benign. CT also plays an important role in staging.	IIb/B
◆ Benign or indeterminate nodules should be followed-up with a repeat CT scan and volumetric assessment. An increase in volume should prompt further investigation or excision.	IIb/B
◆ PET scanning should not be used in the assessment of solitary pulmonary nodules <1cm diameter. PET scanning may provide additional information in nodules thought to be at a low-risk of malignancy. In nodules at a higher risk of malignancy, a definitive tissue diagnosis will be needed.	Ib/A
◆ Bronchoscopy is of value in obtaining a tissue diagnosis in larger lesions that are centrally placed and have a "bronchus sign". Multiple sampling techniques including washings, brushings, biopsy and needle aspiration should be used.	IIb/B
◆ Transthoracic needle biopsy provides the best means to obtain a tissue sample for an indeterminate solitary pulmonary nodule.	IIb/B

References

1. American Cancer Society: Surveillance Research, 2001
2. Patz EF Jr, Rossi S, Harpole DH, Herndon JE, Goodman PC. Correlation of tumour size and survival in patients with stage IA non-small cell cancer. *Chest* 2000; 117: 1568-1571.
3. Martini N, Bains MS, Burt ME, *et al.* Incidence of local recurrence and second primary tumours in resected stage I lung cancer. *J Thorac Cardiovasc Surg* 1995; 109: 120-129.
4. Black WC. Overdiagnosis: an underrecognised cause of confusion and harm in cancer screening. *J Natl Cancer Inst* 2000; 92: 1280-2.
5. Smith IE. Screening for lung cancer: time to think positive. *Lancet* 1999; 354: 86-87.
6. Henschke CI, McCauley DI. Yankelevitz DF, *et al.* Early lung cancer action project: overall design and findings from baseline screening. *Lancet* 1999; 354: 99-105.
7. Cooper JD. Management of the Solitary Pulmonary Nodule: Directed Resection. *Semin Thorac Cardiovasc Surg* 2002; 14(3): 286-291.
8. Quaterman RL, Mcmillan A, Ratcliffe MB, Block MI. Effect of preoperative delay on the prognosis for patients with early stage non-small cell lung cancer. *J Thorac Cardiovasc Surg* 2003; 125(1): 108-114.
9. Geddes DM. The natural history of lung cancer: a review based on rates of tumour growth. *Br J Dis Chest* 1979; 73: 1-17.
10. Patz EF Jr, Rossi S, Harpole DH, Herndon JE, Goodman PC. Correlation of tumour size and survival in patients with stage 1A non-small cell lung cancer. *Chest* 2000; 117: 1568-1571.
11. Martini N, Bains MS, Burt ME, *et al.* Incidence of local recurrence and second primary tumours in resected stage 1 lung cancer. *J Thorac Cardiovasc Surg* 1995; 109: 120-129.
12. Gurney JW. Determining the likelihood of malignancy in solitary pulmonary nodules with Bayesian analysis Pt 1. Theory. *Radiol* 1993; 186: 405-13.
13. Yankelvitz DF, Henschke CI. Derivation for relating calcification and size in pulmonary nodules. *Clin Imaging* 1998; 22: 1-6.
14. Swenson SJ. What is the significance of finding calcifications in pulmonary masses on CT scan? *Am J Roentgenol* 1995; 164: 505-6.
15. Erasmus JJ, Connelly JE, McAdams HP, Roggli VL. Solitary pulmonary nodules: Part 1. Morphologic evaluation for differentiation of benign and malignant lesios. *Radiographics* 2000; 20(1): 43-48.
16. Bateson EM, Abbott EK. Mixed tumours of the lungs, or hamarto-chondromas. A review of the literature and a report of fifteen new cases. *Clin Radiol* 1960: 11: 232.
17. Zerhouni EA, Stitik FP, Siegelmann SS, Naidich DP, Sagel SS, Proto AV, Muhm JR, Walsh JW, Martinez CR, Heelan RT. CT of the pulmonary nodule: a national cooperative study. *Radiology* 1986; 160: 319-27.
18. Mahoney MC, Shipley RT, Corcoran HL, Dickson BA. CT demonstration of calcification in carcinoma of the lung. *Am J Roentgenol* 1990; 154(2): 255-8.
19. Furuya K, Murayama S, Soeda H, Murakami J, Ichinose Y, Yabuuchi H, Katsuda Y, Koga M, Masuda K. New classification of small pulmonary nodules by main

characteristics on high resolution CT. *Acta Radiol* 1999; 40: 496-504.
20. Seemann MS, Seeman O, Luboldt W, *et al.* Differentiation of malignant from benign solitary pulmonary lesions using chest radiography, spiral CT and HRCT. *Lung Cancer* 2000; 29: 105-24.
21. Takashima S, Sone S, Li F, Maruyama Y, Hasegawa M, Matsushita T, Takayama F, Kadoya M. Small solitary pulmonary nodules (<1cm) detected at population-based CT screening for lung cancer: reliable high-resolution CT features of benign lesions. *AJR* 2003; 180: 955-64.
22. Shure D, Fedullo PF. Transbronchial needle aspiration of peripheral masses. *Am Rev Respir Dis* 1983; 140: 473-4.
23. Henschke CI, McCauley DI, Yankelvitz DF, *et al.* Early lung cancer action project: overall design and findings from baseline screening. *Lancet* 1999: 99-105.
24. Woodring JH, Fried AM, Chuang VP. Solitary cavities of the lung: diagnostic implications of cavity wall thickness. *AJR* 1980; 135: 1269-71.
25. Woodring JH, Fried AM. Significance of wall thickness in solitary cavities of the lung: a follow-up study. *AJR* 1983; 140: 473-4.
26. Swensen SJ, Brown LR, Colby TV, Weaver AL, Midthun DE. Lung nodule enhancement at CT: prospective findings. *Radiology* 1996; 201: 447-455.
27. Yamashita K, Matsunobe S, Tsuda T, *et al.* Solitary pulmonary nodules: preliminary study of evaluation with incremental dynamic CT. *Radiology* 1995; 194: 399-405.
28. Zhang M, Kono M. Solitary pulmonary nodules: evaluation of blood flow patterns with dynamic CT. *Radiology* 1997; 205: 471-8.
29. Swensen SJ, Viggiano RW, Midthun DE, *et al.* Lung nodule enhancement at CT: multicenter study. *Radiology* 2000; 214: 73-80.
30. Yankelvitz DF, Reeves AP, Kostis WJ, Zhao B, Henscke CI. Small pulmonary nodules: volumetrically determined growth rates based on CT evaluation. *Radiology* 2000; 217: 251-6.
31. Yankelvitz DF, Henschke CI. Does 2-year stability imply that pulmonary nodules are benign? *Am J Roentgenol* 1997; 168: 325-8.
32. Yankelvitz DF, Reeves AP, Kastis WJ, *et al.* Small pulmonary nodules; volumetrically determind growth rates based on CT evaluation. *Radiology* 2000; 217: 251-6.
33. Bozcuk H, Martin C. Does treatment delay affect survival in non-small cell lung cancer? A retrospective analysis from a single UK center. *Lung Cancer* 2001; 34: 342-52.
34. Gould MK, Maclean CC, Kuschne Wg, *et al.* Accuracy of positron emission tomography for diagnosis of pulmonary nodules and mass lesions: a meta-analysis. *JAMA* 2001; 285: 914-924.
35. Ohno Y, Hatabu H, Takenaka D, Adachi S, Kono M, Sugimara K. Solitary pulmonary nodules; potential role of dynamic MR imaging in management - initial experience. *Radiology* 2002; 224: 503-11.
36. Goldberg-Kahn B, Healy JC, Bishop JW. A comparison of four different strategies in the workup of solitary radiographic lung lesions. *Chest* 1997; 111: 870-6.
37. Swensen SJ, Jett JR, Payne WS, *et al.* An integrated approach to evaluation of the solitary pulmonary nodule. *Mayo Clin Proc* 1990; 65: 173-86.
38. Gaeta M, Pandolgo I, Volta S, *et al.* Bronchus sign on CT in peripheral carcinoma of the lung: value in predicting results of transbronchial biopsy. *AJR* 1991; 157: 1181-85.
39. Dasgupta A, Jain P Aroglia AC, *et al.* Bronchoscopy and needle biopsy techniques for diagnosis and staging of lung cancers. *Chest* 1999; 115: 1237-41.
40. Arroglia AC, Matthay RA. The role of bronchoscopy in lung cancer. *Clin Chest Med* 1993; 14: 87-98.
41. Weisbrod GL. Transthoracic needle biopsy. *World J Surg* 1993; 17: 705-11.
42. Klein JS. Interventional chest radiology. *Current Prob Diagn Radiol* 1992; 13: 11-16.
43. Lacasse Y, Wong E, Guyatt GH, Cook DJ. Transthoracic needle aspiration biopsy for the diagnosis of localised pulmonary lesions: a meta-analysis. *Thorax* 1999; 54: 884-93.
44. Wallace M, Krishnamurthy S, Broemeling L, Gupta S, Ahrar K, Morello F, Hicks M. CT-guided percutaneous fine-needle aspiration biopsy of small (<1cm) pulmonary lesions. *Radiology* 2002; 225: 823-8.
45. Mack MJ, Hazelrigg SR, Landreneau RJ, *et al.* Thoracoscopy for the diagnosis of the indeterminate solitary nodule. *Ann Thorac Surg* 1993; 56: 825-832.
46. Allen MS, Deschamps C, Lee RE, *et al.* Video-assisted thoracoscopic stapled wedge excision for indeterminate pulmonary nodules. *J Thorac Cardiovasc Surg* 1993; 106: 1048-52.

Chapter 9

Bronchopulmonary carcinoid tumours

Aman S Coonar BSc MD MRCP FRCS

Specialist Registrar, Cardiothoracic Surgery

GUY'S AND ST. THOMAS' HOSPITALS, LONDON, UK

Introduction

Carcinoid tumours (neuroendocrine carcinomas) [1] are malignant neoplastic tumours. Langhans [2] first described a gut carcinoid tumour in 1867, and in 1890 Ransom [3] reported symptoms of what is known as the carcinoid syndrome. The term "karzinoide" or "cancer-like" was introduced by Oberndorfer in 1907 [4].

These malignancies may arise anywhere in the body and the commonest primary site is the gastrointestinal tract, which may reflect the relative density of neuroendocrine cells at different sites in the body. Bronchopulmonary carcinoid comprise 10-33% of the total [5,6]. They have been reported in all racial groups and in some series, females are more commonly affected [5,7]. They are commoner in the right lung [5] and occasionally, may be bilateral [8]. They produce symptoms due to local effects, metastases or by the production of chemicals and hormones such as 5-HT (5-hydroxytryptamine), histamine, cortisol and growth hormone [5,9].

Carcinoid cells share histological and molecular characteristics with neuroendocrine cells (amine precursor and decarboxylation cells [APUD], also known as Kulchitsky cells), and these are probably the cells of origin. Their molecular biology is uncertain, but as with other malignancies, there are more molecular abnormalities in the higher-grade lesions [10-13]. There may be a major genetic contribution to aetiology in those tumours that occur as part of the multiple endocrine neoplasia syndromes [14], and in some cases of sporadic atypical carcinoid (AC), mutations in the MEN1 gene have been identified [13].

This chapter will review the quality of evidence that forms the basis for our management of bronchopulmonary carcinoid.

Methodology

A detailed search of on-line databases (Medline from 1966, Embase, Cancerlit) using the principal search terms "carcinoid", "pulmonary" or "lung", and "surgery" generated 544 references. These were scrutinised to identify suitable papers, and leads were followed with references added to the database. Bibliographies of selected references were also searched.

The literature included laboratory reports, population-based cancer registry surveys, retrospectively analysed clinical series, case reports and literature reviews. No prospective randomised trials were found. Papers were inconsistent in their definitions of pathology, surgical methods, follow-up and outcome measures. With respect to the papers reporting clinical management, there is therefore, no level I or II evidence.

This chapter is divided into sections discussing pathology, natural history, surgical management and new developments.

Pathology

Current classification of neuro-endocrine carcinoma: definition and implication

Neuroendocrine carcinoma (NEC) comprise a spectrum of disease ranging from low-grade typical carcinoid (TC) through intermediate-grade atypical carcinoid (AC), to the high-grade categories of large cell neuroendocrine carcinoma (LCNEC) and small cell carcinoma (SCLC).

The current classification was developed to be prognostically useful and was formalised by the WHO in 1999 [11], and the discriminating histological features are shown in Table 1. As with many diseases, there have been differences and controversies in classification, and this has contributed to a difficulty and potential flaw in comparing series and other historical data.

Revisions in pathology create a prognostically useful classification

In 1972, Arrigoni [15] defined atypical carcinoid as a carcinoid tumour with increased mitotic activity with: one mitotic figure per 1-2 high-power fields (HPF) (or 5-10 mitoses/10 HPF); necrosis; nuclear pleomorphism, hyperchromatism, and an abnormal nuclear to cytoplasmic ratio; and areas of increased cellularity with disorganization.

In 1999, this was superceded by a WHO classification [11], and was based on work by Travis [1]. This group presented data on 200 neuroendocrine lung tumours. Surgically resected tumours were studied in 185 cases, and endobronchial biopsy specimens in 15 cases of small cell lung cancer.

Table 1. WHO Histology and grade of lung neuroendocrine tumours (1999) [11].

Histogical type	Grade	Microscopy	Mitoses/2mm^2 (10 HPF)	Necrosis distribution
Typical carcinoid	Low	Carcinoid	<2	None
Atypical carcinoid	Intermediate	Carcinoid	≥2 and <10 or necrosis	Punctate often
Large cell neuroendocrine carcinoma	High	Neuroendocrine morphology and immunohistochemistry, cytological features of large cell carcinoma	>10	Large zones
Small cell carcinoma	High	Small, scant cytoplasm, finely granular nuclear chromatin, absent or faint nucleoli	>10	Large zones

Tumours were evaluated for histological features that may predict prognosis. Survival analyses were performed using the Kaplan-Meier and Cox proportional hazards methods analysing for the variables of average number of mitoses per 10 HPF, necrosis, vascular invasion, pleomorphism, and nucleoli. It was found that prognosis was more accurately determined by defining typical carcinoid tumours as those that had only 0-1 mitoses per 10 HPF. The survival curves are shown in Figure 1.

Impact of change in pathology

The major change between the current [11] and previous classification [15] has been the differentiation between typical and atypical carcinoid. The current classification has more stringent criteria for TC and widened criteria for AC. Therefore, cases categorised before and after re-classification should be considered differently. A prediction of outcome using the new classification would be that prognosis would be improved in the TC group, as some cases would be now upgraded to AC. Similarly, that prognosis would be improved in the AC group, as some cases which previously would have been borderline between TC and AC, will now be graded as AC [1]. It should also be noted that LCNEC was not formally recognised as a separate entity until 1991, and some cases that were originally classified as AC, would now be upgraded to LCNEC [11].

It follows that re-classification may significantly alter the interpretation of outcome, and it may be prudent to consider earlier series in this context. In two recent series, re-classification was performed with up to 20% of cases changing status [16,17].

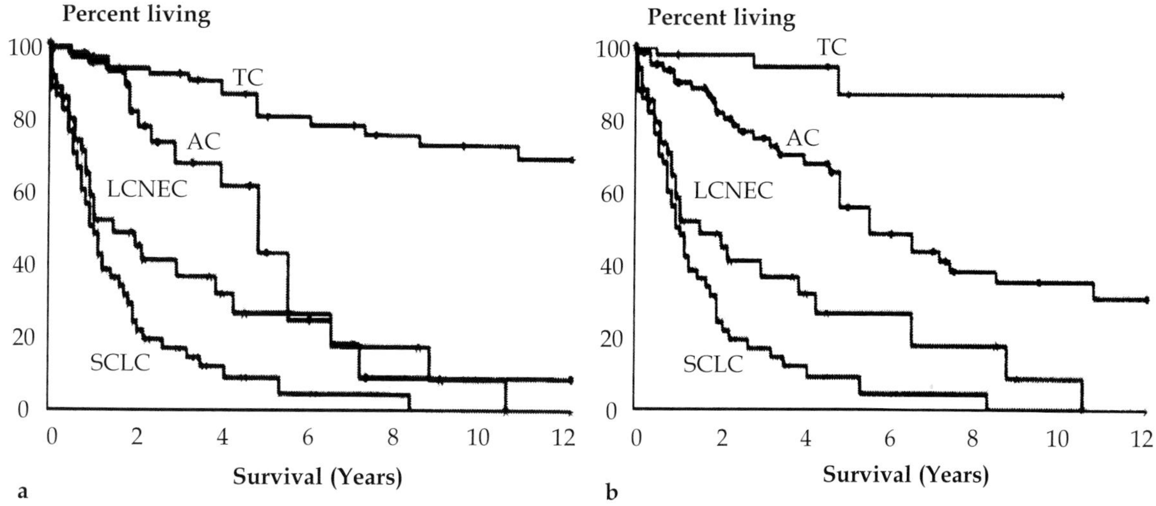

TC = typical carcinoid, AC = atypical carcinoid,
LCNEC = large cell neuroendocrine carcinoma, SCLC = small cell lung cancer

Figure 1. Kaplan-Meier survival curve for 200 neuroendocrine tumours. a) Survival based on classification of neuroendocrine tumours with atypical carcinoid (AC) tumours defined using the Arrigoni criterion of 5-10 mitoses per 2mm^2 (10 high-power fields [HPF]). b) Survival based on classification of neuroendocrine tumours with AC defined by the criteria of 2-10 mitoses per 2mm^2 (10 HPF) or necrosis. *Reproduced with permission from Travis WD, Rush W, Flieder DB, Falk R, Fleming MV, Gal AA, et al. Survival analysis of 200 pulmonary neuroendocrine tumours with clarification of criteria for atypical carcinoid and its separation from typical carcinoid. Am J Surg Pathol 1998; 22(8): 934-44.*

Natural history

Population-based cancer registry surveys

Seven population-based cancer registry surveys were identified [6,7,18-22]. The data from the first two references are incorporated in the third [7]. These are listed in Table 2.

The largest of these investigations was published in 2003 by Modlin and gives epidemiological data on 13,715 carcinoid tumours [7]. This incorporated two large surveys published in 1997 and 1975 [6, 18]. This major work pooled the data from different population-based cancer registries and gives epidemiological evidence about the spectrum of carcinoid tumours in general. 25.3% of the total number of carcinoids were bronchopulmonary, and 0.38% were "endocrine including thymus" carcinoids.

An increase in incidence has been noted and is shown in Table 3. The reasons for this increase in registration are speculative.

Table 2. **Population-based cancer registry surveys.**

Reference	Location	Period	n carcinoid cases	% broncho-pulmonary	% broncho-pulmonary Male:Female	Age adjusted incidence n bp carcinoid /100,000 /year
Modlin [7] 2003 (incorporates [6, 18])	USA	1973-1999	13715	25.3%	0.6:1	(1992-1999) 0.39 (black males) 0.52 (white males) 0.57 (black females) 0.89 (white females)
Hallgrimsson [20] 1989	Iceland	1955-1984	146	15%* 1	0.5:1	0.23 (males) 0.5 (females)
Skuladottir [19] 2002	Denmark	1978-1997	297	NA	1:1	0.37 (males) 0.3 (females)
Newton [21] 1994	UK	1979-1987	3382	18.1* 2	NA	NA for bp alone but the overall incidence of carcinoid increased, and higher rates were seen in females.
Levi [22] 2000	Switzerland	1974-1997	433	18.2* 3	1.2:1	0.46 (males) 0.4 (females)

* 1 A further 3% were of unknown origin and may have contributed to this group.
* 2 In this paper a further category of "disseminated tumour" is recognised. This group was 3.8% of the total, and some may have been bronchopulmonary in origin. This value may be an underestimate.
* 3 This paper uses the term "lung", and an assumption has been made that this refers to bronchopulmonary. A further 10.4% are described as "other" and may also contribute to the bronchopulmonary group.
(bp = bronchopulmonary)

Table 3. Increase in age-related incidence for carcinoid tumours (national US lung cancer incidence for comparison) [7, 23].

	Age-adjusted incidence for bronchopulmonary carcinoid USA n/100,000/year [7]			Age-adjusted incidence for lung cancer USA n/100,000 [23]	
	1969-1971	1973-1991	1992-1999	1973	1999
black males	0.15	0.32	0.39	123.67	112.78
white males	0.22	0.38	0.52	84.83	78.13
black females	0.06	0.37	0.57	23.59	55.47
white females	0.24	0.5	0.89	20.380	51.57

A population-based cancer registry survey from Denmark which has a more homogeneous population, also found an increase in incidence between 1978-1997 of TC, AC and LCNEC from 0.25 to 0.52/100,000 inhabitants/year in men and 0.14 to 0.46/100,000 inhabitants/year in women [19].

Systematic reviews of broncho-pulmonary carcinoid

In 1999, Soga and Yakuwa [5] published their systematic review of 1875 cases of bronchopulmonary carcinoid (1595 TC, 280 AC) (Table 4). This was derived from a total series of 8843 patients with carcinoid who had been registered in the Niigata registry, Japan. This is a database of all patients reported to have carcinoid tumours, and has been generated by performing a systematic review of the world literature from 1945. The authors have published on different aspects of neuroendocrine carcinoma [5,9,24].

Table 4. Source of cases for Soga [5], 1999.

Region	% of cases	n
Worldwide Total	100	1875
Americas	31	572
Europe	30	562
Japan	37	695
Others	2	102
TC	85	1595
AC	15	280

The authors undertook a detailed analysis of the clinical features, management and outcome of these patients. To avoid case duplication their analysis only included those cases from series in which individual identification such as age or sex were included. Reports in which individual patients could not be identified, were excluded. A comparison between TC and AC was performed. In this series, the classification of an individual lesion as TC or AC is as described by the original author. Soga recognises and discusses the dilemma that this raises. The potential error that this introduces has been addressed previously in this chapter. Nevertheless, because of the size of this study and its focus on bronchopulmonary carcinoid, it is an important paper in our understanding of disease natural history, and a number of points are presented below.

Findings by Soga 1999 [5]

In this series there was no statistically significant gender difference, though the disease was commoner in females (male: female = 903:972 ≡ 0.92:1). There were also no gender differences in the proportion with TC vs. AC or overall clinical manifestations. The right lung was more commonly affected than the left (60% vs. 40%). Selected significant differences are shown in Table 5 and the clinical manifestations are shown in Table 6.

Table 5. **Significant differences between TC and AC (p<0.01) [5].**

Feature	TC	AC
Mean age at presentation	46.3 years	54.7 years
Central location	67.8%	36.5%
Tumour >5cm	9.7%	15.7%
Metastases	23.1%	46.4%
Carcinoid syndrome	8.7%	3.9%

Table 6. **Clinical manifestations of bronchopulmonary carcinoid disease [5].**

Clinical feature	%
Not recorded	24.9
Asymptomatic	14.3
Cough	42
Atelectasis	25.4
Fever	23.9
Haemoptysis (and "bloody sputum")	32.5
Dyspnoea	15.6
Chest pain	11.5
Flush	11.4
Diarrhoea	9.9

Table 7. **Frequency and site of metastases [5].**

Cases with metastases	Overall		TC		AC	
	n	%	n	%	n	%
	498	26.6	368	**23.1***	130	**46.4***
Site involved						
Lymph nodes	278	14.8	192	**12***	86	**30.7***
Liver	195	10.4	159	10	36	12.9
Bone	107	5.7	81	5.1	26	9.3
Lung	74	3.9	53	3.3	21	7.5
Adrenal	40	2.1	27	1.7	13	4.6

* TC vs. AC p<0.01

Table 8. **Percentage postoperative survival in patients with bronchopulmonary carcinoid calculated using the Kaplan-Meier method [5].**

Disease	5 years	10 years
All carcinoid	90.2	79.2
TC	93.3	82.1
AC	68.8	58.6
No metastases	98.3	95.4
With metastases	72.8	52.8

Metastases

AC tumours were more likely to be associated with metastases than TC, and for both TC and AC, larger tumours were more likely to be associated with metastases. The commonest site of metastases were lymph nodes, followed by liver, bone, lung and the adrenal glands (Table 7).

Postoperative outcome

In the Soga [5] series, 796/1875 cases were excluded due to a lack of information. From the remainder Kaplan-Meier survival curves were generated comparing TC vs. AC and "no metastases" vs. "with metastases". These are shown in Table 8 and Figure 2.

Surgical management

No randomised controlled trials investigating the role of surgery for the management of carcinoid tumours were identified. Publications comprised retrospectively analysed clinical series and case reports. There have also been recent literature reviews [26-30].

In evaluating these clinical reports, there appears to be a consensus that surgical resection is the main management strategy, and parenchyma preservation is an important consideration. Authors follow a pattern of local or sleeve resection when possible, anatomical resection with lobectomy or pneumonectomy, if clearance cannot be achieved with local resection alone, and lymph node dissection. A clear strategy or recommendation between sampling and more extensive lymphadenectomy is not available. Some authors also describe the use of chemotherapy or radiotherapy as adjunctive treatment, but this is not consistent and there is no published RCT evidence.

In selected cases, endoscopic resection may be successful in clearing the airway. However, a variable amount of residual disease may be identified after subsequent definitive surgical resection [25,26]. Endoscopic resection successfully allowing recovery of the distal lung and so allowing lung-sparing surgery has been described [26]. However, failure due to local recurrence can occur as the tumours may have an important extraluminal component.

Despite the consensus view, there is no level I or II evidence to support it. With this in mind, a focused literature search was performed to identify clinical series that met the following four criteria:-

- Given that the histological criteria had changed in 1999 [11] a clear statement/reference that current WHO criteria was used for histological diagnosis with re-classification when needed.
- TNM and/or stage description stated in paper.
- Clear description of the surgical procedure.
- Outcome including recurrence, disease-free interval and survival.

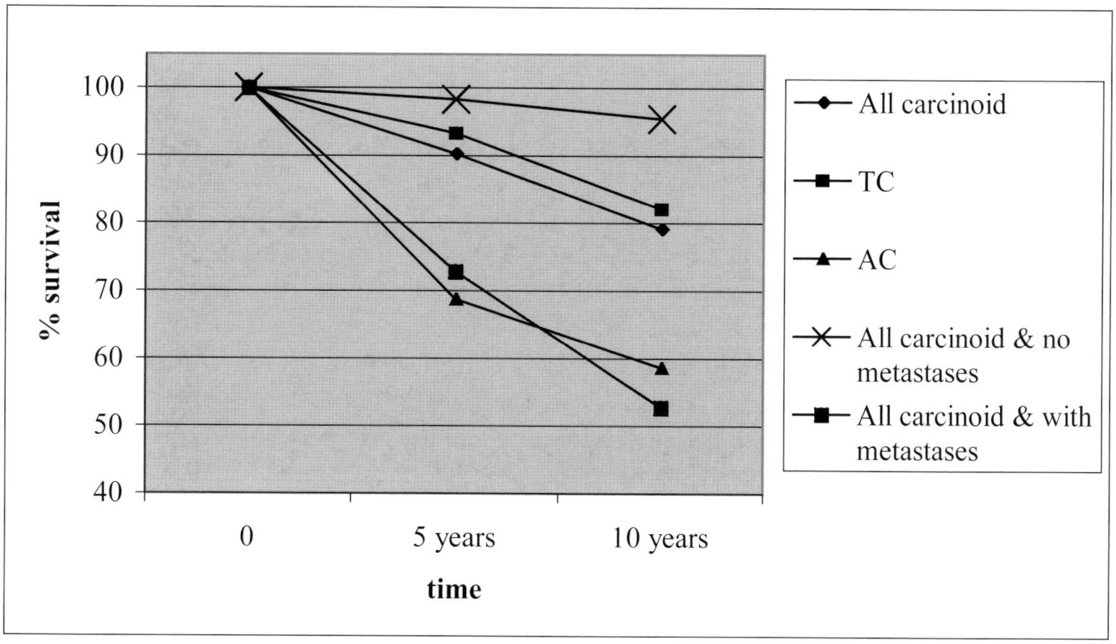

Figure 2. Percentage postoperative survival in patients with bronchopulmonary carcinoid calculated using the Kaplan-Meier method [5].

Table 9. **Clinical series published from 1999 describing surgical management of bronchopulmonary carcinoid.**

Ref	Title	(n) carcinoid	Location	Time period	WHO class-ification [12]	TNM/ stage	Surgery	Outcome	Assessed further	Notes
(17)	The surgical spectrum of pulmonary neuroendocrine neoplasms	77	USA, single centre	1985-1995	Yes in 60/77	No	Yes	Yes (limited)	No	
(27)	Pulmonary carcinoid*: presentation, diagnosis, and outcome in 142 cases in Israel and Review of 640 cases from the literature	142	Israel, 4 centres	1980-1999	No	Partial	Yes	Yes	No	
(28)	**Bronchial carcinoid tumours: surgical management and long-term outcome**	**126**	**Italy, single centre**	**1977-1999**	**Y**	**Y**	**Y**	**Y**	**Y**	**F/u 6-282 months. Survival was related to histology and nodal status. AC tumours more likely to have nodal metastases**
(29)	Sleeve lobectomy for non-small cell lung cancer and carcinoids: results in 160 cases	9	Italy	1965-1999	Not stated	No	No	Yes	No	Paper not designed to investigate carcinoid tumours per se
(30)	Sleeve lobectomy for bronchogenic cancers: factors affecting survival	30	Paris, single centre	1981-2001	Not stated	Yes	Yes	Yes	No	4-180 month follow-up. 5-yr survival 100%, 10-yr survival 92%
(31)	Surgery in bronchial carcinoids: experience with 83 patients	83	Turkey, single centre	1974-2000	Not stated	No	Yes	No	No	
(32)	**The feasibility of conservative resection for carcinoid tumours: is pneumonectomy ever necessary for uncomplicated cases?**	**95**	**UK, single centre**	**20 years to 1999**	**Yes**	**Yes *4**	**Yes**	**Yes**	**Yes**	**Histology >nodal status as predictor of outcome**

Table 9. continued:-

Ref	Title	(n) carcinoid	Location	Time period	WHO classification [12]	TNM/ stage	Surgery	Outcome	Assessed further	Notes
(16)	Typical and atypical pulmonary carcinoids: outcome in patients presenting with regional lymph node involvement	36	USA, single centre	1976-1997	Yes	Yes	No	Yes	Yes	Histology> nodal status as predictor of outcome
(33)	Prognostic factors in neuroendocrine lung tumours: a Spanish multicenter study	304	Spain, 12 centres	1980-1997	No* [5]	Yes	No	Yes	No	Lymph node and distant metastases significantly more common with AC than TC
(34)	**Long-term outcome after resection for bronchial carcinoid tumours**	**139**	**USA, Hong Kong 7 centres**	**1980-1998**	**Yes**	**Yes**	**Yes**	**Yes**	**TC 92% Stage 1 AC 70% Stage 1**	**AC more likely to be more advanced and have higher recurrence rate**

* [4] partial

* [5] This paper used an approximation to the 1999 WHO classification [11]. WHO. Histological typing of lung and pleural tumours. In: *WHO international histological classification of tumours.* 3rd ed. Travis W, Colby T, Corrin B, editors. Springer, Berlin, 1999.

Ten clinical series published after 1999 were identified (Table 9) and three met all criteria (in bold). In general, these papers support the consensus view.

Relative prognostic importance of histology and lymph node status

There is controversy as to the relative importance of histological grade and lymph node metastases in determining prognosis. To address this question Thomas [16] at the Mayo Clinic, specifically investigated the subset of patients who had thoracic lymph node metastases in the absence of other metastatic disease, at the time of surgical resection. From a series of 517 patients with pulmonary carcinoid tumours, 36 were patients who had regional thoracic lymph nodes but without distant disease. Re-classification using current WHO criteria was performed. There were 23 TC and 11 AC. It is important to note that two cases (5.5%) originally classified as atypical carcinoid were reclassified as LCNEC, and a further seven cases (19.6%) changed status.

This paper was selected as it clearly states the pathology reclassified using current WHO criteria and TNM stage for each patient. Although it may be criticised for its small numbers, the differences are striking (Figure 3).

This data suggests that patients with AC + lymph node metastases have a worse prognosis ($p<0.001$) as compared to those with TC + lymph node involvement alone. This in turn suggests that histological grade is a greater determinant of prognosis, and is consistent with other outcome data.

Staging

Again, there is no level I or II evidence to provide a firm recommendation for staging methods. There is a consensus that all patients require CT scanning.

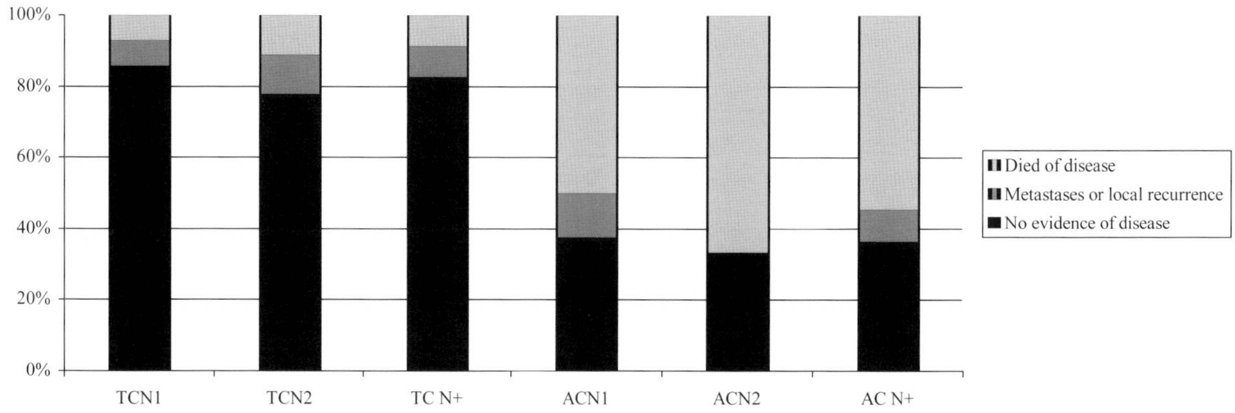

Figure 3. **Outcome (%) by histological grade and nodal status (mean follow-up 78 months).**

^{18}F-deoxyglucose-PET (FDG-PET) competes with glucose for uptake by cells. A FDG-PET scan is useful in detecting tissues with increased metabolic activity and hence, is useful in cancer staging. Recently, the combination of PET and CT has been shown to be superior to either modality alone [35], and better than MRI except for specific circumstances [36]. The relative merits of PET, somatostatin receptor scintigraphy and meta-iodobenzylguanidine (MIBG) scanning for staging carcinoid tumours, is now discussed.

Conventional FDG-PET has been shown to relatively understage carcinoid tumours [37]. Although carcinoid tumours do take up glucose, the carcinoid tumour-host complex is not of high metabolic activity and therefore, even with recent improvements in PET technology [38] FDG-PET is not reported as a common staging investigation. However, most carcinoid tumours express somatostatin receptors. These can be detected by the use of radiolabelled somatostatin analogues, a technique known as somatostatin receptor (SSR) scintigraphy. Belhocine [38] performed a comparison between FDG-PET and SSR scintigraphy and found a significant improvement in staging with the use of the latter (Table 10). However, it is important to be aware that there are cases when carcinoid lesions are PET positive and SSR negative [39].

MIBG is also taken up by neuroendocrine cells and it can be used for staging [40]. New labelled agents for PET scanning are under evaluation and include ^{11}C-5HT [41], ^{18}F-dopa [42] and somatostatin analogues such as 64Cu-TETA-octreotide [43].

Adjunctive treatment

There is no consensus for the routine use of chemotherapy or radiotherapy in the management of bronchopulmonary carcinoid. However, there is interest in the potential of somatostatin analogues such as octreotide or lanreotide. Carcinoid tumours may express somatostatin receptors and the use of

Table 10. **Sensitivity for the detection of carcinoid tumour.**

Reference	Sensitivity PET	Sensitivity SSR scintigraphy
Erasmus, 1998 [37]	14%	NA
Belhocine, 2002 [38]	57% primary 73% mets	86% primary 91% mets

analogues may downregulate these tumours leading to downstaging. These agents may also be of value in the treatment of metastases by reducing tumour bulk, and the palliation of symptoms by reducing release of humorally acting agents [44]. Interferon is also under evaluation [45]. Other agents include conventional chemotherapeutic agents, and radiotherapy with labelled substrates selective for carcinoid tumours (i.e. octreotide, MIBG).

Follow-up

A firm recommendation cannot be made for duration of follow-up or a cost benefit analysis of follow-up. Both local relapse and distant recurrence is recognised, and there are case reports of late recurrence up to 43 years after resection of the primary carcinoid tumour [46].

Haemorrhage after endobronchial biopsy

Several authors mention an increased risk of significant haemorrhage as a complication of endobronchial biopsy. This relates to an impression of increased vascularity of these tumours. To determine a rate for this complication, Dusmet [47] reviewed 13 series to identify 587 endoscopic biopsies of carcinoid tumours. 4/587 (<1%) required thoracotomy for bleeding [48].

Prevention of peri-operative carcinoid syndrome

Carcinoid tumours may secrete a variety of vasoactive substances. The major classes are 5-HT, 5-HT precursors or breakdown products, histamine and glucocorticoid steroids. The lungs are a major site for the clearance of these hormones. If sufficient amounts do reach the systemic circulation, carcinoid syndrome characterised by flushing, vasomotor instability, bronchospasm and diarrhoea, may occur. As mentioned previously, Soga has undertaken an extensive systematic review of the world literature [5]. From the Niigata registry, 748/8867 patients were identified with the syndrome. Of 1871 primary bronchopulmonary cases, 150 (8%) were reported to have the carcinoid syndrome. Because the manifestations of the syndrome are very varied and may be caused by other factors, there is a risk of overdiagnosis. In addition, it was not possible from this series to comment on what proportion of these patients had extrapulmonary metastasis. Soga also reports that the ratio of "carcinoid syndrome in TC" to "carcinoid syndrome in AC" was 8.7%: 3.9% (p<0.01). Carcinoid syndrome appears to be uncommon as a complication of bronchopulmonary carcinoid.

Carcinoid syndrome is described both as a presenting symptom [49], as well as a complication of biopsy, anaesthesia and surgery. There are no RCTs evaluating management. However, expert reviews [49-52] suggest that precautionary measures should include avoidance of histamine release inducing drugs, peri-operative octreotide, other specific mediator antagonists, steroids and aprotinin.

New developments

Clarifying the relative importance of histological grade and stage is likely to require prospective, and in view of the overall incidence, multicentre study. Other important advances in the management of carcinoid tumours are likely to relate to staging methods and the role of adjunctive treatment. Carcinoid tumours with their distinctive biology offer a paradigm for the development of targeted management strategies. This may also impact on the related large cell neuroendocrine cancer and small cell lung cancer. With respect to both staging and treatment, this could exploit somatostatin receptor expression or other neuroendocrine characteristics. Adjunctive treatments may have an important role in the neoadjuvant setting to downstage disease prior to surgery.

Recommendations	Evidence level
◆ Pathological classification changed to improve prognotic accuracy [11,1].	IIa/B
◆ Comparison of series requires classification of pathology by common criteria [16,17].	IIb/B
◆ Cancer registries record an increase in incidence of carcinoid tumours.	IIb/B
◆ The prognosis is better for TC than AC, and better for carcinoid without metastases [5].	III/IV/B/C
◆ Histological grade is a greater determinant of outcome than lymph node status [16].	III/C
◆ Somatostatin receptor scintigraphy is more sensitive in the detection of carcinoid tumours than ^{18}FDG-PET [38]. False negatives may occur with both techniques.	IIb/B
◆ Significant haemorrhage after endobronchial biopsy of carcinoid tumours is uncommon [47].	III/B

References

1. Travis WD, Rush W, Flieder DB, Falk R, Fleming MV, Gal AA, *et al.* Survival analysis of 200 pulmonary neuroendocrine tumors with clarification of criteria for atypical carcinoid and its separation from typical carcinoid. *Am J Surg Pathol* 1998; 22(8): 934-44.
2. Langhans T. Ueber einen drusenpolyp im ileum. *Virchow Arch Pathol Anat Physiol Klin Med* 1867; 38: 559-560.
3. Ransom W. A case of primary carcinoma of the ileum. *Lancet* 1890; 2: 1020-1023.
4. Oberndorfer S. Karzinoide Tumoren des Dunndarms. *Frankf Z Pathol* 1907; 1: 426-429.
5. Soga J, Yakuwa Y. Bronchopulmonary carcinoids: an analysis of 1,875 reported cases with special reference to a comparison between typical carcinoids and atypical varieties. *Ann Thorac Cardiovasc Surg* 1999; 5(4): 211-9.
6. Modlin IM, Sandor A. An analysis of 8305 cases of carcinoid tumors. *Cancer* 1997; 79(4): 813-29.
7. Modlin IM, Lye KD, Kidd M. A 5-decade analysis of 13,715 carcinoid tumors. *Cancer* 2003; 97(4): 934-59.
8. Beshay M, Roth T, Stein R, Schmid RA. Synchronous bilateral typical pulmonary carcinoid tumors. *Eur J Cardiothorac Surg* 2003; 23(2): 251-3.
9. Soga J, Yakuwa Y, Osaka M. Carcinoid syndrome: a statistical evaluation of 748 reported cases. *J Exp Clin Cancer Res* 1999; 18(2): 133-41.
10. Onuki N, Wistuba, II, Travis WD, Virmani AK, Yashima K, Brambilla E, *et al.* Genetic changes in the spectrum of neuroendocrine lung tumors. *Cancer* 1999; 85(3): 600-7.
11. WHO. Histological typing of lung and pleural tumours. In: *WHO international histological classification of tumours.* 3rd ed. Travis W, Colby T, Corrin B, Eds. Springer, Berlin, 1999.
12. Flieder DBMD, Codrington H, Sutedja T, Golding R, van Mourik J, Risse E, *et al.* Neuroendocrine tumors of the lung: recent developments in histopathology 275-280.
13. Debelenko LV, Brambilla E, Agarwal SK, Swalwell JI, Kester MB, Lubensky IA, *et al.* Identification of MEN1 gene mutations in sporadic carcinoid tumors of the lung. *Hum Mol Genet* 1997; 6(13): 2285-90.
14. McKuisik V, *et al.* Online Mendelian Inheritance in Man, OMIM (TM). In: Center for Medical Genetics, Johns Hopkins University (Baltimore, MD) and National Center for Biotechnology Information, National Library of Medicine (Bethesda, MD), 1996. p. World Wide Web URL: http://www.ncbi.nlm.nih.gov/Omim/.
15. Arrigoni MG, Woolner LB, Bernatz PE. Atypical carcinoid tumors of the lung. *J Thorac Cardiovasc Surg* 1972; 64(3): 413-21.
16. Thomas CF, Jr., Tazelaar HD, Jett JR. Typical and atypical pulmonary carcinoids: outcome in patients presenting with regional lymph node involvement. *Chest* 2001; 119(4): 1143-50.
17. Cooper WA, Thourani VH, Gal AA, Lee RB, Mansour KA, Miller JI. The surgical spectrum of pulmonary neuroendocrine neoplasms. *Chest* 2001; 119(1): 14-8.
18. Godwin J. Carcinoid tumors: an analysis of 2837 cases. *Cancer* 1975; 36: 560-569.
19. Skuladottir H, Hirsch FR, Hansen HH, Olsen JH. Pulmonary neuroendocrine tumors: incidence and prognosis of histological subtypes. A population-based study in Denmark. *Lung Cancer* 2002; 37(2): 127-35.
20. Hallgrimsson JG, Jonsson T, Johannsson JH. Bronchopulmonary carcinoids in Iceland 1955-1984. A retrospective clinical and histopathologic study. *Scand J Thorac Cardiovasc Surg* 1989; 23(3): 275-8.
21. Newton JN, Swerdlow AJ, dos Santos Silva IM, Vessey MP, Grahame-Smith DG, Primatesta P, *et al.* The epidemiology of carcinoid tumours in England and Scotland. *Br J Cancer* 1994; 70(5): 939-42.

22. Levi F, Te V-C, Randimbison L, Rindi G, La Vecchia C. Epidemiology of carcinoid neoplasms in Vaud, Switzerland, 1974-97. *British Journal of Cancer* 2000; 83(7): 952-955.
23. SEER - *Surveillance Epidemiology and End Results Program* National Cancer Institute Cancer Statistics Branch Surveillance Research Program Division of Cancer Control and Population Sciences, National Cancer Institute, Bethesda, MD 20892-8316; 2003.
24. Soga J, Yakuwa Y, Osaka M. Evaluation of 342 cases of mediastinal/thymic carcinoids collected from literature: a comparative study between typical carcinoids and atypical varieties. *Ann Thorac Cardiovasc Surg* 1999; 5(5): 285-92.
25. Schreurs AJ, Westermann CJ, van den Bosch JM, Vanderschueren RG, Brutel de la Riviere A, Knaepen PJ. A twenty-five-year follow-up of ninety-three resected typical carcinoid tumors of the lung. *J Thorac Cardiovasc Surg* 1992; 104(5): 1470-5.
26. Sutedja TG, Schreurs AJ, Vanderschueren RG, Kwa B, vd Werf TS, Postmus PE. Bronchoscopic therapy in patients with intraluminal typical bronchial carcinoid. *Chest* 1995; 107(2): 556-8.
27. Fink G, Krelbaum T, Yellin A, Bendayan D, Saute M, Glazer M, *et al.* Pulmonary Carcinoid*: Presentation, Diagnosis, and Outcome in 142 Cases in Israel and Review of 640 Cases From the Literature. *Chest* 2001; 119(6): 1647-1651.
28. Filosso PL, Rena O, Donati G, Casadio C, Ruffini E, Papalia E, *et al.* Bronchial carcinoid tumors: surgical management and long-term outcome. *J Thorac Cardiovasc Surg* 2002; 123(2): 303-9.
29. Terzi A, Lonardoni A, Falezza G, Furlan G, Scanagatta P, Pasini F, *et al.* Sleeve lobectomy for non-small cell lung cancer and carcinoids: results in 160 cases. *Eur J Cardiothorac Surg* 2002; 21(5): 888-93.
30. Fadel E, Yildizeli B, Chapelier AR, Dicenta I, Mussot S, Dartevelle PG. Sleeve lobectomy for bronchogenic cancers: factors affecting survival. *Ann Thorac Surg* 2002; 74(3): 851-8; discussion 858-9.
31. Kurul IC, Topcu S, Tastepe I, Yazici U, Altinok T, Cetin G. Surgery in bronchial carcinoids: experience with 83 patients. *Eur J Cardiothorac Surg* 2002; 21(5): 883-7.
32. El Jamal M, Nicholson AG, Goldstraw P. The feasibility of conservative resection for carcinoid tumours: is pneumonectomy ever necessary for uncomplicated cases? *Eur J Cardiothorac Surg* 2000; 18(3): 301-6.
33. Garcia-Yuste M, Matilla JM, Alvarez-Gago T, Duque JL, Heras F, Cerezal LJ, *et al.* Prognostic factors in neuroendocrine lung tumors: a Spanish Multicenter Study. Spanish Multicenter Study of Neuroendocrine Tumors of the Lung of the Spanish Society of Pneumonology and Thoracic Surgery (EMETNE-SEPAR). *Ann Thorac Surg* 2000; 70(1): 258-63.
34. Ferguson MK, Landreneau RJ, Hazelrigg SR, Altorki NK, Naunheim KS, Zwischenberger JB, *et al.* Long-term outcome after resection for bronchial carcinoid tumors. *Eur J Cardiothorac Surg 2000*; 18(2): 156-61.
35. Antoch G, Stattaus J, Nemat AT, Marnitz S, Beyer T, Kuehl H, *et al.* Non-small cell lung cancer: dual-modality PET/CT in preoperative staging. *Radiology* 2003; 229(2): 526-33.
36. Antoch G. Combined PET and CT whole body imaging superior to MRI in tumor staging. *JAMA* 2003; 290: 3199-3206.
37. Erasmus JJ, McAdams HP, Patz EF, Jr., Coleman RE, Ahuja V, Goodman PC. Evaluation of primary pulmonary carcinoid tumors using FDG PET. *Am J Roentgenol* 1998; 170(5): 1369-73.
38. Belhocine T, Foidart J, Rigo P, Najjar F, Thiry A, Quatresooz P, *et al.* Fluorodeoxyglucose positron emission tomography and somatostatin receptor scintigraphy for diagnosing and staging carcinoid tumours: correlations with the pathological indexes p53 and Ki-67. *Nuclear Medicine Communications* 2002; 23(8): 727-734.
39. Whitaker D, Dussek J. PET scanning in thymic neuroendocrine tumors. *Chest* 2004; 125(6): 2368-9.
40. Hanson MW, Feldman JM, Blinder RA, Moore JO, Coleman RE. Carcinoid tumors: iodine-131 MIBG scintigraphy. *Radiology* 1989; 172(3): 699-703.
41. Eriksson B, Bergstrom M, Orlefors H, Sundin A, Oberg K, Langstrom B. Use of PET in neuroendocrine tumors. *In vivo* applications and in vitro studies. *Q J Nucl Med* 2000; 44(1): 68-76.
42. Hoegerle S, Altehoefer C, Ghanem N, Koehler G, Waller CF, Scheruebl H, *et al.* Whole-body 18F dopa PET for detection of gastrointestinal carcinoid tumors. *Radiology* 2001; 220(2): 373-80.
43. Anderson CJ, Dehdashti F, Cutler PD, Schwarz SW, Laforest R, Bass LA, *et al.* 64Cu-TETA-octreotide as a PET imaging agent for patients with neuroendocrine tumors. *J Nucl Med* 2001; 42(2): 213-21.
44. Filosso PL, Ruffini E, Oliaro A, Papalia E, Donati G, Rena O. Long-term survival of atypical bronchial carcinoids with liver metastases, treated with octreotide. *Eur J Cardiothorac Surg* 2002; 21(5): 913-917.
45. Oberg KP, Fink GMD, Krelbaum TMD, Yellin AMD, Bendayan DMD, Saute MMD, *et al.* Carcinoid tumors: molecular genetics, tumor biology, and update of diagnosis and treatment. *Current Opinion in Oncology* 2001; 14(1): 38-45.
46. Kaiser ED, See RF, Rechdouni AK, Usui Y, Lim JI, Rao NA. Uveal metastasis 43 years after resection of bronchogenic carcinoid. *Br J Ophthalmol* 2002; 86(10): 1191-2.
47. Dusmet ME, McKneally MF. Pulmonary and thymic carcinoid tumors. *World J Surg* 1996; 20(2): 189-95.
48. Stamatis G, Freitag L, Greschuchna D. Limited and radical resection for tracheal and bronchopulmonary carcinoid tumour. Report on 227 cases. *Eur J Cardiothorac Surg* 1990; 4(10): 527-32; discussion 533.
49. Fischer S, Kruger M, McRae K, Merchant N, Tsao MS, Keshavjee S. Giant bronchial carcinoid tumors: a multidisciplinary approach. *Ann Thorac Surg* 2001; 71(1): 386-93.
50. Kulke MH, Mayer RJ. Carcinoid tumors. *N Engl J Med* 1999; 340(11): 858-68.
51. Vaughan DJ, Brunner MD. Anesthesia for patients with carcinoid syndrome. *Int Anesthesiol Clin* 1997; 35(4): 129-42.
52. Warner RR, Mani S, Profeta J, Grunstein E. Octreotide treatment of carcinoid hypertensive crisis. *Mt Sinai J Med* 1994; 61(4): 349-55.

Chapter 10

Surgery in malignant pleural mesothelioma

Simon Swift MB BS BSc MRCS
Specialist Registrar, Thoracic Surgery [1]
David Waller MB BS FRCS (C/Th) FCCP
Consultant Thoracic Surgeon [2]

1 Harefield Hospital, Harefield, Middlesex, UK
2 Glenfield Hospital, Leicester, UK

Introduction

Mesotheliomas are a group of tumours arising from the pleural lining of the thorax. Most mesotheliomas are aggressive soft tissue malignancies. Arising from mesothelial tissue they display a range of histological subtypes, the most common of which are epithelial, sarcomatoid and mixed or biphasic. The risk of developing the malignancy is closely related to asbestos exposure. Asbestos fibre burden in the lung is proportionally related to incidence, with crocidolite fibres (blue asbestos) and amosite (brown asbestos) being higher risk than chrysotile (white asbestos). Damage occurs by oxygen free radical action induced by ferric iron impurities on the fibres [1]. Mesothelioma claims 1600 lives per year in the UK and this is set to increase over the next 15 to 20 years, reaching a peak of 3000 cases per year before predictions suggest a reduction in new cases [2]. This epidemic matches the peak and decline in asbestos imports into the UK by weight in the middle decades of the 20th century with a 40-year lag. It is predicted that 1% of men born in the 1940s will die from mesothelioma [3].

At the time of presentation, most patients have advanced disease and treatment is focused on palliation. The disease progresses rapidly with patients suffering from shortness of breath and refractory chest wall pain as well as other local and systemic symptoms associated with advanced malignancy. Quality of life deteriorates rapidly and survival is very poor with median survival in the range of 5-13 months [4,5]; this range is attributed to the long pre-presentation course of the disease followed by rapid deterioration once the patient becomes symptomatic, survival from diagnosis being a small part of the disease process.

Prognostic factors at presentation that indicate poor survival include: cell type other than epithelial, weight loss greater than 5%, low haemoglobin and abnormal white cell count, thrombocytosis, poor performance status and male sex. There are scoring systems using these factors which successfully stratify patients according to survival [5]. The total pre-operative tumour volume is a useful predictor of T stage and can predict overall survival, with high volumes being associated with nodal spread [6].

The role of thoracic surgery in mesothelioma encompasses diagnosis and palliation, with some centres advocating aggressive surgical management of potentially resectable tumours. Surgeons have employed cytoreductive debulking procedures and radical resections using pleurectomy and extra-pleural-pneumonectomy (EPP), which involves resection of the lung within the pleural envelope with pericardial and diaphragmatic attachments. EPP was first reported for mesothelioma in the 1970s [7] and largely abandoned due to high complication rates and poor outcome. It has been revived recently with advances in surgical technique, peri- and postoperative anaesthetic and intensive care, allowing complex major surgery with acceptable morbidity and mortality. Data on the role of any radical surgery in mesothelioma is not mature, but case cohort analysis suggests some patients may benefit, though more high quality evidence is needed.

Methodology

A formal search was performed using Medline 1966 to 2003, Embase, The Cochrane register of controlled trials and Pubmed. Mesothelioma, surgery, diagnosis, pleurodesis and cytoreduction, pleurectomy, decortication and extra-pleural pneumonectomy/pleuropneumonectomy were used as search terms. Papers returned were assessed in terms of demographics, methodology, inclusion and exclusion criteria and the transparency of the results and conclusion.

Diagnosis

Most patients present with symptoms of breathlessness or chest wall pain [8]. Signs may also include cough, weight loss, respiratory infection and local compression problems such as SVC syndrome. A careful history elicits asbestos exposure in approximately 90%[9] of patients diagnosed with mesothelioma. Plain chest radiography may show pleural plaques, which are commonly calcified and a unilateral pleural effusion.

Pleural fluid cytology is often the first attempt at diagnosis after therapeutic aspiration, though useful diagnostic results are found in only 35% [10] to 45%[11]. A similar rate of diagnosis is produced with blind pleural biopsy with an Abram's type needle [11]. This is partly due to the heterogenous nature of the pleural disease and partly due to the difficulty in histological diagnosis requiring solid tissue to study the tumour architecture. Immunohistochemistry is routinely used in order to differentiate mesothelioma from metastatic adenocarcinoma pleurae, which is particularly difficult with epithelial mesotheliomas. Where histology is reviewed after radical surgery with large tissue blocks, the diagnosis is often changed with one study stating a 21% rate of rediagnosis from mesothelioma to adenocarcinoma [12]. A second study by Blanc *et al* [13] reported on a series of 168 medical thoracoscopies where the diagnosis from closed needle biopsy was changed in 43 of 96 cases. Mesothelioma is a special interest disease in histopathology and specimens are often reviewed by outside second opinion.

Thoracic surgeons are routinely called upon to diagnose suspected malignant recurrent pleural effusions. Some surgeons employ the open technique, performing a mini-thoracotomy and taking a full thickness pleural biopsy. Others will use VATS, which allows assessment of the tumour load within the hemithorax and is often combined with a palliative pleurodesis at the same time.

Staging

Staging of mesothelioma should be performed in all patients to determine resectability. The system commonly used is that produced by the International Mesothelioma Interest Group [14] (IMIG) (Table 1), and is based on the TNM system. There are both prognostic implications and management decisions which can only be made after thorough assessment of the tumour. Initially, imaging should be by CT scan which allows assessment of local disease. An experienced radiologist can stage accurately on the basis of a CT scan, looking at involvement of parietal and visceral pleura, chest wall and pericardial invasion and invasion of vital structures [15]. CT is less good at assessing diaphragmatic invasion, and MRI appears to be better in fine disease staging for operative planning [16].

Mediastinal nodal disease can also be assessed on CT, though it is known that node size is poorly concordant with metastasis [17]. Therefore, any visible

Table 1. IMIG staging.

T1	T1a Tumour limited to the ipsilateral parietal pleura, including mediastinal and diaphragmatic pleura. No involvement of the visceral pleura. T1b Tumour involving the ipsilateral parietal pleura, including mediastinal and diaphragmatic pleura. Scattered foci of tumour also involving the visceral pleura.
T2	Tumour involving each of the ipsilateral pleural surfaces (parietal, mediastinal, diaphragmatic, and visceral pleura) with at least one of the following features:- ◆ Involvement of diaphragmatic muscle. ◆ Confluent visceral pleural tumour (including the fissure) or extension of tumour from visceral pleura into the underlying pulmonary parenchyma.
T3	Describes locally advanced but potentially respectable tumour. Tumour involving all of the ipsilateral pleural surfaces (parietal, mediastinal, diaphragmatic, and visceral pleura) with at least one of the following features:- ◆ Involvement of the endothoracic fascia. ◆ Extension into mediastinal fat. ◆ Solitary, completely respectable focus of tumour extending into the soft tissues of the chest wall. ◆ Nontransmural involvement of the pericardium.
T4	Describes locally advanced technically unresectable tumour. Tumour involving all of the ipsilateral pleural surfaces (parietal, mediastinal, diaphragmatic, and visceral pleura) with at least one of the following features:- ◆ Diffuse extension or multifocal masses of tumour in the chest wall, with or without associated rib destruction. ◆ Direct transdiaphragmatic extension of tumour to the peritoneum. ◆ Direct extension of tumour to one or more mediastinal organs. ◆ Direct extension of tumour into the spine. ◆ Tumour extending through to the internal surface of the pericardium with or without a pericardial effusion; or tumour directly involving the myocardium.

N - Lymph Nodes

Nx	Regional lymph nodes cannot be assessed.
N0	No regional lymph node metastases.
N1	Metastases in the ipsilateral bronchopulmonary or hilar lymph nodes.
N2	Metastases in the subcarinal or the ipsilateral mediastinal lymph nodes, including the ipsilateral internal mammary nodes.
N3	Metastases in the contralateral mediastinal, contralateral internal mammary, ipsilateral, or contralateral supraclavicular lymph nodes.

M - Metastases

Mx	Presence of distant metastases cannot be assessed
M0	No distant metastases
M1	Distant metastases present

Stage		Description
Stage	Ia	T1aN0M0
	Ib	T1bN0M0
Stage	II	T2N0M0
Stage	III	Any T3M0, Any N1M0, Any N2M0
Stage	IV	Any T4, Any N3, Any M1

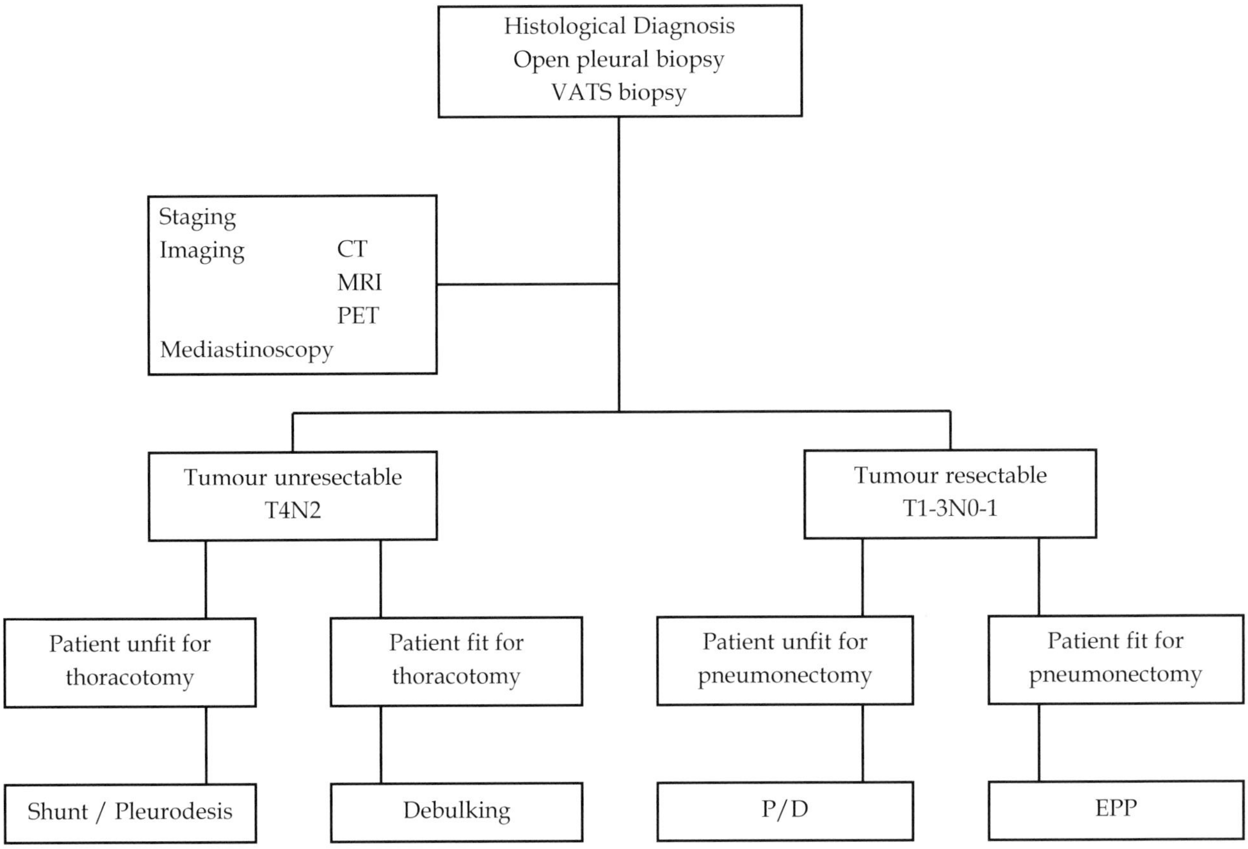

Figure 1. **The role of surgery in mesothelioma.**

node needs further investigation, not just those larger than 1cm as in lung cancer. Positron emission tomography (PET) appears to be a useful technique for excluding mediastinal nodal involvement and is recommended where available in potentially resectable disease [18]. Mediastinoscopy also has an important role, as N2 disease, with involvement of ipsilateral mediastinal (paratracheal, station 4 or subcarinal, station 7) nodes is deemed unresectable due to the poor associated outcome. Nodes within the pleural envelope, stations 1 to 9 [19], are considered N1 disease and allow EPP as they are contained within the resected specimen.

Fitness for surgery

Initial investigations should include a full blood count, electrolytes and renal function, liver function and respiratory function tests. For EPP the British Thoracic Society guidelines on fitness for pneumonectomy [20] are followed requiring a ppo FEV1 of 40% and ppo TLCO of 40%. The cardiac fitness criteria within the guidelines and other points are also followed. For radical surgery WHO performance status is a useful indicator. Most surgeons would only treat WHO stage 0 or 1 patients, since the postoperative recovery period is arduous and requires significant co-operation and effort from the patient.

Decision-making

We follow a simple decision-making algorithm, as outlined in Figure 1.

Management of patients with unresectable disease

Patients who are not fit for radical surgery

Lung mobile

In the worst case scenario of unresectable disease in patients who are not fit for major surgery, simple procedures can significantly improve quality of life by controlling the pleural effusion. Pleurodesis using sterile iodised talc poudrage is the procedure of choice and is easily accomplished by VATS and is often combined with pleural biopsy. This results in life-long effusion control in over 90% of patients [21,22], with major series reporting 0% to 1% mortality. Previous fears of talc-induced ARDS are now lessening with the understanding of the appropriate dose (<5g) and the role of talc granule size being elucidated - small granules as present in US talc cause a higher risk of ARDS compared to large granule sized European talc, where ARDS is an uncommon finding, with no cases reported in most European series.

Lung trapped

In cases where the lung is found to be trapped at thoracoscopy by thickened visceral pleura and the patient is not fit for a larger procedure, the insertion of a pleuro-peritoneal shunt can prevent reaccumulation of a pleural effusion. The Denver Shunt (Denver Biomaterials, Surgimed Inc, Golden, CO.) is placed under direct vision and in a large series, Genc *et al* showed symptomatic relief in more than 95% of a group of 63 patients treated this way with an entrapped lung [23]. The major problem with shunts is that they can become blocked. That was encountered in eight patients in this series (12%) who required re-operation, where five had replacement and three required shunt removal and open drainage. Some surgeons choose an alternative long-term tunnelled catheter such as a PleurX drain (Denver Biomaterials, Surgimed Inc, Golden, CO.), allowing ambulatory care with control of the effusion and breathlessness [24].

In patients fit for major surgery but with unresectable disease (IMIG Stage III N2 and stage IV), debulking surgery has a role in improving quality of life. A recent prospective series looked at 51 consecutive patients presenting with mesothelioma in the UK. In 17 patients (34%), where the lung expanded after drainage of the effusion, a subtotal parietal pleurectomy was performed via VATS. Where the lung was trapped, a parietal and visceral decortication was performed, three by VATS and 31 by thoracotomy. They reported 7.8% 30-day mortality and 13% morbidity with at least three months of symptomatic benefit. This benefit was subsequently offset by increasing mortality in the cohort [25]. The authors gave no data on the effect of debulking on survival. Other series have reported on the role of debulking surgery in patients with advanced disease. Cersoli and collegues[26] report a series of 121 patients where 38 underwent pleurectomy alone, while 16 received pleurectomy followed by adjuvant chemotherapy, with a further 38 patients receiving only chemotherapy. All groups fared better than those treated by effusion control only, with overall median survival of 12 months versus four months in the palliative group. Those treated with surgery plus chemotherapy showed a significant survival advantage, with median survival of 14 months compared to 12.5 months for surgery alone and eight months for chemotherapy alone. These results agree with other series where pleurectomy with adjuvant therapy, both chemotherapy and radiotherapy show significant advantage to surgery alone [27,28,29,30,31].

Port site radiotherapy

In all patients who undergo invasive procedures who are later diagnosed with mesothelioma, there is the possibility of needle track/port site metastasis. The mesothelioma seeds along the site and presents as a hard painful lump on the chest wall, causing considerable trouble to the patient. A randomised controlled trial of local radiotherapy treated half of a group of 40 consecutive patients. A total dose of 21 Gy was given in three fractions within 15 days of thoracoscopy or one month of needle biopsy. In the radiotherapy group, no entry tract metastases formed whereas in the control group, eight of 20 (40%) developed malignant seeding [32]. This is one of the few examples of grade I evidence in the literature; unfortunately, it is not routinely followed.

Management of patients with resectable disease

Patients not fit for pneumonectomy

In those patients who present with early stage disease but are unfit to undergo EPP due to poor lung function, a pleurectomy and decortication (P/D) appears to offer some benefit. The literature consists of a few randomised controlled trials and many cohort studies, as is common in surgical research. P/D is not a standard operation, with different centres using the term to describe a range of radicality from close to a debulking procedure in some cases, to a very radical procedure similar to EPP but sparing lung resection. Some surgeons believe it is not reasonable to sacrifice normal lung in order to achieve complete resection when the benefit of this is unproven and the sequelae are significant to the patient.

Eight published series described P/D alone stating median survival of five [27] to 17 [33] months. Mortality ranged from 0% [34] to 7.8% [25] with morbidity where stated of 16% to 22%. However, most investigators have used surgery as part of a multimodality regime including intra-operative chemotherapy alone [26,27,35,36] or with postoperative chemotherapy [28,37,38]. Median survival times for both are similar and wide-ranging, depending on the series. Overall, there appears to be a net benefit if the patient receives chemotherapy; the additional effect of intra-operative dosing is uncertain. Intra-operative photodynamic therapy (PDT) has been employed, but a recent trial reported a very high mortality rate and many complications [39], but new generations of photosensitisers may be beneficial.

External beam radiotherapy has been used in the adjuvant setting [11], but more recently, intra-operative brachytherapy has been utilised. Adjuvant radiotherapy alone with P/D gave median survival of 10.1 months and no 5-year survival, but when used intra-operatively as well, results are better, with median survival of 18.1 [40] and 21 [29] months, and reasonable long-term survival. Lee *et al* had a mortality rate of 7%, which appears high but in a small series of 26 patients, is not necessarily a reflection of the treatment modality.

P/D as part of trimodality therapy with chemoradiotherapy has been investigated by three large series. The results were disappointing; median survival ranged from eight [11] to 16 [41] months with a more recent series at 10.9 months [42].

Patients fit for pneumonectomy

In patients with resectable disease who are fit to undergo radical surgery, EPP can now be offered with acceptable peri-operative mortality and morbidity. There is no evidence from randomised controlled trials in the literature that overall outcome is improved by aggressive surgery, though some subgroups of patients with favourable prognostic factors appear to benefit.

Aziz and colleagues in Glasgow report a 10-year series of 302 patients referred for management of malignant mesothelioma [34]. Of these, 47 underwent P/D and 64 radical EPP, with intrapleural chemotherapy and adjuvant chemotherapy in 51 of the patients undergoing EPP. In the EPP group, operative mortality was 9% with 21% morbidity. Overall, median survival after EPP was disappointing at 13 months, but for the final 51 patients receiving intra- and postoperative chemotherapy, median survival was 35 months with 48% 3-year and 18% 5-year survival. This improvement in survival is impressive, though many feel that without radiotherapy local control will remain poor, and full trimodality therapy should be the aim. As with other series, survival is dependent on stage with significant difference shown between T1, T2 and T3 stage tumours. Interestingly, nodal spread did not come out as important in their multivariate analysis.

A series of trimodality therapy has been published by Sugarbaker [43] in Boston from an ongoing series with 183 patients at the time of publication. These patients were entered into a protocol of EPP followed by adjuvant chemoradiotherapy. He reports mortality of 3.8% with morbidity of 50%, though a publication on morbidity from later in the series gives a complication rate of 60.4% [44]. This included 44.2% atrial fibrillation, with prolonged intubation (7.9%), vocal cord paralysis (6.7%) and DVT (6.4%) as the next most common problems. Serious morbidity requiring reoperation such as patch dehiscence or haemorrhage, were less common with 6.1% of patients affected. Of the 183 patients entered into the series, follow-up on the 176 who survived the procedure shows overall survival of 38% at two years and 15% at five years, with median survival of 19 months. In the subgroup with best prognostic indicators (epithelial cell type, negative resection margins and node negative mediastinum), using multivariate analysis on their own data, 2-year survival was 68% with 46% 5-year survival and median survival of 51 months.

These impressive survival data catalysed renewed interest in EPP as part of multimodality therapy with chemotherapy and radiotherapy being full and important parts of the treatment plan.

Recently, interest in the feasibility of neoadjuvant chemotherapy has been explored. A Swiss multicentre group found that pre-operative chemotherapy using gemcitabine/cisplatin was feasible and well tolerated and did not compromise surgical resection, though large well organised trials are needed [45]. A group from Toronto showed that induction chemotherapy followed by EPP, then high-dose hemithoracic radiation, is a tolerable regime for selected patients [46] with nine of 18 patients entered completing all three phases of treatment - most withdrawals being due to disease progression at surgery. This echoes a worry by some researchers that though neoadjuvant chemotherapy has benefits, with fitter patients being more likely to receive the full schedule pre-operatively, mesothelioma is relatively insensitive to most agents and resectable disease may progress and become unresectable during chemotherapy. Other researchers feel that progressing during chemotherapy is a poor prognostic indicator on its own and is a useful way to identify patients likely to fare badly.

Conclusions

The role of surgery alone in mesothelioma is only validated in diagnosis and effusion control where biopsy and pleurodesis are well proven. Palliative debulking, either open or VATS, seems to have a quality of life benefit but there is scant evidence to show a survival benefit. Careful consideration should be given to its value in individual patients with sufficient life expectancy to justify surgery.

A recent review of her long-term series by Valerie Rusch serves as a useful summary of the role of radical surgery. Of 306 patients who underwent thoracotomy, with P/D and EPP being employed along with a range of chemo and radiotherapy regimes, four factors came out as significant in a multivariate analysis of prognostic indicators. Early tumour stage (IMIG I/II vs III/IV), cell type (epithelial), use of radiotherapy and use of chemotherapy all came out as significant for a good prognosis, whereas the type of procedure performed did not [47].

This encapsulates the view that surgery alone is not indicated in mesothelioma, but multimodality therapy has a role in selected patients. This is reinforced by Butchart's recent 22-year series [48] in which type of surgery and tumour cell type was not significantly prognostic of long survival but the use of adjuvant therapy was. The authors of this chapter feel extra-pleural pneumonectomy to be a more appropriate procedure than pleurectomy/decortication which cannot be performed if there is lung invasion by the tumour, though this is not reflected in the two studies above and is only weakly evident in the literature. Overall, the quality and number of trials in mesothelioma is poor, with most authors calling for major trials. A trial of palliative chemotherapy for unresectable disease is under way - the MSO-1 trial, which has a three-arm protocol comparing active symptom control with solo Navelbine or the triplet mitomycin/vinblastine/cisplatin. The feasibility study (MESO-1) randomised 100 patients achieving a 59% acceptance rate for randomisation and choosing the EORTC quality of life instrument over the FACT-L questionnaire. The main trial is now recruiting and is expected to complete accrual in four years.

A trial of surgery is proposed in the UK currently; the Mesothelioma and Radical Surgery (MARS) trial, which will test EPP against no EPP in a prospective randomised trial including neoadjuvant chemotherapy and radical hemithoracic irradiation postoperatively. This trial is likely to report in 2010.

Recommendations - Diagnosis	Evidence level
◆ VATS or open biopsy should be performed early in clinically suspicious circumstances.	IIa/B
Recommendations - Palliative surgery	
◆ Talc pleurodesis and shunts are appropriate in most patients who are unfit for radical surgery. In those who are fit, debulking may offer a quality of life advantage. There is minimal evidence to show a survival advantage.	Ib/A
Recommendations - Radical surgery	
◆ Radical surgery has a role in treating appropriately staged patients with malignant mesothelioma. The use of a multimodality approach is to be recommended with trimodality treatment apparently promising. Due to the lack of high quality data showing patient benefit, it is preferable that these patients are entered into appropriately designed randomised controlled trials.	III/B

References

1. Manning CB, Vallyathan V, Mossman BT. Diseases caused by asbestos: mechanisms of injury and disease development. *International Immunopharmacology* 2002; 2(2-3): 191-200.
2. Peto J, Decarli A, La Vecchia C, Levi F, Negri E. The European mesothelioma epidemic. *Br J Cancer* 1999; 79: 666-72.
3. Peto J, Hodgson JT, Matthews FE, Jones JR. Continuing increase in mesothelioma mortality in Britain. *Lancet* 1995; 345(8949): 535-539.
4. Tan C, Swift S, Gilham C, Shaefi S, Fountian W, Peto J, *et al.* Survival in surgically diagnosed patients with malignant mesothelioma in current practice. *Thorax* 2002; 57iii: iii36-iii36.
5. Edwards JG, Abrams KR, Leverment JN, Spyt TJ, Waller DA, O'Byrne KJ. Prognostic factors for malignant mesothelioma in 142 patients: validation of CALGB and EORTC prognostic scoring systems. *Thorax* 2000; 55: 731-735.
6. Pass HI, Temeck BK, Kranda K, Steinberg SM, Feuerstain IR. Pre-operative tumor volume is associated with outcome in malignant pleural mesothelioma. *J Thorac Cardiovasc Surg* 1998; 115: 310-7.
7. Butchart EG, Ashcroft T, Barnsley WC, Holden MP. Pleuropneumonectomy in the Management of Malignant Mesothelioma of the Pleura. Experience with 29 patients. *Thorax* 1976; 31: 15-24.
8. Hillerdahl G. Malignant mesothelioma: review of 4710 published cases. *Br J Dis Chest* 1983; 77: 321-43.
9. Yates DH, Corrin B, Stidolph PN, *et al.* Malignant mesothelioma in south east England: clinicopathological experience of 272 cases. *Thorax* 1997; 52: 507-512.
10. Ruffie P, Feld R, Minkin S, Cormier Y, Boutan-Laroze A, Ginsberg R, Ayoub J, Shepherd FA, Evans WK, Figueredo A, Pater JL, Pringle JF, Kreisman H. Diffuse Malignant Mesothelioma of the Pleura in Ontario and Quebec: A Retrospective Study of 332 Patients. *J Clin Oncol* 1989; 7(8): 1157-1168.
11. Achtazy R, Beba W, Ritschler R, Worn H, Wahlers B, Macha HN, Morgan JA. The diagnosis, therapy and prognosis of diffuse malignant mesothelioma. *Eur J Cardiothorac Surg* 1989; 3: 445-448.
12. Mattson K, Holsti LR, Tammilehto L, Maasilta P, Pyrhonen S, Mantyla M, Kajanti M, Salminen U-S, Rautonen J, Kivisaari L. Multimodality Treatment Programs for Malignant Pleural Mesothelioma Using High Dose Hemithorax Irradiation. *I J Rad Onc Biol Phys* 1992; 24 (4): 643-650.
13. Blanc FX, Atassi K, Bignon J, Housset B. Diagnostic value of medical thoracoscopy in pleural disease: a 6-year retrospective study. *Chest* 2002; 121: 1677-83.
14. Rusch VW. A proposed new international TNM staging system for malignant pleural mesothelioma. *Chest* 1995; 108 (4): 1122-1128.
15. Eibel R, Tuengerthal S, Schoenberg SO. The role of new imaging techniques in diagnosis and staging of malignant pleural disease. *Curr Opin Oncol* 2003; 15: 131-138.
16. Stewart D, Waller D, Edwards J, Jeyapalan K, Entwisle J. Is there a role for pre-operative contrast-enhanced magnetic resonance imaging for radical surgery in malignant pleural

mesothelioma? *Eur J Cardiothorac Surg* 2003 Dec; 24(6): 1019-24.

17. Pilling J, Stewart D, Martin-Ucar A, Muller S, Waller DA. The case for routine cervical mediastinoscopy prior to radical surgery for malignant pleural mesothelioma. *Eur J Cardiothorac Surg* 2004; 25(4): 497-501.
18. Gerbaudo VH, Sugarbaker DJ, Britz-Cunningham S, Di Carli MF, Mauceri C, Treves ST. Assessment of malignant pleural mesothelioma with (18)F-FDG dual-head gamma-camera coincidence imaging: comparison with histopathology. *J Nuc Med* 2002; 43(9): 1144-9.
19. Mountain CF, Dresler CM. Regional lymph node classification for lung cancer staging. *Chest* 1997; 111: 1718-23.
20. British Thoracic Society and Society of Cardiothoracic Surgeons of Great Britain and Ireland. Guidelines on the selection of patients with lung cancer for surgery. *Thorax* 2001; 56: 89-108.
21. Cardillo G, Facciolo F, Carbone L, Regal M, Corzani F, Ricci A, Di Martino M, Martelli M. Long-term follow-up of video-assisted talc pleurodesis in malignant recurrent pleural effusions. *Eur J Cardiothorac Surg* 2002; 21(2): 302-5.
22. Schulze M, Bohle AS, Kurdow R, Dohrmann P, Henne-Bruns D. Effective treatment of malignant pleural effusions by minimal invasive thoracic surgery: thoracoscopic talc pleurodesis and pleuroperitoneal shunts in 101 patients. *Ann Thorac Surg* 2001; 71: 1809-12.
23. Genc O, Petrou M, Ladas G, Goldstraw P. The long-term morbidity of pleuroperitoneal shunts in the management of recurrent malignant effusions. *Eur J Cardiothorac Surg* 2000: 18: 143-146.
24. Putnam JB Jr, Walsh GL, Swisher SG, Roth JA, Suell DM, Vaporciyan AA, Smythe WR, Merriman KW, DeFord LL, Cerfolio RJ, Jude JR. Outpatient management of malignant pleural effusion by a chronic indwelling pleural catheter. *Ann Thorac Surg* 2000; 69: 369-375.
25. Martin-Ucar AE, Edwards JG, Rengajaran A, Muller S, Waller DA. Palliative surgical debulking in malignant mesothelioma Predictors of surgical and symptom control. *Eur J Cardiothorac Surg* 2001; 20 (2001): 1117-1121.
26. Ceresoli GL, Locati DL, Ferreri AJM, Cozzarini C, Passoni P, Melloni G, Zannini P, Bolognesi A, Villa E. Therapeutic outcome according to histologic subtype in 121 patients with malignant pleural mesothelioma. *Lung Cancer* 2001; 34: 279-287.
27. Huncharek M, Kelsey K, Mark E, Muscat J, Choi N, Carey R, Christiani D. Treatmetn and Survival in Diffuse Malignant Pleural Mesothelioma: a Study of 83 Cases from the Massachusetts General Hospital. *Anticancer Res* 1996; Vol 16; 1256-8.
28. Rusch VW, Saltz I, Venkaratnam E, Ginsberg R, McCormack P, Burt M, Markman M, Kelsen D. A Phase II Trial of Pleurectomy/Decortication Followed by Intrapleural and Systemic Chemotherapy for Malignant Plaural Mesothelioma. *J Clin Oncol* 1994; 12: 1156-1163.
29. Hilaris B, Dattatreyudu N, Kwong E, Kutcher G, Martini N. Pleurectomy and Intraoperative Brachytherapy and Postoperative Radiation in the Treatment of Malignant Pleural Mesothelioma. *Int J Rad Oncol Biol Phys* 1984: 10: 325-331.
30. Waller DA, Morritt GN, Forty J. Video-assisted thoracoscopic pleurectomy in the management of malignant pleural effusion. *Chest* 1995; 107: 1454-1456.
31. Grossebner MW, Arifi AA, Goddard M, Ritchie AJ. Mesothelioma - Vats Biopsy and lung mobilization improves diagnosis and palliation. *Eur J Cardiothorac Surg* 1999; 16 Dec (6): 619-23.
32. Boutin C, Rey F, Viallat J-R. Prevention of malignant seeding after invasive diagnostic procedures in patients with pleural mesothelioma: a randomized trial of local radiotherapy. *Chest* 1995; 108: 754-758.
33. Soysal O, Karaoglanoglu N, Demircan S, Topcu S, Tastepe I, Kaya S, Unlu M, Cetin G. Pleurectomy/decortication for palliation in malignant pleural mesothelioma: results of surgery. *Eur J Cardiothorac Surg* 1997; 11: 210-213.
34. Aziz T, Jilaihawi A, Prakash D. The management of malignant pleural mesothelioma: single center experience in 10 years. *Eur J Cardiothorac Surg* 2002; 22: 298-305.
35. Allen KB, Faber LP, Warren WH. Malignant Plaural Mesothelioma. Extrapleural Pneumonectomy and Pleurectomy. *Chest Surg Clin N Am* 1994; 4: 113-126.
36. Hasturk S, Tastepe I, Unlu M, Cetin G, Baris YI. Combined Chemotherapy in Pleurectomised Malignant Mesothelioma Patients. *J Chemother* 1996; 8 pt 2: 159-164.
37. Colleoni M, Sartori F, Calabro F, Nelli P, Vicario G, Sgarbossa G, Gaion F, Bortolotti L, Toniolo L, Manente P. Surgery followed by intracavitary plus systemic chemotherapy in malignant pleural mesothelioma. *Tumori* 1996; 82: 53-56.
38. Sauter ER, Langer C, Coia LR, Goldberg M, Keller SM. Optimal Management of Malignant Mesothelioma After Subtotal Pleurectomy: Revisiting the Role of Intrapleural Chemotherapy and Postoperative Radiation. *J Surg Oncol* 1995; 60: 100-105.
39. Pass HI, Temeck BK, Kranda K. Phase III randomized trial of surgery with or without photodynamic therapy and postoperative immunochemotherapy for malignant pleural mesothelioma. *Ann Surg Oncol* 1997; 66: 1128-1133.
40. Lee TT, EverettDL, Shu H-KG, Jahan TM, Roach M, Speight JL, Cameron RB, Phillips TL, Chan A, Jablons DM. Radical pleurectomy/decortication and intraoperative radiotherapy followed by conformal radiation with or without chemotherapy for malignant pleural mesothelioma. *J Thorac Cardiovasc Surg* 2002; 124 (6): 1183-1189.
41. McCormack PM, Nagasaki F, Hilaris BS, Martini N. Surgical Treatment of Pleural Mesothelioma. *J Thorac Cardiovasc Surg* 1982; 84: 834-842.
42. Alberts AS, Falkson G, Goedhals L, Vorobiaf DA, Van Der Mewe CA. Malignant pleural mesothelioma: a disease unaffected by current therapeutic maneuvers. *J Clin Oncol* 1988; 6: 527-535.
43. Sugarbaker DJ, Flores RM, Jacklitsch MT, Richards WG, Strauss GM, Corson JM, DeCamp MM, Swanson SJ, Bueno R, Lukanich JM, Baldini EH, Mentzer SJ. Resection margins, extrapleural nodal status, and cell type determine postoperative long-term survival in trimodality therapy of malignant pleural mesothelioma: results in 183 patients. *J Thorac Cardiovasc Surg* 1999; 117: 54-65.

44. Sugarbaker DJ, Richards W, Jaklitsch M, Lukanich J, Mentzer S, Colson Y, Chang M, Linden P, Bueno R. Prevention, early detection and management of complications following 328 consecutive extrapleural pneumonectomies. Presented AATS 2003.
45. Stanel RA, Weder W, Ballabeni P, Jermann M, Kestenholtz P, Jorger M, Stupp R,Vogt P, Migrone W, Betticher D. Neoadjuvant chemotherapy followed by pleuropneumonectomy for pleural mesothelioma: a multicenter phase II trial of SAKK. Presented 10th World Conference on Lung Cancer, 10-14 August 2003, Vancouver, Canada.
46. de Perrot M, Ginsberg RJ, Payne D, Bezjak A, Reid R, Shepherd FA, Darling G, Waddell TK, Keshavjea S, Johnston MR. A phase II trial of induction chemotherapy followed by extrapleural pneumonectomy and high-dose hemithoracic radiation for malignant pleural mesothelioma. Presented 10th World Conference on Lung Cancer, 10-14 August 2003, Vancouver, Canada.
47. Rusch VW, Venkatraman E, Rosenzweig KE, Krug LM. Adjuvant therapy, stage, tumor histology impact prognosis after resection of malignant pleural mesothelioma. Presented 10th World Conference on Lung Cancer, 10-14 August 2003, Vancouver, Canada.
48. Rahman M, Payne N, Lester J, de la Santa PM, Gibbs AR, Butchart EG. Comparison of pleurectomy/decortication and pleuropneumonectomy in the treatment of mesothelioma: a 22 year experience. Presented 10th World Conference on Lung Cancer, 10-14 August 2003, Vancouver, Canada.

Chapter 11

The management of (spontaneous) pneumothorax

Carol Tan MB ChB MRCS(Eng)
Specialist Registrar, Thoracic Surgery

GUY'S AND ST THOMAS' HOSPITALS, LONDON, UK

Introduction

Pneumothorax is air in the pleural space between the lung and the chest wall. The adjective "spontaneous" is used to distinguish those occurring without a precipitating traumatic event such as rib fracture, penetrating injury, central venous needles, or ventilator barotrauma. Spontaneous pneumothoraces are further classified into primary and secondary pneumothoraces. Primary pneumothorax occurs in otherwise healthy individuals due to the rupture of subpleural blebs and bullae characteristically found at the apex of the lungs. It is seen from mid teens up to the early thirties, in males more than females (Figure 1). It runs in families and is characteristically found in tall, lean individuals. Secondary spontaneous pneumothorax means that it is secondary to lung disease. Chronic obstructive airways disease is the commonest, but the visceral pleura is a very thin and delicate structure and any lung disease that breaches it can present as pneumothorax, including TB, Wegner's granulomosis, lymphangiolyomyomatosis (LAM), Langerhans histiocytosis; in fact, the list is endless. Recently, marijuana smoking has been blamed for cases, but since the denominator for the habit is unknown, this is speculative at present.

Physiologic mechanisms keep the pleural space free of gas and fluid, and under negative pressure. This negative pressure is due to the tendency of the elastic lung to collapse and the tendency for the relatively rigid chest wall to expand. When there is a breach in the visceral pleura, air passes from the lung into the pleural space until the pressure gradient equalizes or until the communication is sealed. During quiet spontaneous breathing when the whole cycle is at negative pressure, the crowding of the peripheral alveoli is sufficient to limit the flow of air. Pneumothorax results in varying degrees of breathlessness and typically, pleuritic chest pain. Haemothorax and tension pneumothorax where the mediastinum is pushed to the contralateral side, can also occur.

There is extensive variation in practice amongst clinicians in the management of this relatively common condition[1-4] and optimal management remains controversial. Not only is there a need to consider the immediate treatment to evacuate the air from the pleural space to allow re-expansion of the lung, a definitive procedure to prevent recurrence may also need to be addressed.

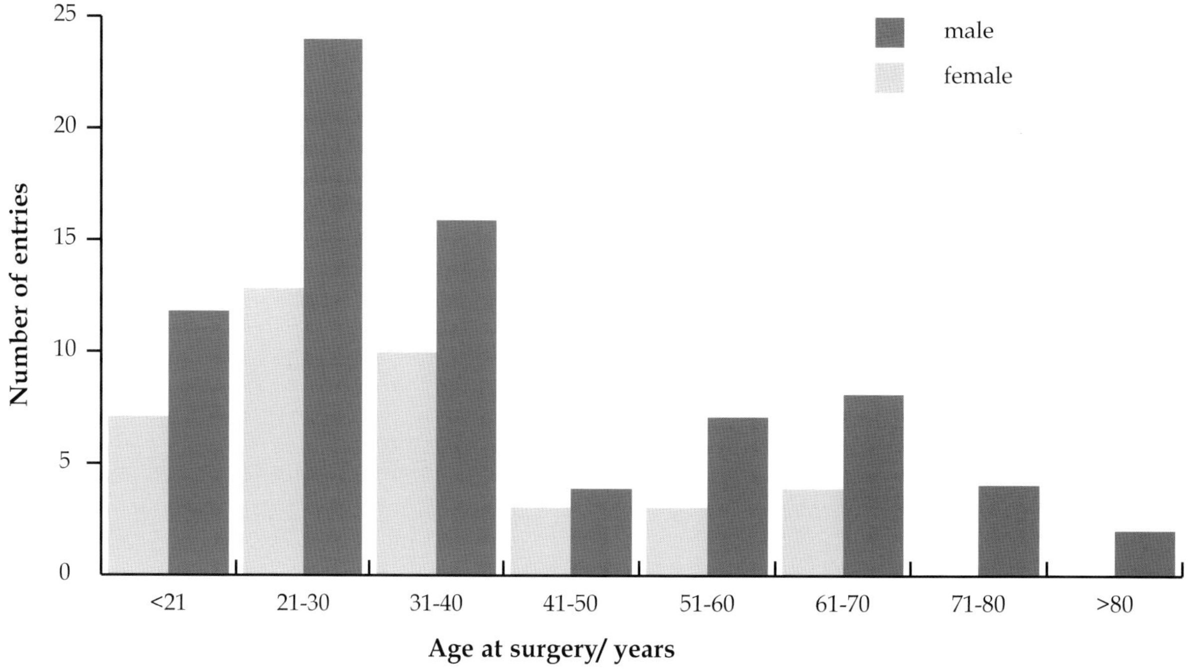

Figure 1. **Pneumothorax surgery 2004: 127 cases operated in Guy's Hospital.**

Management in the "acute" presentation varies widely, and may include one or more of the following: observation, needle aspiration, small or large bore chest tube drainage. The choice of method is often dependent on criteria such as size of the pneumothorax, the presence or absence of symptoms, the presence or absence of underlying lung disease, and on the practitioner's experience of each technique. Similarly, there is wide variation in the practice of recurrence prevention with different criteria (for example, the number of previous episodes, unilateral or bilateral, failure of primary treatment) and techniques (medical or surgical pleurodesis, "key-hole" or open surgery) being employed. This chapter summarizes the available evidence for management of spontaneous pneumothorax at both levels.

Methodology

The Medline database was searched using the following strategy and employing a search filter.

	Search History	Results
1	PNEUMOTHORAX/su, th [Surgery, Therapy]	2674
2	Incidence.mp. or exp mortality/ or follow-up studies.mp. or Mortality (sh) or Prognos: (tw) or Predict: (tw) or Course (tw)	1251771
3	1 and 2	377
4	PLEURODESIS/	419
5	2 and 4	111
6	5 not 3	80
7	3 or 6	457

Table 1. **Studies where outcome of observation is reported.**

Author (year)	Level of evidence	Total no. of patients	Patient characteristics	No. observed	Characteristics of observed patients	Outcome of observation
Alfageme (1994)	IIb	183	1° and 2° spontaneous pneumothorax; 1st and recurrent episodes	32 (38 episodes)	Pneumothorax size <20%	28 patients available for follow-up 10 (36%) recurred, 7 of these within first year
Vernejoux (2001)	IIb	65	Spontaneous pneumothorax	6	Not reported	Recurrence in 1 patient
Hart (1983)	III	236	Spontaneous pneumothorax; 1st episode	108	Not reported	Lung re-expanded in all cases, recurrence in 23 patients (21%)
O'Rourke (1989)	III	130	1° and 2° spontaneous pneumothorax; 1st and recurrent episodes	49	Mild symptoms; pneumothorax size 5-50%, most <15%	Worsening symptoms /pneumothorax progression in 9 2 deaths from tension pneumothorax Recurrence in 13/40 (32.5%) patients
Selby (1994)	III	37	Spontaneous pneumothorax	14	Pneumothorax size 10% (5-30%)	2 failures of observation alone (1 required chest tube, 1 aspiration)

Results

All titles and abstracts, where initially available, were reviewed. Papers found at the first search totalled 318. The majority of these papers were case series reporting management and outcome of patients with pneumothorax. Level I evidence for the management of pneumothorax was found in only 15 randomised control trial publications which will be further described below. Where the use of certain practices is widespread and no level I evidence is available, the evidence was sought from other studies.

Observation as the initial management

The British Thoracic Society (BTS) recommends observation for small, closed, mildly symptomatic pneumothorax. There are no RCTs comparing observation alone with other treatment modalities. There are many reports where observation alone is used as the initial management of pneumothorax in a proportion of the study population [5-11], but only five reporting the outcome from observation alone (Table 1). Two of these are prospective studies[10,11]. The first is a non-randomised prospective study of 213 spontaneous pneumothorax episodes, where 38 episodes in 32 patients were managed by observation alone where the pneumothorax size was less than 20% [10]. Included in this group were patients with secondary spontaneous pneumothorax (9/38) as well as those with previous history of pneumothorax (13/38). Recurrence in this group of patients was 36%, with the recurrence time range between 22 days to 17 months. The second study included six of 65 patients presenting with their first spontaneous pneumothorax who underwent observation only [11]. Of these six patients, there was one recurrence.

Table 2. **RCTs of needle aspiration versus tube drainage of pneumothorax.**

Author (year)	Patients	N	Group 1	Group 2	Outcome
Harvey (1994)	1° spontaneous pneumothorax; 1st and recurrent	73	Simple aspiration (35)	Intercostal drain (38)	No significant difference in pain during procedure. Longer hospital stay and greater daily pain with intercostal tube drains. 28/35 patients aspirated successfully No significant difference in recurrence at 1 year
Andrivet (1995)	1st or 2nd spontaneous pneumothorax	61	Needle aspiration (33)	Thoracic drainage (28)	Significantly higher success rate with drain than aspiration No significant difference in recurrence at 90 days
Noppen (2002)	1st 1° spontaneous pneumothorax	60	Manual aspiration (27)	Chest tube drainage (33)	No significant difference in immediate success, or at 1 week 48% aspiration group did not need hospital stay versus 100% No significant difference in recurrence at 1 year

Criteria used or the characteristics of patients observed, are not comparable in these studies, and are often based on the pneumothorax size or symptoms of the patient. Initial resolution of the pneumothorax is reported in most cases but with a risk of recurrence. Observation as an initial management is appropriate in small (say <20%) and asymptomatic cases and avoids an unnecessary invasive procedure. Although not included in reports in a way that can be analyzed, the time since onset influences management. If the onset of the pneumothorax was hours or days earlier and the clinical situation is stable, conservative management is easier to recommend than if the patient presents soon (less than an hour) after the onset and the pneumothorax may still be enlarging. The most critical factor in this group of patients is the unrecognised development of continual air leak from the breached pleura which can quickly progress to a tension pneumothorax with risk of sudden death.

Short wave diathermy for small pneumothoraces

When the decision is made to observe a small, stable pneumothorax, the gas in the pleural space should gradually become absorbed over a period of days to weeks, resulting in resolution of the pneumothorax. Some authors have looked at ways of accelerating the resolution of such small pneumothoraces. There was one RCT of 22 patients which tested the use of short wave diathermy to the affected side of the chest [12]. The authors hypothesized that a change in temperature of the pleural cavity and the increased blood flow of the pleural capillary caused by high frequency waves of electromagnetic radiation in short wave diathermy, may increase the rate of absorption of gas from the pleural cavity. In the study, the maximum size of pneumothorax was 45% and all patients were asymptomatic. Although a significantly shorter time to resolution of pneumothorax was reported in the treatment group, the necessity for intervention is questionable in this group of asymptomatic patients with small pneumothoraces.

Recurrence was not reported and compared in the study. We found no further reports of this intervention in the literature.

Needle aspiration or chest tube drainage

Three RCTs of 194 patients compare the use of needle aspiration with chest tube drainage in the management of primary pneumothorax (Table 2) [13-15]. Only patients with spontaneous pneumothorax were included in these studies, but two excluded patients with recurrent episodes. In all three studies, there was no significant difference in long-term outcome/ recurrence (at 90 days or one year), but one study reported significantly higher immediate success with a chest drain than with aspiration. Chest tube drainage was however, associated with greater pain and longer hospital stay, while a proportion of patients who had their pneumothorax aspirated were successfully treated as outpatients.

Ambulatory management

Where needle aspiration fails to re-expand the lung, usually because there is an ongoing air leak from a breach in the visceral pleura, chest tube drainage becomes necessary. The major disadvantage of conventional chest tube drainage is the need to connect the tube to an underwater seal device, resulting in hospitalisation and a restriction in mobility. One way of getting round this problem is to connect a one-way valve to the end of the chest tube. The thoracic vent, Heimlich valve and flutter valve are such devices frequently used and reported in the literature. There was however, only one RCT [16] comparing a one-way valve device (thoracic vent) with conventional intercostal tube drainage. Thirty patients were included in this study which reported no significant differences in the rate of re-expansion and complications between groups, but the patients treated with the thoracic vent had less pain, and 70% of them were managed successfully on an outpatient basis. We found a further seven publications reporting outcome in the use of one-way valves (Table 3) [17-23]. Success rates range from 73 to 93%, with most being managed successfully in the outpatient setting.

Intrapleural analgesia

The intensity of pain caused by the presence of an intrapleural chest drain may be sufficient to immobilize the patient. Regular analgesia with paracetamol and non-steroidal anti-inflammatory drugs are often required. When this fails to control pain, narcotics or other means of delivering analgesics may become necessary. One RCT of 22 patients compared the use of intrapleural bupivacaine at 8-hour intervals with a placebo (saline) during the period of chest tube drainage [24]. Visual analogue pain scale scores were found to be significantly lower in those receiving bupivacaine within five minutes of injection and for up to four hours after.

Bedside chemical pleurodesis

The consensus view [25] is that preventative treatment of primary spontaneous pneumothorax is not appropriate at the first episode, because in two thirds of cases there is no recurrence. After a second ipsilateral episode or the first contralateral episode, the BTS guidelines recommend preventive management. The instillation of a chemical into the pleural place leads to inflammation and the formation of adhesions between the two layers of pleurae. This can be performed at the bedside through a chest tube or surgically at thoracoscopy. Three RCTs compared the outcome of bedside pleurodesis with pleural drainage through a chest tube only (Table 4) [26-28]. All report a reduction in recurrence of pneumothorax with pleurodesis. In particular, the study by Almind *et al*, consisting of 96 subjects, showed a reduction in recurrence at a mean follow-up time of 4.6 years from 13 to 8% after the first episode of pneumothorax, if bedside talc slurry was used [27]. Tetracycline did not appear to have the same long-term result in two of the three studies showing no significant difference in late recurrence.

Surgical management

Surgical management introduces two potential advantages in the prevention of recurrent pneumothorax. Firstly, the lung and pleura can be inspected and any bullous areas or breach in the parietal pleura can be dealt with by staple resection,

Table 3. Valved devices as an alternative to underwater seal drains.

Author (year)	Level of evidence	N	Patient characteristics	Method	Outcome
Ikeda (1994)	III	111	Spontaneous pneumothorax	Chest tube + suction; outpatient flutter valve if air leak stops	72.9% (81) success. 19 hospitalised (14 air leaks, 5 wound pains) 11 admitted following failed outpatient management
Campisi (1997)	III	14	Spontaneous pneumothorax	Chest tube and Heimlich flutter valve	3 overnight admissions All subsequently managed successfully as outpatient
Niemi (1999)	III	76	Spontaneous pneumothorax	19 patients treated with Heimlich flutter valve, 57 with standard under-water seal drain	Drainage time and hospitalisation time shorter in Heimlich group
Varela (1994)	III	72	Pneumothorax	Chest tube (2.2mm internal diameter) equipped with Heimlich valve	Full lung expansion in 93% 10.7% recurrence
Minami (1992)	III	71	Spontaneous pneumothorax	Small bore catheter + Heimlich	84.5% success.
Samelson (1991)	III	16	Spontaneous, traumatic or iatrogenic pneumothorax	Thoracic vent	Resolution after mean 2.5 days No immediate recurrences
Mercier (1976)	III	226	Spontaneous pneumothorax	Observation, chest tube +/- flutter valve, surgery	167 managed as successfully as outpatient (45 observed, 122 intercostal tube + flutter valve); 59 hospitalised (42 surgical treatment)

electrocautery or ligation. Secondly, a procedure which creates pleurodesis can be performed. Treatment options include pleurectomy, pleural abrasion with a scourer, or introduction of a chemical agent as with the bedside procedure. The advantage with surgical introduction of the chemical agent is that it can be sprayed over the pleural surfaces under direct vision ensuring a more uniform covering than may be achieved by bedside pleurodesis. We found two RCTs which compared the use of a minimally invasive operation, often termed video-assisted thoracoscopic surgery (VATS), with pleural drainage through a chest tube (Table 5) [29,30]. The trial by Abdala *et al* randomising patients to treatment by chest tube drainage or VATS with management of the ruptured bleb, showed a reduction in recurrence with the latter treatment [29]. Tschopp's multicentre trial of 108 patients compared the short and long-term efficacy of thoracoscopic talc insufflation under local anaesthesia with chest tube drainage [30]. Although there was no significant difference in the duration of chest tube drainage and hospital stay, and the group undergoing thoracoscopy had more early pain, thoracoscopy had better immediate and long-term outcome with respect to recurrences.

Table 4. RCTs of talc or tetracycline pleurodesis for pneumothorax compared with chest tube drainage alone

Author (year)	Patient characteristics	N	Group 1	Group 2	Group 3	Outcome
Light (1990)	Spontaneous pneumothorax	229	Tube drainage (116)	Tube drainage + tetracycline (113)		Recurrence rate lower in tetracycline group during 5-year study period. Tetracycline associated with chest pain
Almind (1989)	1st spontaneous pneumothorax	96	Tube drainage (34)	Tube drainage + tetracycline (33)	Tube drainage + talc (29)	No significant difference in hospital + drain time, infection, persistent pneumothorax, in-hospital relapse. Recurrence at mean follow-up (4.6 years) were 13%, 13% & 8% in groups 1, 2 & 3
van den Brande (1989)	1st 1° spontaneous pneumothorax	20	Tube drainage (10)	Tube drainage + tetracycline (10)		Early recurrence reduced by tetracycline. No significant difference with late recurrence

Table 5. RCTs comparing VATS with chest tube drainage.

Author (year)	Patient characteristics	N	Group 1	Group 2	Outcome
Abdala (2001)	Spontaneous pneumothorax	40	VATS + management of bleb	Chest tube drainage	Shorter hospital stay and less analgesic with VATS No recurrence or prolonged air leaks with VATS
Tschopp (2002)	1° spontaneous pneumothorax	108	VATS talc (61)	Chest tube drainage (47)	No significant difference in drainage and hospital duration. Higher recurrence with drainage only (34% v 5% at 5 years). Higher postoperative pain with VATS, but not significant at 1 month

Surgical approach

Prior to the advent of VATS and more recently, improvements in its technology, the surgical approach would have been by thoracotomy. This was most frequently done through an axillary thoracotomy, although the lateral approach or an approach through the auscultatory triangle, was also sometimes used. VATS allows access into the thoracic cavity producing less tissue trauma than the larger thoracotomy incision. There are two RCTs comparing surgical approach (Table 6) [31,32]. Waller *et al* compared VATS with posterolateral thoracotomy, demonstrating less postoperative decline in lung function, less pain, and shortened hospital stay with VATS [31]. Follow-up in this study was up to 20 months and during this time there was 2/30 and 1/30 recurrent pneumothorax in the VATS and thoracotomy groups. Sekine *et al*

Table 6. **RCTs comparing VATS approach with thoracotomy.**

Author (year)	Patient characteristics	N	Group 1	Group 2	Outcome
Waller (1994)	Persistent air leak or recurrent pneumothorax; 1° or 2°	60	VATS, bullectomy, apical pleurectomy (30)	Posterolateral thoracotomy, bullectomy, apical pleurectomy (30)	Greater postoperative decline in lung function with thoracotomy Less postoperative pain and shorter hospital stay with VATS 4 primary treatment failures with VATS versus 1 thoracotomy - all had 2° pneumothorax
Sekine (1999)	Spontaneous pneumothorax	38	VATS bullectomy (20)	Axillary thoracotomy bullectomy (18)	Higher PaO_2 with VATS up to day 4. Alveolar-arterial O_2 tension gradient less with VATS to day 4. Pain and peripheral atelectasis more with thoracotomy

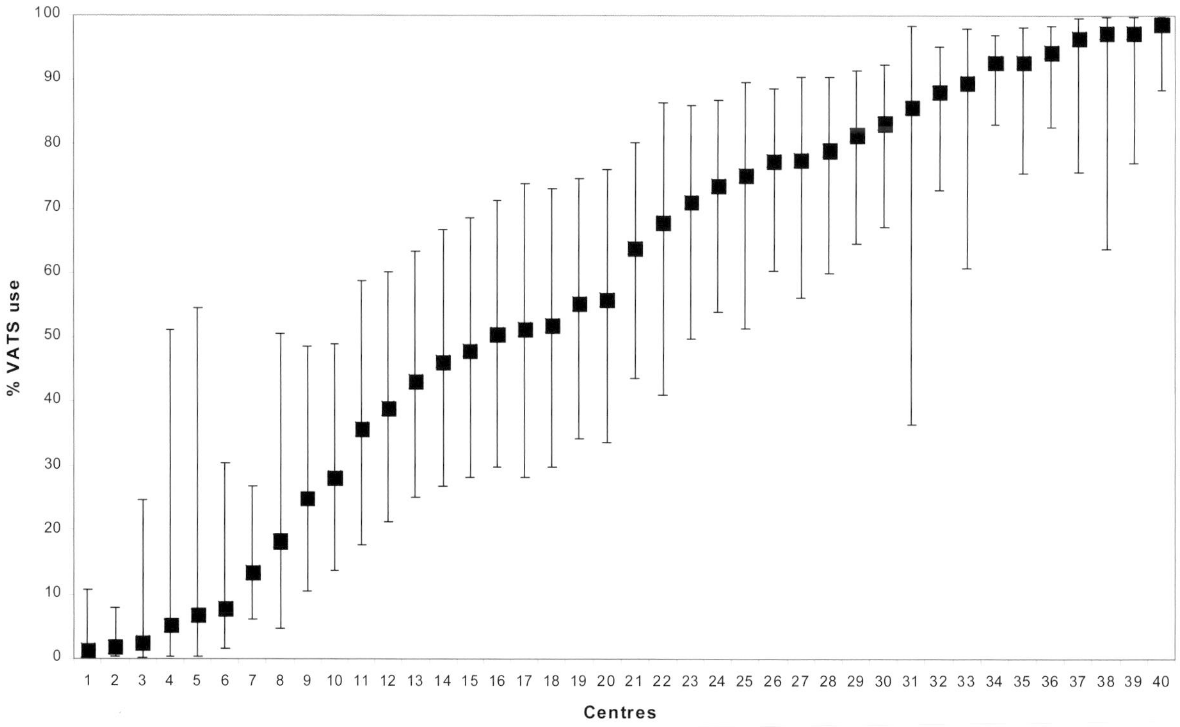

Figure 2. **UK register VATS: thoracotomy for pneumothorax (data 2000-2002 on about 2,000 operations). Sedrakyan *et al* in preparation for publication.**

Table 7. RCTs of suction versus no suction on chest drains.

Author (year)	Patient characteristics	N	Group 1	Group 2	Outcome
So (1982)	1° and 2° spontaneous pneumothorax	53	Suction on intercostal drainage (30)	No suction; intercostal drainage (23)	57% success with suction versus 50% No significant difference
Ayed (2003)	Pneumothorax; undergoing VATS apical pleurectomy	100	Suction (50)	Underwater seal after brief suction (50)	7/50 prolonged air leak with suction, 1/50 in underwater seal group. Shorter chest tube days and hospital stay in group 2

compared VATS with the axillary approach, assessing gas exchange and atelectasis on chest radiographs postoperatively and showed a significant benefit with VATS [32]. Traditionally, surgical therapy would be offered after the second or third occurrence. With the availability of a less intrusive surgical approach like VATS, an intervention is more likely to be offered earlier, after the second pneumothorax episode. In the UK, VATS is widely available, but the surgical practice varies widely (Figure 2) from 0% to 100%.

Suction versus no suction

There is no agreement on the routine use of suction on underwater seal chest drains. Advocators of suction use believe that a low negative pressure artificially generated in the pleural space aids in the re-expansion of the collapsed lung, while others believe that an air leak may be prolonged by holding the "hole" (breach in the pleura) open with suction. Two RCTs address this dilemma (Table 7). So *et al* [33] randomised 53 patients with spontaneous pneumothorax treated by intercostal catheter drainage to underwater seal suction drainage or underwater seal alone. No significant advantage was demonstrated with suction. The second RCT of 50 patients addressed the issue in patients following thoracoscopy with blebectomy and pleurectomy [34]. Patients were randomised to receive either underwater seal suction drainage or underwater seal alone after an initial two hours of suction. There were significantly more patients with prolonged air leak, as well as a prolonged chest tube drainage and hospital time, in the underwater seal suction drainage. These are two small, incomparable studies, suggesting the need for further research in this area.

Timing of drain removal

In the same study, So *et al* addressed the timing of chest drain removal by randomly allocating patients to two further groups: early, as soon as the lung was re-expanded, or late, two days following lung re-expansion [33]. No difference in success rate was demonstrated with success rates of 52% and 53% respectively. The authors have partly attributed their low success rates to the small size of the tube (13FG), which may have become blocked by fluid or kinked. There are however, no RCTs suggesting that large bore tubes are more effective than small ones in the management of pneumothorax.

Recommendations	Evidence level
◆ Observation as an initial management of pneumothorax is appropriate in small (say <20%) and asymptomatic cases and avoids an unnecessary invasive procedure.	IIb/B
◆ Simple needle aspiration and chest tube insertion for spontaneous pneumothorax in patients with normal lungs have similar long-term outcome, but chest tube insertion is associated with greater discomfort and pain.	Ib/A
◆ The use of ambulatory systems (one-way valves) is acceptable and an effective way of managing pneumothorax, and reduces hospital stay.	Ib/A
◆ Pleurodesis at the bedside reduces the recurrence rate of pneumothorax when compared with chest tube drainage alone.	Ib/A
◆ Surgical treatment by VATS reduces the recurrence rate of pneumothorax when compared to chest tube drainage alone. (But there are no RCTs comparing bedside pleurodesis with VATS pleurodesis)	Ib/A
◆ The VATS approach offers a significant advantage to thoracotomy in the immediate postoperative period, with no compromise to long-term outcome.	Ib/A

References

1. Sutherland M, Burdon J, Hart D. Primary spontaneous pneumothorax: treatment practices in Australia. *Respirology* 2000; 5: 277-80.
2. Yeoh JH, Ansari S, Campbell IA. Management of spontaneous pneumothorax - a Welsh survey. *Postgrad Med J* 2000; 76: 496-9.
3. Soulsby T. British Thoracic Society guidelines for the management of spontaneous pneumothorax: do we comply with them and do they work? *J Accid Emerg Med* 1998; 15: 317-21.
4. Baumann MH, Strange C. The clinician's perspective on pneumothorax management. *Chest* 1997; 112: 822-8.
5. Chee CB, Abisheganaden J, Yeo JK, Lee P, Huan PY, Poh SC, *et al.* Persistent air-leak in spontaneous pneumothorax - clinical course and outcome. *Respir Med* 1998; 92: 757-61.
6. Weissberg D, Refaely Y. Pneumothorax: experience with 1,199 patients. *Chest* 2000; 117: 1279-85.
7. Hart GJ, Stokes TC, Couch AH. Spontaneous pneumothorax in Norfolk. *Br J Dis Chest* 1983; 77: 164-70.
8. O'Rourke JP, Yee ES. Civilian spontaneous pneumothorax. Treatment options and long-term results. *Chest* 1989; 96: 1302-6.
9. Selby CD, Sudlow MF. Deficiencies of management of spontaneous pneumothoraces. *Scott Med J* 1994; 39: 75-7.
10. Alfageme I, Moreno L, Huertas C, Vargas A, Hernandez J, Beiztegui A. Spontaneous pneumothorax. Long-term results with tetracycline pleurodesis. *Chest* 1994; 106: 347-50.
11. Vernejoux JM, Raherison C, Combe P, Villanueva P, Laurent F, Tunon de Lara JM, *et al.* Spontaneous pneumothorax: pragmatic management and long-term outcome. *Respir Med* 2001; 95: 857-62.
12. Ma Y, Li J, Liu Y. Short wave diathermy for small spontaneous pneumothorax. *Thorax* 1997; 52: 561-6.
13. Andrivet P, Djedaini K, Teboul JL, Brochard L, Dreyfuss D. Spontaneous pneumothorax. Comparison of thoracic drainage vs immediate or delayed needle aspiration. *Chest* 1995; 108: 335-9.
14. Harvey J, Prescott RJ. Simple aspiration versus intercostal tube drainage for spontaneous pneumothorax in patients with normal lungs. British Thoracic Society Research Committee. *BMJ* 1994; 309: 1338-9.
15. Noppen M, Alexander P, Driesen P, Slabbynck H, Verstraeten A. Manual aspiration versus chest tube drainage in first episodes of primary spontaneous pneumothorax: a multicenter, prospective, randomized pilot study. *Am J Respir Crit Care Med* 2002; 165: 1240-4.
16. Roggla M, Wagner A, Brunner C, Roggla G. The management of pneumothorax with the thoracic vent versus conventional intercostal tube drainage. *Wien Klin Wochenschr* 1996; 108: 330-3.
17. Ikeda M, Yamane Y, Hagiwara N, Ohnumi K, Hasuike M. [Outpatient drainage treatment for simple spontaneous pneumothorax]. *Nihon Kyobu Shikkan Gakkai Zasshi* 1994; 32: 763-7.
18. Campisi P, Voitk AJ. Outpatient treatment of spontaneous pneumothorax in a community hospital using a Heimlich flutter valve: a case series. *J Emerg Med* 1997; 15: 115-9.

19. Niemi T, Hannukainen J, Aarnio P. Use of the Heimlich valve for treating pneumothorax. *Ann Chir Gynaecol* 1999; 88: 36-7.
20. Varela G, Arroyo A, Larru E, Diaz-Hellin V, Gamez P. [The treatment of pneumothorax by small-caliber drainage without a water seal]. *Arch Bronconeumol* 1994; 30: 185-7.
21. Minami H, Saka H, Senda K, Horio Y, Iwahara T, Nomura F, *et al.* Small caliber catheter drainage for spontaneous pneumothorax. *Am J Med Sci* 1992; 304: 345-7.
22. Samelson SL, Goldberg EM, Ferguson MK. The thoracic vent. Clinical experience with a new device for treating simple pneumothorax. *Chest* 1991; 100: 880-2.
23. Mercier C, Page A, Verdant A, Cossette R, Dontigny L, Pelletier LC. Outpatient management of intercostal tube drainage in spontaneous pneumothorax. *Ann Thorac Surg* 1976; 22: 163-5.
24. Engdahl O, Boe J, Sandstedt S. Interpleural bupivacaine for analgesia during chest drainage treatment for pneumothorax. A randomized double-blind study. *Acta Anaesthesiol Scand* 1993; 37: 149-53.
25. Henry M, Arnold T, Harvey J. BTS guidelines for the management of spontaneous pneumothorax. *Thorax* 2003; 58: ii39-ii52.
26. Light RW, O'Hara VS, Moritz TE, McElhinney AJ, Butz R, Haakenson CM, *et al.* Intrapleural tetracycline for the prevention of recurrent spontaneous pneumothorax. Results of a Department of Veterans Affairs cooperative study. *JAMA* 1990; 264: 2224-30.
27. Almind M, Lange P, Viskum K. Spontaneous pneumothorax: comparison of simple drainage, talc pleurodesis, and tetracycline pleurodesis. *Thorax* 1989; 44: 627-30.
28. van den BP, Staelens I. Chemical pleurodesis in primary spontaneous pneumothorax. *Thorac Cardiovasc Surg* 1989; 37: 180-2.
29. Abdala OA, Levy RR, Bibiloni RH, Viso HD, De Souza M, Satler VH. [Advantages of video-assisted thoracic surgery in the treatment of spontaneous pneumothorax]. *Medicina* (B Aires) 2001; 61: 157-60.
30. Tschopp JM, Boutin C, Astoul P, Janssen JP, Grandin S, Bolliger CT, *et al.* Talcage by medical thoracoscopy for primary spontaneous pneumothorax is more cost-effective than drainage: a randomised study. *Eur Respir J* 2002; 20: 1003-9.
31. Waller DA, Forty J, Morritt GN. Video-assisted thoracoscopic surgery versus thoracotomy for spontaneous pneumothorax. *Ann Thorac Surg* 1994; 58: 372-6.
32. Sekine Y, Miyata Y, Yamada K, Yamada H, Yasukawa T, Saitoh Y, *et al.* Video-assisted thoracoscopic surgery does not deteriorate postoperative pulmonary gas exchange in spontaneous pneumothorax patients. *Eur J Cardiothorac Surg* 1999; 16: 48-53.
33. So SY, Yu DY. Catheter drainage of spontaneous pneumothorax: suction or no suction, early or late removal? *Thorax* 1982; 37: 46-8.
34. Ayed AK. Suction versus water seal after thoracoscopy for primary spontaneous pneumothorax: prospective randomized study. *Ann Thorac Surg* 2003; 75: 1593-6.

Chapter 12

Pleurodesis for malignant effusion

Carol Tan MB ChB MRCS (Eng)
Specialist Registrar, Thoracic Surgery

GUY'S AND ST THOMAS' HOSPITALS, LONDON, UK

Introduction

There is a constant physiological production and re-absorption of pleural fluid in health. In the parietal pleura, where hydrostatic pressure exceeds the osmotic force, there is a net efflux of fluid as governed by Starling forces. The pulmonary capillaries have a hydrostatic pressure, which in health is less than osmotic pressure, and are responsible for 90% of absorption from the pleural space. The lymphatics of the mediastinum and diaphragm actively take up protein and clear about 10% of the pleural fluid. Where there is malignant disease of the pleural or mediastinal lymphatics there is disturbance of this physiological flux. There is a tendency for the protein content of pleural fluid to rise from the normal of 10-20 grams per litre due to failure of the lymphatic mechanism or an increased leak from malignant involvement of the pleura, or both effects. This further upsets the normal balance in favour of accumulation of fluid in the pleural space. In fact, pleural accumulation is probably a more correct term than effusion, because the rate of fluid production is not necessarily the abnormality.

The clinical consequence is breathlessness: its severity depends on the volume of fluid and the respiratory reserve. Aspiration of a litre or so of fluid is dramatically effective in relieving breathlessness in many patients. The symptomatic relief can be maintained if the pleural space is obliterated by pleurodesis. The principles underlying management are widely agreed. If the fluid resolves as the underlying disease is treated (for example chemotherapy for lymphoma) then pleurodesis is not justified. However, if it persists and recurs after aspiration, pleurodesis is an option.

Pleurodesis has been common practice since the 1960s with a very large variety of agents being used. In the UK Thoracic Surgery Register for the last five years for which reports are available (1998 to 2002), there have been 492, 690, 932, 1071, and 977 cases per year treated by surgeons [1]. When performed by thoracic surgeons the method is almost always to insufflate talc powder at video-assisted thoracoscopic surgery (VATS). An unknown, but probably large number, are managed at the bedside by oncological, respiratory and general physicians.

Although the technique is widely practised and there have been many publications on the management of malignant effusion, there is a wide variation in indications and techniques employed.

Despite a fair degree of uniformity in how these cases are managed by surgeons, the agents used by physicians include talc slurry, but also tetracycline, bleomycin and other anti-neoplastic agents, Corynebacterium parvum, and any number of other irritants and pro-inflammatory drugs. It is clear that to some extent there is a mixed intention with most strategies, aimed at simply creating inflammation, while others include the objective of killing intrapleural cancer. Some clinicians drain to dryness and instill the agent; some leave a tube until daily drainage diminishes, and there are various practices for duration of drainage, drain size, and management of the drain. To find the evidence for current practice we have performed a systematic review [2]. In this chapter we will summarize the areas of practice for which there is evidence.

Methodology

Medline, PubMed, World of Science, Embase and Cochrane were searched. After excluding papers that did not contribute to evidence, there were 227, but for the purposes of this chapter we have been more selective in our bibliography. Level I evidence is provided by 46 publications and we will concentrate mainly on those.

There is level IV evidence in the form of British Thoracic Society guidelines [3].

Results

Pleurodesis

Agents used to achieve pleurodesis

Systematic review

A previous systematic review [4] incorporating the literature up to 1992 and a Cochrane Review [5] concluded that talc was the most effective (and cheapest) agent for pleurodesis.

RCT

We found reports on 33 different agents used for pleurodesis (Figure 1). Talc was the commonest agent studied followed by tetracycline and bleomycin. Sixteen agents were reported in a single study each. Talc is the longest standing and most frequently studied.

There are 37 RCTs comparing agents [6-42]. Seven of them compare an agent with drainage alone [6-12], and 11 studies feature talc [11-21]. Included in these studies are a spread of doses and different techniques. The studies and results where talc was tested are summarised in Table 1. Talc has consistently been found to be the better agent wherever compared and to have the additional merit of being cheaper.

Method of administration

There were three RCTs comparing the same agent applied by thoracoscopy versus bedside techniques in a total of 141 randomised patients. Two employed talc [43,44] and one tetracycline [45] (Table 2). Where talc was used it was by dry powder insufflation during a VATS procedure, either under general anaesthesia or local anaesthesia with sedation, while talc slurry was used in the bedside method. In one study [44], there were fewer recurrences following thoracoscopic talc insufflation, but no significant difference was found in outcome in the other two studies. Cost was in favour of the bedside method in one study [43].

VATS +/- pleurodesis

There are many reports on the use of VATS to obtain tissue diagnosis and/or achieve pleurodesis. A variety of agents are used, but most surgeons use talc. The summary message is that claimed efficacy rates (complete and partial response) range from 82% to 100% by various criteria; some are by symptom relief, some radiological, and some combinations of the two [46]. Many of these patients were offered VATS with the dual intent of biopsy for tissue diagnosis and pleurodesis which in clinical practice would justify performing the more invasive surgical technique, given similar outcomes for pleurodesis.

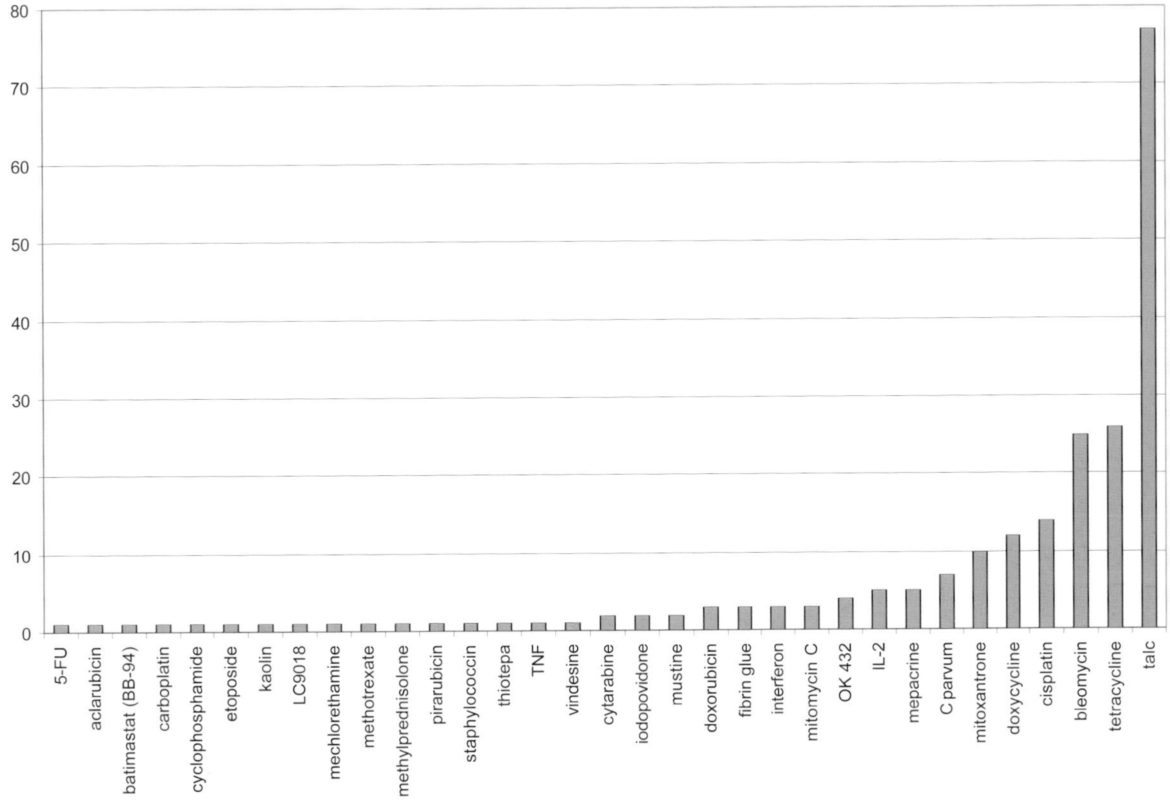

Figure 1. **Number of references versus agent.**

Bedside pleurodesis using talc slurry

We have established that the evidence supports talc as the best agent, but that bedside administration (which is by talc slurry rather than dry powder insufflation, also known as poudrage) is as effective. Both prospective non-randomised studies and retrospective series claim success (complete and partial responses) of about 80-100%, based on the larger series [47,48]. This finding is in line with the RCT evidence.

Other agents used at bedside

There are both well-designed prospective and retrospective case series, in which agents other than talc are tested at the bedside. Although some report 100% response to pleurodesis [49], many of these studies are small with different inclusion criteria, making the results difficult to interpret and summarise.

Distribution of sclerosing agent

There is a belief that when talc is insufflated into the chest with the lung collapsed (VATS), it has the advantage that the talc is evenly distributed over the pleural surface. Similarly, tetracycline can be sprayed

Table 1. **RCTs where talc tested (NR = not recorded).**

Study, year	Age	Longest F/U (months)	Comparison groups	N	Recurrence /no success	Pain	Fever	Other complications	Conclusions
Fentiman 1983	53	17	Talc insufflation	20	2	NR	NR	3	Talc better
			Mustine	17	8	NR	NR	3	
Hamed 1989	54	24 (median)	Talc insufflation	10	0	NR	NR	NR	Talc better
			Bleomycin	15	5	NR	NR	NR	
Lynch 1996	60	6 (median)	Bleomycin	14	4	4	5	NR	No statistical difference
			Talc slurry	17	9	4	8	NR	
			Tetracycline	15	7	7	6	NR	
Noppen 1997	61	Until death	Bleomycin	12	3	0	3	0	No difference, but talc cheaper
			Talc slurry	14	3	0	5	0	
Zimmer 1997	66	8	Bleomycin	14	3	Pain score 2.4	NR	0	Talc better, but not statistical; cheaper
			Talc slurry	19	2	Pain score 3.1	NR	3 wound infection	
Diacon 2000	67	6	Bleomycin	17	11	Visual analogue scale recorded	2	1 nausea	Talc better
			Talc insufflation	15	2		2	1 shoulder pain	
Ong 2000	63	1	Bleomycin	20	6	2	4	0	Talc better
			Talc slurry	18	2	0	1	0	
Haddad 2004	58	6	Talc slurry	37	10	NR	NR	3	No statistical difference
			Bleomycin	34	11	NR	NR	3	
Fentiman 1986	52	12 (minimum)	Talc insufflation	12	1	NR	NR	NR	Talc better
			Tetracycline	21	11	NR	NR	NR	
Sorensen 1984	62	24	Talc slurry	9	0	pain in all, not prolonged	NR	1 septicaemia	Talc better
			Pleural drain	12	5		NR		
Leverenz 2000	61	NR	Talc slurry	33	5	NR	NR	NR	Continuous drain better
			Continuous drain	28	0	NR	NR	NR	

onto the pleura at VATS. To ensure a similar dispersion with bedside techniques, it has been the custom to roll and tip the patient from time-to-time following instillation of the agent. There is level I evidence in two RCTs that these physical manoeuvres make no difference to the distribution of the agents (Table 3) [50,51]. One of the studies also demonstrated no significant difference in survival, duration of chest tube or fluid recurrence. Two studies, one using ^{99m}Tc-sestamibi-labelled talc suspension [51] and the other ^{99m}Tc-colloid [52] showed no improvement in distribution or outcome due to rolling. This removes one argument in favour of VATS as opposed to bedside techniques.

Tube size

We found one RCT with 18 patients comparing the size of chest tube used for drainage and instillation of sclerosant [53]. Although placement of the larger tube was at diagnostic thoracoscopy, and the smaller percutaneously, there was no significant difference in outcome.

Table 2. **RCTs of bedside versus thoracoscopy (NR = not recorded).**

Study, year	Age	Longest F/U (months)	Agent	Comparison groups	N	Recurrence /no success	Pain	Fever	Other complications	Conclusions
Evans 1993	57	60	Tetracycline	Bedside	14	8	NR	NR	NR	No significant difference
				Thoracoscopy	15	9	NR	NR	NR	
Yim 1996	63	16	Talc	Bedside slurry	29	3	NR	NR	2	No significant difference; bedside cheaper
				Thoracoscopic insufflation	28	1	NR	NR	3	
Manes 2000	NR	12 or till death	Talc	Bedside slurry	29	8	7	10	2	Fewer recurrence with thoracoscopy
				Thoracoscopic insufflation	26	1	0	6	1 empyema	

Table 3. **RCTs of rotation versus no rotation (NR = not recorded).**

Study, year	Age	Longest F/U (months)	Agent	Comparison groups	N	Recurrence /no success	Pain	Fever	Other complications	Conclusions
Dryzer 1993	63	12	Tetracycline, minocycline or doxycycline	Rotation	19	5	NR	NR	NR	No significant difference
				No rotation	21	7	NR	NR	NR	
Mager 2002	67	1	Radiolabelled talc	Rotation	10	2	NR	NR	NR	No significant difference
				No rotation	10	1	NR	NR	NR	

We found studies where the question of the use of small tubes was addressed. These included patients in whom the tube was placed radiologically and/or outpatient drain management protocols were employed. Sclerosant practice varied. The evidence is not easy to summarise, but success rates in excess of 90% are being reported [54,55]. Smaller tubes may be more comfortable, but further evaluation in prospectively designed trials with larger numbers is required.

Short protocols

Three studies looked at duration of chest drainage following instillation of the sclerosant (Table 4) [56-58]. Where two methods are equally effective, a protocol that shortens or obviates the need for hospital admission should be preferred. One RCT [56] showed that similar results were obtained (80% success), but with a much shorter median chest tube time of two days in the short protocol group as opposed to seven days in the control group. An RCT so far presented only in abstract form concurs with this finding [59].

Table 4. Short protocols.

Study	Year	Design	N	Method	Results
Villanueva	1994	RCT	25	Group 1, n=15 (standard) - tube suction drainage until lung expanded and <150ml/day drained Tetracycline instilled. Tube removed when <150ml/day Group 2, n=10 (short) - tube suction drainage Tetracycline instilled within 24 hour Tube removed the next day	NSD in pleurodesis success (80%) Duration of chest tube shorter for group 2
Spiegler	2003	Prospective case series	38	Catheter inserted into space. When CXR shows fluid completely drained, talc slurry or bleomycin instilled (within 2hrs). Tube clamped for 90 min, than drained for 2hrs before removal	Complete response in 48%, partial 31%, 21% failure
Hsu	1998	Prospective case series	26	Ultrasound guided insertion of small bore catheter. When fluid drained completely and lung re-expanded on CXR, bleomycin instilled. Catheter removed after 2 hrs	41% complete response, 36% partial, 23% failure 71% completed procedure in 2 days

Other surgical techniques

Pleurectomy

We found five papers. Four are retrospective case series [60-63] and one was a prospective study of 19 patients [64] reporting on pleurectomy as a means of palliating symptoms. These include a series of mesothelioma [63] and others in which tumour debulking and decortication were part of the procedure. Prolonged air leak is amongst the complications suggesting that tumour was removed from the visceral pleura. This falls outside palliative pleurodesis as intended in this review. Palliation of symptoms of the order of 85% to 100% was reported, but this form of surgery is much more major and should only be considered in patients considered to have a commensurately long expectation of life to justify it.

Shunts

We found four reports of retrospectively analysed case series of pleuroperitoneal shunts, usually used where the lung failed to expand fully after drainage of the effusion [65-68]. In one series, 160 of 360 patients referred with malignant effusion were managed by a pleuroperitoneal shunt with a 15% shunt complication rate [67]. The groups are not readily comparable because there was declared case selection. Trapped lung was managed by shunting when pleurodesis was expected to fail after inspection of the lung at VATS.

Trapped lung

The indication for an indwelling pleuroperitoneal shunt (Denver shunt) or a long-term drain, is if the lung will not expand because it is "trapped", that is to say held down in a non-inflated state by cancer or fibrin peel. Two retrospective studies have looked at the consequences and outcome of this condition [69,70]. The evidence was that this was a stable tolerated state. In the absence of a control group, no strong claim can be made for benefit.

Diagnostic techniques

Biochemical characteristics of the effusion

Much has been made of various chemical characteristics of effusion in making the diagnosis of the underlying cause. These include protein content, glucose, pH, and LDH which are included in Light's criteria for distinguishing exudates from transudates [71]. In general, transudates (low protein) are associated with heart failure and hypoalbuminaemia, while exudates (high protein) are characteristic of infection. Most malignant effusions are intermediate in protein content and highly variable in other respects. The diagnosis hinges on the clinical context, cytology of the effusion and histology of the pleura. The chemical characteristics of the fluid are of little diagnostic value, if the question being asked is simply whether or not the effusion is malignant.

Diagnostic yield by cytology and various techniques of pleural biopsies

Many studies report on pathological diagnostic yield because the management of pleural effusion may hinge on being certain that it is a manifestation of disseminated malignancy. Cytology of the effusion may clinch the diagnosis in up to 46% of patients [72], but up to a 86% yield was reported in one series with repeated sampling [73]. VATS allows the direct visualisation of the pleura and is the most specific method for pleural involvement. In the absence of a prior diagnosis, it may be chosen for that reason alone with pleurodesis being an adjunct, rather than being preferred as a means of pleurodesis in its own right. Furthermore, in some instances (breast in particular), the effusion and the pleura are free of cancer. The lesion creating an effusion is usually lymphatic obstruction in the mediastinum.

Predictors of outcome and survival

Predictors of technical success

Researchers have sought to find features of the effusion, in particular biochemical characteristics which might determine success or failure. Many have measured pleural pH and although some have found a difference, the overall conclusion is that it is not predictive. Elastance was suggested as a means of detecting trapped lung [74], but it has not been adopted in other reports.

Predictors of survival after pleurodesis

The value of a palliative intervention is in part determined by how long the patient has left to live. Probably the single biggest determinant of survival is likely to be the underlying pathology. Analysis of pleural biochemistry may be a determinant in that low pH and low glucose are believed to reflect tumour activity and therefore, bulk. There is some evidence for this belief [75,76].

Tumour types

Cancers of the breast, lung, pleura and ovary feature most numerously in clinical series of malignant pleural effusion. Results of pleurodesis vary, but effusions due to breast cancer appear to have better rates of success than lung cancer [77], especially if the lung is trapped, for example by a central tumour obstructing the bronchus. Many reports are an unreliable source of information for likely survival by disease, but median survival times measured in months for lung cancer [78] and into years for breast cancer [77,79], are characteristic of the known expectation of life for these diseases. Since the benefit of a palliative pleurodesis is the product of the degree of benefit and the length for which that benefit is appreciated, knowledge of life expectancy might be a deciding factor in deciding whether an intervention is justified.

Conclusions

There was only one previous systematic review which captured literature up to 1992 [4] and now a Cochrane review [5]. The headline conclusion, that talc is the most effective and cheapest agent, is the same as ours. The evidence then and now is that bleomycin is less effective than either talc or tetracycline and considerably more expensive. Nevertheless, we know it is still in clinical use and included in a research protocol reporting in 2003. On the evidence we could make a firm recommendation that talc is the agent of choice, whichever technical procedure is employed.

Case reports have attributed pneumonitis to talc. There is also some evidence on the variability in particle size [80] and it is postulated that it might be the cause of the variable clinical reporting of pneumonitis. We found 36 cases of pneumonitis following talc pleurodesis in the literature from case reports and retrospective case series. In patients with malignant disease and lungs collapsed due to effusion, the cause and effect relationship is unconvincing. In a small randomised trial of 19 patients, Maskell *et al* studied ^{99m}Tc-DTPA lung clearance (a sensitive marker of lung inflammation) in the contralateral lung and found a significant difference between talc and tetracycline, suggesting a greater systemic inflammatory response with talc [81]. There was also a higher rise in CRP and a greater fall in oxygen saturation in the patients who received talc slurry. None of these patients developed respiratory failure. Perhaps the success of talc as a sclerosant is attributed to the greater inflammatory response it induces. It should be noted that there were many patients in prospective studies, randomised and non-randomised, about 1000 patients in the UK have the procedure in surgical hands, and we perform this procedure in 120 patients a year. We are inclined to reject these alerts in the face of the volume of evidence to the safety of talc. For the large proportion of patients who benefit from the procedure, we advocate talc as the agent of choice.

Where compared directly one with the other, VATS had a marginal advantage over bedside techniques, but with increased cost implications. We would comment that the patients included in these RCTs were selected patients without a trapped lung, giving the best opportunity for success. Furthermore, the bedside pleurodesis performed in these studies was to a specific protocol within a formal study. VATS is likely to be performed in a well controlled environment, whereas we would speculate that in clinical practice the bedside techniques tend to be performed on a more *ad hoc* basis. If a recommendation were based on this evidence, the standard of administration of the bedside technique would have to be maintained to trials standard.

An interesting finding is that the belief that rolling the patient about the bed has an important benefit in dispersing talc, can be rejected on good evidence. Beyond that, the evidence found in the review is of diminishing quality as we progress through the evidence tables.

Recommendations	**Evidence level**
◆ Talc is the most effective agent.	Ia/A
◆ Within RCTs, VATS offers some advantage over bedside methods when talc is used.	Ia/A
◆ Early removal of the tube is as effective as protracted drainage.	Ib/A
◆ There is no advantage in rolling the patient to disperse the agent.	Ib/A
◆ The size of chest drain used does not alter outcome.	Ib/A

References

1. UK Thoracic Surgical Register. www.scts.org . 2004.
2. Tan C, Swift S, Browne J, Treasure T. A systematic review of the evidence for management of malignant pleural effusion. IN DRAFT FORM 2004.
3. Antunes G, Neville E, Duffy J, Ali N. BTS guidelines for the management of malignant pleural effusions. *Thorax* 2003; 58 Suppl 2: ii29-ii38.
4. Walker-Renard PB, Vaughan LM, Sahn SA. Chemical pleurodesis for malignant pleural effusions. *Ann Intern Med* 1994; 120: 56-64.
5. Shaw P, Agarwal R. Pleurodesis for malignant pleural effusions. *Cochrane Database Syst Rev* 2004; CD002916.
6. Mejer J, Mortensen KM, Hansen HH. Mepacrine hydrochloride in the treatment of malignant pleural effusion. A controlled randomized trial. *Scand J Respir Dis* 1977; 58: 319-23.
7. Putnam JB Jr., Light RW, Rodriguez RM, Ponn R, Olak J, Pollak JS, *et al.* A randomized comparison of indwelling pleural catheter and doxycycline pleurodesis in the management of malignant pleural effusions. *Cancer* 1999; 86: 1992-9.
8. North SA, Au HJ, Halls SB, Tkachuk L, Mackey JR. A randomized, phase III, double-blind, placebo-controlled trial of intrapleural instillation of methylprednisolone acetate in the management of malignant pleural effusion. *Chest* 2003; 123: 822-7.
9. Zaloznik AJ, Oswald SG, Langin M. Intrapleural tetracycline in malignant pleural effusions. A randomised study. *Cancer* 1983; 51: 752-5.
10. Groth G, Gatzemeier U, Haussingen K, Heckmayr M, Magnussen H, Neuhauss R, *et al.* Intrapleural palliative treatment of malignant pleural effusions with mitoxantrone versus placebo (pleural tube alone). *Ann Oncol* 1991; 2: 213-5.
11. Sorensen PG, Svendsen TL, Enk B. Treatment of malignant pleural effusion with drainage, with and without instillation of talc. *Eur J Respir Dis* 1984; 65: 131-5.
12. Leverenz A, Heckmayr M, Tischer-Neuhauss R, Gatzemeier U. Intrapleural palliative treatment of malignant pleural effusions with talcum versus placebo (pleural tube alone). *Lung Cancer* 2000; 29A: 274.
13. Diacon AH, Wyser C, Bolliger CT, Tamm M, Pless M, Perruchoud AP, *et al.* Prospective randomized comparison of thoracoscopic talc poudrage under local anesthesia versus bleomycin instillation for pleurodesis in malignant pleural effusions. *Am J Respir Crit Care Med* 2000; 162: 1445-9.
14. Haddad FJ, Younes RN, Gross JL, Deheinzelin D, Suzuki I. Prospective randomised trial of pleurodesis with talc slurry versus bleomycin in patients with symptomatic malignant pleural effusions. *Am J Respir Crit Care Med* 2001; 163(5 Suppl), A901.
15. Ong KC, Indumathi V, Raghuram J, Ong YY. A comparative study of pleurodesis using talc slurry and bleomycin in the management of malignant pleural effusions. *Respirology* 2000; 5: 99-103.
16. Zimmer PW, Hill M, Casey K, Harvey E, Low DE. Prospective randomized trial of talc slurry vs bleomycin in pleurodesis for symptomatic malignant pleural effusions. *Chest* 1997; 112: 430-4.
17. Noppen M, Degreve J, Mignolet M, Vincken W. A prospective, randomised study comparing the efficacy of talc slurry and bleomycin in the treatment of malignant pleural effusions. *Acta Clin Belg* 1997; 52: 258-62.
18. Lynch T, Kalish L, Mentzer SJ, Decamp M, Strauss G, Sugarbaker DJ. Optimal therapy of malignant pleural effusions: Report of a randomised trial of bleomycin, tetracycline, and talc and a meta-analysis. *Int J Oncol* 1996; 8: 183-90.
19. Hamed H, Fentiman IS, Chaudary MA, Rubens RD. Comparison of intracavitary bleomycin and talc for control of pleural effusions secondary to carcinoma of the breast. *Br J Surg* 1989; 76: 1266-7.
20. Fentiman IS, Rubens RD, Hayward JL. Control of pleural effusions in patients with breast cancer. A randomized trial. *Cancer* 1983; 52: 737-9.
21. Fentiman IS, Rubens RD, Hayward JL. A comparison of intracavitary talc and tetracycline for the control of pleural effusions secondary to breast cancer. *Eur J Cancer Clin Onc* 1986; 22: 1079-81.
22. Nio Y, Nagami H, Tamura K, Tsubono M, Nio M, Sato M, *et al.* Multi-institutional randomized clinical study on the comparative effects of intracavital chemotherapy alone versus immunotherapy alone versus immunochemotherapy for malignant effusion. *Br J Cancer* 1999; 80: 775-85.
23. Patz EF, Jr., McAdams HP, Erasmus JJ, Goodman PC, Culhane DK, Gilkeson RC, *et al.* Sclerotherapy for malignant pleural effusions: a prospective randomized trial of bleomycin vs doxycycline with small-bore catheter drainage. *Chest* 1998; 113: 1305-11.
24. Sartori S, Trevisani L, Neilsen I, Tassinari D, Abbasciano V. Intracavitary bleomycin versus interferon in the management of malignant pleural effusions. *Chest* 1998;113:1145.
25. Tattersall M, Fox R, Woods R, Kefford R. Intracavitary adriamycin nitrogen mustard and tetracycline in the control of malignant effusions: a randomised study. *Medical Journal of Australia* 1980; 2: 447-8.
26. Kessinger A, Wigton RS. Intracavitary bleomycin and tetracycline in the management of malignant pleural effusions: A randomised study. *J Surg Oncol* 1987; 36: 81-3.
27. Emad A, Rezaian GR. Treatment of malignant pleural effusions with a combination of bleomycin and tetracycline. A comparison of bleomycin or tetracycline alone versus a combination of bleomycin and tetracycline. *Cancer* 1996; 78: 2498-501.
28. Martinez-Moragon E, Aparicio J, Rogado MC, Sanchis J, Sanchis F, Gil-Suay V. Pleurodesis in malignant pleural effusions: a randomized study of tetracycline versus bleomycin. *Eur Respir J* 1997; 10: 2380-3.
29. Schmidt M, Schaarschmidt G, Chemaissani A. [Pleurodesis in malignant pleural effusion: bleomycin versus mitoxantrone.]. *Pneumologie* 1997; 51: 367-72.
30. Bjermer L, Gruber A, Sue-Chu M, Sandstrom T, Eksborg S, Henriksson R. Effects of intrapleural mitoxantrone and

mepacrine on malignant pleural effusion - a randomised study. *Eur J Cancer* 1995; 31A: 2203-8.
31. Salomaa E, Pulkki K, Helenius H. Pleurodesis with doxycycline or corynebacterium parvum in malignant pleural effusion. *Acta Oncologica* 1995; 34: 117-21.
32. Loutsidis A, Bellenis I, Argiriou M, Exarchos N. Tetracycline compared with mechlorethamine in the treatment of malignant pleural effusions. A randomized trial. *Respir Med* 1994; 88: 523-6.
33. Koldsland S, Svennevig JL, Lehne G, Johnson E. Chemical pleurodesis in malignant pleural effusions: a randomised prospective study of mepacrine versus bleomycin. *Thorax* 1993; 48: 790-3.
34. Ruckdeschel JC, Moores D, Lee JY, Einhorn LH, Mandelbaum I, Koeller J, *et al.* Intrapleural therapy for malignant pleural effusions. A randomized comparison of bleomycin and tetracycline. *Chest* 1991; 100: 1528-35.
35. Masuno T, Kishimoto S, Ogura T, Honma T, Niitani H, Fukuoka M, *et al.* A comparative trial of LC9018 plus doxorubicin and doxorubicin alone for the treatment of malignant pleural effusion secondary to lung cancer. *Cancer* 1991; 68: 1495-500.
36. Luh KT, Yang PC, Kuo SH, Chang DB, Yu CJ, Lee LN. Comparison of OK-432 and mitomycin C pleurodesis for malignant pleural effusion caused by lung cancer. A randomized trial. *Cancer* 1992; 69: 674-9.
37. Gust R, Kleine P, Fabel H. [Fibrin glue and tetracycline pleurodesis in recurrent malignant pleural effusions. A randomized comparative study]. *Med Klin* 1990; 85: 18-23.
38. Hillerdal G, Kiviloog J, Nou E, Steinholtz L. Corynebacterium parvum in malignant pleural effusion. A randomized prospective study. *Eur J Respir Dis* 1986; 69: 204-6.
39. Leahy BC, Honeybourne D, Brear SG, Carroll KB, Thatcher N, Stretton TB. Treatment of malignant pleural effusions with intrapleural Corynebacterium parvum or tetracycline. *Eur J Respir Dis* 1985; 66: 50-4.
40. Bayly T, Kisner DL, Sybert A, MacDonald JS, Tsou E, Schein PS. Tetracycline and quinacrine in the control of malignant pleural effusions. A randomised trial. *Cancer* 1978; 41: 1188-92.
41. Won SO, Choi J, Yong SK, Yong HD, Tae WJ, Mann HJ. Intrapleural doxycycline and bleomycin in the management of malignant pleural effusions: a randomised study. *Tuberculosis and Respiratory Diseases* 1997; 44: 85-92.
42. Ostrowski MJ, Priestman TJ, Houston RF, Martin WMC. A randomised trial of intracavitary bleomycin and corynebacterium parvum in the control of malignant pleural effusions. *Radiotherapy and Oncology* 1989; 14: 19-26.
43. Yim AP, Chan AT, Lee TW, Wan IY, Ho JK. Thoracoscopic talc insufflation versus talc slurry for symptomatic malignant pleural effusion. *Ann Thorac Surg* 1996; 62: 1655-8.
44. Manes N, Rodriguez-Panadero F, Bravo JL, Hernandez H, Alix A. Talc pleurodesis. Prospective and randomised study. Clinical Follow-up. *Chest* 2000; 118(4):131S.
45. Evans TR, Stein RC, Pepper JR, Gazet JC, Ford HT, Coombes RC. A randomised prospective trial of surgical against medical tetracycline pleurodesis in the management of malignant pleural effusions secondary to breast cancer. *Eur J Cancer* 1993; 29A: 316-9.
46. Aelony Y, King R, Boutin C. Thoracoscopic talc poudrage pleurodesis for chronic recurrent pleural effusions. *Ann Intern Med* 1991; 115: 778-82.
47. Jacobi CA, Wenger FA, Schmitz-Rixen T, Muller JM. Talc pleurodesis in recurrent pleural effusions. *Langenbecks Arch Surg* 1998; 383: 156-9.
48. Kennedy L, Rusch VW, Strange C, Ginsberg RJ, Sahn SA. Pleurodesis using talc slurry. *Chest* 1994; 106: 342-6.
49. Matsuzaki Y, Shibata K, Yoshioka M, Inoue M, Sekiya R, Onitsuka T, *et al.* Intrapleural perfusion hyperthermo-chemotherapy for malignant pleural dissemination and effusion. *Ann Thorac Surg* 1995; 59: 127-31.
50. Dryzer SR, Allen ML, Strange C, Sahn SA. A comparison of rotation and non-rotation in tetracycline pleurodesis. *Chest* 1993; 104: 1763-6.
51. Mager HJ, Maesen B, Verzijlbergen F, Schramel F. Distribution of talc suspension during treatment of malignant pleural effusion with talc pleurodesis. *Lung Cancer* 2002; 36: 77-81.
52. Baas P, Neijens VH, Olmos RA, Hoefnagel CA. Distribution of 99mTc colloid in the thoracic cavity of patients with malignant pleural effusions. *Lung Cancer* 1997; 17: 239-47.
53. Clementsen P, Evald T, Grode G, Hansen M, Krag JG, Faurschou P. Treatment of malignant pleural effusion: pleurodesis using a small percutaneous catheter. A prospective randomized study. *Respir Med* 1998; 92: 593-6.
54. Chen YM, Shih JF, Yang KY, Lee YC, Perng RP. Usefulness of pig-tail catheter for palliative drainage of malignant pleural effusions in cancer patients. *Support Care Cancer* 2000; 8: 423-6.
55. Pollak JS, Burdge CM, Rosenblatt M, Houston JP, Hwu WJ, Murren J. Treatment of malignant pleural effusions with tunneled long-term drainage catheters. *J Vasc Interv Radiol* 2001; 12: 201-8.
56. Villanueva AG, Gray AW, Jr., Shahian DM, Williamson WA, Beamis JF, Jr. Efficacy of short-term versus long-term tube thoracostomy drainage before tetracycline pleurodesis in the treatment of malignant pleural effusions. *Thorax* 1994; 49: 23-5.
57. Hsu WH, Chiang CD, Chen CY, Kwan PC, Hsu JY. Ultrasound-guided small-bore Elecath tube insertion for the rapid sclerotherapy of malignant pleural effusion. *Jpn J Clin Oncol* 1998; 28: 187-91.
58. Spiegler PA, Hurewitz AN, Groth ML. Rapid pleurodesis for malignant pleural effusions. *Chest* 2003; 123: 1895-8.
59. Davies CWH, Chapman S, Reza T, Thomas J. Efficacy of short (24 hours) versus longer (72 hours) chest drainage after talc pleurodesis for malignant pleural effusion. ERS. 2003.
60. Fry WA, Khandekar JD. Parietal pleurectomy for malignant pleural effusion. *Ann Surg Oncol* 1995; 2: 160-4.
61. Martini N, Bains MS, Beattie EJ, Jr. Indications for pleurectomy in malignant effusion. *Cancer* 1975; 35: 734-8.
62. Harvey JC, Erdman CB, Beattie EJ. Early experience with videothoracoscopic hydrodissection pleurectomy in the treatment of malignant pleural effusion. *J Surg Oncol* 1995; 59: 243-5.

63. Soysal O, Karaoglanoglu N, Demiracan S, Topcu S, Tastepe I, Kaya S, *et al.* Pleurectomy/decortication for palliation in malignant pleural mesothelioma: results of surgery. *Eur J Cardiothorac Surg* 1997; 11: 210-3.
64. Waller DA, Morritt GN, Forty J. Video-assisted thoracoscopic pleurectomy in the management of malignant pleural effusion. *Chest* 1995; 107: 1454-6.
65. Petrou M, Kaplan D, Goldstraw P. Management of recurrent malignant pleural effusions. The complementary role talc pleurodesis and pleuroperitoneal shunting. *Cancer* 1995; 75: 801-5.
66. Reich H, Beattie EJ, Harvey JC. Pleuroperitoneal shunt for malignant pleural effusions: a one-year experience. *Semin Surg Oncol* 1993; 9: 160-2.
67. Genc O, Petrou M, Ladas G, Goldstraw P. The long-term morbidity of pleuroperitoneal shunts in the management of recurrent malignant effusions. *Eur J Cardiothorac Surg* 2000; 18: 143-6.
68. Schulze M, Boehle AS, Kurdow R, Dohrmann P, Henne-Bruns D. Effective treatment of malignant pleural effusion by minimal invasive thoracic surgery: thoracoscopic talc pleurodesis and pleuroperitoneal shunts in 101 patients. *Ann Thorac Surg* 2001; 71: 1809-12.
69. Boland GW, Gazelle GS, Girard MJ, Mueller PR. Asymptomatic hydropneumothorax after therapeutic thoracentesis for malignant pleural effusions. *Am J Roentgenol* 1998 ;170: 943-6.
70. Chang YC, Patz EF, Jr., Goodman PC. Pneumothorax after small-bore catheter placement for malignant pleural effusions. *Am J Roentgenol* 1996; 166: 1049-51.
71. Light RW, Macgregor MI, Luchsinger PC, Ball WC, Jr. Pleural effusions: the diagnostic separation of transudates and exudates. *Ann Intern Med* 1972; 77: 507-13.
72. Canto A, Arnau A, Galbis J, Martin E, Guijarro R, Fernandez A, *et al.* [The so-called malignant pleural effusion: a new review of direct data obtained with diagnostic pleuroscopy]. *Arch Bronconeumol* 1996; 32: 453-8.
73. Sahn SA, Good JT, Jr. Pleural fluid pH in malignant effusions. Diagnostic, prognostic, and therapeutic implications. *Ann Intern Med* 1988; 108: 345-9.
74. Lan RS, Lo SK, Chuang ML, Yang CT, Tsao TC, Lee CH. Elastance of the pleural space: a predictor for the outcome of pleurodesis in patients with malignant pleural effusion. *Ann Intern Med* 1997; 126: 768-74.
75. Rodriguez-Panadero F, Lopez MJ. Low glucose and pH levels in malignant pleural effusions. Diagnostic significance and prognostic value in respect to pleurodesis. *Am Rev Respir Dis* 1989; 139: 663-7.
76. Rodriguez-Panadero F, Lopez-Mejias J. Survival time of patients with pleural metastatic carcinoma predicted by glucose and pH studies. *Chest* 1989; 95: 320-4.
77. Halasz L, Szentkereszty Z, Furka A, Kiss S, Kollar S. [Surgical treatment of pleural metastases in breast cancer]. *Magy Seb* 2002; 55: 265-7.
78. Werner-Wasik M, Scott C, Cox JD, Sause WT, Byhardt RW, Asbell S, *et al.* Recursive partitioning analysis of 1999 Radiation Therapy Oncology Group (RTOG) patients with locally-advanced non-small-cell lung cancer (LA-NSCLC): identification of five groups with different survival. *Int J Radiat Oncol Biol Phys* 2000; 48: 1475-82.
79. Uschinsky K, Kruger M, Hassler K, Engelmann C. [Thoracic surgery relevant indications for adjuvant and/or palliative measures in breast carcinoma]. *Zentralbl Chir* 1998; 123 Suppl 5: 122-4.
80. Ferrer J, Villarino MA, Tura JM, Traveria A, Light RW. Talc preparations used for pleurodesis vary markedly from one preparation to another. *Chest* 2001; 119: 1901-5.
81. Maskell N, Gleeson F, Jones E, Davies R. Talc but not tetracycline pleurodesis induces hypoxaemia and increased DTPA clearance from the contralateral lung. *Am J Resp & Crit Care Med* 2002; 165: B11-B12.

Chapter 13

Surgical treatment of thoracic empyema

Ani C Anyanwu MD MSc FRCS
Specialist Registrar, Cardiothoracic Surgery [1]
Parag Jaiswal MRCS
Senior House Officer, Cardiothoracic Surgery [2]
Tom Treasure MD MS FRCS
Professor of Cardiothoracic Surgery [2]

1 Harefield Hospital, Harefield, Middlesex, UK
2 Guy's and St Thomas' Hospitals, London, UK

Introduction

Empyema thoracis is one of the earliest thoracic diseases to be described and successfully treated; indeed, the principles of treatment were first outlined by Hippocrates and other Greek physicians. Hippocrates is said to have taught drainage by rib trephination [1], but apparently his teaching and understanding of the importance of drainage was forgotten. Surprisingly, there is no consensus on treatment of empyema, with wide variation in opinion between thoracic surgeons and physicians, and, amongst thoracic surgeons, a wide range of practice (Figure 1). Our task in this chapter is to reflect the published evidence, such as it is.

Empyema is the collection of purulent fluid in the pleural cavity and usually occurs secondary to pneumonia, but is also a consequence of infection introduced by trauma or medical interventions of any type including needle aspiration, tube drainage or surgery. In contemporary medical parlance, the term empyema is used for any pleural collection which is deemed to be infected. The criteria in medical texts are that there are "organisms in the fluid, an increase in polymorphs and a fall in pH and glucose" [2]. A more surgical definition of empyema is based on the macroscopic pathological appearance of frank pus with grossly thickened visceral and parietal pleura, which may eventually heal by fibrosis [3]. The thickening is due to inflammation and the deposition of fibrin and it is this layer on top of the normally very thin visceral pleura which is the "cortex" in the operation of decortication. This clarification is important because any form of open drainage depends on the development of this thickness of the visceral layer and its adhesion to the parietal layer. In the pre-antibiotic era, when open drainage was the norm, one of the methods used was to take daily aspirates to ensure that the pus was thickening as an indication of the pleural thickening [4] (Figure 2). Only when the pus was sufficiently thickened could drainage be undertaken as this was an indication that "the lung would hold up" and that the patient would not die from total collapse of the lung and paradoxical movement of the mediastinum [5].

Empyema as seen by thoracic surgeons, is the final common end-point of any contaminated pleural effusion or haemothorax, whether the infection is introduced by nature (as part of the original process as in para- or synpneumonic effusion complicating

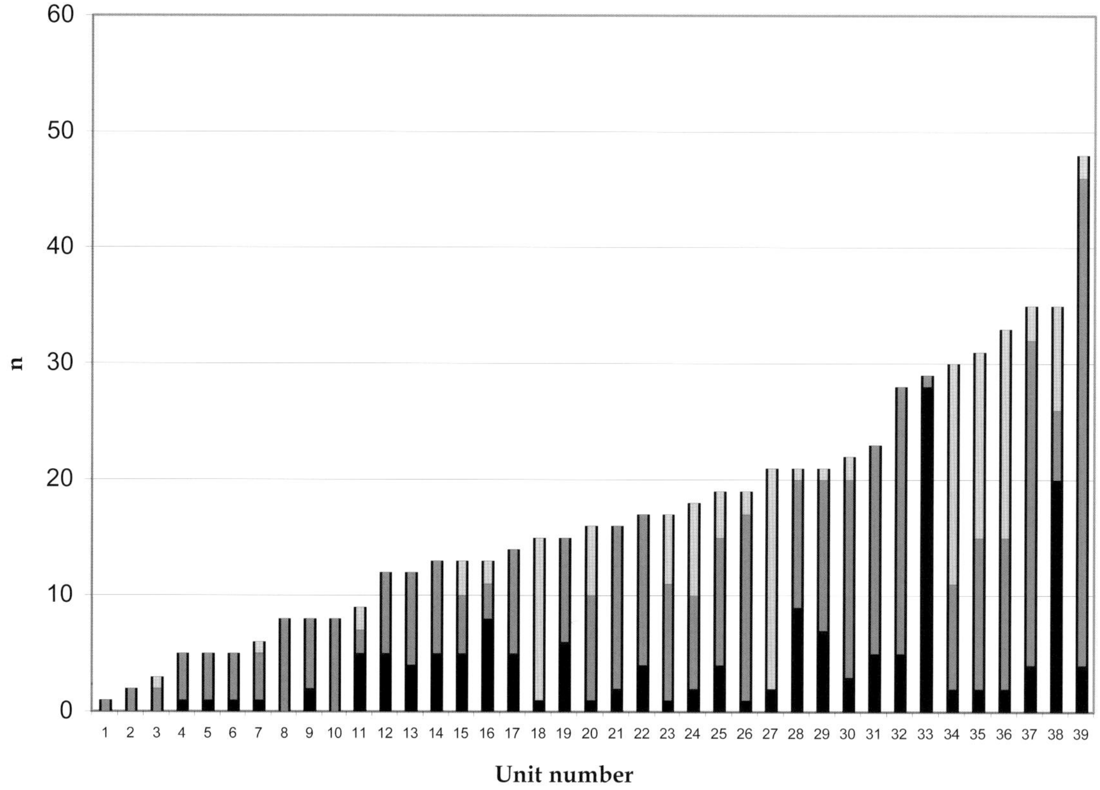

Figure 1. **Operations for empyema reported to a national registry in 2001/02 by 39 thoracic surgical units in the United Kingdom and Ireland. Black columns (below) - rib resections, dark grey (middle) - decortication, and pale grey (above) - video-assisted thoracoscopy. The predominant operation used to treat empyema varies from centre to centre. Source: *Society of Cardiothoracic Surgeons of Great Britain and Ireland Thoracic Surgical Register.* * The units are ranked by total annual caseload for clarity.**

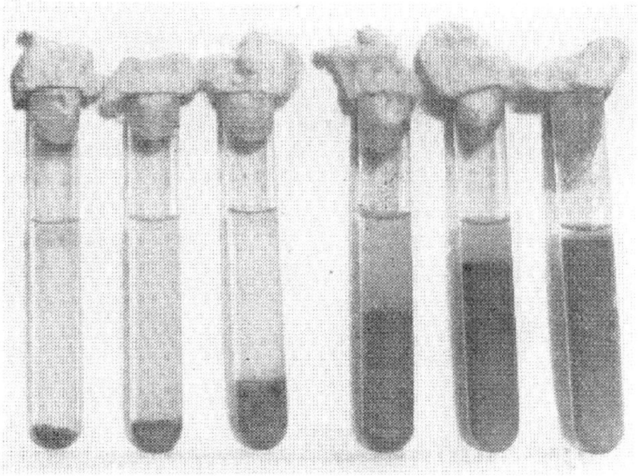

Figure 2. **Illustration of solid matter increasing as a proportion of daily aspirates of pus from an empyema [4].**

streptococcal pneumonia), trauma (for example on the assailant's knife) or iatrogenically, following drainage or surgery. It is this common end-stage of empyema with established pus, a fibrinous or fibrous cortex, and parietal pleural thickening, that is usually seen in thoracic surgical practice. In this chapter we confine ourselves to the evidence on the management of "surgical" empyema and focus primarily on post-pneumonic empyema (that is complicating bacterial pneumonia), which is the predominant aetiology in the current era. See later under "classification of empyema" for a more detailed consideration of these distinctions. Experience in management of other forms of empyema such as tuberculous, post-traumatic and post-surgical, is more limited as is the available evidence.

Table 1. Characteristics of identified studies.

First author	Location, year of study	Study type	N	N treated with surgery	Surgical treatments	Level of evidence
Angelillo-Mackinlay [14]	Buenos Aires, Argentina, Argentina, 1985-96	Prospective with historical controls	86	86	Decortication (33) VATS (53)	III
Cassina [15]	Zurich, Switzerland, 1993-6	Retrospective case series	45	45	VATS (45)	IV
De Souza [16]	Denver, US, 1993-8	Retrospective case series	58	19	Decortication (19)	IV
Ferguson [17]	Multicentre, UK, 1986-90	Prospective cohort	119	52	Rib resection (24) Decortiation (28)	III
Forty [18]	Cambridge, UK, 1985-89	Retrospective case series	53	53	Rib resection (6) Decortication (47)	IV
Galea [19]	Nottingham, UK, 1987-92	Retrospective case series	107	72	Rib resection (50) Decortication (22)	III
Lawrence [11]	Harefield, UK, 1993-6	Retrospective case series	44	44	VATS (42) Decortication (2)	IV
LeMense [20]	Charleston, US, 1989-93	Retrospective case series	43	23	Decortication (21) Eloesser flap (2)	IV
Mandal [21]	Los Angeles, US, 1973-1997	Prospective cohort	179	76	Decortication (76)	IV
Striffeler [12]	Bern, Switzerland, 1992-6	Retrospective case series	67	67	VATS (67)	IV
Thourani [6]	Atlanta, US, 1975-2001	Retrospective case series	78	78	Eloesser flap (78)	IV
Thourani [22]	Atlanta, US, 1990-7	Retrospective case series	77	29	Decortication (17) Eloesser flap (8) Muscle interposition (4)	IV
Waller [13]	Leicester, UK, 1990s	Prospective with historical control	48	48	Decortication (12) VATS (36)	III

Methodology

Although a relatively common surgical disease, there are few large series in the literature on the surgical management of empyema. We searched MEDLINE (search term "empyema") for the years 1988 to 2003 seeking original articles on empyema that included a cohort of 40 or more patients. We chose not to consider papers before 1988 because at this time video-assisted thoracoscopic treatment of empyema had not been widely introduced. We excluded papers which exclusively considered non-surgical approaches to management and also those that predominantly dealt with restricted empyema subgroups such as tuberculous or post-surgical. To be included, papers must have presented data on at least one of two chosen outcomes (mortality and freedom from further interventions) on a minimum of 15 patients undergoing a surgical technique. Thirteen papers fulfilled our criteria for inclusion: three prospective cohort studies and ten retrospective case series. Only two papers directly compared different surgical techniques. We did not identify any randomised trials. Studies are detailed in Table 1. For most of the studies, patients treated with a given surgical technique were few (<30) and the study period spanned several years.

Surgical methods for treating empyema

Principal methods identified in the literature were:-

- Video-assisted thoracic surgery (VATS).
- Rib resection techniques (including a modification of the Eloesser flap [6]).
- Thoracotomy and decortication.

There were some small series or case reports of other surgical approaches in the literature, but none of these contained a sufficient number of patients to allow meaningful deduction. Some papers have compared surgery with tube thoracostomy. Tube thoracostomy is usually undertaken in a non-surgical setting and does not typically feature as a surgical alternative for empyema management (see below).

Classification of empyema

In understanding the various approaches to treating empyema, the natural history of the disease has to be understood. Empyema is a spectrum from thin fluid, with a mobile lung, where empyema is defined on the basis of pus cells in a pleural effusion [2], to well developed chronic fibrous inflammation [3]. Most authorities recognise classification of empyema into three groups:-

- Exudative. Thin fluid with white cells on microscopy. Lung re-expands when drained.
- Fibrinopurulent. Deposition of fibrin strands with fluid loculation. Lung will expand if most fluid pockets can be drained, and loculi and adhesions broken down.
- Organising or chronic empyema. Thick exudates with formation of a thick rind over visceral pleura preventing lung expansion.

Classification often relies on radiological demonstration of loculations or visceral peel. Although this classification is commonly used, in practice, the presentation is not always clear-cut and the differentiation between the fibrinopurulent and organising stage is often made at surgery.

Outcomes

For the purpose of this chapter, the primary outcome of interest for surgical treatment is resolution of empyema. Most authors have defined this by the absence of further intervention. Also important is treatment (or disease) associated mortality and duration of treatment (i.e. of hospitalisation). Quality of life (QoL) would be the ideal method of measuring the outcome of empyema treatment (as different treatment methods have implications for both short and long-term quality of life). We found no studies that included formal QoL data.

Results

As most studies were retrospective, patients were defined by the treatment they received and not by the stage of the empyema. Any series of patients undergoing a specified surgical approach could have included patients in two or more stages of empyema. It was therefore, often not possible to definitively delineate the effect of a given treatment on different stages of empyema. For simplicity, we have presented the results by empyema stage and made assumptions that patient treatments were indeed defined by their stage of disease.

Exudative empyema

Most workers would agree that surgery is not indicated in this stage of the disease. The treatment for this condition is non-operative and includes antibiotic therapy, needle aspiration, radiologically guided catheter drainage, and tube thoracostomy. Fibrinolysis offers no advantage [7]. Some exudative empyemas may go on to require surgery if they progress to a fibropurulent stage, despite initial treatment.

Fibrinopurulent empyema

Treatment options for this stage of empyema include tube thoracostomy, VATS, rib resection, and thoracotomy with decortication.

Tube thoracostomy

As initial management of empyema is often undertaken by chest physicians, it is likely that most patients would have undergone initial non-operative management prior to surgical referral. We have therefore, assumed that surgery is considered only after first-line treatment has failed. However, occasionally, patients already in a fibrinopurulent stage, may present to surgeons having had no prior attempts at drainage, or where prior drainage was ineffective or inadequate. In such cases, initial tube thoracostomy by the thoracic surgeon may be a reasonable option.

In a systematic review of empyema treatment, Colice and colleagues reviewed outcomes from 13 studies in which tube thoracostomy was the primary treatment for empyema and found that 40% failed treatment and required further intervention [8]. If tube thoracostomy is undertaken as a primary measure by a thoracic surgeon then this failure rate should be borne in mind. Tube thoracostomy should therefore, only be undertaken in the surgical setting if the radiology is favourable and should not unnecessarily delay definitive surgery.

VATS as an initial management may have a role in primary treatment of empyema (as an alternative to initial tube thoracostomy) as it provides superior drainage in loculated empyema. The superiority of VATS over thoracostomy for drainage of multi-loculated empyema has to be balanced against the necessity for general anaesthesia, the morbidity of VATS, and the effectiveness (in over 50% of cases) of thoracostomy as primary treatment in empyema. Although one group has undertaken a randomised trial comparing VATS with thoracostomy and fibrinolysis as primary treatment for empyema [9], their study included only 20 patients, limiting useful generalisation. The use of VATS as primary treatment for empyema (in lieu of thoracostomy) cannot currently be recommended as there is absence of robust supporting data in the literature.

Choice of surgical treatment

We have assumed that tube thoracostomy has been previously undertaken or is not a viable option. Table 2 summarises data on alternative approaches to surgical management of fibrinopurulent empyema.

Rib resection

Rib resection is the oldest of the available techniques for treating empyema. It is well described by Paget in 1896 [10] as a form of open drainage. For it to be done safely, the lung had to be already widely adherent so that it would "hold up". Those constraints do not apply in an era of general anaesthesia with positive pressure ventilation and a sealed underwater or vacuum drainage system, so rib resection is now also applied to earlier "less mature" stages of empyema. It is less invasive than a standard thoracotomy and has an advantage that it may be applied to very sick patients who cannot tolerate a prolonged operation as required for the VATS and thoracotomy approaches. The literature suggests that rib resection leads to successful resolution of empyema in over 90% of patients in whom it is applied (Table 2). However, although the results may seem comparable to that of thoracotomy and decortication, it is likely that series reporting the latter, reflect a more advanced stage of disease. Rib resection in the hands of thoracic surgeons is recommended for surgical treatment of fibrinopurulent empyema and is effective for the majority of patients.

Video-assisted thoracic surgery

Video-assisted thoracic surgery successfully treats empyema in about 75% of patients to which it is applied (Table 2). However, a quarter of patients who undergo VATS empyema drainage will go on to require further surgery (usually thoracotomy and decortication) at either the same setting or at a future date. Based on the confidence intervals (see Table 2), it seems likely that VATS has the lowest cure rate of the three surgical approaches, if applied to all patients regardless of stage. However, considering that VATS is successful in three-quarters of patients, it is a viable option to open decortication, as it can help avoid thoracotomy. Some surgeons do a preliminary thoracoscopy prior to planned open

Table 2. **Outcome of empyema treatment for the three surgical techniques.**

First author							
Technique	**N**	**Deaths**	**%**	**Failures^**	**%**	**Hospital Stay* (days)**	**Chest drain* (days)**
VATS							
Angelillo-Mackinlay [14]	53	1	2	3	6	10.6	4.3
Cassina [15]	45	0	0	8	18	10.7	7.1
Lawrence [11]	42	0	0	12	29	NA	NA
Striffeler [12]	67	3	4	19	28	12.3	4.1
Waller [13]	36	2	6	15	42	NA	NA
All studies	**243**	**6**	**2.5**	**57**	**23.5**		
95% CI			**0.1-5.3**		**18.3-28.8**		
Rib resection							
Ferguson [17]	24	2	8	2	8	11 median	NA
Galea [19]	50	7	14	2	4	21	NA
Thourani [6]#	78	4	5	0	0	16	NA
All studies	**152**	**13**	**8.6**	**4**	**2.6**		
95% CI			**4.6-14.2**		**0.1-6.6**		
Thoracotomy and decortication							
Angelillo-Mackinlay [14]	33	1	3	4	12	11.6	6.1
De Souza [16]	19	NA	0	1	5	17.9	11.0
Ferguson [17]	28	0	0	NA	NA	12 median	NA
Forty [18]	47	5	11	3	6	13 median	7 median
Galea [19]	22	4	18	0	0	18.0	NA
LeMense [20]	22	0	0	1	5	19.3	NA
Mandal [21]	76	1	1.3	9	12	14.0	NA
Thourani [22]	17	1	6	NA	0	17.0	NA
All studies	**264**	**12**	**4.5**	**18**	**6.8**		
95% CI			**2.4-7.8**		**4.1-10.1**		

^ = Includes immediate (conversion to alternate technique) and subsequent re-intervention.
* = Mean unless otherwise stated.
# = Eloesser flap.
NA = Not available
CI = Confidence interval

decortication and if favourable, continue the procedure thoracoscopically. The main benefits of the VATS approach in this setting are possibly shorter duration of hospitalisation and shorter requirement for chest drainage. VATS is also perceived by some to be less invasive, more cosmetic, less painful and associated with less morbidity, when compared to thoracotomy*. Video-assisted thoracoscopy is a preferred alternative to routine thoracotomy for fibrinopurulent empyema. There are however, insufficient data to recommend this technique over rib resection.

Thoracotomy and decortication

Decortication is as effective as rib resection techniques in success rate for resolution of empyema and has the advantage that it is applicable to even advanced stages of disease. Thoracotomy allows pulmonary procedures (such as resection) or additional procedures to obliterate the empyema cavity if required and is the technique most likely to result in complete re-expansion of the lung. Decortication is superior to the VATS approach in terms of resolution of empyema, although it may have a higher mortality and morbidity. The higher mortality (Table 2) is probably largely a reflection of the severity of the disease, but may also reflect, to at least some degree, the invasiveness of the procedure. It is the most invasive surgical approach for empyema treatment, requiring a large thoracotomy, extensive tissue debridement, substantial blood loss, and inevitable and sometimes protracted air leak. For this reason, although thoracotomy is effective, it cannot be recommended for first-line treatment for most fibrinopurulent empyemas. Its use as primary treatment of fibrinopurulent empyema should probably be reserved for those cases where the other two approaches cannot be successfully applied. Decortication is the procedure of choice when previous surgery has failed to successfully treat empyema (except where previous surgery was decortication; in that instance, rib resection may also be applied).

* although widely perceived as benefits of VATS, these are not substantiated by randomised data.

Chronic organizing empyema

Thoracotomy and decortication is the treatment of choice for this stage of disease as lung expansion cannot otherwise be achieved. In some patients where lung expansion is thought unachievable, or thoracotomy thought to be risky, rib resection techniques may be applied. Some workers have systematically applied VATS to all empyemas and have found that VATS was futile where there was a fibrous peel on the lung and conversion to thoracotomy was necessary [11-13]. VATS is therefore, not recommended in advanced empyema, if there is formation of a fibrous peel.

Cost-effectiveness

Because of lack of data, recommendations based on cost-effectiveness cannot be made. No studies have compared the cost-effectiveness of the various surgical approaches. Although several workers have detailed durations of hospitalisation, these cannot be directly equated to resource consumption.

Risks

Available data in the literature do not allow any recommendations that incorporate the risks of the surgical approaches. Mortality was the only adverse event consistently recorded in the literature. As authors generally did not differentiate between deaths caused by the infective process and those directly related to surgical intervention, we could not usefully compare the mortality risk for the surgical approaches. Whilst some authors have used hospital stay as a surrogate for morbidity, this cannot be usefully relied upon, as factors other than morbidity, such as disease stage and surgical approach influence duration of hospitalisation.

Quality of papers

The majority of the papers we reviewed were retrospective and thus subject to various forms of bias and error. Of the 13 papers, seven indicated that they had reported a series of consecutive patients. Only six stated how they had selected patients for a given surgical technique (and this was typically down to surgeon preference). Nine papers did not give any information on patients who presented in the same period who were not treated surgically. Only three papers reported that they had actively followed-up patients for outcomes. No papers provided details of previous treatment prior to surgery, and none provided sufficient information on patient characteristics and stage of empyema. Finally, no authors defined their criteria for performing rescue therapy (i.e. the stage at which it was accepted that surgery had failed and re-intervention was required). Re-intervention was itself undefined and it is not clear what this entailed, for example whether this encompassed all interventions including new tube thoracostomy. The final points are particularly important as most papers defined successful surgical treatment as freedom from re-intervention. Overall, the studies are not sufficiently robust and while they represent the best available evidence, they cannot be regarded as definitive evidence.

Conclusions

Despite centuries of interest in empyema, it remains one of the most understudied surgical diseases. We were unable to identify any level I studies, or level II studies of sufficient quality. The lack of good quality studies probably reflects in part the heterogeneity of the disease and the presentation of patients in varying stages of the disease. Additionally, as initial treatment is often undertaken by chest physicians, patients have often been subjected to weeks of unsuccessful intervention, the nature, degree and duration of which, is varied depending on local practice and physician preference. For similar reasons, the non-randomised case series on which this chapter is based, are subject to flaws and largely reflect the local practice and preferences of the authors' hospitals. Heterogeneity may be partly overcome by large numbers, but few workers have accumulated sufficient numbers to allow meaningful analysis. These limitations restrict the strength of our recommendations and are reflected in the variation of practice shown in Figure 1. There are not sufficient published data to define which patients would be more likely to benefit from one treatment method over another. Until more robust data are available, it remains likely that surgeon preference will remain the overriding factor in the choice of approach to surgical management of empyema.

Recommendations	Evidence level
◆ Exudative empyema should be treated medically by aspiration or tube thoracostomy.	III/B
◆ Fibrinopurulent empyema is most successfully treated surgically.	IV/C
◆ Rib resection provides an effective cure for the majority of fibrinopurulent empyemas.	III/B
◆ VATS can effectivley treat 75% of empyemas, but has a higher failure rate compared to rib resection.	III/B
◆ Thoractomy and decortication provides definitive treatment of empyema and is the treatment of choice for chronic empyemas and where earlier surgery has failed.	III/B

References

1. Hurt R. *The History of Cardiothoracic Surgery from Early Times*. Parthenon Publishing Group, Carnforth, Lancashire, UK, 1996.
2. Millard FJC, Pepper JR. Pleural disease. In: *Repiratory Medicine*. Brewis R, Corrin B, Geddes D, Gibson GJ, Eds. Saunders, London, 1995: 1554-79.
3. Barrett NR. The pleura: with special reference to fibrothorax. *Thorax* 1970; 25: 515-24.
4. Brock R. Some points in the treatment of empyema. *Guy's Hospital Gazette* 1933; December 9th: 1-18.
5. Brock R. Treatment of non-tuberculous empyema. *Proc R Soc Med* 1947; 40: 7-11.
6. Thourani VH, Lancaster RT, Mansour KA, Miller JI, Jr. Twenty-six years of experience with the modified eloesser flap. *Ann Thorac Surg* 2003; 76: 401-5.
7. Davies R, Maskell N, Nunn A. Primary result from the UK MRC/BTS randomised trial of streptokinase v placebo in pleural infection (the MRC/BTS MIST trial, ICTN 39138989). *In press*, 2004.
8. Colice GL, Curtis A, Deslauriers J, Heffner J, Light R, Littenberg B, *et al*. Medical and surgical treatment of parapneumonic effusions: an evidence-based guideline. *Chest* 2000; 118: 1158-71.
9. Wait MA, Sharma S, Hohn J, Dal Nogare A. A randomized trial of empyema therapy. *Chest* 1997; 111: 1548-51.
10. Paget S. *The Surgery of the Chest*. John Wright and Co, Bristol, 1896.
11. Lawrence DR, Ohri SK, Moxon RE, Townsend ER, Fountain SW. Thoracoscopic debridement of empyema thoracis. *Ann Thorac Surg* 1997; 64: 1448-50.
12. Striffeler H, Gugger M, Im H, V, Cerny A, Furrer M, Ris HB. Video-assisted thoracoscopic surgery for fibrinopurulent pleural empyema in 67 patients. *Ann Thorac Surg* 1998; 65: 319-23.
13. Waller DA,.Rengarajan A. Thoracoscopic decortication: a role for video-assisted surgery in chronic postpneumonic pleural empyema. *Ann Thorac Surg* 2001; 71: 1813-6.
14. Angelillo-Mackinlay T, Lyons GA, Piedras MB, Angelillo-Mackinlay D. Surgical treatment of postpneumonic empyema. *World J Surg* 1999; 23: 1110-3.
15. Cassina PC, Hauser M, Hillejan L, Greschuchna D, Stamatis G. Video-assisted thoracoscopy in the treatment of pleural empyema: stage-based management and outcome. *J Thorac Cardiovasc Surg* 1999; 117: 234-8.
16. De Souza A, Offner PJ, Moore EE, Biffl WL, Haenel JB, Franciose RJ, *et al*. Optimal management of complicated empyema. *Am J Surg* 2000; 180: 507-11.
17. Ferguson AD, Prescott RJ, Selkon JB, Watson D, Swinburn CR. The clinical course and management of thoracic empyema. *QJM* 1996; 89: 285-9.
18. Forty J, Yeatman M, Wells FC. Empyema thoracis: a review of a 41/2 year experience of cases requiring surgical treatment. *Respir Med* 1990; 84: 147-53.
19. Galea JL, De Souza A, Beggs D, Spyt T. The surgical management of empyema thoracis. *J R Coll Surg Edinb* 1997; 42: 15-8.
20. LeMense GP, Strange C, Sahn SA. Empyema thoracis. Therapeutic management and outcome. *Chest* 1995; 107: 1532-7.
21. Mandal AK, Thadepalli H, Mandal AK, Chettipally U. Outcome of primary empyema thoracis: therapeutic and microbiologic aspects. *Ann Thorac Surg* 1998; 66: 1782-6.
22. Thourani VH, Brady KM, Mansour KA, Miller JI, Jr., Lee RB. Evaluation of treatment modalities for thoracic empyema: a cost-effectiveness analysis. *Ann Thorac Surg* 1998; 66: 1121-7.

Chapter 14

Lung Volume Reduction Surgery (LVRS)

Donald C Whitaker FRCS (Ed)
Specialist Registrar, Cardiothoracic Surgery [1]
Robert J Cerfolio MD FACS
Associate Professor of Cardiothoracic Surgery [2]

1 Guy's and St Thomas' Hospitals, London, UK
2 University of Alabama, Birmingham, Alabama, USA

Introduction

Patients with diffuse, smoking-related, end-stage emphysema have a poor quality of life and reduced survival. The only treatment for these patients has been pulmonary rehabilitation combined with medical treatment. Lung volume reduction surgery (LVRS) and lung transplantation are the two main surgical options available to improve quality of life of patients with severe emphysema. This chapter examines the evidence to assess if LVRS leads to an improvement in the quality of life, survival and other outcome measures, when compared to continued medical therapy alone.

This chapter treats LVRS as a distinct entity from bullectomy. The initial work of Cooper [1] as well as subsequent randomised trials of LVRS discussed herein tend to exclude patients with simple giant bullae. However, there is now evidence that excising the more bullous areas of heterogeneous emphysema is beneficial, giving rise to potential confusion with bullectomy. It is possible that attempts are being made to "rebrand" bullectomy with the more fashionable term LVRS, but this should be resisted in order to avoid confusion. On the other hand it is possible that there is a genuine spectrum of pathological substrate between simple giant bullae and heterogeneous diffuse emphysema.

LVRS, also known as reduction pneumoplasty or partial pneumectomy, is a particularly interesting example of evidence collection. Although Brantigan [2] initially proposed the idea of reducing lung volume in emphysematous patients with hyperinflated lungs, in order to improve lung mechanics in 1957, his initial surgical results were poor and the technique did not become accepted. LVRS was re-introduced in the USA in 1993 by Cooper [1]. His initial series showed an 82% improvement in FEV1 following LVRS [1] in selected patents. After the presentation of several small case series in 1994 and 1995, there was a rapid and widespread adoption of the technique, especially in the USA. This occurred because retrospective, highly selected series showed a benefit favouring LVRS. However, as small centres began to perform LVRS, the morbidity, mortality and financial costs were high. Because of the large number of potential patients and the large expense associated with LVRS, Medicare (the main payer of medical care in the United States in patients older than 65 years) declined reimbursement for surgeons and hospitals for patients undergoing LVRS. They insisted that a large, prospective, randomised multi-institutional controlled trial (RCT) be performed in order to generate scientific proof that this operation was beneficial. Some American surgeons argued that the large number of case series that showed benefit with LVRS made RCTs, (in which half the patients would not receive LVRS) unethical. In contrast, a Cochrane [3] review in 1999 stated that there was insufficient evidence to support the use of LVRS outside a RCT. There is good evidence that LVRS is of definite benefit in properly selected patients for up to 24 months after surgery. Further study is needed to determine long-term benefits, to further refine selection criteria, to investigate mechanisms of improvement and establish which surgical approach and techniques are best.

Methodology

Pubmed 1996-2003 was searched with the term "lung volume reduction surgery". Of 458 articles returned, 213 were relevant. There were:-

- 133 original articles (6 reporting RCTs).
- 66 reviews/editorials.
- 14 letters.

Randomised controlled trials of LVRS versus medical therapy

Although there have been many case series published relating to LVRS, they comprise a low level of evidence and therefore, they will not be discussed in this chapter. Each case series can be evaluated on its merits, but there is always the cumulative effect of selection and publication bias. One should be extremely wary about making an evidence base of highly selected case series for any problem, especially without control groups. Moreover, it could be argued that it is the accompanying pulmonary rehabilitation that benefits the patients rather than the surgery itself. It is important to have a randomly assigned control group who receive the same intensive pulmonary rehabilitation, which is given to those patients who receive LVRS. This allows one to separate these two treatments. Most weight is therefore given to the following five RCTs [4-9] (the NETT trial is reported twice).

Inclusion criteria (Table 1) and surgical and medical treatments (Table 2) are first discussed with regard to all five studies. The outcomes are then discussed separately and in more detail, although a summary for comparison is given in Table 3.

Inclusion criteria

Table 1 shows that all studies had strict inclusion and exclusion criteria such that only between 17% (Goldstein) and 32% (NETT) of patients screened were actually included. Goldstein's study is the first RCT in which only patients with heterogeneous disease were enrolled as they were thought to be most likely to benefit and this accounts for their low inclusion rate. The authors of the NETT trial on the other hand state that an important goal of their study was to identify patient selection criteria for LVRS and so all patients who might benefit from LVRS were included, thus leading to a relatively higher inclusion rate. Although there is considerable variation in entry criteria between the studies, all have strictly defined quantitative definitions of hyperinflation of the lungs. Most exclude asthmatic patients, those with a high $PaCO_2$ or pulmonary artery pressure and also, those over 75 years of age or who have not stopped smoking.

Surgical and medical treatments

There is no uniformity of treatment in the five RCTs. Most include a period of pulmonary rehabilitation before randomisation, but Pompeo's study does not. The control medical treatment is not always detailed but in most cases, seems to be a mixture of physiotherapy and intensive medical therapy. A variety of surgical methods are detailed with some studies using exclusively VATS or median sternotomy approaches and others, a mixture of both. All use stapled resection of the lung with or without buttressing. It is interesting that although all the studies except that of Criner did not allow cross-over

Table 1. Randomised controlled trials entry criteria.

Name	Criner	Pompeo	Geddes	Goldstein	Fishman (NETT)
Date	1999	2000	2000	2003	2003
Screened	200	237	174	328	3777
n	37	60	48	55	1218
n/screened (%)	19	25	28	17	32
Dyspnoea	NYHA 3-4	Dyspnoea score>3	NA	NA	NA
Hyperinflation	FEV1<30% FRC or TLC>120%	FEV1<40% RV>180% TLC>120%	FEV1>500mls	FEV1<40% FEV1/FVC<0.7 TLC>120%	FEV1<45% RV>150% TLC>100%
Asthma/ Bronchitis	NA	No sputum, bronchiectasis or asthma	No asthma	No asthma	NA
Emphysema	Hyperinflation on CXR and diffuse bullous emphysema on HRCT	Diffuse bullous and non-bullous severe heterogeneous emphysema on HRCT	No isolated bullae, no restriction on pattern or distribution of emphysema	Heterogeneity of emphysema on CT or VQ scan	HRCT evidence of bilateral emphysema
Perfusion scan	Areas of decreased perfusion	NA	NA	NA	NA
Oxygenation	PaO_2/FiO_2<150	NA	O_2 use <18hrs/day	NA	Requiring <6L O_2 to maintain O_2 sats >90% with exercise
Ventilation	Self-ventilating	NA	NA	NA	NA
$PaCO_2$ (kPa)	NA	7.3	6	6.6	8
DLCO	NA	>20% pred	NA	NA	NA
Pulmonary pressure	Mean <35mmHg	Peak systolic <50mmHg	NA	Systolic <42mmHg Mean <35mmHg	NA
Weight (BMI)	<70% predicted	18-29	NA	NA	<31.1
Age (years)	NA	<75	<75	<75	NA
Psychology	Assessed	NA	NA	NA	NA
Smoking (x months cessation)	6	4	NA	6	4
Anaesthetic risk	NA	ASA </=3	NA	NA	Approval of anaesthetist sought
Other exclusions	Cardiovascular disease	Unstable angina Ventricular arrythmia Neoplasia with life expectancy <12 months	Previous thoracic surgery >10mg steroids per day	Previous thoracic surgery or pleural disease	Previous transplant, lobectomy, LVRS or median sternotomy >20mg steroids per day

NA = criteria not applied; NYHA = New York Heart Association dyspnoea score; FEV1 = forced expiratory volume in 1 second; FRC = functional residual capacity; TLC = total lung capacity; RV = residual volume; CXR = chest x-ray; CT = computed tomography; HRCT = high resolution computed tomography; VQ = ventilation perfusion.

Table 2. Surgical and medical treatments in the randomised controlled trials.

Name	Pre-randomisation treatment	Surgical treatment	Control medical treatment	Cross-over allowed?
Criner	8 weeks pulmonary rehabilitation for all patients	Bilateral LVRS via median sternotomy. Stapled resection of 20-40% of the volume of each lung	3 months pulm rehab	Yes, 13 of 18 patients in the medical arm crossed over after pulmonary rehab
Pompeo	No patients in the surgical arm had pre-operative pulmonary rehab	Unilateral or bilateral VATS Stapled resection of 20-30% lung vol	6 weeks pulm rehab	No
Geddes	All patients had intensive pulmonary rehabilitation before randomisation	Bilateral lung resection via VATS or median sternotomy Stapled resections were buttressed with bovine pericardium or fibrin glue	Continued medical treatment for 12 months	No, but 6 of 21 medical patients had surgery after the trial analysis
Goldstein	All patients had 6 weeks of rehabilitation	VATS mainly, some median sternotomies, 20-30% reduction in lung volume, bilateral where possible	Continued medical treatment for 12 months	No
Fishman (NETT)	All patients had 6 to 10 weeks of pulmonary rehabilitation	VATS (30%) or median sternotomy (70%) bilateral stapled wedge excision of 20-35% of each lung	Continued medical treatment for 24 months	No, but 33 of 610 patients in the medical group underwent LVRS outside the study

from medical to surgical groups during the study period, a significant number of medically allocated patients ended up having surgery after the study in Geddes and the NETT study.

Outcomes

Criner 1999

After three months of rehabilitation, patients were allowed to cross over to the surgical group. Thirteen of 18 patients in the medical arm did cross over. Although this cross-over method precludes analysis of longer-term differences between the groups, it may have been necessary to encourage patients to enrol. The main outcome measures were functional status, gas exchange, symptom limited maximal exercise performance and 6-minute walk distance. Unfortunately, most of the analysis did not actually compare treatment and control groups, but compared pre-to postoperative changes in the LVRS group. After the initial 8-week pulmonary rehab program, pulmonary function tests remained unchanged compared to the baseline data. However, there was a trend toward a higher 6-minute walk distance (p=0.14) and an increase in maximal exercise test (p=0.001). In the pulmonary rehabilitation group, there was a trend towards higher maximal oxygen consumption only. The LVRS group had a significant increase in their FVC (2.79 +/- 0.59 versus 2.36 +/- 0.55L, p <0.001) and FEV1 (0.85 +/- 0.3 versus 0.65 +/- 0.16L, p <0.005). Similarly, the patients randomised to LVRS also experienced a significant reduction in TLC (6.53 +/- 1.3 versus 7.65 +/- 2.1L, p <0.001) and residual volume (RV) (3.7 +/- 1.2 versus 4.9 +/- 1.1 L, p <0.001). In addition, $PaCO_2$ decreased significantly three months post-LVRS compared with $PaCO_2$ eight weeks post-rehabilitation. Six-minute walk distance, total exercise time, and VO_2 max were higher after LVRS but did not reach statistical significance. However, when 13 patients who crossed over from the medical to the surgical arm, were included in the analysis, the increases in 6-minute walk distance (337 +/- 99 versus 282 +/- 100m, p<0.001) and VO_2 max

Table 3. **Outcomes in the randomised controlled trials.**

		Criner	Pompeo	Geddes	Goldstein	Fishman (NETT)
When assessed		3 months	3 and 6 months	3,6,12 and 24 months	3,6,9 and 12 months	6,12 and 24 months
Mortality (%)	LVRS	9.4 overall, LVRS	6.6	21	14.3	26
	Control	vs control not stated	3.3 (ns)	12 (ns)	3.7 (ns)	26
Pulmonary function tests	LVRS	Increased FEV1 and FVC, decreased TLC and RV	Increased FEV1 and FVC, decreased RV and FVC	Increased FEV1 and FVC (temporary)	Decreased TLC, RV FRC, increased FEV1	Increased FEV1
	Control	No change	No change	Deterioration	No change	No change
Gas exchange	LVRS	Decreased $paCO_2$ Increased $paCO_2$	$paCO_2$ unchanged	NA	TLCO unchanged	NA
	Control	No change	Increase sig less	NA	TLCO unchanged	NA
Maximal exercise performance	LVRS	Increased(a)	Increased	NA	NA	Max perf increased by more tha 15 W in 15%
	Control	No change	Increase sig less	NA	NA	Max perf increased by more tha 15 W in 3%
6-minute walk distance	LVRS	Increased(a)	Increased	NA	Increased	Increased
	Control	No change	Increase sig less	NA	Decreased	Decreased
Shuttle walking distance	LVRS	NA	NA	Increased (temporary)	NA	NA
	Control	NA	NA	Deterioration	NA	NA
Quality of life	LVRS	NA	NA	Increased (temporary)	25% failure	Improved
	Control	NA	NA	Deterioration	63% failure	No change

(a) = only when cross-over patients included in the analysis

(13.8 +/- 4 versus 12.0 +/- 3 ml/kg/min, $p < 0.01$) three months post-LVRS, were statistically higher when compared with post-rehabilitation data. Both groups had an increased quality of life as measured by the Sickness Impact Profile. Thus, although short-term benefits were seen in this trial, it is difficult to fully assess how LVRS compares to medical treatment. Significance was only achieved when the cross-over patients were included in analysis. There were three (9.4%) postoperative deaths, and one patient died before surgery (2.7%). Mortality rates were not compared between the two groups.

Pompeo 2000

These authors found that LVRS and rehabilitation both improved some outcomes at six months, but that there was a significantly greater benefit in the LVRS group for dyspnoea index, FEV1, FVC, RV, PaO_2, 6-minute walk test and incremental treadmill test. Only LVRS improved lung function measures with a mean 0.46l and 0.42l increase in FEV1 and FVC and a 1.4l decrease in RV. The greater difference between groups compared to Criner's study may be explained by the lack of pre-treatment rehabilitation on Pompeo's study. Although 1-month morbidity was higher in the LVRS group, it was lower when compared to the rehab group at six months. The short-term follow-up limits this study. After the 6-month trial period, 12 patients in the rehab group opted for LVRS within two years making further comparison difficult to decipher.

Geddes 2000

The primary outcome measures were mortality, FEV1 change, shuttle walking distance and quality of life (Short Form 36 - a general rather than disease-specific questionnaire) at three, six and 12 months after randomisation. There were three deaths in the medical group and five in the LVRS group (not found to be a statistically significant difference). The study was underpowered to adequately determine differences in mortality. In the medical group, most measures decreased over 12 months. However, LVRS was found to increase FVC, shuttle walking distance and SF36 compared to medical management. FEV1 was improved at three months after LVRS, but declined back towards baseline in a similar fashion to the decline in FEV1 seen in the medical group. This suggested that LVRS produced a short-term benefit in quality of life, but it did not alter the ultimate course of the disease. Another interesting feature of this study was that five of the 19 surviving surgical patients had no benefit at all. These five patients were reported to have similar baseline features to those patients who had improvement apart from having more diffusely distributed emphysema on a pre-operative CT scan. These patients with homogenous emphysema were less likely to benefit from LVRS than those with heterogeneous emphysema. This finding additionally illustrates how examining group averages for continuous variables, can show an apparent improvement in a group, yet mask a significantly large subgroup which has no improvement at all. Individual patient responses to a treatment may be hidden by the overall effect to a group of patients.

Fishman (NETT) 2001

This was a preliminary report. Its sole purpose was to warn physicians of the high LVRS operative mortality in patients with FEV1 less than 20% predicted and either a CO transfer factor less than 20% of predicted or a homogeneous distribution of emphysema. This report therefore supported the findings of Geddes described above. It also found a high operative mortality in patients with a transfer factor less than 30% predicted and those with diffuse emphysema. Furthermore, those patients that survived the operation did not seem to have much benefit.

Goldstein 2003

This study was not powerful enough to detect a difference in mortality. However, it did show an improvement in patient reported health-related quality of life in all four CRQ (Chronic Respiratory Questionnaire) domains: dyspnoea, emotional function, fatigue and mastery (defined as a patient's sense of being in control of their lives and their health problems). Treatment failure was defined as death or a functional decline on the CRQ from which the patients did not recover. LVRS was shown to greatly reduce the likelihood of treatment failure over the 12-month follow-up period. Failure occurred in 7/28 (25%) of LVRS patients and 17/27 (63%) of medical patients. This is arguably the most robust outcome measure since the purpose of LVRS is to palliate and improve quality of life. However, the relationship between lung function and quality of life is unclear since the former is a multi-faceted concept. This is an extremely important finding in a well controlled prospective randomised trial that supports the fact the LVRS improves the quality of life when compared to pulmonary rehabilitation alone.

Fishman (NETT) 2003

This is an important study in which 17 centres participated. It presents the main results of the NETT trial. The NETT trial is the largest RCT so far published and also, has the greatest length of follow-up. The main outcomes were mortality (all causes) and maximal exercise tolerance at two years. Importantly, baseline measurements were made after the rehab (unlike other studies). Patients were classified as having homogeneous or heterogeneous distribution of emphysema on a CT scan. HRCT scans were used to systematically score a patient's emphysema as one of four types. One type was called heterogeneous upper lobe predominance. It was compared to the three others that were combined for the final analysis. The other three types were called non-upper lobe predominance and they included:-

- homogenous or diffuse emphysema;
- lower lobe emphysema, including patients with alpha 1 antitrypsin deficiency; and
- emphysema of the superior segment of the lower lobe.

Because early surgical mortality can appear to make the surgical survivors appear healthier, the authors chose to use binary classification of outcomes such as improvement or no improvement that would take into account those patients who had died. The 90-day mortality was significantly higher in the LVRS group (7.9% versus 1.3%) when all patients were included in the analysis. Surprisingly, a 30-day operative mortality was not reported. However, when the 140 patients that had been previously identified as very high-risk (patients that few informed general thoracic surgeons would have operated on in the first place) were eliminated from the analysis, the 30-day operative mortality was only 2.2% and the 90-day mortality was 5.3%. This compares to a 0.2% mortality in the medical arm. There was no statistically significant difference in mortality between patients who underwent VATS when compared to those that had a median sternotomy. However, despite this early surgical mortality, the total mortality was the same in both the LVRS and medical groups by two years. Exercise capacity increased by more than 10w in 28%, 22%, and 15% of LVRS patients at six, 12 and 24 months respectively, compared to 4%, 5% and 3% in the medical group. LVRS patients had significantly greater improvements in 6-minute walk distance, FEV1, degree of dyspnoea and general and health-related quality of life. When one stratifies patients according to the distribution of emphysema and maximal exercise capacity after rehab, four subgroups were found. Patients with low exercise capacity and predominantly upper lobe emphysema, showed the greatest and most sustained improvement in all symptomatic and physiological variables. They also had a lower mortality compared to similar patients treated medically. Patients with non-upper lobe predominance and a preserved exercise capacity did poorly. The other two groups (non-upper lobe/poor exercise capacity and upper lobe/preserved exercise capacity) had similar mortality when treated medically or by LVRS, but showed significant improvement in spirometry and exercise capacity.

Patient selection

One of the most important factors in LVRS surgery is careful patient selection (Table 4). The surgical procedure carries a significant operative risk, especially in poorly chosen patients and only offers benefit in selected patients as well. By resecting the areas with little function and reducing the overall hyper-expansion, other areas of healthy pulmonary parenchyma function better. Improvement in lung elastic recoil results in more rapid and complete expiratory flow [10]. This is the theoretical concept that supports selecting patients with heterogeneity of emphysema. One needs to select patients who are likely to benefit in terms of function and quality of life and exclude those who have an unacceptably high risk of morbidity and mortality. However, this simple concept is complicated by the fact that there is evidence of an overlap between these two patient groups. For example, the higher the volume of emphysema the greater the mortality, but the greater the gain in exercise capacity in those who survive surgery [11,12]. A balance is needed as with diffusing capacity of the lung for carbon monoxide (DLCO) when a value below 60% predicted indicates the patient will benefit, but a value below 20% indicates a very high risk of dying. Patients and surgeons will have differing degrees of risk aversion depending on their symptoms and desired lifestyle, so there can be no simple algorithm of selection criteria applicable to all patients.

In the initial report in 1995 [1] of a series of 20 patients, the inclusion criteria were severe COPD, distended thorax and significant functional limitation, despite maximal medical therapy. Patients with simple giant bullae, or who still smoked or had alpha 1 antitrypsin deficiency were excluded. Using selection criteria of heterogeneous emphysema with target areas for resection, age <75, FEV1 <35% predicted, RV >250% predicted, $PaCO_2$ <7.3kPa (55mmHg) and ability to participate in a pulmonary rehab program, Cooper's group reported a 4% 90-day mortality in a series of 150 patients [13]. Selection criteria have been refined considerably since then even though some criteria are based on the physiological principles discussed, while others remain arbitrary and have no supporting evidence.

The more recent RCTs have not replicated the impressive physiological and clinical results of the earlier uncontrolled case series. It has been suggested that this may be due to more liberal selection criteria in the RCTs. However, the RCTs did actually identify particularly high-risk patients who should avoid LVRS as well as identify definite subsets of patients who are most likely to benefit.

Table 4. Suggested selection criteria for LVRS.

Clinical determinants	
Include	**Exclude**
Severe emphysema	Age over 70 to 80 years
Marked dyspnoea with maximal medical therapy	Hypercapnia
Nutritional status 70-130% ideal body weight	Pulmonary hypertension
Able to undergo pulm rehab	Still smoking
	Severe comorbidity
	Alpha-1-antitrypsin deficiency
Physiologic testing	
Include	**Exclude**
Hyperinflation (TLC >130%)	
Airflow obstruction (FEV1 <35%)	
TLCO <60%	TLCO <20%
Radiology	
Include	**Exclude**
Heterogeneous emphysema (severe)	Diffuse emphysema
Flattened diaphragms (sign of hyperinflation)	

Pulmonary function tests to diagnose emphysema

There is a heterogeneous spectrum of patients with "chronic obstructive airways disease" ranging from patients with pure emphysema to those with asthmatic bronchitis. All of these patients tend to be dyspnoeic and have reduced airflow on simple spirometry. Phlthesmography is therefore essential to select patients with reduced airflow due to emphysema and air trapping rather than due to reactive airways. Patients with emphysema tend to have trapped gas volumes of greater than two litres and diffusion capacities for carbon monoxide of less than 50-60%.

Pattern of emphysema

Once it has been established that the patient has emphysema, the two tests useful to determine the pattern of emphysema are the CT scan, especially the high resolution CT scan and the quantitative ventilation perfusion (V/Q) scan. The CT gives a qualitative picture of structure and will indicate heterogeneity of emphysema. The V/Q scan gives additional information about lung function and how this varies between the zones of the lungs. McKenna *et al* [14], as far back as 1997, suggested that the most important selection criteria for LVRS was a bilateral upper lobe heterogeneous pattern of emphysema on a chest computed tomography and lung perfusion scan. This has been a consistent finding in the literature in both case series and RCTs [15]. McKenna *et al* [14] examined the results of a cohort of 154 patients selected on the basis of having heterogeneous emphysema. The pattern of emphysema was classified as upper lobe, lower lobe or diffuse. The upper lobe group has a significantly greater improvement in FEV1. However, McKenna *et al* were unable to find any association between other clinical or physiological factors and outcome. They concluded that once patients had been selected on the basis of heterogeneous emphysema, other selection criteria were unnecessary. Geddes' RCT [7] has confirmed that patients with diffuse emphysema tend not to benefit from LVRS.

Nutritional status

In a prospective observational study of 51 patients, Mazolewski *et al* [16] found that approximately half of the patients had a lower than normal body mass index and this group needed more prolonged ventilatory support following LVRS. They also had a longer hospital stay. It is suggested that patients outside 70-130% of predicted BMI are at particularly high risk.

Age

The life expectancy of candidates for LVRS should be such that they benefit from surgery. For this reason most patients over 75 have been excluded. There is however, little evidence to justify this. Glaspole *et al* [17] reviewed the pre-operative characteristics of 89 patients having LVRS and found that the only predictors for mortality and morbidity were age and operative time. Age greater than 70 was associated with a significantly increased mortality (odds ratio of 9).

Hypercapnia

There is conflicting evidence with regard to treating patients with hypercapnia. Most of the early case series excluded patients with a $paCO_2$ >6.7-8 kPa [14]. Szekely *et al* [18], in a retrospective review of 47 consecutive patients, found that a $paCO_2$ greater than 6kPa or a 6-minute walk test of less than 200m predicted a high mortality (6/16=38%) compared to 0/25. O'Brien *et al* [19] prospectively examined morbidity, mortality, quality of life (QOL), and physiologic outcome, including spirometry, gas exchange, and exercise performance in 15 patients with a resting $PaCO_2$ of >6kPa compared to 31 patients with a $PaCO_2$ of <6kPa. Both groups improved significantly and there was no difference in mortality suggesting that a $PaCO_2$ >6kPa should not be a contraindication to LVRS. This is supported by data from Wisser *et al* [20] who retrospectively compared 22 patients with hypercapnia having LVRS to 58 patients without hypercapnia. Although 30-day mortality was higher in the hypercapnia group (9.1% versus 5.2%), this was not statistically significant due to the small numbers in the study.

DLCO

As previously discussed, the randomised studies provide the strongest evidence that a low DLCO predicts a high mortality [4,7] although in some case series it has not been found to be a significant determinant [17,21,22].

Timing of surgery

The optimum timing of surgery has not been studied and is not known. As the patient ages and lung function decreases, operative risk will increase. However, if surgery is performed too early then there may be no worthwhile gain. The physiologic benefits of LVRS are well described but the actual mechanics that lead to that benefit are controversial. Further studies are needed that examine pulmonary mechanics, elastic recoil and diaphragmatic function.

Types of LVRS

There are several different surgical techniques available for performing LVRS. Although stapled resection with buttressing via VATS or median sternotomy seems to predominate, there is no high-grade evidence that supports one as better than the other.

Laser vs stapling

McKenna (1996) compared stapled lung resection to laser (Nd; YAG) bullectomy in 72 patients receiving unilateral VATS LVRS [23] in a prospective randomised trial. Laser treatment was associated with a significantly higher rate of delayed pneumothorax. Postoperative dependency on supplemental oxygen was 87.5% in the laser group and 52% in the stapled group (p=0.02). The mean postoperative improvement in FEV1 at six months was significantly greater for the patients undergoing the staple technique (32.9% vs 13.4%, p=0.01) than for the laser treatment group. Laser treatment seems to have subsequently been abandoned.

Bilateral vs unilateral

There are a number of studies comparing bilateral and unilateral surgery but none have been randomised. An early study by McKenna [24] compared the results of 166 consecutive patients who underwent unilateral (n=87) or bilateral (n=79) VATS LVRS. The early mortality was the same but the physiological outcome in terms of FEV1 was not as good in the unilateral group. Although it is difficult to give this study much weight since it was a retrospective analysis, its findings are provocative.

Another small retrospective review [25] compared 28 patients who had unilateral LVRS because of asymmetric disease distribution, previous thoracic surgery or concomitant tumour resection to 64 patients having bilateral LVRS. Unilateral LVRS gave similar improvements in exercise capacity and dyspnoea as the bilateral procedure. Peri-operative mortality and actuarial survival to 24 months was similar. Although improvements in spirometric indices of pulmonary function were less in patients undergoing unilateral LVRS, this study showed that equivalent functional benefits were possible. A similarly designed study by Kotloff *et al* [26] found better short-term functional outcome in bilateral compared to unilateral LVRS. Serna *et al* [27] suggest that survival at two years is better in bilateral LVRS (86.4%) compared to unilateral VATS (72.6%) in another retrospective review. Naunheim *et al* [28] in a larger review of 673 patients found no difference in 3-year mortality between unilateral and bilateral VATS LVRS. The groups were not however, matched for age and other pre-operative variables. Most recently, Oey *et al* [29] prospectively collected data on 65 patients who were eligible for bilateral LVRS. The effect of LVRS on spirometry was compared in 26 patients having bilateral LVRS via sternotomy or VATS and 39 having LVRS via unilateral VATS. They found that the spirometric benefit was the same in both groups, but the bilateral group had a significantly higher morbidity. Therefore, although there is a theoretical advantage to bilateral surgery as it retains the symmetry of chest wall dynamics, there is no evidence to support this surgical approach. A true comparison of unilateral and bilateral surgery still awaits a randomised trial.

Bilateral vs staged unilateral

Hazelrigg *et al* [30] compared prospectively in a non-randomised study 50 patients having staged VATS LVRS to 29 patients having bilateral LVRS via a median sternotomy. The results were the same in the two groups in terms of lung function although the staged group had a significantly better improved 6-minute walking distance six months post surgery. The mortality was higher (13.8% vs 6%) in the median sternotomy group. This difference did not reach statistical significance as the study was underpowered. Overall, the results of this study are unhelpful. Soon *et al* [31] in a non-randomised study found that staged VATS at a median interval of nine months did not improve upon the benefit conferred by unilateral benefit, but did prolong the duration of the benefit by a year. Again randomised studies are needed.

VATS vs median sternotomy

One study compares the two approaches. Kotlof *et al* [32] compared 40 patients receiving bilateral LVRS by VATS by one surgeon with 80 patients receiving bilateral LVRS via median sternotomy by another surgeon over the same period of time in the same institution. The results at six months were comparable for pulmonary function and exercise tolerance. However, there was a significant reduction in the rate of respiratory failure in the VATS group, so this minimally invasive approach may be more suitable for high-risk patients. Again, randomised studies are needed.

Buttressing vs no buttressing

The reintroduction of LVRS probably owes much to the use of the buttressing of stapled suture lines. Buttressing has been shown in randomised studies to reduce the incidence of air leaks. In a randomised controlled trial of 123 patients having unilateral stapled LVRS, Hazelrigg *et al* [33] compared bovine pericardial buttressing to no buttressing. Those patients with buttressing had their drains removed after a mean of 7.9 days compared to 10.4 in the control group (p=0.04) with a corresponding reduction in the length of hospital stay. A multicentre randomised controlled trial of 65 patients compared bilateral VATS LVRS with and without buttressing the staple lines with bovine pericardium. Stammerberger *et al's* study [34] found that there was a significantly shorter median air leak time and drainage time in those patients with pericardial buttressing. Hospital stay was however, the same in both groups.

Buttressing with collagen or bovine pericardium

A study in 1997 [35] compared bovine pericardium to the less expensive bovine collagen in patients having bilateral VATS LVRS. Each of 57 patients acted as his own control with the two types being used on opposite sides. No differences were seen in the mean time to chest drain removal or the incidence of air leaks beyond seven days. Since the time to chest drain removal is heavily skewed and not normally distributed, it is not clear why these two studies used means rather than medians. It has been noted that in LVRS patients who go on to lung transplant have dense and often vascularised adhesions especially when bovine pericardium has been used [36]. It has therefore been suggested that bovine pericardium be used with caution in younger patients who may later become lung transplant candidates [34].

Recommendations	Evidence level
◆ LVRS benefits select patients with emphysema (see selection recommendations).	Ib/A
◆ Patients with heterogeneous (particularly upper lobe) emphysema are more likely to benefit.	Ib/A
◆ Patients with FEV1 less than 20% predicted and either a CO transfer factor less than 20% predicted or a homogeneous distribution of emphysema have a high mortality.	Ib/A
◆ Stapled resection is superior to laser.	Ib/A
◆ Buttressing of staple lines with bovine pericardium or collagen reduces air leak.	Ib/A

References

1. Cooper JD, Trulock EP, Triantafillou AN, Patterson GA, Pohl MS, Deloney PA, *et al.* Bilateral pneumectomy (volume reduction) for chronic obstructive pulmonary disease. *J Thorac Cardiovasc Surg* 1995; 109: 106-16.
2. Brantigan OC. Surgical treatment of pulmonary emphysema. *Md State Med J* 1957; 6: 409-414.
3. Hensley M, Coughlan JL, Gibson P. Lung volume reduction surgery for diffuse emphysema. *Cochrane Database Syst Rev* 2000; CD001001.
4. Patients at high risk of death after lung-volume-reduction surgery. *N Engl J Med* 2001; 345: 1075-83.
5. Criner GJ, Cordova FC, Furukawa S, Kuzma AM, Travaline JM, Leyenson V, *et al.* Prospective randomized trial comparing bilateral lung volume reduction surgery to pulmonary rehabilitation in severe chronic obstructive pulmonary disease. *Am J Respir Crit Care Med* 1999; 160: 2018-27.
6. Fishman A, Martinez F, Naunheim K, Piantadosi S, Wise R, Ries A, *et al.* A randomized trial comparing lung-volume-reduction surgery with medical therapy for severe emphysema. *N Engl J Med* 2003; 348: 2059-73.
7. Geddes D, Davies M, Koyama H, Hansell D, Pastorino U, Pepper J, *et al.* Effect of lung-volume-reduction surgery in patients with severe emphysema. *N Engl J Med* 2000; 343: 239-45.
8. Goldstein RS, Todd TR, Guyatt G, Keshavjee S, Dolmage TE, van Rooy S, *et al.* Influence of lung volume reduction surgery (LVRS) on health-related quality of life in patients with chronic obstructive pulmonary disease. *Thorax* 2003; 58: 405-10.
9. Pompeo E, Marino M, Nofroni I, Matteucci G, Mineo TC. Reduction pneumoplasty versus respiratory rehabilitation in severe emphysema: a randomized study. Pulmonary Emphysema Research Group. *Ann Thorac Surg* 2000; 70: 948-53.
10. Gelb AF, Zamel N, McKenna RJ, Jr., Brenner M. Mechanism of short-term improvement in lung function after emphysema resection. *Am J Respir Crit Care Med* 1996; 154: 945-51.
11. Rogers RM, Coxson HO, Sciurba FC, Keenan RJ, Whittall KP, Hogg JC. Preoperative severity of emphysema predictive of improvement after lung volume reduction surgery: use of CT morphometry. *Chest* 2000; 118: 1240-7.
12. Wisser W, Klepetko W, Kontrus M, Bankier A, Senbaklavaci O, Kaider, A *et al.* Morphologic grading of the emphysematous lung and its relation to improvement after lung volume reduction surgery. *Ann Thorac Surg* 1998; 65: 793-9.
13. Cooper JD, Patterson GA, Sundaresan RS, Trulock EP, Yusen RD, Pohl MS, *et al.* Results of 150 consecutive bilateral lung volume reduction procedures in patients with severe emphysema. *J Thorac Cardiovasc Surg* 1996; 112: 1319-29.
14. McKenna RJ, Jr., Brenner M, Fischel RJ, Singh N, Yoong B, Gelb AF, *et al.* Patient selection criteria for lung volume reduction surgery. *J Thorac Cardiovasc Surg* 1997; 114: 957-64.
15. Hamacher J, Bloch KE, Stammberger U, Schmid RA, Laube I, Russi EW, *et al.* Two years' outcome of lung volume reduction surgery in different morphologic emphysema types. *Ann Thorac Surg* 1999; 68:1792-8.
16. Mazolewski P, Turner JF, Baker M, Kurtz T, Little AG. The impact of nutritional status on the outcome of lung volume reduction surgery: a prospective study. *Chest* 1999; 116: 693-6.
17. Glaspole IN, Gabbay E, Smith JA, Rabinov M, Snell GI. Predictors of perioperative morbidity and mortality in lung volume reduction surgery. *Ann Thorac Surg* 2000; 69: 1711-6.
18. Szekely LA, Oelberg DA, Wright C, Johnson DC, Wain J, Trotman-Dickenson B, *et al.* Preoperative predictors of operative morbidity and mortality in COPD patients undergoing bilateral lung volume reduction surgery. *Chest* 1997; 111: 550-8.
19. O'Brien GM, Furukawa S, Kuzma AM, Cordova F, Criner GJ. Improvements in lung function, exercise, and quality of life in hypercapnic COPD patients after lung volume reduction surgery. *Chest* 1999; 115: 75-84.
20. Wisser W, Klepetko W, Senbaklavaci O, Wanke T, Gruber E, Tschernko E, *et al.* Chronic hypercapnia should not exclude patients from lung volume reduction surgery. *Eur J Cardiothorac Surg* 1998; 14: 107-12.
21. Chatila W, Furukawa S, Criner GJ. Acute respiratory failure after lung volume reduction surgery. *Am J Respir Crit Care Med* 2000; 162: 1292-6.
22. Szekely LA, Oelberg DA, Wright C, Johnson DC, Wain J, Trotman-Dickenson B, *et al.* Preoperative predictors of operative morbidity and mortality in COPD patients undergoing bilateral lung volume reduction surgery. *Chest* 1997; 111: 550-8.
23. McKenna RJ, Jr., Brenner M, Gelb AF, Mullin M, Singh N, Peters H, *et al.* A randomized, prospective trial of stapled lung reduction versus laser bullectomy for diffuse emphysema. *J Thorac Cardiovasc Surg* 1996; 111: 317-21.
24. McKenna RJ, Jr., Brenner M, Fischel RJ, Gelb AF. Should lung volume reduction for emphysema be unilateral or bilateral? *J Thorac Cardiovasc Surg* 1996; 112: 1331-8.
25. Argenziano M, Thomashow B, Jellen PA, Rose EA, Steinglass KM, Ginsburg ME, *et al.* Functional comparison of unilateral versus bilateral lung volume reduction surgery. *Ann Thorac Surg* 1997; 64: 321-6.
26. Kotloff RM, Tino G, Palevsky HI, Hansen-Flaschen J, Wahl PM, Kaiser LR, *et al.* Comparison of short-term functional outcomes following unilateral and bilateral lung volume reduction surgery. *Chest* 1998; 113: 890-5.
27. Serna DL, Brenner M, Osann KE, McKenna RJ, Jr., Chen JC, Fischel RJ, *et al.* Survival after unilateral versus bilateral lung volume reduction surgery for emphysema. *J Thorac Cardiovasc Surg* 1999; 118: 1101-9.
28. Naunheim KS, Kaiser LR, Bavaria JE, Hazelrigg SR, Magee MJ, Landreneau RJ, *et al.* Long-term survival after thoracoscopic lung volume reduction: a multi-institutional review. *Ann Thorac Surg* 1999; 68: 2026-31.
29. Oey IF, Waller DA, Bal S, Singh SJ, Spyt TJ, Morgan MD. Lung volume reduction surgery - a comparison of the long-

term outcome of unilateral vs. bilateral approaches. *Eur J Cardiothorac Surg* 2002; 22: 610-4.
30. Hazelrigg SR, Boley TM, Magee MJ, Lawyer CH, Henkle JQ. Comparison of staged thoracoscopy and median sternotomy for lung volume reduction. *Ann Thorac Surg* 1998; 66: 1134-9.
31. Soon SY, Saidi G, Ong ML, Syed A, Codispoti M, Walker WS. Sequential VATS lung volume reduction surgery: prolongation of benefits derived after the initial operation. *Eur J Cardiothorac Surg* 2003; 24: 149-53.
32. Kotloff RM, Tino G, Bavaria JE, Palevsky HI, Hansen-Flaschen J, Wahl PM, *et al.* Bilateral lung volume reduction surgery for advanced emphysema. A comparison of median sternotomy and thoracoscopic approaches. *Chest* 1996; 110: 1399-406.
33. Hazelrigg SR, Boley TM, Naunheim KS, Magee MJ, Lawyer C, Henkle JQ, *et al.* Effect of bovine pericardial strips on air leak after stapled pulmonary resection. *Ann Thorac Surg* 1997; 63: 1573-5.
34. Stammberger U, Klepetko W, Stamatis G, Hamacher J, Schmid RA, Wisser W, *et al.* Buttressing the staple line in lung volume reduction surgery: a randomized three-center study. *Ann Thorac Surg* 2000; 70: 1820-5.
35. Fischel RJ, McKenna RJ, Jr. Bovine pericardium versus bovine collagen to buttress staples for lung reduction operations. *Ann Thorac Surg* 1998; 65: 217-9.
36. Klepetko W. Surgical aspects and techniques of lung volume reduction surgery for severe emphysema. *Eur Respir J* 1999; 13: 919-25.

Chapter 15

Pulmonary transplantation

Joseph Zacharias FRCS (C/Th)
Consultant Cardiothoracic Surgeon [1]
Stephan Schueler MD FRCS
Professor and Consultant in
Cardiothoracic Surgery & Transplantation [2]

1 Blackpool Victoria Hospital, Blackpool, UK
2 Freeman Hospital, Newcastle upon Tyne, UK

Introduction

Since the first series of successful lung transplants carried out in the early 1980s, lung transplantation has now become established as the best option for patients with failing medical therapy. The International Society for Heart and Lung Transplantation (ISHLT) registry reported that almost 15,000 lung transplants have been done worldwide with more than 1500 done annually. As with many interventions for extreme situations, we went from the first experimental series to the establishment of lung transplantation, without a randomised trial between medical therapy and lung transplantation. Hence, the evidence on which most decisions in lung transplant surgery are made is based on case series rather than randomised controlled trials. There is a wealth of information gathered over the past two decades in large registries such as the United Network for Organ Sharing registry (UNOS), and the ISHLT registry. Some aspects of lung transplantation have been investigated by randomised trials and these have been highlighted later. For ease of reading we have tried to segregate the current best evidence into that available for patient selection, donor selection and donor lung preservation, and procedure selection.

Recipient selection

In all cases of progressive pulmonary disease that has failed medical therapy, lung transplantation could be considered. The difficulty arises in predicting the progress of the condition to a situation where the benefits from transplantation are outweighed by the surgical and immunosuppression risks. Conceptually, we think in terms of putting a patient on the waiting list for a donor lung when the predicted survival approaches the expected waiting time to transplantation.

The common indications can be grouped into four broad categories of end-stage lung disease: obstructive, restrictive, suppurative and vascular [1]. In 1998, the ISHLT, the American Thoracic Society and the American Society of Transplant Physicians published guidelines for the selection of lung transplant recipients [2]. This is reproduced in Table1 along with additional considerations that since 1998, have been shown to be associated with a worse prognosis in specific patient groups [3]. This evidence was mainly based on registry details and case series.

Obstructive lung disease

Initial studies observing patients with a diagnosis of COPD over 15 years showed a mean survival of about five years with good correlation with worsening forced expiratory volume in one second (FEV1) [4]. Other groups have highlighted the increase in mortality with lower body mass index, oxygen therapy, lower FEV1 [5] and dyspnoea scores [6]. Prior to referral for transplantation in patients with emphysema, other modalities must be considered. Latterly, this had included lung volume reduction surgery (LVRS). The recently reported randomised controlled trial comparing LVRS to medical therapy showed that LVRS does yield a survival advantage for patients with both predominantly upper-lobe emphysema and low base-line exercise capacity [7]. This is dealt with more fully in Chapter 14.

Patients should be referred for transplantation based on published guidelines, taking into consideration other markers of poor prognosis, such as nutritional status, lean body mass and dyspnoea. Patients with emphysema affecting the upper lobe and poor exercise capacity should be considered for LVRS, rather than referral for transplantation, although ultimately, some of these patients will be considered for transplantation.

Suppurative lung disease

In a retrospective analysis of patients with cystic fibrosis, a FEV1 <30% predicted, hypoxaemia, hypercapnia and age were related to higher one and 2-year mortality [8]. Further case series have shown a link between rate of decline of FEV1 and mortality [9]. However, contradictory data from a large retrospective study suggested that rate of decline should not be considered in transplant evaluation [10]. Pulmonary artery hypertension [11] and nutritional status [12] have also been linked with survival in case series. Chronic colonisation with *Burkholderia cepacia* (previously called *Pseudomonas cepacia*) has been associated with an approximately eight-fold increase in mortality [13]. Long-term outcome is also adversely affected [14]. In children, colonisation by *Pseudomonas aeruginosa* is also associated with higher mortality and morbidity [15].

A retrospective multivariate analysis conducted on 11,000 patients led to the development of a ten variable model that included FEV1, age, gender, weight, pancreatic function, diabetes, and type of infection. In subgroups transplantation was noted to confer survival benefits [16]. This is yet to be studied prospectively. A multicentre trial would be required to answer the question as to the appropriate management of patients colonised with multi drug-resistant organisms.

Pulmonary fibrosis

Though a less common disease compared to the above two, fibrosis has a relentlessly short course to respiratory failure. It is commonly primary (cryptogenic or familial) or part of a systemic disease (sarcoidosis, scleroderma, lymphangioleiomyomatosis (LAM) and histiocytosis X). A survival benefit was demonstrated in this group from lung transplantation [17] within 90 days of surgery. The challenge in this disease is to refer patients for transplantation prior to deterioration, as the majority of patients do not survive to receive transplantation.

The factors affecting prognosis of cryptogenic pulmonary fibrosis were studied prospectively by Schwartz *et al*, and male gender, higher FEV1/ FVC ratio, lower FVC, total lung capacity and DLCO were associated with an increased mortality at five years [18]. Histological factors have also been correlated with worsening prognosis [19]. A scoring system and survival model taking into consideration clinical, radiological and physiological findings has been developed, which may help to predict 2-year mortality and thus, timing for transplantation [20].

Pulmonary hypertension

Registry details suggest a survival benefit from transplantation for primary and secondary pulmonary hypertension [2]. The risk factors for worse prognosis, listed in Table 1, include dyspnoea (NYHA) class IV, mean PA pressure >60mmHG, increased mean right atrial pressure, cardiac index <2L/min/m^2, and decreased DLCO [21]. Other factors such as raised

Table 1. Disease-specific indications for transplantation candidate selection. *Reproduced with permission from the International Society for Heart and Lung Transplantation. Maurer J, Frost A, Estenne M, et al. International guidelines for selection of lung transplant candidates. J Heart Lung Transplant 1998; 17: 703-709.*

Obstructive lung disease

- FEV1 <25% predicted without reversibility
- Dyspnoea score >grade IV
- $PaCO_2$ ≥55mmHg and/or Cor pulmonale
- Preference to patients on oxygen therapy
- BMI <20
- DLCO <20%

Cystic fibrosis/bronchiectasis

- FEV1 ≤30% predicted or
- FEV1 >30% with:
- Increased number of hospitalizations
- Rapid fall in FEV1: increased rate in deterioration of FEV1 >1.8 FEV1 % predicted/yr
- Massive haemoptysis
- Increased cachexia
- $PaCO_2$ >55mmHg
- PaO_2 <55 mmHg
- Poor 6-min walk
- Young female with rapid deterioration

Pulmonary fibrosis

- Symptomatic and progressive disease
- Abnormal pulmonary function without symptoms
- Vital capacity <60-70% predicted
- DLCO corrected <50-60% predicted

Pulmonary hypertension

- NYHA III or IV despite vasodilator therapy
- Plasma Von Willebrand Factor Ag activity
- Cardiac index <2L/min/m^2
- Right atrial pressure >15mmHg
- Mean pulmonary artery pressure >55 mmHg
- Six-minute walk <332m
- Failure to respond to prostacyclin therapy after 3 months

Eisenmenger syndrome

- Progressive symptoms: NYHA III or IV

uric acid levels [22], a 6-minute walk test less than 332 meters [23] and ECG changes of pulmonary hypertension [24] were also markers of poor prognosis.

Novel modalities of treatment ranging from pulmonary vasodilators [25] to pulmonary thrombo-endarterectomy [26] have been reported as treatment options prior to referral to transplantation. These have never been compared to transplantation in RCTs.

In patients with pulmonary hypertension secondary to congenital heart defects (Eisenmenger syndrome), the survival post-transplantation is better compared to patients with primary pulmonary hypertension [27]. As transplantation is the only available treatment, patients are referred for surgery when they are symptomatic.

Donor selection and donor organ preservation

Lung transplantation is limited by the supply of donor organs. These limitations mandate optimal use of this scarce resource. A change to some form of assumed consent for organ donation would have the greatest impact on the availability of organs, but that requires legislative changes. At the current time, the use of donor lungs depends on the applied acceptance criteria, keeping in mind that the quality of transplanted organs has a significant impact on outcome. Individual opinion and reasonable sense helped establish the early lung specific donor criteria [28,29]. With increasing experience these criteria have undergone a continuous process of redefining.

The current upper age limit for lung donors is 55 years. A number of centres are willing to accept otherwise ideal donors up to the age of 65 years [30] without worsening of outcomes. The interaction between donor age and an extended ischaemic time was predictive of higher mortality at one year in an analysis of 136 transplants [31]. Ischaemic time of less than eight hours of the donor lungs itself, was not associated with an adverse outcome [32]. A general prerequisite of a clear chest radiograph is not a necessity for donor lung procurement and many groups have shown good results with selective usage of lungs with abnormal radiographs [33]. Most donor teams now examine the airway bronchoscopically for evidence of aspiration or pneumonia. In the presence of purulent sputum or extensive tracheobronchitis the lungs are often turned down, though purulent secretions on its own has not been shown to impact short-term results [34] with appropriate antibiotic prophylaxis. The presence of organisms in the washing after broncho-alveolar lavage has been shown to carry a poorer early and medium-term result [35].

A smoking history of more than 20 pack years in itself is not considered a contraindication to lung procurement [33]. These donors must be carefully evaluated for signs of emphysema or other pulmonary changes on their chest radiograph. Previously, chest wall or lung trauma was considered to be a contraindication to transplantation. Lately, many groups have shown good results using lungs with mild contusion [30,33,34], and if there are gross changes in a single lung, the contralateral lung can be used successfully for transplantation [36]. Despite this widening of acceptance criteria many lungs currently rejected may be suitable for transplantation. Ware *et al* and Fischer *et al* assessed rejected lungs on the basis of their physiology, microbiology and histology and found a large proportion would have been suitable for transplantation [37,38]. There is a need for a prospective assessment of selection criteria

Active therapeutic manipulations have led to use of donor lungs previously thought unusable. Appropriate fluid management, antibiotic therapy, physiotherapy, bronchoscopy and toilet and changes in ventilatory settings have led to improvements in donor lung function [39]. Recipient outcomes have been noted to be comparable to donors with standard criteria [40]. This form of donor management is not widely practised for logistic reasons, but does hold promise in expanding the pool of lungs available for transplantation. Another attempt at widening the donor pool has been the usage of organs from non-heart beating donors [41]. The experience has been limited to a few centres, but unpublished results from our centre and others, appear to get comparable results to standard donors. Split lung techniques have also been recommended to increase the usage of lungs that might be oversized for the recipient [42]. The procedure is most useful in children and small adults who are unable to wait for an appropriate sized donor.

Despite the widely reproduced success of lung transplantation, ischaemia/reperfusion induced lung injury remains a significant cause of early morbidity and mortality after transplantation. Apart from the early effects it has been correlated with an increased risk of acute rejection and organ dysfunction in the longer-term. The goal of ideal lung preservation is to reduce the incidence of ischaemia/reperfusion injury and ultimately improve graft outcomes. We have summarised the available evidence for using the current lung preservation strategy and also looked at options available to prevent or treat ischaemia/reperfusion injury.

In 1998, a survey reported that most lung transplant units used either Euro-Collins or University of Wisconsin solution [43] for lung preservation. It was also found that a proportion were not satisfied with the quality of graft preservation. Historically, Euro-Collins was developed for kidney preservation and the University of Wisconsin solution for liver preservation [44]. Some units had previously also used donor core cooling on bypass as a means of organ preservation [45]. This produced good results, but for logistic reasons it lost favour and was only used in one unit by the 1998 survey [43]. In the early '90s, an extracellular type solution with Low-Potassium Dextran (LPD) was developed specifically for lung preservation. Laboratory and animal studies showed superior and prolonged organ preservation compared to Euro-Collins solution [46]. A commercially available LPD-glucose solution is Perfadex (Vitrolife, Sweden) which has been shown, when compared to historical controls, to produce significantly better lung function post-transplantation compared to Euro-Collins solution [47,48,49], though this has not been reproduced in all centres [50]. A prospective randomised trial is required to prove the possible advantage of one preservation solution over the other. Despite the lack of more rigorous evidence, there is a trend for more units to switch to using the LPD-glucose as the lung preservation fluid in their transplant programmes [44].

As previously mentioned, reperfusion injury still has a major impact on early graft function and affects nearly 15% of all lung transplants. Clinical studies in the prevention or treatment of reperfusion injury are limited. Most publications are based on case series. A few randomised controlled trials have been reported. The pulmonary artery pressure during the initial ten minutes of reperfusion is of prime importance as endothelial permeability is elevated, leukocyte sequestration and pulmonary oedema can occur [51]. Controlled reperfusion has been shown to have advantages when used in the clinical setting [52] when compared to historical controls. Inhaled nitric oxide has been used clinically to treat ischaemia/reperfusion injury, as it decreases pulmonary artery pressures without affecting systemic pressures. A randomised, double-blind, placebo-controlled trial of inhaled nitric oxide administered to lung transplant patients failed to show significant differences in immediate oxygenation, time to extubation or 30-day mortality [53]. Inhaled nitric oxide may be useful in the treatment of established reperfusion injury, but its role in prevention has not been demonstrated.

Activation of the complement system after reperfusion may lead to cellular injury through direct or indirect mechanisms. The activation of complement fragments C3 and C5 is essential for the activation of the complement cascade and the generation of the membrane attack complex, which leads to direct cell lysis [54]. Complement receptor-1 is a cloned complement antagonist which is available in the soluble form. It suppresses complement activation by inhibiting C3 and C5 convertases. It has been shown in the animal model to improve oxygenation in the transplanted lung when administered before reperfusion [55]. A multicentre, randomised, double-blind trial that included 59 lung transplant recipients, demonstrated a significantly earlier extubation time in patients given soluble complement receptor-1 before reperfusion, when compared to the control group [56]. Another potent mediator of inflammation is platelet activating factor (PAF). PAF exerts its biological effects by activating the PAF receptors, which consequently activate leukocytes, stimulate platelet aggregation and induce release of cytokines. The administration of PAF receptor antagonists during ischaemic storage and after reperfusion, has been shown to improve lung function in experimental studies [57]. A recent prospective, randomised trial looking at high-dose (eight patients), low-dose of PAF antagonists (eight patients) and placebo (eight patients) in the flush solution, and after reperfusion, showed a trend towards better oxygenation and a better chest radiograph score in the two groups receiving PAF antagonists [58]. Experimental studies and clinical observations have found exogenous surfactant to also have a beneficial effect in ischaemia / reperfusion injury [59,60]. These above modalities show encouraging results, but need to be investigated in larger multicentre co-operative trials to test their real impact on clinical practice.

Procedure selection

The procedures available to a surgeon when faced with a patient in impending respiratory failure are single lung transplantation, bilateral lung transplantation and heart lung transplantation. The complexity and familiarity of the operation, the time taken, the associated morbidity and the appropriate allocation of scarce organs all influence the final choice of procedure. Again there are no RCTs that dictate choice of procedure, despite some uncertainty in particular subgroups of patients. Most of the evidence available is in the form of registry data or based on large case series. The evidence available for choice of procedure in the disease groups is summarised below.

Obstructive lung disease

Patients with emphysema form the largest group considered for single lung transplantation. Increasingly, they are being considered for bilateral lung transplantation. Early reports suggested better early results with a single lung transplant [61], due to the high incidence of early complications associated with two bronchial anastomoses. However, there is now evidence of better lung function, quality of life and long-term survival with bilateral lung transplantation without an increase in early postoperative complications [62]. The ISHLT registry shows an apparent advantage of two lungs over one in patients from about three years post-transplantation [63]. In the presence of a source of sepsis in a lung a bilateral transplant is clearly required. In most other cases, a single lung transplant is the indicated procedure, though if two organs are available it would be advantageous from the individual patient perspective [64].

Fibrotic lung disease

These patients were the initial successes in single lung transplantation [65] which remains the procedure of choice. Most studies have shown good long-term outcomes in this group with single lung transplantation. The only reason for bilateral lung transplantation is the presence of an infective focus in the remaining lung. A study looking at patients on the waiting list compared to patients post-transplantation have shown a survival benefit with single lung transplantation [66].

Septic lung disease

Most of the patients in this category suffer from cystic fibrosis or bronchiectasis. As the disease is likely to affect both lungs to some extent these patients will generally require a bilateral lung transplant to avoid leaving a septic focus in the native lung in the presence of immunosuppression. Recent reports have confirmed good long-term results with bilateral lung transplants in this subgroup of patients [67]. Heart/lung transplantation has been advocated by certain groups with greater experience in this procedure with comparable short and long-term results [68]. Though no randomised comparison has been published regarding choice of procedure, centres with experience in both procedures have shown a comparable outcome in selected patients [69]. Normal functioning hearts explanted from recipients of a heart-lung block are used as a "domino" heart transplant. These hearts have been shown to have a good long-term recipient outcome with a lesser attrition rate [70]. The accepted procedure of choice in most units for patients with septic lung disease is a bilateral lung transplant. In children and small adults who may not survive long enough for a cadaveric lung transplant, living lobar transplantation holds promise [71]. Experience of this procedure is limited to few centres at present.

Pulmonary vascular disease

In patients with pulmonary hypertension, lung transplantation has been shown to provide acceptable long-term results with resolution of high pulmonary vascular resistance. The early mortality in this subgroup is still higher than other patients, but long-term results are good [72,73]. The appropriate procedure of choice between single lung transplants and double lung transplants has not been investigated in a prospective fashion. Bilateral lung transplants appear to have a better medium-term outcome in primary pulmonary hypertension [74]. It is less clear in secondary pulmonary hypertension. If the high pulmonary pressures have adversely affected the right heart, these patients will benefit from heart/lung transplantation, which in the modern era has a very acceptable early mortality in some centres [75]. A recent retrospective review of registry details on patients operated for Eisenmenger's syndrome appeared to suggest a better early and late result with heart/lung transplantation [76]. These improved results were more likely depending on the complexity of the intracardiac pathology. It is accepted that most patients with pulmonary vascular disease will not need a heart transplant, as a lower post-transplantation pulmonary resistance would allow better cardiac function in the presence of normal cardiac anatomy.

Recommendations	Evidence level
◆ As lung transplantation has been successfully practised only for the last two decades it is still a sub-speciality in its infancy. Most decisions are made on registry details and good quality retrospective studies.	IIa & IIb/B
◆ Multicentre randomised trials need to be carried out in this sub-speciality, particularly looking at organ preservation techniques and choice of procedure for specific disease conditions.	

References

1. Smith CM. Patient selection, evaluation and preoperative management for lung transplant candidates. *Clin Chest Med* 1997; 18(2): 183-97.
2. Maurer JR, Frost AE, Estenne M, Higenbottam T, Glanville AR. International guidelines for the selection of lung transplant candidates. *Transplantation* 1998; 66(7): 951-6.
3. Yu AD, Garrity ER, Recipient selection. *Chest Surg Clin N Am* 2003; 13; 405-428.
4. Travers GA, Cline MG, Burrows B. Predictors of mortality in chronic obstructive pulmonary disease. *Am Rev Respir Dis* 1979; 119: 895-902.
5. Gray-Donald K, Gibbons L, Shapiro SH, Macklem PT, Martin JG. Nutritional status and mortality in chronic obstructive pulmonary disease. *Am J Respir Crit Care Med* 1996; 153(3): 961-6.
6. Nishimura K, Izumi T, Tsukino M, Oga T. Dyspnea is a better predictor of 5-year survival than airway obstruction in patients with COPD. *Chest* 2002; 121(5): 1434-40.
7. Fishman A, Martinez F, Naunheim K, Piantadosi S, Wise R, Ries A, Weinmann G, Wood DE. National Emphysema Treatment Trial Research Group. A randomized trial comparing lung-volume-reduction surgery with medical therapy for severe emphysema. *N Engl J Med* 2003; 348(21): 2059-73.
8. Kerem E, Reisman J, Corey M, Canny GJ, Levison H. Prediction of mortality in patients with cystic fibrosis. *N Engl J Med* 1992; 326(18): 1187-91.
9. Milla CE, Warwick WJ. Risk of death in cystic fibrosis patients with severely compromised lung function. *Chest* 1998; 113(5): 1230-4.
10. Liou TG, Adler FR, Cahill BC, FitzSimmons SC, Huang D, Hibbs JR, Marshall BC. Priorities for lung transplantation among patients with cystic fibrosis. *JAMA* 2002; 287(12): 1523-4.
11. Vizza CD, Yusen RD, Lynch JP, Fedele F, Alexander Patterson G, Trulock EP. Outcome of patients with cystic fibrosis awaiting lung transplantation. *Am J Respir Crit Care Med* 2000; 162: 819-25.
12. Sharma R, Florea VG, Bolger AP, Doehner W, Florea ND, Coats AJ, Hodson ME, Anker SD, Henein MY. Wasting as an independent predictor of mortality in patients with cystic fibrosis. *Thorax* 2001; 56(10): 746-50.
13. Ledson MJ, Gallagher MJ, Jackson M, Hart CA, Walshaw MJ. Outcome of *Burkholderia cepacia* colonisation in an adult cystic fibrosis centre. *Thorax* 2002; 57(2): 142-5.
14. De Perrot M, Chaparro C, McRae K, Waddell TK, Hadjiliadis D, Singer LG, Pierre AF, Hutcheon M, Keshavjee S. Twenty-year experience of lung transplantation at a single center: Influence of recipient diagnosis on long-term survival. *J Thorac Cardiovasc Surg* 2004; 127(5): 1493-501.
15. Nixon GM, Armstrong DS, Carzino R, Carlin JB, Olinsky A, Robertson CF, Grimwood K. Clinical outcome after early *Pseudomonas aeruginosa* infection in cystic fibrosis. *J Pediatr* 2001; 138(5): 699-704.
16. Liou TG, Adler FR, Cahill BC, FitzSimmons SC, Huang D, Hibbs JR, Marshall BC. Survival effect of lung transplantation among patients with cystic fibrosis. *JAMA* 2001; 286(21): 2683-9.
17. Hosenpud JD, Bennett LE, Keck BM, Edwards EB, Novick RJ. Effect of diagnosis on survival benefit of lung transplantation for end-stage lung disease. *Lancet* 1998; 351(9095): 24-7.
18. Schwartz DA, Helmers RA, Galvin JR, Van Fossen DS, Frees KL, Dayton CS, Burmeister LF, Hunninghake GW. Determinants of survival in idiopathic pulmonary fibrosis. Am *J Respir Crit Care Med* 1994; 149(2 Pt 1): 450-4.
19. Nicholson AG, Fulford LG, Colby TV, du Bois RM, Hansell DM, Wells AU. The relationship between individual histologic features and disease progression in idiopathic pulmonary fibrosis. *Am J Respir Crit Care Med* 2002; 166(2): 173-7.
20. King TE Jr, Tooze JA, Schwarz MI, Brown KR, Cherniack RM. Predicting survival in idiopathic pulmonary fibrosis: scoring system and survival model. *Am J Respir Crit Care Med* 2001; 164(7): 1171-81.
21. Ewert R, Wensel R, Opitz C, Habedank D, Lodziewski S, Hummel M, Knosalla C, Kapell S, Dandel M, Hetzer R; Berlin Pulmonary Hypertension Group. Prognosis in patients with primary pulmonary hypertension awaiting lung transplantation. *Transplant Proc* 2001; 33(7-8): 3574-5.
22. Nagaya N, Uematsu M, Satoh T, Kyotani S, Sakamaki F, Nakanishi N, Yamagishi M, Kunieda T, Miyatake K. Serum uric acid levels correlate with the severity and the mortality of primary pulmonary hypertension. *Am J Respir Crit Care Med* 1999; 160(2): 487-92.
23. Miyamoto S, Nagaya N, Satoh T, Kyotani S, Sakamaki F, Fujita M, Nakanishi N, Miyatake K. Clinical correlates and prognostic significance of six-minute walk test in patients with primary pulmonary hypertension. Comparison with cardiopulmonary exercise testing. *Am J Respir Crit Care Med* 2000; 161(2 Pt 1): 487-92.
24. Bossone E, Paciocco G, Iarussi D, Agretto A, Iacono A, Gillespie BW, Rubenfire M. The prognostic role of the ECG in primary pulmonary hypertension. *Chest* 2002; 121(2): 513-8.
25. Ghofrani HA, Wiedemann R, Rose F, Schermuly RT, Olschewski H, Weissmann N, Gunther A, Walmrath D, Seeger W, Grimminger F. Sildenafil for treatment of lung fibrosis and pulmonary hypertension: a randomised controlled trial. *Lancet* 2002; 360(9337): 895-900.
26. Jamieson SW, Kapelanski DP, Sakakibara N, Manecke GR, Thistlethwaite PA, Kerr KM, Channick RN, Fedullo PF, Auger WR. Pulmonary endarterectomy: experience and lessons learned in 1,500 cases. *Ann Thorac Surg* 2003; 76(5): 1457-62.
27. Hopkins WE, Ochoa LL, Richardson GW, Trulock EP. Comparison of the hemodynamics and survival of adults with severe primary pulmonary hypertension or Eisenmenger syndrome. *J Heart Lung Transplant* 1996; 15: 100-5.
28. Patterson GA, Cooper JD. Status of lung transplantation. *Surg Clin North Am* 1988; 68(3): 545-58.

29. Griffith BP, Zenati M. The pulmonary donor. *Clin Chest Med* 1990; 11(2): 217-26.
30. Bhorade SM, Vigneswaran W, McCabe MA, Garrity ER. Liberalization of donor criteria may expand the donor pool without adverse consequence in lung transplantation. *J Heart Lung Transplant* 2000; 19(12): 1199-204.
31. Meyer DM, Bennett LE, Novick RJ, Hosenpud JD. Effect of donor age and ischemic time on intermediate survival and morbidity after lung transplantation. *Chest* 2000; 118(5): 1255-62.
32. Fiser SM, Kron IL, Long SM, Kaza AK, Kern JA, Cassada DC, Jones DR, Robbins MC, Tribble CG. Influence of graft ischemic time on outcomes following lung transplantation. *J Heart Lung Transplant* 2001; 20(12): 1291-6.
33. Aigner C, Seebacher G, Klepetko W. Lung transplantation. Donor selection. *Chest Surg Clin N Am* 2003; 13(3): 429-42.
34. Whiting D, Banerji A, Ross D, Levine M, Shpiner R, Lackey S, Ardehali A. Liberalization of donor criteria in lung transplantation. *Am Surg* 2003; 69(10): 909-12.
35. Avlonitis VS, Krause A, Luzzi L, Powell H, Phillips JA, Corris PA, Gould FK, Dark JH. Bacterial colonization of the donor lower airways is a predictor of poor outcome in lung transplantation. *Eur J Cardiothorac Surg* 2003; 24(4): 601-7.
36. Puskas JD, Winton TL, Miller JD, Scavuzzo M, Patterson GA. Unilateral donor lung dysfunction does not preclude successful contralateral single lung transplantation. *J Thorac Cardiovasc Surg* 1992; 103(5): 1015-7
37. Ware LB, Wang Y, Fang X, Warnock M, Sakuma T, Hall TS, Matthay M. Assessment of lungs rejected for transplantation and implications for donor selection. *Lancet* 2002; 360(9333): 619-20.
38. Fisher AJ, Donnelly SC, Pritchard G, Dark JH, Corris PA. Objective assessment of criteria for selection of donor lungs suitable for transplantation. *Thorax* 2004; 59(5): 434-437.
39. Gabbay E, Williams TJ, Griffiths AP, Macfarlane LM, Kotsimbos TC, Esmore DS, Snell GI. Maximizing the utilization of donor organs offered for lung transplantation. *Am J Respir Crit Care Med* 1999;160(1):265-71.
40. Straznicka M, Follette DM, Eisner MD, Roberts PF, Menza RL, Babcock WD. Aggressive management of lung donors classified as unacceptable: excellent recipient survival one year after transplantation. *J Thorac Cardiovasc Surg* 2002; 124(2): 250-258.
41. Steen S, Sjoberg T, Pierre L, Liao Q, Eriksson L, Algotsson L. Transplantation of lungs from a non-heart-beating donor. *Lancet* 2001; 357(9259): 825-9.
42. Aigner C, Mazhar S, Jaksch P, Seebacher G, Taghavi S, Marta G, Wisser W, Klepetko W. Lobar transplantation, split lung transplantation and peripheral segmental resection - reliable procedures for downsizing donor lungs. *Eur J Cardiothorac Surg* 2004; 25(2): 179-83.
43. Hopkinson DN, Bhabra MS, Hooper TL. Pulmonary graft preservation: a worldwide survey of current clinical practice. *J Heart Lung Transplant* 1998; 17(5): 525-31.
44. de Perrot M, Keshavjee S. Lung transplantation. Lung preservation. *Chest Surg Clin N Am* 2003; 13(3): 443-62.
45. Schueler S, De Valeria PA, Hatanaka M, Cameron DE, Bando K, Zeebley M, Hutchins GM, Reitz BA, Baumgartner WA. Successful twenty-four-hour lung preservation with donor core cooling and leukocyte depletion in an orthotopic double lung transplantation model. *J Thorac Cardiovasc Surg* 1992; 104(1): 73-82.
46. Keshavjee SH, Yamazaki F, Yokomise H, Cardoso PF, Mullen JB, Slutsky AS, Patterson GA. The role of dextran 40 and potassium in extended hypothermic lung preservation for transplantation. *J Thorac Cardiovasc Surg* 1992; 103(2): 314-25.
47. Fischer S, Matte-Martyn A, De Perrot M, Waddell TK, Sekine Y, Hutcheon M, Keshavjee S. Low-potassium dextran preservation solution improves lung function after human lung transplantation. *J Thorac Cardiovasc Surg* 2001; 121(3): 594-6.
48. Struber M, Wilhelmi M, Harringer W, Niedermeyer J, Anssar M, Kunsebeck A, Schmitto JD, Haverich A. Flush perfusion with low potassium dextran solution improves early graft function in clinical lung transplantation. *Eur J Cardiothorac Surg* 2001; 19(2): 190-4.
49. Muller C, Furst H, Reichenspurner H, Briegel J, Groh J, Reichart B. Lung procurement by low-potassium dextran and the effect on preservation injury. Munich Lung Transplant Group. *Transplantation* 1999; 68(8): 1139-43.
50. Aziz TM, Pillay TM, Corris PA, Forty J, Hilton CJ, Hasan A, Dark JH. Perfadex for clinical lung procurement: is it an advance? *Ann Thorac Surg* 2003; 75(3): 990-5.
51. Pierre AF, DeCampos KN, Liu M, Edwards V, Cutz E, Slutsky AS, Keshavjee SH. Rapid reperfusion causes stress failure in ischemic rat lungs. *J Thorac Cardiovasc Surg* 1998; 116(6): 932-42.
52. Alvarado CG, Poston R, Hattler BG, Keenan RJ, Dauber J, Griffith B, McCurry KR. Effect of controlled reperfusion techniques in human lung transplantation. *J Heart Lung Transplant* 2001; 20(2): 183-184.
53. Meade MO, Granton JT, Matte-Martyn A, McRae K, Weaver B, Cripps P, Keshavjee SH; Toronto Lung Transplant Program. A randomized trial of inhaled nitric oxide to prevent ischemia-reperfusion injury after lung transplantation. *Am J Respir Crit Care Med* 2003; 167(11): 1483-9.
54. Zhou W, Farrar CA, Abe K, Pratt JR, Marsh JE, Wang Y, Stahl GL, Sacks SH. Predominant role for C5b-9 in renal ischemia/reperfusion injury. *J Clin Invest* 2000; 105(10): 1363-71.
55. Schmid RA, Zollinger A, Singer T, Hillinger S, Leon-Wyss JR, Schob OM, Hogasen K, Zund G, Patterson GA, Weder W. Effect of soluble complement receptor type 1 on reperfusion edema and neutrophil migration after lung allotransplantation in swine. *J Thorac Cardiovasc Surg* 1998; 116(1): 90-7.
56. Zamora MR, Davis RD, Keshavjee SH, Schulman L, Levin J, Ryan U, Patterson GA. Complement inhibition attenuates human lung transplant reperfusion injury: a multicenter trial. *Chest* 1999; 116(1 Suppl): 46S.
57. Kawahara K, Tagawa T, Takahashi T, Akamine S, Nakamura A, Yamamoto S, Muraoka S, Tomita M. The effect of the

platelet-activating factor inhibitor TCV-309 on reperfusion injury in a canine model of ischemic lung. *Transplantation* 1993; 55(6): 1438-9.

58. Wittwer T, Grote M, Oppelt P, Franke U, Schaefers HJ, Wahlers T. Impact of PAF antagonist BN 52021 (Ginkolide B) on post-ischemic graft function in clinical lung transplantation. *J Heart Lung Transplant* 2001; 20(3): 358-63.
59. Novick RJ, MacDonald J, Veldhuizen RA, Wan F, Duplan J, Denning L, Possmayer F, Gilpin AA, Yao LJ, Bjarneson D, Lewis JF. Evaluation of surfactant treatment strategies after prolonged graft storage in lung transplantation. *Am J Respir Crit Care Med* 1996; 154(1): 98-104.
60. Struber M, Hirt SW, Cremer J, Harringer W, Haverich A. Surfactant replacement in reperfusion injury after clinical lung transplantation. *Intensive Care Med* 1999; 25(8): 862-4.
61. Low DE, Trulock EP, Kaiser LR, Pasque MK, Dresler C, Ettinger N, Cooper JD. Morbidity, mortality, and early results of single versus bilateral lung transplantation for emphysema. *J Thorac Cardiovasc Surg* 1992; 103(6): 1119-26.
62. Sundaresan RS, Shiraishi Y, Trulock EP, Manley J, Lynch J, Cooper JD, Patterson GA. Single or bilateral lung transplantation for emphysema? *J Thorac Cardiovasc Surg* 1996; 112(6): 1485-94
63. Hosenpud JD, Bennett LE, Keck BM, Fiol B, Boucek MM, Novick RJ. The Registry of the International Society for Heart and Lung Transplantation: sixteenth official report - 1999. *J Heart Lung Transplant* 1999; 18(7): 611-26.
64. Force SD, Choong C, Meyers BF. Lung transplantation for emphysema. *Chest Surg Clin N Am* 2003; 13(4): 651-67.
65. Cooper JD, Pearson FG, Patterson GA, Todd TR, Ginsberg RJ, Goldberg M, DeMajo WA. Technique of successful lung transplantation in humans. *J Thorac Cardiovasc Surg* 1987; 93(2): 173-81.
66. Thabut G, Mal H, Castier Y, Groussard O, Brugiere O, Marrash-Chahla R, Leseche G, Fournier M. Survival benefit of lung transplantation for patients with idiopathic pulmonary fibrosis. *J Thorac Cardiovasc Surg* 2003; 126(2): 469-75.
67. Coloni GF, Venuta F, Ciccone AM, Rendina EA, De Giacomo T, Filice MJ, Diso D, Anile M, Andreetti C, Aratari MT, Mercadante E, Moretti M, Ibrahim M. Lung transplantation for cystic fibrosis. *Transplant Proc* 2004; 36(3): 648-50.
68. Yacoub MH, Gyi K, Khaghani A, Dyke C, Hodson M, Radley-Smith R, Banner NR. Analysis of 10-year experience with heart-lung transplantation for cystic fibrosis. *Transplant Proc* 1997; 29(1-2): 632.
69. Vricella LA, Karamichalis JM, Ahmad S, Robbins RC, Whyte RI, Reitz BA. Lung and heart-lung transplantation in patients with end-stage cystic fibrosis: the Stanford experience. *Ann Thorac Surg* 2002; 74(1): 13-7.
70. Anyanwu AC, Banner NR, Radley-Smith R, Khaghani A, Yacoub MH. Long-term results of cardiac transplantation from live donors: the domino heart transplant. *J Heart Lung Transplant* 2002; 21(9): 971-5.
71. Starnes VA, Bowdish ME, Woo MS, Barbers RG, Schenkel FA, Horn MV, Pessotto R, Sievers EM, Baker CJ, Cohen RG, Bremner RM, Wells WJ, Barr ML. A decade of living lobar lung transplantation: recipient outcomes. *J Thorac Cardiovasc Surg* 2004; 127(1): 114-22.
72. Mendeloff EN, Meyers BF, Sundt TM, Guthrie TJ, Sweet SC, de L, Shapiro S, Balzer DT, Trulock EP, Lynch JP, Pasque MK, Cooper JD, Huddleston CB, Patterson GA. Lung transplantation for pulmonary vascular disease. *Ann Thorac Surg* 2002; 73(1): 209-17.
73. De Perrot M, Chaparro C, McRae K, Waddell TK, Hadjiliadis D, Singer LG, Pierre AF, Hutcheon M, Keshavjee S. Twenty-year experience of lung transplantation at a single center: influence of recipient diagnosis on long-term survival. *J Thorac Cardiovasc Surg* 2004; 127(5): 1493-501.
74. Conte JV, Borja MJ, Patel CB, Yang SC, Jhaveri RM, Orens JB. Lung transplantation for primary and secondary pulmonary hypertension. *Ann Thorac Surg* 2001; 72(5): 1673-9.
75. Reichart B, Gulbins H, Meiser BM, Kur F, Briegel J, Reichenspurner H. Improved results after heart-lung transplantation: a 17-year experience. *Transplantation* 2003; 75(1): 127-32.
76. Waddell TK, Bennett L, Kennedy R, Todd TR, Keshavjee SH. Heart-lung or lung transplantation for Eisenmenger syndrome. *J Heart Lung Transplant* 2002; 21(7): 731-7.

Chapter 16

Coronary revascularisation: chronic stable angina

Paul J Sheridan MB ChB MRCP PhD
Specialist Registrar, Cardiology
David Crossman MD FRCP FESC FACC
Professor of Cardiology

NORTHERN GENERAL HOSPITAL, SHEFFIELD, UK

Introduction

Coronary artery disease represents a substantial health burden in the developed world. In the UK, more than 1.4 million people suffer with angina with a greater prevalence in older age groups. The prevalence of angina in men and women between the ages of 55 and 75 years in the UK is estimated to be 9% and 5%, respectively [1]. The diagnosis of angina is associated with a significant reduction in 10-year survival [2], and the associated morbidity with substantial health costs [1]. Beyond pharmacotherapy, revascularisation by coronary artery bypass grafting (CABG) or percutaneous coronary intervention (PCI) may offer symptomatic and/or prognostic benefits. Presently, over ½ million bypass graft operations and 1½ million PCI procedures are performed worldwide each year.

Methodology

A MEDLINE database search for English language articles from 1966 through to 2003 was performed using subject headings "revascularisation", "bypass graft", "angioplasty", "coronary stent", "coronary artery disease" and "stable angina". The search yielded three meta-analyses, 67 randomised controlled trials, 101 non-randomised controlled trials or observational studies, 50 review papers and three practice guidelines. Search results were individually evaluated to determine appropriateness and in order to deselect duplicated data. Publications were also identified from bibliographies of retrieved articles and from expert knowledge of the field. If individuals or institutions had authored updates of previous articles, the earlier publications were also deselected.

Initial experience: coronary revascularisation vs medical therapy

Randomised Controlled Trials (RCTs)

Mathur *et al* published the first prospective RCT comparing surgical revascularisation to medical therapy [3]. This small single centre report pertained to 72 patients with refractory angina and represented a small cohort derived from the first of three larger multicentre RCTs. These were the Veterans Administration Coronary Artery Bypass Surgery Co-operative Study (VA study) [4-6], the European Coronary

Table 1. Original multicentre randomised controlled trials: medical therapy vs surgical revascularisation.

	VA study	European study	CASS trial
No. randomised patients	686	768	780
Enrolment period	1972-1974	1973-1976	1975-1979
Age criteria	-	<65	<65
Male (%)	100	100	90.3
Coronary disease	>50% stenosis in ≥1 epicardial artery	>50% stenosis in ≥2 epicardial artery	>70% stenosis in ≥1 epicardial artery
Angina status	No angina - 0% NYHA I - 3% NYHA II - 39% NYHA III - 55% NYHA IV - 3%	No angina - 0% CCS I/II - 57% CCS III - 42% N/A - 1%	No angina - 22% CCS I - 15% CCS II - 59% CCS III/IV - 0% Non-exertional - 4%
Left ventricular function	LVEF <50% in 55%	LVEF >50% in 100%	LVEF >50% in 74%; 35-50% in 21%
Operative mortality	5.60%	3.60%	1.40%

NYHA = New York Heart Association; CCS = Canadian Cardiac Society; LVEF = Left Ventricular Ejection Fraction

Surgery Study (ECSS) [7-10] and the Coronary Artery Surgery Study (CASS) [11-13]. The enrolment characteristics of these studies are detailed in Table 1.

Together, these disparate studies amount to 2234 randomised patients. All of these patients were male with the exception of 10% in CASS. Only the VA study permitted inclusion of patients older than 65 years. Left ventricular function was variable between the trials. In the VA study, patients with decompensated heart failure in the previous three weeks were excluded. However, further limitations were not applied which resulted in 55% of enrolled patients having impaired left ventricular function (ejection fraction ≤50%). In contrast, the ECSS and CASS trial excluded patients with an ejection fraction <50% and <35%, respectively.

Published studies have reported intention-to-treat analyses of these trials, i.e. outcomes dependent on the assigned randomisation strategy, rather than the less statistically rigorous methods of treatment-received or cross-over analyses. This has amounted to a reduction in statistical power, but parallels the process of clinical decision-making most closely.

Left main coronary disease

All three studies demonstrated improved 5-year survival for patients with left main coronary artery (LMCA) stenosis greater than 50% who were randomised to surgery rather than medical therapy. Only the VA study randomised a sufficient number of patients to reach statistical significance (80% vs 64%, p=0.016) [14]. Similar trends were observed in the ECSS (93% vs 62%) and CASS trial (100% vs 83%), but insufficient numbers were recruited to reach statistical significance. Pathophysiologically, one might expect disease in the LAD proximal to the first septal perforator and proximal to the first obtuse marginal in the circumflex artery to behave identically to left main disease; this has been termed left main equivalent (LMEQ) disease [15]. Although observational studies concur with this hypothesis, there are no randomised controlled studies to support this, owing to the rarity of these angiographic findings in the absence of disease elsewhere [15]. Nevertheless, long-term follow-up demonstrated a median survival in patients with LMEQ disease treated by CABG or medical therapy of 13.1 years and 6.2 years (p=<0.001), respectively. This benefit appeared to be limited to those individuals with LV ejection fractions <50% and under the age of 65 years [16].

Symptomatic myocardial ischaemia

Not surprisingly, all three studies demonstrated significant symptomatic benefit with revascularisation compared to medical therapy. Revascularisation produces both greater freedom from angina and in those who are not rendered asymptomatic, reduces the severity of their symptoms; with the former outcome having a more marked difference between the two treatment groups than the latter.

In the European study, the incidence of freedom from angina at one, two and three years was 58%, 55% and 49% in the surgical group compared to 15%, 16% and 20% in the medically treated group [7]. This symptomatic benefit appears greatest in the earliest years, but is eroded by the end of the first decade such that at the 10-year follow-up in the CASS trial, the proportion of patients who were symptom-free, as well as the number of anti-anginal medications used, was similar in both groups [13].

Overall survival

Only the European study [7] demonstrated a significant survival benefit with surgery compared to medical therapy at five years, 93.5% vs 84.1% (p<0.001). Although not statistically significant, similar trends in overall 5-year survival rate were observed in the VA study [5] and CASS trial [12], 82% vs 80% and 95% vs 92%, respectively. In the European study, a survival advantage in patients assigned to surgical intervention persisted, albeit diminishing in magnitude, and remained significant for up to 12 years, 70.6% vs 66.7% (p=0.04) [9].

Subgroup analyses

Since surgical revascularisation is associated with an appreciable peri-operative risk (see Table 1) and an overall prognostic advantage was demonstrated in only one of these three landmark trials, it is essential to separate groups of patients that will gain most, prognostically, by revascularisation from those in which the risks of surgery are not offset by a significant prognostic gain.

With the small number of patients in these studies, subgroup analyses should be interpreted with caution. Notwithstanding, all three studies revealed significant mortality benefits in high-risk patients assigned to surgery. Surgical revascularisation conferred the greatest benefit, and this benefit persisted longest, in the highest risk patients. At seven years in the VA study, patients assigned to revascularisation with triple vessel disease had a non-significant 75% vs 63% survival advantage, and those with LV dysfunction had a *"barely"* significant 74% vs 63% (p=0.049) survival advantage, compared to patients assigned to conservative treatment. This benefit in both groups was blunted at 11 years [5]. However, surgical revascularisation in the group with both triple vessel disease and impaired LV dysfunction was highly significant at seven years (76% vs 52%, p=0.002) and remained significant at 11 years (50% vs 38%, p=0.026) [5].

In the ECSS [8], in addition to left main and triple vessel disease, LAD disease proximal to the first septal perforator was identified as a marker of high mortality risk. For example, 5-year survival of two vessel disease assigned to surgery was 91.6% and 87.5% with medical therapy (p=NS). In the 60% of these patients with LAD disease proximal to the first perforator, survival rates at five years were 96% vs 82%, respectively, and at eight years 87.8% and 78.7%, respectively; however, the small numbers involved mean these differences were not statistically significant [7-10].

Multivariate analysis of the European study identified other predictors of improved survival with surgical revascularisation, including an abnormal resting electrocardiogram, >1.5mm ST segment depression at peak exercise, peripheral vascular disease and age >53 years [8].

In the CASS trial, overall 10-year survival was not significantly different for patients assigned to surgery or medical therapy (82% and 79%, respectively). However, in the cohort (1/5th) of patients with an ejection fraction <50%, surgical revascularisation was associated with a significantly enhanced survival compared to medical therapy, 80% vs 59% (p=0.01), respectively.

In contrast to the VA study and ECSS, this survival advantage in the CASS study was not attenuated with time. There are explanations for the convergence of the survival curves arising from factors within the medical patients and the surgical group of patients. First, in the group assigned to medical therapy, anti-anginal medications associated with improved prognosis including ß-blockers, were more frequently continued (eg. VA study 68% vs 39%); and secondly, throughout follow-up progressively more patients assigned to medical therapy crossed over to surgical intervention (eg. by 11 years 38% in the VA study and 36% in ECSS). In the group assigned to surgical revascularisation, convergence with the medical group over time might be exaggerated by progression of their native arterial disease, and failure of their venous conduit grafts (10-30% in the first year). With respect to the latter point, the maintained survival advantage observed in the CASS trial corresponds with, and may be attributed to, the highest use of internal thoracic artery grafts (16% vs 3% in the VA study) in these trials.

Meta-analyses

There are no published meta-analyses comparing the outcomes of surgical revascularisation and conservative therapy in the three multicentre trials.

Non-randomised clinical data

The relatively small number of patients randomised in the trials alluded to were drawn from much larger registries of patients, the results of which have been extensively published as observational studies. Although these studies are prone to bias, the larger numbers involved lend greater statistical power to subgroup analysis and have largely reinforced the findings of subgroup analyses from the randomised trials. From these papers, further information relating to the role of revascularisation with respect to coronary anatomy, left ventricular function and their respective clinical surrogates, has been derived.

Coronary anatomy

Of more than 20,000 patients listed in the CASS registry, over 5,000 were found to have significant coronary artery disease. In those patients treated medically, 4-year survival was dependent on the extent of coronary disease - 92%, 84% and 68%, for single, double and triple vessel disease, respectively. Revascularisation benefited patients with the highest risk coronary anatomy. In this regard, left main coronary artery (LMCA) stenosis >50% was the most important prognostic determinant (3-year survival 91% with revascularisation and 69% without), but more mild LMCA disease only conferred prognostic importance with concomitant coronary artery disease [17]. In the context of single vessel disease, the left anterior descending artery exerted greater prognostic influence than either the circumflex or right coronary arteries [18]. The severity of stenosis was also correlated with mortality [18]. The 5-year and 15-year survival rates for a significant LAD stenosis were 69% and 46%. In the context of left dominant coronary anatomy, stenosis in the circumflex artery was associated with a less favourable prognosis than LAD disease, 60% and 20% at the five and 15-year time points, similar to the survival observed with two vessel disease [18]. In contrast to symptomatic coronary disease, observational data from CASS indicate that in the presence of silent myocardial ischaemia, revascularisation does not confer a survival advantage with either one or two vessel disease [19].

Left ventricular function

Prognosis appears more strongly driven by left ventricular function. The respective survivals for patients with one, two and three vessel disease and preserved LV systolic function was 94%, 91% and 79% at four years, whilst for those with impaired LV function, were 67%, 61% and 42% [20]. Not surprisingly, clinical markers of left ventricular function carry predictive value including signs and symptoms of congestive heart failure, increased cardiothoracic ratio on a chest radiograph and LVEDP >20mmHg [18]. Surgery for coronary artery disease significantly attenuates mortality in patients with LVEDP >30mmHg or electrocardiographic abnormalities including left ventricular hypertrophy or intraventricular conduction delays [18].

Contemporary experience: coronary revascularisation

Coronary revascularisation: coronary artery bypass grafting vs percutaneous coronary intervention

The symptomatic and prognostic advantages observed with surgical revascularisation in the earliest studies were offset by the high rate of procedure-related complications. For example, in the first major surgery/conservative treatment trial, the VA study, the peri-operative myocardial infarction rate was 9.9% and the 30-day mortality rate was 5.6% [5]. Despite these rates falling in subsequent trials, presumably, due to increased experience, these factors handicapped the outcomes from this strategy.

In 1977, Andreas Gruentzig pioneered percutaneous balloon angioplasty to treat coronary stenoses and percutaneously revascularise the subtended myocardium [21]. Plain Old Balloon Angioplasty (POBA), as it has become known to distinguish it from coronary angioplasty with stenting, was complicated by acute coronary dissection, a complication that was associated with a frequent requirement for emergency CABG. This risk has been largely obviated by the development of coronary stenting [22], and there has been a concomitant reduction in the rates of emergency CABG to rates less than 0.5%. Stents, because of this and other advantages, have revolutionised the practice of percutaneous coronary intervention (PCI). Stenting is undertaken in approximately 90% of all PCI cases. These developments as well as year-on-year improvements in the equipment used now, allow cardiologists to attempt revascularisation comparable in extent to that achieved with bypass grafting, by percutaneous coronary intervention (PCI).

Thirteen studies that included patients with stable coronary disease were found where percutaneous and surgical revascularisations were compared (Table 2). The nine earliest studies (RITA [23], ERACI-I [24], Lausanne [25], GABI [26], CABRI [27], EAST [28], MASS [29], BARI [30] and the French Monocentric study [31]) used almost exclusively POBA in the group randomised to receive percutaneous revascularisation, whereas in the later four studies (ERACI-II [32], ARTS [33], SoS [34] and AWESOME [35], coronary stenting was predominantly used. All of the balloon angioplasty studies enrolled patients with multivessel disease, except for MASS and the Lausanne study that enrolled patients with isolated left anterior descending artery stenoses (Table 2.)

Randomised controlled trials: plain old balloon angioplasty vs coronary artery bypass surgery

These studies, taken together, reported follow-up data between one and five years and failed to demonstrate a significant difference in survival in groups assigned to either strategy. Only one trial, the French Monocentric study [31], demonstrated a significant difference in Q wave myocardial infarctions during the follow-up period. Six of the multivessel disease trials [23-25,27,28,30,31] using POBA reported angina status, and apart from the German study [26], all confirmed a lower incidence of angina following surgical revascularisation. In four of these, RITA [21], EAST [26], ERACI-I [24] and the French study [31], the difference was reported as statistically significant, although in the Argentine trial, the significance at six months was lost at three years. In the largest of these studies, RITA [23], the incidence of freedom from symptoms at 2.5 years in the PCI group was 60% compared to 79% in the surgical group, an absolute difference of nearly 20%. Commensurate with the increased prevalence of angina following percutaneous therapy, all nine POBA studies reported up to a 10-fold increase in revascularisation procedures in patients assigned to percutaneous revascularisation. In the two studies that enrolled the greatest numbers of patients with CSA, RITA [21] and CABRI [27], revascularisation procedures were performed in >1/3 assigned to PCI, whereas less than 4% required revascularisation following CABG. The

Table 2. Multicentre randomised controlled trials: surgical revascularisation vs percutaneous revascularisation.

Trail	Entry crrteria	Enrolled	Date	CABG details	PCI details
RITA	≥1 lesion supplying >20% LV, occluded vessels included, no requirement for complete RV	1011	1988-91	74% ITA, 97% of planned RV achieved, 1.2% peri-operative death	100% POBA, 7% multi-staged procedure, 87% of planned RV achieved
ERACI-I	≥2 lesions in ≥2arteries with LVEF >35%. Complete RV possible with either strategy	127	1988-90	Peri-operative mortalty 4.7%	100% POBA
Lausanne	Isolated proximal LAD stenosis and preserved LV function	134	1989-93	100% left ITA with 98% procedural success	100% POBA, 3% required emergencey CABG and 3% coronary stenting
GABI	Angina (CCS II-IV) and ≥2 lesions of >70% stenosis in ≥2 arteries. Occlusions excluded.	359	1986-91	37% ITA	100% POBA, 86% revascularisation, 30% multi-staged procedures
EAST	≥2 lesions in ≥2arteries with LVEF >50%	392	1985-86	Complete RV 98%	Complete revascularisation 77%
CABRI	Symptomatic multivesseal disease (vessel diam.>2mm) and LVEF>35%	1054 (85% CSA)	1988-92	82% of lesions bypassed 81% patients received ≥1 arterial graft	53.5% lesions bypassed, 29% complete RV
MASS	Single vessel proximal LAD disease and normal LV	214	1988-91	100% left ITA	100% POBA. Procedural success 96%
BARI	Symptomatic multivesseal disease	1829 (1/3-CSA)	1988-91	82% ITA, 91% revascularisation	57% revascularisation
French Monocentric	Multivessel disease >70% Occlusions excluded. Complete RV of 2 arterial territories feasible	152 "few" CSA	1989-93	58% ITA. Complete RV 92.1%	100% POBA. Bail out stenting alone used Complete RV 84.2%
ERACI-II	Two vessel (diam. ≥3mm) disease (>70% plus >50%) and LVEF>35%. Up to one occlusion permitted. CCS III/IV or UA	450 (>10% CSA)	1996-98	88.5% ITA. Complete RV 85%. Peri-operative mortality 5.7%	99% >1 coronary stent Complete RV 50.2% 28% GpIIb/IIIa inhibitor
ARTS	≥2 lesions in ≥2arteries LVEF>35%. Complete RV achievable with either strategy	1205 (755 -CSA)	1997-98	93% ≥1 arterial graft, 84% complete RV	89% coronary stents, 70% complete RV, Gp IIb/IIIa inhibitor used
SoS	≥1 lesion	988	1996-99	81% ITA, 11% BITA, 1% radial	77% coronary stents, 8% GpIIb/IIIa, 94% revascularisation
AWESOME	High risk patients with refractory/unstable angina	454	1995-2000	70% Left ITA, 3.4% right ITA, 2.8% radial artery graft, 5% procedural mortality	54% coronary stents, 11% Gp IIb/IIIa inhibitor, 1% procedural mortality

RITA = Randomised Intervention Treatment of Angina; ERACI =Argentine Randomised Trial of PTCA vs CABG; GABI = German Angioplasty Bypass Surgery Investigation; EAST = Emory Angioplasty Versus Surgery Trial; CABRI = Coronary Angioplasty Versus Bypass Revascularisation Investigation; MASS = Medicine, Angioplasty or Surgery Study; BARI = Bypass Angioplasty Revascularisation Investigation; ARTS = Arterial Revascularisation Therapies Trial; SOS = Stent or Surgery trial; AWESOME = Angina With Extremely Serious Operative Mortality Evaluation.

Table 2. Continued.

	Death			MI			RV			Angina free		
Follow-up	CABG	PCI	P	CABG	PCI	P	CABG	PCI	P	CABG	PCI	P
2.5 years	3.6%	3.1%	NS	5.2%	6.7%	NS	4.0%	37.0%	<0.001	78.5%	59.7%	0.007
3 years	4.7%	9.5%	NS	7.8%	7.8%	NS	6.3%	37.0%	0.001	96.8%	95.2%	NS†
2.5 years	1.0%	0.0%	NS	3.0%	11.7%	NS	3.0%	25.0%	<0.01	89.0%	77.0%	NS
1 year	5.1%	0.5%	N/A	7.3%	3.8%	N/A	4.0%	43.0%	N/A	71.0%	74.0%	NS
3 years	6.2%	7.1%	NS	19.6%	14.6%	NS	14.0%	63.0%	<0.001	88.0%	80.0%	0.039
1 year	2.7%	3.9%	NS	3.5%	4.9%	NS	3.5%	36.5%	N/A	75.0%	67.0%	N/A
2 years	2.9%	5.7%	NS	2.7%	0.0%	N/A	0.0%	30.0%	N/A	72.7%	64.7%	N/A
5 years	10.7%	13.7%	NS	11.7%	10.9%	NS	8.0%	54.0%	<0.001	N/A	N/A	N/A
5 years	10.5%	13.0%	NS	1.3%	5.2%	<0.01	9.0%	29.0%	<0.01	53.0%	21.1%	<0.01
18 months	7.5%	3.1%	0.017	6.3%	2.3%	<0.001	4.8%	16.8%	0.01	N/A	N/A	N/A
1 year	2.8%	2.5%	NS	4.8%	6.2%	NS	3.8%	21.0%	<0.01	89.5%	78.9%	<0.001
2 years	2.0%	5% *13/22 cardiac*	0.001	8.0%	5.0%	NS	6.0%	21.0%	<0.01	79.0%	66.0%	<0.001
5 years	27.0%	22.0%	NS	4.0%	6.0%	NS	5.0%	12.0%	NS	60.0%	56.0%	NS‡

LV = Left Venticle; PCI = Percutaneous Coronary Intervention; LVEF = Left Ventricular Ejection Fraction; ITA = Internal Thoracic Artery; POBA = Plain Old Balloon Angioplasty; CABG = Coronary Artery Bypass Grafting; LAD = Left Anterior Descending Artery; RV = Revascularisation; CSA = Chronica Stable Angina.
† Significant difference at 1 year in favour of CABG (61% vs 82%), ‡ Freedom from unstable angina.

results were comparable to those of the larger BARI study [30], 54% vs 8%; however, only one third of patients enrolled had CSA.

These POBA studies though representing a huge effort of clinical investigation, because of the rise in stenting and the impact of technology and adjunctive pharmacological therapy, are of largely historical interest. They do show, however, the very low mortality rate of contemporary CABG surgery.

Randomised controlled trials: coronary stenting vs coronary artery bypass surgery

With respect to the four studies in which coronary stenting was widely used, the overall findings of two of these, the ERACI-II [32] and AWESOME [35] studies, can not easily be extended to patients with CSA. In ERACI-II trial >90% patients enrolled presented with unstable angina, and AWESOME recruited patients with refractory myocardial ischaemia who were considered to be at very high surgical risk. The findings of ARTS [33] and SoS [34] parallel those of the earlier POBA trials and demonstrate that surgical revascularisation confers significantly greater relief from symptoms of angina or need for subsequent revascularisation compared to coronary stenting. In the SoS study [34], 66% of patients assigned to PCI and 79% of those assigned to surgery were free of angina at one year (p=<0.0001). In ARTS [34], the corresponding incidences were 78.9% and 89.5%, respectively (p=<0.001). In both of these studies, 21% of patients assigned to PCI required further revascularisation, lower than the rates observed in earlier POBA studies and commensurate with the 30-50% reduction in angiographic restenosis associated with stenting compared to POBA [36-39]. Notably, the similar rates of revascularisation are observed despite the follow-up period of ARTS being one year and SoS, two years. This observation can be explained by the natural history of in-stent restenosis which generally manifests within six months of the percutaneous procedure. There was no significant difference in the incidence of myocardial infarction. However, in SoS, there appeared to be a significant mortality benefit associated with surgery (2% vs 5%, p=<0.001), though the study was not powered for this interpretation because of the overall very low death rate.

Meta-analyses: percutaneous coronary intervention vs coronary artery bypass grafting

Three meta-analyses [40-42] were identified comparing surgical and percutaneous (either POBA or coronary stenting) revascularisation. The most recent of these papers [40] examined long-term, in addition to short- and intermediate-term outcomes with each strategy, and supersedes the earlier analyses. Death, non-fatal myocardial infarction, revascularisation (CABG and/or PCI) and angina were evaluated at one, three, five and eight years following assignment to bypass grafting or percutaneous revascularisation in 7964 patients. At the 5-year time-point there was a significant absolute risk reduction in death of 1.9% (p=<0.01) in favour of surgery, equating to one life saved for every 53 surgical procedures performed. There was a survival advantage at one, three or eight years with CABG, but this was small and not statistically significant. Subsequent PCI or CABG was more common in patients assigned to percutaneous revascularisation at all time-points. Most of these were necessary within the first year following the index procedure, but continued to accumulate, albeit at a slower rate, in patients assigned to PCI rather than CABG from one to eight years. The percentage of patients with angina was also significantly more frequent in this group up to five years; however, the difference between the groups narrowed with time, and by eight years, there was no significant difference. The superiority of surgical revascularisation was less clear cut, when only the studies which compared CABG to coronary stenting were considered. In fact, the non-significant survival advantage in favour of surgery was reversed in favour of PCI with coronary stenting, and there was a significant 2.9% absolute risk reduction of non-fatal myocardial infarction at three years (p=<0.01). Angina and revascularisation remained significantly higher in the PCI group with stenting, but had converged closer to the incidence rates in the CABG group owing to the lower rate of restenosis.

Non-randomised clinical data

Percutaneous revascularisation: demographics

The number of women or individuals older than 65 years in revascularisation trials has been small. Men and women shared identical prognostic profiles in the CASS registry [18]. In the TIME trial [43], that exclusively enrolled patients with symptomatic myocardial ischaemia >75 years old and randomised them to conservative therapy or angiography, followed by an appropriate revascularisation strategy, an invasive strategy was associated with improved quality of life, and reduced hospital admissions with unstable angina. There was also a non-significant 50% reduction in mortality.

Several studies have highlighted the increased incidence of complications associated with percutaneous and surgical revascularisation in elderly patients [44-47]. Surgical revascularisation in one registry [44] was associated with an increased risk of in-hospital death in patients >80years compared to those below, 8.1% vs 3.0%. The risks of stroke are more than doubled [44] and prolonged hospital stays are common [45]. Many elderly patients also require simultaneous valve surgery further increasing the operative risks [45]. Similarly, the outcomes of PCI in elderly patients are less favourable with greater incidence of myocardial infarctions and subsequent procedures, although observational data indicates procedural success remains high [46,47]. Therefore, careful appraisal of the risk: benefit ratio is justified, especially if the clinical significance of a small prognostic benefit is unclear or manifests beyond the expected life expectancy of the patient.

Percutaneous revascularisation: diabetes

A subgroup analysis [30] of 353 randomised patients with diabetes by the BARI investigators, revealed a prognostic benefit for those patients assigned to surgical revascularisation. At five years, the survival rate of patients assigned to PCI and CABG, was 65.5% and 80.6% (p=0.003), respectively. At seven years, the survival gap widened (55.7% vs 76.4%). Latterly, a 2-year follow-up of 122 diabetic patients from CABRI [48] and an 8-year follow-up of 59 diabetic patients from EAST [49], confirmed these findings. However, the effect observed in the BARI study has been shown to be largely driven by a potent advantage in a small group of 50 patients with diabetes who suffered a Q wave myocardial infarction during the follow-up period [50]. Eighty percent of diabetics who had been assigned to PCI and had a myocardial infarction during the follow-up period, subsequently died. Surgery protected diabetics from this effect, reducing the respective mortality rate to just 17%, similar to the respective rate in the non-diabetic cohort [50].

There is no evidence that diabetics with multivessel disease benefit prognostically from surgical revascularisation, rather than contemporary PCI. Only 15% (n=142) of patients enrolled in the SoS trial were diabetic and although a detailed subgroup analysis has not been published, there was no difference in incidence of revascularisation procedures between diabetic and non-diabetic patients (25% and 20%, p=0.54). The ARTS trial included 208 patients with diabetes and an analysis [51] demonstrated no significant difference in survival or myocardial infarction between patients assigned to either strategy at either one or three years [52]. Moreover, in the AWESOME study [35, 53] which enrolled very high-risk patients with poor LV function and recent MI, 80% of whom had multivessel disease including the left anterior descending artery, a revascularisation strategy did not influence survival in the subgroup of patients with diabetes. In ARTS, repeat revascularisation at one year was more common in the stent group rather than the CABG group (22.3% vs 3.1%, p<0.001) and higher than the rate in the non-diabetic group assigned to PCI (14.6%). Whether these findings would be replicated in the modern era of more aggressive antiplatelet therapy, however, remains unclear. Meta-analysis of abciximab usage in patients undergoing PCI suggests that rates of death at the time of PCI are equivalent between diabetics who received Reopro and non-diabetics who did or did not receive abciximab [54].

Extent of revascularisation

Secondary analysis [55] of the ARTS trial has also indicated that completeness of revascularisation is important in predicting event-free survival, which is largely determined by the need for a repeat revascularisation procedure. Similar to RITA, GABI and ERACI-I, patients were enrolled in ARTS if equivalent revascularisation was possible with either strategy. Complete revascularisation was achieved in 84.1% of patients assigned to surgery and 70.5% assigned to PCI ($p<0.05$). Incomplete revascularisation had little effect on surgically treated patients, whilst in those assigned to PCI, it was associated in a 5-fold increase in surgical revascularisation at one year from 2% to 10% ($p=<0.05$). In two studies that did not set out to achieve equivalent revascularisation, CABRI [56] and BARI [57], similar findings have been made after 1-year follow-up. Irrespective of whether equivalent revascularisation was deemed possible or not, almost all of the studies indicate complete revascularisation is achieved more often with surgery than PCI. Thus, in-stent restenosis and incomplete treatment of the coronary disease account for the associated increase in morbidity with PCI. Both the extent of arterial disease and the number of occlusions have been found to be angiographic predictors of incomplete revascularisation [55]. In clinical practice, the presence of ostial or bifurcation lesions, lesions within very tortuous vessels and diffuse disease, will also impact on the feasibility of revascularisation percutaneously, and presumably, translate in to a less favourable outcome with PCI, although this has not been formally examined.

Optimal contemporaneous revascularisation strategy

With the exception of left main stem disease, surgical revascularisation does not produce superior survival or freedom from subsequent myocardial infarction compared to equivalent revascularisation by a percutaneous approach. Surgery, however, does improve freedom from angina and the need for a second revascularisation procedure. An initial percutaneous strategy is more cost-effective due to the higher initial costs of surgery. Despite the greater subsequent need for repeat procedures following PCI, the cost remains lower than that for CABG surgery. One example [33] from the stent era presented by the ARTS trialists, indicated that the mean cost of surgical revascularisation would be more than $10,000; $4,000 greater than PCI. Even after 12 months, the period within which most repeat procedures are performed for restenosis, the difference only narrowed to $3,000. Moreover, longer-term cost-effectiveness may swing further back in favour of PCI, due to the increased rate of revascularisation in the second decade following surgery because of the high attrition rate associated with vein graft conduits [6]. It is likely that percutaneous revascularisation in the post-ARTS trial era may produce superior freedom from symptoms and lower re-intervention rates, approximating even closer to those of surgery. The difference should narrow with the use of more aggressive anti platelet agents, clopidogrel [58] and glycoprotein IIb/IIIa inhibitors [59], but more markedly by the development of drug eluting stents (DES) which potently suppress the development of in-stent restenosis. In the past, the high procedural success of PCI has been offset by the relatively high incidence of restenosis resulting in recurrence of symptoms and the need for further procedures. The impact of this can be demonstrated by comparing two similar trials. The RITA (using POBA) and SoS (using coronary stents) trials both enrolled approximately 1000 patients and followed-up patients for similar periods. In both studies, angina-free status was reported by 79% of patients assigned to surgery; however, the transition to stents in the PCI group improved this proportion from 59% to 66%. The need for a repeat procedure fell more markedly from 37% to 21%, converging with those of surgery (4%). Thus, although stenting only modestly (30-50%) reduced the incidence of restenosis compared to POBA, it was associated with a commensurate improvement in clinical outcome following PCI.

Recently, two anti-proliferative agents, Sirolimus [60] and Paclitaxel [61], have been delivered to the coronary vasculature by deployment of a DES, and have been shown to reduce neointima growth by >90% compared to bare metal stents. A commensurate reduction in angina symptoms and repeat procedures can be expected with DES. Interestingly, DES stents appear to reduce the incidence of restenosis to the same degree in all examined subgroups [60], including diabetics in whom restenosis occurs more frequently (and consequently poorer outcomes). Whether the advent of DES guarantees equivalent long-term outcomes with PCI and surgery in diabetics will be revealed in the ongoing CARDia trial in Europe, which will enroll 600 diabetic patients with multivessel disease and randomise them to CABG, bare metal stents with abciximab or DES and abciximab [62].

Perhaps the most difficult area of contemporary contextualisation of the available evidence is our understanding of the benefit of CABG versus current medical therapy. Since the CABG vs. medical therapy trials, very major advances in medical therapy that impact on survival have been made. These include the widespread use of aspirin, statin drugs and ACE inhibitors. Whilst the benefits of these drugs would be equal between the CABG and medical groups (if they were equally prescribed), if there was even a slight decrease in overall mortality, it is difficult to imagine that the statistically small advantages in prognosis gained in the subset analyses of the CASS and European studies would remain.

Conclusions

The indications for surgical revascularisation in coronary artery disease are evolving from criteria based on simple angiographic criteria. Patients with challenging coronary disease, that is not amenable to equivalent revascularisation by a percutaneous approach and those patients in whom the success of PCI is difficult to guarantee (eg. occlusions, ostial and bifurcation lesions), surgery still remains attractive as an initial strategy, supported by evidence.

On evidence to date, at least in the first few years, surgical revascularisation results in superb symptomatic benefit, better than PCI without drug eluting stents. Contemporary PCI will close this gap, but to what extent, remains unclear at the time of writing. Regardless, for some patients repeat percutaneous procedures might be considered an acceptable alternative to surgery. The technological advances in percutaneous revascularisation mean that surgery is increasingly being reserved for the most challenging patients with the most extensive coronary disease. Bilateral Internal Mammary Artery (BIMA) grafts or Total Arterial Revascularisation (TAR) have been reported to show improved graft survival and might transform surgery into a single definitive procedure; however, there are no prospective randomised data to support this notion [63]. If arterial conduits do fulfil their promise and surgical risks remain low, surgical revascularisation might become cost-effective in the longer-term.

Recommendations	Evidence level
◆ Revascularisation should be considered for patients with:- LMCA stenosis >50%; three vessel disease; two vessel disease including proximal LAD stenosis >50%; symptomatic myocardial ischaemia refractory to optimal medical therapy; silent myocardial ischaemia subtending a substantial portion of the left ventricular wall.	Ia/A
◆ Surgical revascularisation should be considered if equivalent revascularisation is unlikely to be achieved by a percutaneous strategy.	Ib/A

References

1. Pepine CJ, Cohn PF, Deedwania PC, Gibson RS, Handberg E, Hill JA, *et al.* Effects of treatment on outcome in mildly symptomatic patients with ischemia during daily life. The Atenolol Silent Ischemia Study (ASIST). *Circulation* 1994; 90(2): 762-8.
2. Lampe FC, Whincup PH, Wannamethee SG, Shaper AG, Walker M, Ebrahim S. The natural history of prevalent ischaemic heart disease in middle-aged men. *Eur Heart J* 2000; 21(13): 1052-62.
3. Mathur VS, Guinn GA, Anastassiades LC, Chahine RA, Korompai FL, Montero AC, *et al.* Surgical treatment for stable angina pectoris. Prospective randomized study. *N Engl J Med* 1975; 292(14): 709-13.
4. Murphy ML, Hultgren HN, Detre K, Thomsen J, Takaro T. Treatment of chronic stable angina. A preliminary report of survival data of the randomized Veterans Administration cooperative study. *N Engl J Med* 1977; 297(12): 621-7.
5. Eleven-year survival in the Veterans Administration randomized trial of coronary bypass surgery for stable angina. The Veterans Administration Coronary Artery Bypass Surgery Cooperative Study Group. *N Engl J Med* 1984; 311(21): 1333-9.
6. Peduzzi P, Kamina A, Detre K. Twenty-two-year follow-up in the VA Cooperative Study of Coronary Artery Bypass Surgery for Stable Angina. *Am J Cardiol* 1998; 81(12): 1393-9.
7. Prospective randomised study of coronary artery bypass surgery in stable angina pectoris. Second interim report by the European Coronary Surgery Study Group. *Lancet* 1980; 2(8193): 491-5.
8. Long-term results of prospective randomised study of coronary artery bypass surgery in stable angina pectoris. European Coronary Surgery Study Group. *Lancet* 1982; 2(8309): 1173-80.
9. Varnauskas E. Twelve-year follow-up of survival in the randomized European Coronary Surgery Study. *N Engl J Med* 1988; 319(6): 332-7.
10. Coronary-artery bypass surgery in stable angina pectoris: survival at two years. European Coronary Surgery Study Group. *Lancet* 1979; 1(8122): 889-93.
11. Coronary artery surgery study (CASS): a randomized trial of coronary artery bypass surgery. Quality of life in patients randomly assigned to treatment groups. *Circulation* 1983; 68(5): 951-60.
12. Alderman EL, Bourassa MG, Cohen LS, Davis KB, Kaiser GG, Killip T, *et al.* Ten-year follow-up of survival and myocardial infarction in the randomized Coronary Artery Surgery Study. *Circulation* 1990; 82(5): 1629-46.
13. Rogers WJ, Coggin CJ, Gersh BJ, Fisher LD, Myers WO, Oberman A, *et al.* Ten-year follow-up of quality of life in patients randomized to receive medical therapy or coronary artery bypass graft surgery. The Coronary Artery Surgery Study (CASS). *Circulation* 1990; 82(5): 1647-58.
14. Takaro T, Hultgren HN, Lipton MJ, Detre KM. The VA cooperative randomized study of surgery for coronary arterial occlusive disease II. Subgroup with significant left main lesions. *Circulation* 1976; 54(6 Suppl): III107-17.
15. Chaitman BR, Davis KB, Kaiser GC, Mudd G, Wiens RD, Ng GS, *et al.* The role of coronary bypass surgery for "left main equivalent" coronary disease: the Coronary Artery Surgery Study registry. *Circulation* 1986; 74(5 Pt 2): III17-25.
16. Caracciolo EA, Davis KB, Sopko G, Kaiser GC, Corley SD, Schaff H, *et al.* Comparison of surgical and medical group survival in patients with left main equivalent coronary artery disease. Long-term CASS experience. *Circulation* 1995; 91(9): 2335-44.
17. Chaitman BR, Fisher LD, Bourassa MG, Davis K, Rogers WJ, Maynard C, *et al.* Effect of coronary bypass surgery on survival patterns in subsets of patients with left main coronary artery disease. Report of the Collaborative Study in Coronary Artery Surgery (CASS). *Am J Cardiol* 1981; 48(4): 765-77.
18. Proudfit WJ, Bruschke AV, MacMillan JP, Williams GW, Sones FM, Jr. Fifteen year survival study of patients with obstructive coronary artery disease. *Circulation* 1983; 68(5): 986-97.
19. Weiner DA, Ryan TJ, McCabe CH, Chaitman BR, Sheffield LT, Ng G, *et al.* Comparison of coronary artery bypass surgery and medical therapy in patients with exercise-induced silent myocardial ischemia: a report from the Coronary Artery Surgery Study (CASS) registry. *J Am Coll Cardiol* 1988; 12(3): 595-9.
20. Mock MB, Ringqvist I, Fisher LD, Davis KB, Chaitman BR, Kouchoukos NT, *et al.* Survival of medically treated patients in the coronary artery surgery study (CASS) registry. *Circulation* 1982; 66(3): 562-8.
21. Gruentzig A. Results from coronary angioplasty and implications for the future. *Am Heart J* 1982; 103(4 Pt 2): 779-83.
22. Sigwart U, Puel J, Mirkovitch V, Joffre F, Kappenberger L. Intravascular stents to prevent occlusion and restenosis after transluminal angioplasty. *N Engl J Med* 1987; 316(12): 701-706.
23. Coronary angioplasty versus coronary artery bypass surgery: the Randomized Intervention Treatment of Angina (RITA) trial. *Lancet* 1993; 341(8845): 573-80.
24. Rodriguez A, Mele E, Peyregne E, Bullon F, Perez-Balino N, Liprandi MI, *et al.* Three-year follow-up of the Argentine Randomized Trial of Percutaneous Transluminal Coronary Angioplasty Versus Coronary Artery Bypass Surgery in Multivessel Disease (ERACI). *J Am Coll Cardiol* 1996; 27(5): 1178-84.
25. Goy JJ, Eeckhout E, Moret C, Burnand B, Vogt P, Stauffer JC, *et al.* Five-year outcome in patients with isolated proximal left anterior descending coronary artery stenosis treated by angioplasty or left internal mammary artery grafting. A prospective trial. *Circulation* 1999; 99(25): 3255-9.
26. Hamm CW, Reimers J, Ischinger T, Rupprecht HJ, Berger J, Bleifeld W. A randomized study of coronary angioplasty compared with bypass surgery in patients with symptomatic multivessel coronary disease. German Angioplasty Bypass Surgery Investigation (GABI). *N Engl J Med* 1994; 331(16): 1037-43.
27. First-year results of CABRI (Coronary Angioplasty versus Bypass Revascularisation Investigation). CABRI Trial Participants. *Lancet* 1995; 346(8984): 1179-84.

28. King SB, 3rd, Lembo NJ, Weintraub WS, Kosinski AS, Barnhart HX, Kutner MH, *et al.* A randomized trial comparing coronary angioplasty with coronary bypass surgery. Emory Angioplasty versus Surgery Trial (EAST). *N Engl J Med* 1994; 331(16): 1044-50.
29. Hueb WA, Bellotti G, de Oliveira SA, Arie S, de Albuquerque CP, Jatene AD, *et al.* The Medicine, Angioplasty or Surgery Study (MASS): a prospective, randomized trial of medical therapy, balloon angioplasty or bypass surgery for single proximal left anterior descending artery stenoses. *J Am Coll Cardiol* 1995; 26(7): 1600-5.
30. Comparison of coronary bypass surgery with angioplasty in patients with multivessel disease. The Bypass Angioplasty Revascularization Investigation (BARI) Investigators. *N Engl J Med* 1996; 335(4): 217-25.
31. Carrie D, Elbaz M, Puel J, Fourcade J, Karouny E, Fournial G, *et al.* Five-year outcome after coronary angioplasty versus bypass surgery in multivessel coronary artery disease: results from the French Monocentric Study. *Circulation* 1997; 96(9 Suppl): II-1-6.
32. Rodriguez A, Bernardi V, Navia J, Baldi J, Grinfeld L, Martinez J, *et al.* Argentine Randomized Study: Coronary Angioplasty with Stenting versus Coronary Bypass Surgery in patients with Multiple-Vessel Disease (ERACI II): 30-day and one-year follow-up results. ERACI II Investigators. *J Am Coll Cardiol* 2001; 37(1): 51-8.
33. Serruys PW, Unger F, Sousa JE, Jatene A, Bonnier HJ, Schonberger JP, *et al.* Comparison of coronary-artery bypass surgery and stenting for the treatment of multivessel disease. *N Engl J Med* 2001; 344(15): 1117-24.
34. Coronary artery bypass surgery versus percutaneous coronary intervention with stent implantation in patients with multivessel coronary artery disease (the Stent or Surgery trial): a randomised controlled trial. *Lancet* 2002; 360(9338): 965-70.
35. Morrison DA, Sethi G, Sacks J, Henderson W, Grover F, Sedlis S, *et al.* Percutaneous coronary intervention versus coronary artery bypass graft surgery for patients with medically refractory myocardial ischemia and risk factors for adverse outcomes with bypass: a multicenter, randomized trial. Investigators of the Department of Veterans Affairs Cooperative Study #385, the Angina With Extremely Serious Operative Mortality Evaluation (AWESOME). *J Am Coll Cardiol* 2001; 38(1): 143-9.
36. Serruys PW, de Jaegere P, Kiemeneij F, Macaya C, Rutsch W, Heyndrickx G, *et al.* A comparison of balloon-expandable-stent implantation with balloon angioplasty in patients with coronary artery disease. Benestent Study Group. *N Engl J Med* 1994; 331(8): 489-95.
37. Serruys PW, van Hout B, Bonnier H, Legrand V, Garcia E, Macaya C, *et al.* Randomised comparison of implantation of heparin-coated stents with balloon angioplasty in selected patients with coronary artery disease (Benestent II). *Lancet* 1998; 352(9129): 673-81.
38. Savage MP, Fischman DL, Rake R, Leon MB, Schatz RA, Penn I, *et al.* Efficacy of coronary stenting versus balloon angioplasty in small coronary arteries. Stent Restenosis Study (STRESS) Investigators. *J Am Coll Cardiol* 1998; 31(2): 307-11.
39. Betriu A, Masotti M, Serra A, Alonso J, Fernandez-Aviles F, Gimeno F, *et al.* Randomized comparison of coronary stent implantation and balloon angioplasty in the treatment of *de novo* coronary artery lesions (START): a four-year follow-up. *J Am Coll Cardiol* 1999; 34(5): 1498-506.
40. Hoffman SN, TenBrook JA, Wolf MP, Pauker SG, Salem DN, Wong JB. A meta-analysis of randomized controlled trials comparing coronary artery bypass graft with percutaneous transluminal coronary angioplasty: one- to eight-year outcomes. *J Am Coll Cardiol* 2003; 41(8): 1293-304.
41. Sim I, Gupta M, McDonald K, Bourassa MG, Hlatky MA. A meta-analysis of randomized trials comparing coronary artery bypass grafting with percutaneous transluminal coronary angioplasty in multivessel coronary artery disease. *Am J Cardiol* 1995; 76(14): 1025-9.
42. Pocock SJ, Henderson RA, Rickards AF, Hampton JR, King SB, 3rd, Hamm CW, *et al.* Meta-analysis of randomised trials comparing coronary angioplasty with bypass surgery. *Lancet* 1995; 346(8984): 1184-9.
43. Trial of invasive versus medical therapy in elderly patients with chronic symptomatic coronary-artery disease (TIME): a randomised trial. *Lancet* 2001; 358(9286): 951-7.
44. Alexander KP, Anstrom KJ, Muhlbaier LH, Grosswald RD, Smith PK, Jones RH, *et al.* Outcomes of cardiac surgery in patients > or = 80 years: results from the National Cardiovascular Network. *J Am Coll Cardiol* 2000; 35(3): 731-8.
45. Kolh P, Kerzmann A, Lahaye L, Gerard P, Limet R. Cardiac surgery in octogenarians; peri-operative outcome and long-term results. *Eur Heart J* 2001; 22(14): 1235-43.
46. Thompson RC, Holmes DR, Jr., Grill DE, Mock MB, Bailey KR. Changing outcome of angioplasty in the elderly. *J Am Coll Cardiol* 1996; 27(1): 8-14.
47. Lefevre T, Morice MC, Eltchaninoff H, Chabrillat Y, Amor M, Juliard JM, *et al.* One-month results of coronary stenting in patients > or = 75 years of age. *Am J Cardiol* 1998; 82(1): 17-21.
48. Kurbaan AS, Bowker TJ, Ilsley CD, Sigwart U, Rickards AF. Difference in the mortality of the CABRI diabetic and nondiabetic populations and its relation to coronary artery disease and the revascularization mode. *Am J Cardiol* 2001; 87(8): 947-50; A3.
49. King SB, 3rd, Kosinski AS, Guyton RA, Lembo NJ, Weintraub WS. Eight-year mortality in the Emory Angioplasty versus Surgery Trial (EAST). *J Am Coll Cardiol* 2000; 35(5): 1116-21.
50. Seven-year outcome in the Bypass Angioplasty Revascularization Investigation (BARI) by treatment and diabetic status. *J Am Coll Cardiol* 2000; 35(5): 1122-9.
51. Abizaid A, Costa MA, Centemero M, Abizaid AS, Legrand VM, Limet RV, *et al.* Clinical and economic impact of diabetes mellitus on percutaneous and surgical treatment of multivessel coronary disease patients: insights from the Arterial Revascularization Therapy Study (ARTS) trial. *Circulation* 2001; 104(5): 533-8.
52. Legrand VM, Serruys PW, Unger F, van Hout BA, Vrolix MC, Fransen GM, *et al.* Three-year outcome after coronary stenting versus bypass surgery for the treatment of multivessel disease. *Circulation* 2004; 109(9): 1114-20.

53. Sedlis SP, Morrison DA, Lorin JD, Esposito R, Sethi G, Sacks J, *et al.* Percutaneous coronary intervention versus coronary bypass graft surgery for diabetic patients with unstable angina and risk factors for adverse outcomes with bypass: outcome of diabetic patients in the AWESOME randomized trial and registry. *J Am Coll Cardiol* 2002; 40(9): 1555-66.
54. Bhatt DL, Marso SP, Lincoff AM, Wolski KE, Ellis SG, Topol EJ. Abciximab reduces mortality in diabetics following percutaneous coronary intervention. *J Am Coll Cardiol* 2000; 35(4): 922-8.
55. van den Brand MJ, Rensing BJ, Morel MA, Foley DP, de Valk V, Breeman A, *et al.* The effect of completeness of revascularization on event-free survival at one year in the ARTS trial. *J Am Coll Cardiol* 2002; 39(4): 559-64.
56. Kurbaan AS, Bowker TJ, Ilsley CD, Rickards AF. Impact of postangioplasty restenosis on comparisons of outcome between angioplasty and bypass grafting. Coronary Angioplasty versus Bypass Revascularisation Investigation (CABRI) Investigators. *Am J Cardiol* 1998; 82(3): 272-6.
57. Whitlow PL, Dimas AP, Bashore TM, Califf RM, Bourassa MG, Chaitman BR, *et al.* Relationship of extent of revascularization with angina at one year in the Bypass Angioplasty Revascularization Investigation (BARI). *J Am Coll Cardiol* 1999; 34(6): 1750-9.
58. Mehta SR, Yusuf S, Peters RJ, Bertrand ME, Lewis BS, Natarajan MK, *et al.* Effects of pretreatment with clopidogrel and aspirin followed by long-term therapy in patients undergoing percutaneous coronary intervention: the PCI-CURE study. *Lancet* 2001; 358(9281): 527-33.
59. Topol EJ, Mark DB, Lincoff AM, Cohen E, Burton J, Kleiman N, *et al.* Outcomes at 1 year and economic implications of platelet glycoprotein IIb/IIIa blockade in patients undergoing coronary stenting: results from a multicentre randomised trial. EPISTENT Investigators. Evaluation of Platelet IIb/IIIa Inhibitor for Stenting. *Lancet* 1999; 354(9195): 2019-24.
60. Moses JW, Leon MB, Popma JJ, Fitzgerald PJ, Holmes DR, O'Shaughnessy C, *et al.* Sirolimus-eluting stents versus standard stents in patients with stenosis in a native coronary artery. *N Engl J Med* 2003; 349(14): 1315-23.
61. Hong MK, Mintz GS, Lee CW, Song JM, Han KH, Kang DH, *et al.* Paclitaxel coating reduces in-stent intimal hyperplasia in human coronary arteries: a serial volumetric intravascular ultrasound analysis from the Asian Paclitaxel-Eluting Stent Clinical Trial (ASPECT). *Circulation* 2003; 107(4): 517-20.
62. Smith D. The CARDia trial protocol. *Heart* 2003; 89(10): 1125-6.
63. Taggart DP, D'Amico R, Altman DG. Effect of arterial revascularisation on survival: a systematic review of studies comparing bilateral and single internal mammary arteries. *Lancet* 2001; 358(9285): 870-5.

Chapter 17

Revascularisation in acute coronary syndrome

Nick G Bellenger BSc MD MRCP
Specialist Registrar, Cardiology
Nicholas P Curzen PhD FRCP
Consultant Interventional Cardiologist

WESSEX CARDIOTHORACIC CENTRE, SOUTHAMPTON, UK

Introduction

"Acute coronary syndrome" (ACS) is now the leading cause for emergency hospital admission. Of the patients with ACS, those with an ST elevation myocardial infarction (STEMI) are now considered clinically distinct from those with either unstable angina or non-ST elevation myocardial infarction (NSTEMI). Together, this represents an enormous health burden with 150,000 admissions for acute MI in the UK annually, and an incidence of ACS in England and Wales of 115,000 new patients per year. The prognosis for ACS is not benign. United Kingdom registry data reveal at six months after admission for non-STEMI ACS there is a 12.2% rate of death or non-fatal MI, and a 30% rate of death, MI, refractory angina or readmission for unstable angina [1]. The aims of treatment strategies in both STEMI and ACS include stabilisation of the atheromatous plaque, restoration of coronary blood flow and alleviation of any flow-limiting stenosis. A variety of medical therapies are available, increasingly in association with mechanical coronary revascularisation strategies which include percutaneous intervention (PCI) and coronary artery bypass graft surgery (CABG). The evolution of revascularisation has been rapid in recent years and technological developments in PCI have led to an increase in the number of these procedures being undertaken in the UK, so that the latest figures demonstrate a ratio approaching 2:1 comparing PCI with CABG (Figure 1). This has coincided with a very large increase in the number of patients with ACS undergoing early angiography and revascularisation on the grounds of improved prognosis. Increasingly, patients with this group of conditions will be dealt with by interventional cardiologists: already the majority of out-of-hours coronary revascularisation in the UK takes place in the catheter lab rather than the operating theatre. This chapter will firstly review the evidence base for revascularisation in STEMI, cardiogenic shock and then focus specifically on ACS.

Revascularisation in STEMI

In STEMI there is coronary thrombus formation on a disrupted or fissured coronary atherosclerotic plaque, leading to vessel occlusion. A number of pharmacological agents have been shown to play a key role in counterbalancing the many factors involved in progressive platelet and thrombus propagation, distal embolisation and re-occlusion of the coronary artery. Fundamental to any treatment, however, is to

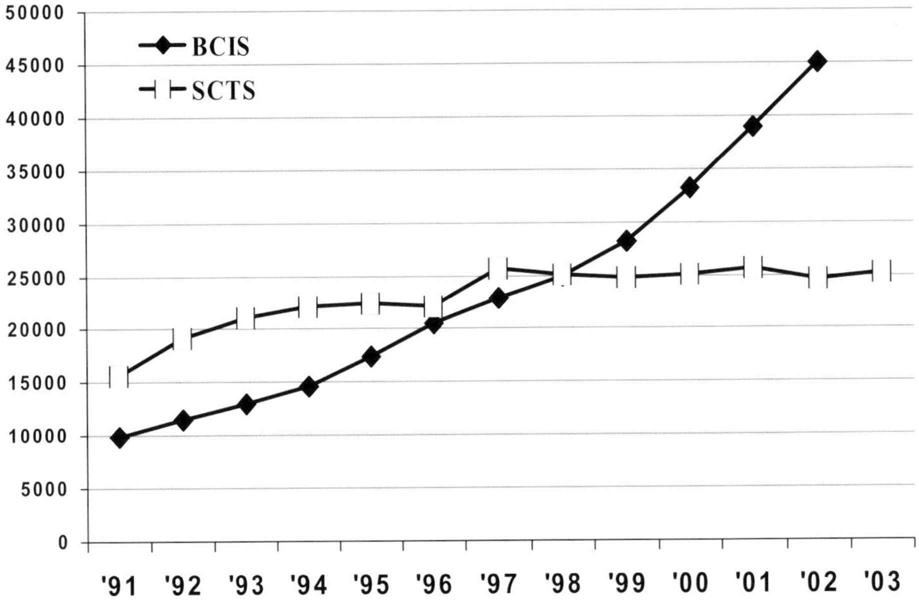

Figure 1. **Rates of PCI versus isolated CABG in the UK. BCIS British Cardiovascular Intervention Society; SCTS Society of Cardiothoracic Surgeons of Great Britain and Ireland.**

re-open the occluded artery. Conventional aspirin plus thrombolytic therapy is successful in only a limited number of patients (<60% achieving TIMI III flow), and a significant proportion of patients are denied this therapy because of contraindications (principally related to bleeding). There is, in any case, a 1% risk of cerebral haemorrhage. This has led to increased interest in mechanical revascularisation. Bypass surgery has little to offer in this setting. There are no randomised trials of early surgery vs medical treatment in STEMI, but data from North American and UK databases suggest that CABG in the early phase of myocardial infarction is associated with a significant mortality (18-20%) [2,3]. By contrast, percutaneous intervention has proved itself to be an attractive and effective treatment in these patients.

Primary PCI

There is now irrefutable evidence from randomised trials that, when compared to thrombolysis, primary PCI offers a higher rate of infarct-related artery (IRA) patency, a lower incidence of intracranial bleeding and a reduction in hospital stay and overall cost, but most important of all, attenuated LV dysfunction and overall mortality [4,5] (Figure 2).

An overview of the results of ten comparisons of primary PCI versus thrombolysis confirmed a lower mortality (4.4% versus 6.5%, $p<0.05$), resulting in two lives saved per 100 treated with PCI [6]. The combination of death and non-fatal MI was more profound, 11.9% versus 7.2%, $p<0.05$. Procedural success rate, even in studies with low stent usage, were greater than 90%. Such short-term benefits are reflected in a longer-term trend, with a mortality at five years post-PCI of 13% versus 24% for thrombolysis, in a randomised trial of 395 patients [7]. The non-fatal MI at five years was 6% (PCI) versus 22%, with a lower rate of readmission for ischaemia and heart failure. Furthermore, few of these patients were treated with intracoronary stents that may be expected to reduce the readmission rate still further as demonstrated by recent data [8]. With the advent of more efficacious adjuvant medical therapy, including pharmacological pre-treatment on the way to the catheter laboratory, even better results may be expected in the future.

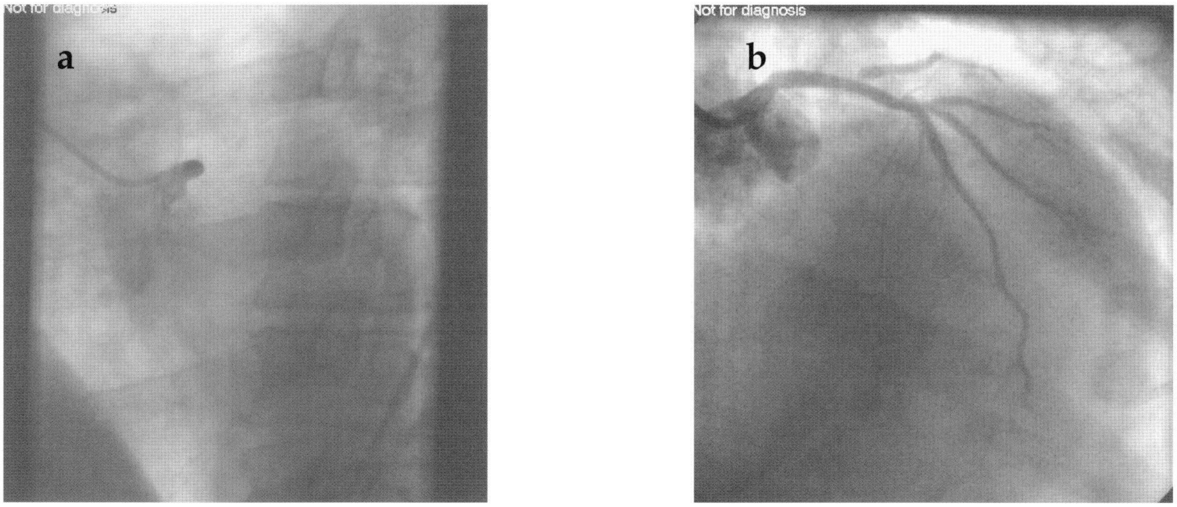

Figure 2. **Primary PCI with disobliteration and stenting of left main stem coronary in the context of acute MI with cardiogenic shock. a) Left coronary artery on arrival. b) Left coronary artery after the LMS has been re-opened and a 3x18mm stent deployed. An intra-aortic balloon pump was also inserted. The patient went home several days later.**

Rescue PCI

Until sufficient infrastructure is in place to provide a comprehensive primary angioplasty service, many patients will still be treated with aspirin and thrombolysis. This treatment fails to achieve arterial patency in 15-40% of patients, and fails to achieve TIMI III flow in 40-50% [9]. Controversy still exists regarding the best treatment of this group who have “failed thrombolysis”. This represents a high-risk group with a 30-day mortality of over 15% who may receive repeat thrombolysis, for which there are no supportive data, or rescue angioplasty. Until recently, the evidence for this latter approach has been limited to a few small studies, which have not shown consistent results [10,11]. Rescue angioplasty is currently one of the commonest reasons for out of hours PCI in many centres in the UK. There are however, no evidence-based practice guidelines, and the rate of intervention for this condition varies extensively from centre to centre. Whilst ongoing angina appears a clear-cut indication for rescue PCI, failure of ST elevation to resolve, without pain, is fraught with the potential for doing more harm than good. The recent early data from the REACT study [12] suggest that rescue PCI is a beneficial strategy, but further data are required. Perhaps, more than any other commonly performed emergency PCI, this raises an important question about the conventional concept of "surgical cover" for modern PCI. The vast majority of rescue PCI is performed in a setting where no formal surgical back-up has either been requested or is available. In many cases, the patient experiencing a catastrophic PCI complication would be deemed inoperable due to excessive risk.

Rescue CABG

There are no randomised trials of surgery in the setting of failed thrombolysis. But overall, PCI offers a substantially lower risk than CABG in this setting because of the combined influences of evolving myocardial infarction, active thrombolysis and antiplatelet therapy. If surgery is required (for LMS or multivessel disease not amenable to total percutaneous revascularisation), this is generally delayed with target vessel PCI and the use of an intra-aortic balloon pump to stabilize the patient.

Revascularisation in cardiogenic shock

The leading cause of death in patients hospitalised for MI is cardiogenic shock. The high-risk nature of the condition often leads to conservative management, thereby denying the patient the potential for a more successful outcome, particularly from PCI (Figure 2) [13].

The GUSTO I trial contains the largest prospectively identified registry of patients with cardiogenic shock: 2972 patients with an overall mortality of 55% [14]. The 30-day mortality of patients undergoing CABG was 29% and for those undergoing PCI was 22%. Other non-randomised data also suggest that the outcome is better in patients treated by revascularisation, but of course interpretation is limited by the selected nature of the group [13]. The SHOCK trial [15] randomly allocated 302 patients with cardiogenic shock to early revascularisation (PCI or CABG) (defined as within six hours of presentation) or medical treatment. The results showed no differences in the primary end-point of 30-day mortality between the groups (47% vs 56%). A significant mortality benefit in the revascularisation group was, however, identified at six months (50% mortality revascularisation vs 63% medical, $p<0.05$). It should be noted though, that this was not a primary end-point of the study, but it nevertheless represents 13 additional lives saved per 1000 patients treated [16]! The 1-year mortality in the patients undergoing PCI with an occluded infarct-related artery was 39% in those with a successful procedure, but was 85% if PCI failed to restore good flow ($p=0.001$). Outcome was clearly associated with improvement in TIMI flow rate. Restoration of coronary blood flow as early as possible is thus a major predictor of outcome in cardiogenic shock. The data in those less than 75 years suggests that 20 additional lives would be saved in six months by early revascularisation. The SMASH trial [17] comparing initial strategy of PCI with medical treatment also showed a high mortality for both groups (69% vs 78%) and this trial was stopped early. Further evidence for benefit of early revascularisation in cardiogenic shock comes from the primary PCI registry of ALKK [18]. Nine thousand four hundred and twenty-two procedures were registered over six years, 14.2% in the context of cardiogenic shock. In-hospital mortality was dependent on the TIMI flow achieved: TIMI III 38%, TIMI II 66%, TIMI 0-I 78%.

The differences in outcome between registry and randomised data could be explained by the inevitable selection bias in the former. The outcome of cardiogenic shock remains poor. Most interventional cardiologists consider the available data suggest that many of these patients should undergo emergency angiography and, where technically feasible, PCI. The place for CABG surgery is likely to be limted.

Revascularisation in non-ST elevation acute coronary syndromes

A number of studies are available in which patients with NSTEMI were randomised to medical treatment or early angiography and revascularisation. Such studies can be divided into two broad groups. TIMI IIIB and VANQWISH are historical studies in the sense that certain factors, specifically the trial design and angioplasty with virtually no stents or modern adjuvant pharmacological therapy, make their findings difficult to interpret. FRISC II, TACTICS TIMI and RITA 3 are contemporary studies, although, with the increasing use of platelet inhibitors and drug eluting stents, even these data may now not be a good reflection of PCI practice. It is, nevertheless, the contemporary studies that have revolutionised the way general physicians and cardiologists manage these patients. Furthermore, important lessons have been learnt from the historical studies.

TIMI IIIB

This multicentre trial enrolled 1473 patients with unstable angina and objective signs of ischaemia or documented coronary disease and randomised them to either invasive or conservative strategies [19]. Angiography was undertaken 18-24 hours after randomisation and revascularisation was by means of either immediate PCI, with no stent, in 41% or CABG as soon as possible, but up to six weeks. By six weeks 49% of the conservative group had required revascularisation, making interpretation of the study difficult. The primary end-point of composite death, MI and positive stress test at six weeks was reached in

16.2% of the invasive group and 18.1% in the conservative group (p=0.33). At one year, the incidence of death and MI was similar in the two groups (10.8% vs 12.25, p=0.4), although repeat hospital admissions remained significantly lower in the invasive group (26% vs 33%, p<0.005).

VANQWISH

Nine hundred and twenty patients with an evolving non-Q wave MI and a level of creatine kinase MB isoenzymes that was more than 1.5 times the upper limit of normal for the hospital were enrolled into this multicentre randomised trial of early revascularisation versus medical therapy with revascularisation for refractory ischaemia [20]. Forty-four percent of the invasive group received revascularisation, as did 33% of the medical group, again making interpretation difficult. The primary composite end-point of death or MI was reached in 29.9% of the invasive group and 26.9% of the conservative group (p=0.35) at a mean of 23 months follow-up.

The in-hospital mortality in the CABG patients was 12% in this study. This result is likely to have lowered enthusiasm for urgent in-patient surgery in these patients, many of whom were in fact high-risk compared to the contemporary studies in which surgical mortality was lower.

The number of patients with one of the primary end-point components and the number who died were significantly higher in the invasive-strategy group (36 vs 15 patients, p=0.004 for the primary end-point at hospital discharge; 21 vs 6 patients; p=0.007 for death at one month and results were similar at one year.

FRISC II

Two thousand four hundred and fifty-seven patients with class IIIb unstable angina and ST depression of at least 1mm or T wave inversion and/or cardiac enzyme rise (57% of patients with TnT rise) were randomly assigned to invasive or conservative strategy and to three months of either dalteparin or placebo using a factorial design [21]. Randomisation occurred within 72 hours and patients were revascularized within ten days. At six months there was a significant difference in the primary composite outcome of death or MI (9.4% invasive vs 12.1% conservative, p=0.031). Furthermore, there was a significant reduction of 4.2% of the combined end-point at two years (12.1% vs 16.3%). Hospital admissions were also significantly reduced over two years in the invasive group (44.8% vs 64.5%, p<0.001). It is important to note that 43% of the conservative group underwent revascularisation within one year, a finding that elegantly demonstrates the natural history of this condition.

TACTICS TIMI

In TACTICS TIMI [22], 2220 patients with non-STEMI ACS (56% with TnT rise) recruited between 1997 and 1999 were treated with intravenous glycoprotein IIb/IIIa (GPIIb/IIIa) antagonists for 48 hours and then randomised to medical or invasive treatment. The primary composite end-point of death, MI or re-hospitalisation for ACS at six months was significantly less in the invasive group (15.9% vs 19.4%, p=0.025). The patients that derived the most benefit from early intervention were those of high or even intermediate risk (positive troponin, elderly, diabetes, post-infarction, ST depression on ECG). There was an absolute reduction of 10% in those patients with a raised troponin. The low-risk patients, however, derived similar benefit from PCI or CABG. The marked reduction in MI seen in this study when compared to FRISC II may be due to the increased use of GPIIb/IIIa antagonists (only 10% of PCI patients in FRISC II).

RITA 3

The objective of this study was to test early angiography (<72hrs) and revascularisation against a conservative strategy of medical treatment with angiography for refractory angina or ischaemia [23]. This multicentre randomised trial recruited 1810 patients with class IIIb unstable angina and ST depression, transient ST elevation, T wave inversion, old Q waves or known coronary artery disease. Patients with CK rise were excluded. The primary end-point of death, non-fatal MI or refractory angina at four months occurred in significantly fewer patients in the early invasive group and the early conservative group (9.6% vs 14.5%, p=0.001). This difference was maintained at one year (p=0.003). Compared to the high-risk patients in TACTICS where most of the benefit was derived from a reduction in MI and re-hospitalisation for recurrent ischaemia, the moderate-risk patients in RITA 3 had a 54% reduction in refractory ischaemia (4.4% vs 9.3%, p<0.0001) which drove the significant primary end-point results. The rates of death and MI in both groups were similar.

ISAR-COOL

In the light of growing evidence for the benefit of early revascularisation, a number of strategies for delivering this service have been explored. This includes community pre-treatment with agents such as GPIIb/IIIa inhibitors, expansion in the number of local PCI centres or transfer from district hospitals to major PCI centres. The key to this strategy is the timing of intervention. The trials attempting to answer this question have thrown further light on the central question of the benefit of intervention itself.

In ISAR-COOL, 410 patients with non-STE ACS were randomised to immediate PCI (mean 2.4 hours) or a period of 72-120 hours of pre-treatment with aspirin, clopidogrel, tirofiban and heparin [24]. The primary end-point of death or non-fatal MI at 30 days was significantly reduced in the early PCI group (5.9% vs 11.6%, p=0.04), with excess MIs occurring prior to catheterisation. This not only reinforces the benefit of revascularisation, but also suggests that a cooling-off period prior to catheterisation is counterproductive. This very early intervention time causes considerable logistical problems, and a more realistic strategy may be initial pre-treatment with revascularisation being performed within 24 hrs. This intermediate time was not tested by ISAR-COOL, but the results of TACTICS, with a low event rate (4.7%) after pre-treatment and intervention at <48hrs, would tend to support this more realistic strategy.

A review of modern practice

PCI: stents

Until the mid 1990s, PCI was based on balloon angioplasty. Whilst this had been shown to be superior to medical treatment alone in CAD, the initial success rate was less than current practice, with a far greater degree of acute closure (around 10%), and a restenosis rate of up to 50%, classically occurring in the first six months. Since then, the introduction of bare metal stents has had a significant impact on both procedural success and a reduction of restenosis to between 15-20%. This trial data is supported by BCIS audit data of UK intervention that demonstrates an increase in angioplasty from 1992 to 1998 from 11,575 to 24,661 (113%) with the reduction in re-intervention for restenosis (from 11.6% to 5.2%) being inversely proportional to the increase in stent use (2.7% to 69%) [25]. As a result, the National Institute of Clinical Excellence (NICE) recommends the routine use of stents. Stent deployment is now routine in over 90% of procedures in most high volume centres because of the improved clinical outcome. By contrast, stent utilisation in the quoted studies was relatively low. It is highly likely that the unequivocal benefit would be enhanced by more universal stent deployment as well as by the application of other adjunctive technologies. The addition of drug eluting stents (DES) to PCI options is likely to substantially improve medium and long-term outcome in ACS patients as it has been shown to do in other patient groups.

PCI: GPIIb/IIIa antagonists

The binding of fibrinogen and other adhesive proteins to adjacent platelets via the GPIIb/IIIa integrin serves as the final common pathway of platelet thrombus formation. A large number of trials have demonstrated that GPIIb/IIIa inhibitors reduce the frequency of ischaemic complications during and after PCI [26,27,28]. Indeed, the use of these agents was responsible for the reduction in very early events seen in TACTICS compared to FRISC II. The administration of these agents should begin as soon as possible and continued during the intervention to achieve maximum benefit. Once again, NICE recommendations support the use of GPIIb/IIIa antagonists in the setting of ACS. The use of these agents in the era prior to TACTICS was limited. Furthermore, data from trials such as EPISTENT suggest that diabetic patients derive particular prognostic benefit from abciximab in terms of reduced mortality and in-stent restenosis [28].

PCI: clopidogrel

It is now standard practice for ACS patients to receive treatment with both aspirin and clopidogrel prior to and following PCI. Clopidogrel is a thienopyridine that inhibits platelet activation via the adenosine diphosphonate (ADP) pathway. The CURE study randomised 12,562 patients with ACS to aspirin and clopidogrel or aspirin alone, and found a 20% relative risk reduction in the combined end-point of cardiovascular death, MI or stroke (9.3% vs 11.4%, p<0.001) [30]. This benefit was at the cost of a 1% increase in major bleeding. PCI-CURE was a prospectively designed observational study looking at the 2658 patients in CURE that underwent PCI for refractory unstable angina [31]. The primary end-point of composite cardiovascular death, MI or target vessel revascularisation at 30 days was significantly reduced by the use of clopidogrel (4.5% vs 6.4%, p=0.03). Long-term administration (nine months) of clopidogrel after PCI was associated with a lower rate of cardiovascular death, myocardial infarction, or any revascularisation (p=0.03), and of cardiovascular death or myocardial infarction (p=0.047). Overall, (including events before and after PCI) there was a 31% reduction in cardiovascular death or myocardial infarction (p=0.002). Patients in these studies discussed here, were not routinely receiving clopidogrel. The evidence, therefore, supports the routine use of clopidogrel in ACS, with or without PCI. This raises an important clinical dilemma for the cardiac surgeon. Patients with ACS are routinely treated with clopidogrel as part of their medical management. Up to around 20% of such patients referred for angiography are then referred for CABG surgery. The data, however, suggest that the risk of bleeding complications is significantly higher in patients on clopidogrel. Re-operation for bleeding is known to be associated with a significant increase in peri-operative mortality and morbidity and there is evidence that this drug should be withheld for 5-7 days prior to CABG [32]. Despite these data, surgical practice in this area is heterogenous. Some centres routinely stop clopidogrel for 5-7 days, whereas others operate without stopping it at all. There is theoretical concern about stopping such an agent, proven to reduce acute ischaemic event rates, in patients with ACS awaiting CABG.

PCI: drug eluting stents

The long-term success of coronary stenting has been hampered by in-stent restenosis as a result of exaggerated healing in the form of neointimal proliferation. The risk of in-stent restenosis is associated with diabetes, vessel calibre, lesion length, plaque burden, presence of dissections, number of stents, stent diameter and configuration of multiple stents. The recent emergence of drug eluting stents has revolutionized the prevention of restenosis [33]. These stents can be coated in a variety of slow-release preparation anti-proliferative drugs. Currently, the two devices already available are the sirolimus-eluting Cypher stent (Cordis, J&J) and the paclitaxel-eluting Taxus stent (Boston Scientific). Both these stents have shown a dramatic reduction in in-stent restenosis [34,35]. Drug eluting stents were not used in any of the trials mentioned in this chapter, and to date have not been formally tested in the specific setting of ACS. Nevertheless, the available data demonstrate large reductions in restenosis rates across all subgroups of patients tested and trial data in patients with both STEMI and other ACS will be available shortly.

CABG

The studies presented did not specifically analyse the results of the subgroup of patients undergoing CABG. The VANQWISH trial reported a high hospital mortality (11.6%) for the patients undergoing early revascularisation (median eight days from randomisation). In this study, the operative mortality was 3.4% in the patients undergoing CABG at a median of 28 days. The operative mortality for early surgical revascularisation was 2.1% in FRISC II and 3.6% in TACTICS TIMI and mortality for delayed revascularisation was 1.7% and 1.9% respectively. It is not possible to unravel the operative mortality of CABG in the two groups in RITA 3, but the overall CABG mortality was 3.0%. The striking difference in operative mortality in patients with early CABG in VANQWISH could be explained by the fact that all patients enrolled in this trial had a significant CK-MB rise compatible with non-Q myocardial infarction. In FRISC II the data on CK/CK-MB cannot be unravelled and it is reported that 43% of patients did not have an enzyme rise. In TACTICS TIMI, 44% of patients did not have cardiac enzyme rise and 37% had a small CK/CK-MB rise. The RITA 3 study excluded patients with CK/CK-MB rise. New data are now needed to assess accurately the risk of early CABG in ACS patients in order to provide uniformity of practice.

The current perspective

Trial data unequivocally confirm the superiority of primary PCI over thrombolysis in ST-elevation MI. Government initiatives are now directed at facing the considerable logistic challenge of offering this therapy to the UK population.

The available evidence now supports early revascularisation in patients with NSTEACS. The challenge for the management of NSTEACS in current UK practice is to achieve revascularisation within the evidence-based time frame. National and international guidelines recommend early angiography and revascularisation for high-risk NSTEACS patients [36]. Unfortunately, it proves impossible to deliver this therapy within the time frame upon which the evidence is based (1-7 days) in the majority of patients. This has led to inequity of access for patients in some hospitals compared with patients in invasive centres [37] and has incurred substantial bed wastage for patients awaiting transfer to revascularisation centres [38].

With time, more accurate risk stratification will enable the early invasive strategy to be directed at those who are at highest risk and who therefore, gain the most benefit. Preliminary data already reveal the promise of inflammatory markers (such as HS-CRP, IL-6, CD40 ligand [36]) that reflect the process within the coronary artery rather than the damage incurred by the myocardium, which is what the troponin level tells us.

Trial acronyms

- CURE: Clopidogrel in Unstable angina to prevent Recurrent Events study.
- EPISTENT: Evaluation of Platelet IIb/IIIa Inhibitor for Stenting Trial.
- FRISC II: Fragmin and Fast Revascularization during InStability in Coronary artery disease.
- GUSTO: Global Utilization of Streptokinase and t-PA for Occluded Arteries.
- ISAR-COOL: Intracoronary Stenting and Antithrombotic Regimen.
- PCI-CURE: Percutaneous Intervention Clopidogrel in Unstable angina to prevent Recurrent Events study.
- REACT: Rescue Angioplasty or Conservative Therapy.
- RITA 3: Randomised Interventional Trial of unstable Angina 3.
- SHOCK: Should We Emergently Revascularize Occluded Coronaries for Cardiogenic Shock.
- SMASH: Swiss Multicenter Angioplasty for Shock trial.
- TACTICS TIMI: Treat Angina with Aggrastat and determine Cost of Therapy with an Invasive or Conservative Strategy.
- TIMI: Thrombolysis in Myocardial Infarction.
- TIMI IIIb: Thrombolysis in Myocardial Infarction IIIb.
- VANQWISH: Veterans Affairs Non-Q-Wave Infarction Stratification in Hospital.

Recommendations	Evidence level
♦ Acute coronary syndromes are the commonest group of conditions leading to acute hospital admission.	III/B
♦ Despite advances in pharmacological therapy, early revascularisation (within 1-7 days) has been shown to be of considerable benefit in the majority of such patients	Ia/A
♦ In ST-elevation MI, early primary angioplasty is unequivocally superior to thrombolysis in terms of mortality and LV dysfunction.	Ia/A
♦ In cardiogenic shock, randomised trial data are sparse. One trial showed a small survival benefit at six months for patients undergoing revascularisation.	Ia/A
♦ In non ST-elevation ACS, data demonstrate that an early revascularisation strategy is associated with outcome benefit compared to optimal medical therapy alone.	Ia/A

References

1. Collinson J, Flather MD, Fox KA, *et al.* Clinical outcomes, risk stratification and practice patterns of unstable angina and myocardial infarction without ST elevation: Prospective Registry of Acute Ischaemic Syndromes in the UK (PRAIS-UK). *Eur Heart J* 2000; 21: 1450-7.
2. Curtis JJ, *et al.* Impact of unstable angina on operative mortality with coronary revascularization at varying time intervals after MI. *J Thorac Cardiovasc Surg* 1991: 102: 867-73.
3. Keogh BE, Kinsman R. National Adult Cardiac Surgical Database Report 2000-2001. The Society of Cardiothoracic Surgeons of Great Britain and Ireland.
4. Grines CL, Browne KF, Marco J, *et al*, for the Primary Angioplasty in Myocardial Infarction Study Group. A comparison of immediate angioplasty with thrombolytic therapy for acute myocardial infarction. *N Engl J Med* 1993; 328: 673-9.
5. Keeley EC, Grines CL. Primary coronary intervention for acute myocardial infarction. *JAMA* 2004; 29: 736-9.
6. Weaver WD, Simes RJ, Betriu A, *et al* Comparison of primary angioplasty and intravenous thrombolytic therapy for acute myocardial infarction: a quantitative overview. *JAMA* 1997; 278: 2093-8.
7. Zijlstra F, Hoorntie JCA, de Boer MJ, *et al.* Long-term benefit of primary angioplasty as compared with thrombolytic therapy for acute MI. *N Engl J Med* 1999; 341: 1413-9.
8. Stone GW, Brodie BR, Griffin JJ, *et al* Clinical and angiographic follow-up after primary stenting in acute myocardial infarction: the Primary Angioplasty in Myocardial Infarction (PAMI) stent pilot trial. *Circulation* 1999; 99: 1548-54.
9. de Belder MA. Acute myocardial infarction: failed thrombolysis. *Heart* 2001: 85: 104-12.
10. Califf RM, Topol EJ, Stack RS, *et al*, for the TAMI Study group. Evaluation of combination thrombolytic therapy and timing of cardiac catheterization in acute MI. Results of thrombolysis and angioplasty in myocardial infarction-phase 5 randomised trial. TAMI study group. *Circulation* 1991; 83: 1543-56.
11. Ellis SG, da Silva ER, Heyndrickx GR, *et al*, for the RESCUE Investigators. Randomized comparison of rescue angioplasty with conservative management of patients with early failure of thrombolysis for acute MI. *Circulation* 1994; 90: 2280-84.
12. Gershlick A on behalf of REACT Investigators. Oral presentation. British Cardiac Society 2004.
13. Gacioch GM, Ellis SG, Lee L, *et al.* Cardiogenic shock complicating acute myocardial infarction: the use of coronary angioplasty and the integration of the new support devices into patient management. *J Am Coll Cardiol* 1992; 19: 647-53.
14. Holmes DR Jr, Bates ER, Kleiman NS, *et al.* Contemporary reperfusion therapy for cardiogenic shock: the GUSTO-I trial experience. The GUSTO-I Investigators. Global Utilization of Streptokinase and Tissue Plasminogen Activator for Occluded Coronary Arteries. *J Am Coll Cardiol* 1995; 26: 668-74.
15. Hochman JS, Sleeper LA, Webb JG, *et al.* Early revascularization in acute MI complicated by cardiogenic shock. SHOCK Investigators. Should we emergently revascularize occluded coronaries for cardiogenic shock. *N Engl J Med* 1999; 341: 625-34.
16. Williams SG, Wright DJ, Tan LB. Management of cardiogenic shock complicating acute myocardial infarction; towards evidence-based medical practice. *Heart* 2000; 83: 621-626.
17. Urban P, *et al.* A randomized evaluation of early revascularization to treat shock complicating acute myocardial infarction. The Swiss Multicenter trial of Angioplasty for SHock. *Eur Heart J* 1999; 20: 1030-1038.

18. Zeymer U, Vogt A, Zahn R, *et al.* Predictors of in-hospital mortality in 1333 patients with acute MI complicated by cardiogenic shock treated with primary PCI: results of the Arbeitsgemeinschaft Leitende Kardiologische Krankenhausarzte (ALKK). *Eur Heart J* 2004; 25: 322-8.
19. Anderson HV, Cannon CP, Stone PH, *et al.* One year results of the Thrombolysis in Myocardial Infarction (TIMI) IIIB clinical trial. A randomized comparison of tissue-type plasminogen activator versus placebo and early invasive versus early conservative strategies in unstable angina and non-Q wave MI. *J Am Coll Cardiol* 1995; 26: 1643-50.
20. Boden WE, O'Rourke RA, Crawford MH, *et al.* Outcomes in patients with acute non-Q-wave MI randomly assigned to an invasive as compared with a conservative management strategy. Veterans Affairs Non-Q-Wave Infarction Strategies in Hospital (VANQWISH) Trial Investigators. *N Engl J Med* 1998; 338: 1785-92.
21. Invasive compared to non-invasive treatment in unstable coronary-artery disease: FRISC II prospective randomised multi-center study. Fragmin and Fast Revascularization during InStability in Coronary artery disease Investigators. *Lancet* 1999; 354: 708-15.
22. Cannon CP, Weintraub WS, Demopoulos LA, *et al.* TACTICS (Treat Angina with Aggrastat and determine Cost of Therapy with an Invasive or Conservative Strategy) - Thrombolysis In Myocardial Infarction 18 Investigators. Comparison of early invasive and conservative strategies in patients with unstable coronary syndromes treated with glycoprotein IIb/IIIa inhibitor tirofiban. *N Engl J Med* 2001; 344: 1879-87.
23. Fox KA, Poole-Wilson PA, Henderson RA, *et al.* Randomised Interventional trial of unstable Angina (RITA) Investigators. Interventional versus conservative treatment for patients with unstable angina or non-ST elevation MI: the British Heart Foundation RITA 3 randomised trial. *Lancet* 2002; 360: 743-51.
24. Neumann FS, Kastrati A, Pogats-Murray G, *et al.* Evaluation of prolonged antithrombotic pretreatment ("cooling-off" strategy) before intervention in patients with unstable coronary syndromes: a randomised controlled trial. *JAMA* 2003; 290: 1593-9.
25. Gershlick AH. Role of stenting in coronary revascularization. *Heart* 2001; 86: 104-12.
26. Topol EJ, Moliterno DJ, Herrmann HC, *et al.* Comparison of two platelet glycoprotein IIb/IIIa inhibitors, tirofiban and abciximab, for the prevention of ischaemic events with percutaneous coronary revascularization. *N Engl J Med* 2001; 344: 1888-94.
27. Anderson KM, Califf RM, Stone GW, *et al.* Long-term mortality benefit with abciximab in patients undergoing percutaneous coronary intervention. *J Am Coll Cardiol* 2001; 37: 2059-65.
28. Braunwald ME, Antman EM, Beasley JW, *et al.* ACC/AHA guideline update for the management of patients with unstable angina and non-ST segment elevation myocardial infarction. *Circulation* 2002; 106: 1893-900.
29. Steinhubl SR, Ellis SG, Wolski K, *et al.* Ticlopidine pretreatment before coronary stenting is associated with sustained decrease in adverse cardiac events: data from the Evaluation of Platelet IIb/IIIa Inhibitor for Stenting (EPISTENT) Trial. *Circulation* 2001; 103: 1403-9.
30. The CURE Investigators. Effects of clopidogrel in addition to aspirin in patients with acute coronary syndromes without ST segment elevation. *N Engl J Med* 2001; 345: 494-502.
31. Mehta SR, Yousef S, Peters RJG, *et al.* Effects of pre-treatment with clopidogrel and aspirin followed by long-term therapy in patients undergoing PCI: the PCI-CURE study. *Lancet* 2001; 358: 527-33.
32. ACC/AHA 2002 Guideline Update for the Management of Patients with Unstable Angina and Non-ST-Segment Elevation Myocardial Infarction. A Report of the American College of Cardiology/American Heart Association Task Force on Practice Guidelines (Committee on the Management of Patients With Unstable Angina). http://www.acc.org/clinical/guidelines/unstable/incorporated.
33. Devadathan S, Curzen N. Drug-eluting stents: a new era in interventional cardiology. *Geriatric Medicine* 2003; 33: 89-95.
34. Sousa E, Serruys P, Costa M. New Frontiers in Cardiology. Drug-Eluting Stents: Part I. *Circulation* 2003; 107: 2274-2279.
35. Sousa E, Serruys P, Costa M. New Frontiers in Cardiology. Drug-Eluting Stents: Part II. *Circulation* 2003; 107: 2383-2389.
36. Archbold RA, Curzen N. The role of revascularisation in the management of non-ST elevation acute coronary syndromes: who should you refer? *Clin Med* 2004; 4: 32-35.
37. Miller C, Lipscomb K, Curzen N. Are district general hospital patients with unstable angina at a disadvantage? *Postgrad Med J* 2003; 79: 93-8.
38. Bellenger NG, Eichhofer J, Crone D, Curzen N. Hospital stay in patients with non-ST-elevation acute coronary syndromes. *Lancet* 2004; 363: 1399-400.

Chapter 18

Different conduits in coronary surgery

Shafi Mussa MA MRCS

Specialist Registrar, Cardiothoracic Surgery [2]

David P Taggart MD (Hons) PhD FRCS

Professor of Cardiovascular Surgery [1*]

Consultant Cardiothoracic Surgeon [2]

1 University of Oxford, Oxford, UK

2 John Radcliffe Hospital, Oxford, UK

Introduction

Most patients undergoing coronary surgery in the UK receive three bypass grafts, usually as a combination of arterial and venous conduits [1]. A wide choice of conduits can be used to construct coronary artery bypass grafts. Venous conduits include long saphenous vein, short saphenous vein and cephalic vein. Arterial conduits include the left and right internal thoracic arteries, the radial artery, the gastroepiploic artery and the inferior epigastric artery. There have also been attempts to use synthetic conduits with very limited success.

For each type of conduit, performance is judged on two main criteria: graft patency following surgery, and clinical outcome. The most widely reported method of assessing graft patency is catheter-based contrast angiography. Intuitively one would expect that graft patency would relate to clinical outcomes, and there is published data to substantiate this [2]. Clinical outcomes following coronary bypass grafting are commonly presented as survival rates and as freedom from Major Adverse Cardiac Events (MACE) such as myocardial infarction, and requirement for re-intervention (angioplasty, redo surgery). Both angiographic and clinical end-points can be measured at specific time intervals following surgery, and enable the comparison of different conduits.

However, a multitude of factors influence graft patency and will thus impact on clinical performance. In particular, graft inflow and distal run-off are important considerations, as well as the inherent biological characteristics of the conduit including endothelial function, and smooth muscle contractility. It is likely that even the most meticulously harvested, best quality conduit will perform poorly as a graft if the inflow and/or the distal run-off are compromised. Historically, superior patency of left internal thoracic artery (ITA) and saphenous vein graft conduits has been demonstrated on grafting to the left anterior descending artery versus non-left anterior descending targets [3,4]. However, more recent data suggest that patency rates of ITA grafts are independent of coronary target site [5]. Thus, the previous speculation that the comparatively large myocardial muscle mass supplied by the left anterior descending artery and its branches results in extensive run-off, with consequent superior graft patency, is now called into question. Conduits placed on coronary targets with low-grade stenoses will be subject to competitive flow from the

* from Oct 2004

native coronary artery, and may have poorer patency rates as a result.

It is thus important to select the most appropriate conduit according to the nature and extent of coronary disease, giving due consideration to other patient-specific factors such as age, comorbidity, and conduit availability. This chapter explores the current evidence for the use of different conduits in coronary surgery.

Methodology

Current literature for different conduits in coronary surgery was reviewed commencing with an electronic database search (Pubmed) using the terms "coronary artery bypass graft", "survival", "patency" and then individual search terms pertaining to the conduit of choice eg. "saphenous vein". This strategy was supplemented by an expert knowledge of the literature, and a further hand search and review of citations within key papers. All citations were available by electronic search, except data retrieved from the *National Adult Cardiac Surgical Database Report* available from the Society of Cardiothoracic Surgeons of Great Britain and Ireland.

Venous conduits

Long saphenous vein

First used by Sabiston to bypass a failed right coronary artery endarterectomy in 1962, the technique of end-to-side coronary anastomosis using long saphenous vein was refined and then described by Favoloro in 1968 [6]. The relative ease of harvest and plentiful supply of autologous long saphenous vein has resulted in wide use of this conduit for the construction of coronary bypass grafts. However, soon after this technique became established, routine angiographic follow-up revealed that venous bypass grafts were susceptible to occlusive disease [7]. Early occlusion of venous grafts (within 30 days of surgery) occurs most commonly due to thrombosis either resulting from poor blood flow down grafts with limited distal run-off, or surgical manipulation of the conduit causing injury to the endothelium and other components of the vessel wall, with subsequent disruption to thromboregulatory pathways [8]. Grafts studied after surgical removal or at post-mortem revealed that late occlusive disease occurred as a result of atherosclerotic processes, with observation of intimal fibrous plaque, foam cell and smooth muscle cell infiltration [9].

FitzGibbon and colleagues established a grading system enabling a consistent classification of the angiographic features of venous bypass grafts [10].

1. Grade A = perfect patency.
2. Grade B = graft narrowed to <50% of grafted artery, at any point in the course of the graft.
3. Grade O = graft occluded.

The same group then reported angiographic follow-up of 403 venous bypass grafts ten years after surgery, and demonstrated 41% of grafts to be occluded, 7% of grafts patent but diseased (Grade B), and 52% to be perfectly patent (Grade A) [11]. Further studies at a mean of 15 years following CABG revealed that 50% of 353 venous grafts were occluded, 10% were patent but diseased, and 40% were perfectly patent [12]. The possibility remains that the true long-term patency rate of venous grafts may indeed have been lower, as only those patients surviving to ten years were able to undergo repeat coronary angiography, and that some deaths in this patient cohort may have been attributable to graft occlusion and its sequelae.

Further observations from these studies revealed that the majority of Grade B grafts imaged less than one year after surgery were classified as such due to technical defects at the distal anastomosis, whereas grafts imaged later after surgery were more likely to be classified as Grade B because they displayed atherosclerotic disease in the trunk of the graft. Ten years following surgery, occlusion rates of venous grafts to the left anterior descending and diagonal arteries were reduced compared to grafts to the other coronary systems. This finding may be attributable to poorer run-off of the right coronary and marginocircumflex systems and also the increased technical difficulty in grafting the inferior and posterior surfaces of the heart.

Short saphenous vein and upper limb veins

Lack of sufficient quantity of good quality long saphenous vein due to varicosities, previous surgery or phlebitis has necessitated the use of alternative venous conduits, namely short saphenous, cephalic and basilic veins. These conduits are not used commonly and thus, there is little data addressing long-term patency and clinical outcome in patients that have undergone CABG utilising these conduits. Stoney and colleagues reported 57% angiographic patency of 56 upper limb vein grafts in 28 patients, at a mean angiographic follow-up time of two years [13]. This is considerably lower than the reported patency rates for long saphenous vein grafts at a similar interval from surgery [12]. The particularly poor performance of upper limb venous grafts has limited their use to exceptional circumstances only. There have been no studies to specifically examine patency rates of short saphenous vein.

Current perspective

Occlusive disease of venous bypass grafts remains a major limitation of coronary artery bypass surgery. However, many of these studies are based on cohorts of patients that underwent coronary bypass surgery in its first or second decade, and can be considered outdated.

Refinements in both surgical technique (eg. improved harvesting techniques, avoidance of conduit distension at suprasystemic pressures), and postoperative medical therapy may contribute to improved performance of venous grafts in contemporary coronary surgery. The early use of aspirin after surgery has resulted in improvement in vein graft patency rates at one year after surgery [14]. The use of HMG CoA Reductase inhibitors or statins, has led to reduced progression of venous graft disease in the medium-term [15]. However, there are no data to confirm that these refinements improve graft patency in the long-term. An up-to-date assessment of venous bypass graft disease would be welcomed.

Arterial conduits

Internal thoracic artery

After early contributions by Vineberg and Kolessov, it was Green who was the first successful advocate of the left internal thoracic artery as a conduit for coronary artery surgery [6]. The left ITA was under-utilised as a conduit in the early 1970s, the conduit of choice being autologous saphenous vein. However, a small number of surgeons continued to use the left ITA.

Accumulating information with respect to venous bypass graft disease led surgeons to investigate the angiographic patency of ITA grafts. Early evidence was conflicting, with some reports suggesting little advantage in using the ITA as a conduit instead of saphenous vein, as the angiographic patency at six months was similar to those of venous grafts [16]. Lytle and colleagues retrospectively used data from serial coronary angiograms in 501 patients post-CABG to investigate saphenous vein and ITA patency in the longer-term. They demonstrated superior patency of ITA grafts (93%) versus saphenous vein grafts (46%) at a mean follow-up time of 7.5 years [17]. These findings were confirmed by other groups [18].

A major change in practice occurred following publication of a seminal article from Loop and associates [19]. In a retrospective observational study they compared clinical outcomes and angiographic findings between 2306 patients who received a single ITA to the left anterior descending artery with supplementary vein grafts and 3265 patients who received only venous grafts. Mean follow-up time was 8.7 years. They demonstrated that 10-year actuarial survival was improved by approximately 10% in all patients receiving ITA grafts to the left anterior descending artery compared with those patients receiving venous grafts, notwithstanding the total number of grafts performed. Placement of a left ITA graft also improved the 10-year actuarial survival of patients with poor left ventricular function by 15% compared to those patients receiving exclusively venous grafts. The use of an ITA graft also improved freedom from major adverse cardiac events.

Ten years later, Cameron and colleagues published a retrospective study comparing 479 patients with a single ITA graft to 4888 patients with exclusively saphenous vein grafts over a 15-year follow-up period [20]. Multivariate analysis (to account for the differences between the two groups) revealed the use of an ITA graft to be an independent predictor of improved survival in all patients, as well as in subgroups of patients over 65, those with impaired left ventricular function and both males and females.

In summary, despite the lack of data from prospective randomised trials, abundant and compelling evidence has ensured the wide acceptance of the left ITA as the conduit of choice to the diseased left anterior descending artery.

Bilateral internal thoracic arteries

The positive results achieved with the use of the left ITA, and the apparent biological similarity between the left and right ITAs, intuitively leads to the assumption that the use of two ITA conduits may provide additional benefits over the conventional strategy of a single ITA and supplementary saphenous vein grafts. This led several groups to investigate the use of bilateral ITA grafting as a strategy for myocardial revascularisation. The technique was already in use in a small number of centres; the indications being for patients whose venous conduits were either poor in quality (due to varicose veins or previous venous thrombotic disease), lacking in sufficient quantity (previous varicose vein surgery or previous use for vascular or cardiac procedures), or for a carefully selected group of patients with an appropriate distribution of coronary atherosclerosis.

Angiographic patency of bilateral ITA grafts in several different studies has been consistently good at varying time intervals after surgery. Endo and colleagues reassessed 1083 patients within 2-3 weeks of CABG, and demonstrated that 97% of bilateral ITA grafts were widely patent [21]. Calafiore and associates reported 99% perfect patency of bilateral ITAs at 18 months [22]. Dion and colleagues demonstrated no difference in angiographic patency (93-97%) between left and right ITAs anastomosed to both left anterior descending and circumflex targets in 161 patients followed-up to a mean of 7.5 years [5]. Buxton and associates reported that right ITA conduits performed better if grafted to branches of the left coronary artery, and if grafted to coronary arteries with high-grade stenoses [23].

Does the superior patency of ITA conduits translate to improved clinical outcomes? Currently, there are no randomised controlled trials of single versus bilateral ITA grafting. The majority of the data is derived from observational studies, most of which are underpowered to show any additional survival benefit over patients receiving a single ITA graft, due to small numbers, poor case matching and short follow-up times.

However, Lytle and colleagues compared clinical outcomes in a retrospective, non-randomised study of patients undergoing elective primary CABG, either with a single ITA graft (8123 patients) or with bilateral ITA grafts (2001 patients) over a mean follow-up period of ten years [24]. As the patient cohort was not randomised, multivariable risk factor analysis and propensity score matching was used to account for heterogeneity and selection bias between the two groups. They reported a survival advantage (bilateral ITA 79% versus single ITA 72%), and improved freedom from re-operation or cardiac re-intervention (bilateral ITA 77% versus single ITA 62%), in those patients who underwent bilateral ITA grafting compared to single ITA grafting, after 12 post-operative years [24]. Also noted was an increasing benefit of bilateral ITA grafting with time. Subgroup analysis demonstrated improved survival for diabetic patients, and patients with impaired left ventricular function, undergoing bilateral ITA grafting compared to those receiving a single ITA graft. In a smaller study with shorter follow-up, Endo and associates retrospectively compared 7-year clinical outcomes following single (688 patients) versus bilateral (443 patients) ITA grafting [21]. They demonstrated improved freedom from redo CABG and myocardial infarction, but no survival benefit at seven years for the bilateral ITA group. Hazard ratios for death were lower for those patients receiving bilateral ITA grafts under the age of 71, and those patients with moderate or better (>40%) pre-operative left ventricular ejection fraction. Subgroup analysis, specifically addressing outcomes in diabetic patients, revealed that diabetic patients with moderate or better left ventricular function had 10-year freedom from death, redo CABG or recurrent myocardial infarction rates that were significantly higher than non-diabetic patients [25]. This benefit did not extend to those with poor left ventricular function.

In possibly the single most powerful study to date, a meta-analysis of seven studies comparing bilateral to single ITA grafting, encompassing a total of 11,269 single ITA versus 4,693 bilateral ITA patients matched for age, gender, left ventricular function and diabetes mellitus, has revealed improved survival for patients undergoing bilateral ITA grafting [26]. The combined hazard ratio, weighted for the number of patients in each study (larger studies therefore had more bearing on the final result), was 0.81 (95% confidence interval 0.70-0.94) in favour of bilateral ITA grafting. However, despite the large number of patients in this meta-analysis, the data should be interpreted with caution as none of the studies were randomised. The meta-analysis, while well conducted, is not a substitute for a prospective randomised controlled trial of single ITA versus bilateral ITA grafting.

The benefits of bilateral ITA grafting must be weighed against the potential risks. The perceived increased risk of sternal wound complications due to the relative devascularisation of the sternum is the major objection to the use of both ITAs. Lytle and colleagues noted a 2.5% incidence of sternal wound complications in the bilateral ITA group, significantly greater than the 1.4% incidence of wound complications in the single ITA group [24]. This finding was confirmed by Calafiore [22]. Some studies have demonstrated an association between diabetes mellitus and sternal dehiscence in patients undergoing bilateral ITA grafting [27]. Skeletonisation of the ITA is thought to preserve sternal blood supply compared to pedicled harvest. Matsa and associates retrospectively reviewed 765 patients (231 diabetics) undergoing bilateral skeletonised ITA grafting, and noted that the sternal wound complication rate was not significantly greater in the diabetic patients, compared to the non-diabetic patients [28]. They did however, demonstrate a 15% incidence of sternal wound complications in obese, diabetic females. However, this paper does not indicate the proportion of patients receiving bilateral ITA grafts of all the patients undergoing coronary surgery in their unit, and how they were selected. At most, the available evidence suggests that using skeletonised ITA conduits may reduce the incidence of sternal wound complications in diabetic patients.

There have also been concerns about increased incidence of respiratory and myocardial injury, although there is good evidence to refute this [29, 30]. Other issues are a perceived increase in operation time as each ITA can not be harvested simultaneously, and the greater technical challenge of using bilateral ITAs. However, the promise of improved patient outcomes should encourage surgeons to persevere with this strategy. Indeed, a postal survey of UK consultant cardiothoracic surgeons revealed that most would opt for bilateral ITA grafting if they were to undergo CABG [31].

Alternative arterial conduits

The high incidence of venous bypass graft disease and the spectacular results achieved with the internal thoracic arteries have led surgeons to explore the use of other arterial conduits for coronary artery bypass grafting. Approximately 20% of patients undergoing isolated CABG in the UK now receive two or more arterial conduits and approximately 75% of patients undergoing first time CABG in 2001 required three or more bypass grafts [1]. There are frequent instances when a third arterial conduit may be required or occasions when the use of bilateral ITAs is not appropriate, resulting in the need for an alternative arterial conduit. Options for the alternative arterial conduit are the radial artery (RA), gastroepiploic artery (GEA) and inferior epigastric artery (IEA).

Radial artery

The radial artery was first used as an aortocoronary graft by Carpentier in 1971 [32]. Subsequent angiographic studies of radial artery bypass grafts at several centres had shown patency rates of between 35-50% up to ten months after surgery [33,34]. Suggested reasons for the low patency rate were vasospasm and intimal hyperplasia, and the RA was abandoned as a bypass conduit. The discovery of patent RA grafts up to 18 years following surgery [35], a low incidence of atherosclerosis in the *in situ* artery [36], together with attractive handling characteristics, availability in sufficient length to reach any distal coronary target, relative ease of harvest, and low morbidity related to harvest, formed the basis for the re-emergence of the RA as a conduit for CABG [37].

Acar and colleagues then demonstrated 29 out of 31 patent RA grafts (93.5%) after a mean follow-up period of 9.2 months [35]. The improved patency rate was attributed to a reduction in mechanical trauma during harvest and the use of pharmacological measures to prevent vasospasm intra- and postoperatively.

Further studies have confirmed and extended these early results (Table 1). Although these results are encouraging, the data must be interpreted with caution. All of the studies were retrospective analyses. The percentage of grafts used that were followed-up with angiography in these studies varies from 3.4% [38] to 92% [39]. Thus the quoted patency rates in some of the studies are based on a relatively small proportion of all RA grafts constructed, and do not necessarily reflect the RA patency rates for the entire study population. The assumption that asymptomatic patients are likely to have more patent grafts is logical, but does not enable extrapolation of graft patency rates to the entire cohort. The recent study by Possati with 92% angiographic follow-up to almost nine years, contains the least number of patients, but provides the most compelling data to date.

Three prospective randomised controlled trials comparing RA to other conduits with the intention of complete angiographic follow-up are currently in progress. The results of two of these studies, the Radial Artery Patency Study (RAPS) and Radial artery versus Saphenous Vein Patency study (RSVP), are keenly awaited [43]. Recently, Buxton and associates, have reported the interim (5-year) results of the Radial Artery Patency and Clinical Outcome (RAPCO) study, a prospective randomised trial comparing RA to saphenous vein grafts and free right ITA grafts [44]. All patients received left ITA grafts to the left anterior descending artery, and were then randomised to receive either a RA or a right ITA to a secondary target in patients under 70, and either a RA or saphenous vein graft to a secondary target in patients over 70. They have demonstrated comparable 5-year actuarial angiographic patency rates between RA and right ITA of 95% versus 100%, and between RA and saphenous vein of 87% versus 94%.

The concept of competitive flow suggests that graft blood-flow is influenced by native coronary blood-flow, with poorer flow in conduits anastomosed to native vessels with higher flows. Royse and colleagues demonstrated that blood flow through composite arterial grafts (LITA-RA T-graft) fell by 44% upon re-introduction of native coronary flow [45]. Grafted conduits may therefore fare better in conditions of poor native coronary flow, typified by high-grade coronary stenoses. Indeed, there is accumulating evidence that grafting the RA to coronary targets with moderate stenoses (<70%) results in reduced anastomotic patency [46]. Moran and colleagues studied 51 RA grafts in 50 patients approximately one year after CABG, demonstrating 35 perfectly patent and ten occluded grafts. Nine of the occluded grafts had been anastomosed to target coronary vessels with <70% stenosis. Multivariate analysis confirmed that the degree of native coronary artery stenosis was a strong predictor of RA graft patency. More recently, Maniar and associates reported similar findings, but

Table 1. Radial artery patency for CABG – summary of published data.

Author	No of RA conduits used	No of RA conduits reassessed (*anastomoses)	% of original grafts grafts reassessed	% Angiographic patency (FitzGibbon Grade A)	Length of follow-up (years)
Acar *et al* [40]	910	64	7	83	5.6±1.1
Possati *et al* [41]	325	62	19	87	4.9±0.5
Iaco *et al* [42]	164	*91	47	95	4.0±2.3
Tatoulis *et al* [38]	8420	280 (*369)	3	90	1.2±0.9
Possati [39]	91	84	92	88	8.8±0.8

also noted that angiographic patency rates were lower in RA grafts to the right coronary artery compared to the left anterior descending artery [47]. Possati and colleagues have also demonstrated that the majority of occluded RA grafts in their study had been anastomosed to coronary targets with less than 70% stenosis, but found that the target vessel location did not influence graft patency [39].

The major concern with the use of the RA is an enhanced tendency for vasospasm due to its muscular wall [48] and an abundance of receptors [49] for circulating vasoactive mediators that may be present following cardiac surgery [50]. The occurrence of conduit vasospasm in the peri-operative or immediate postoperative period may be inconsequential, but could potentially lead to peri-operative myocardial infarction and its sequelae. Prevention of vasospasm is thus an important part of the management strategy if RA conduits are to be employed. The use of topical agents during surgery, followed by oral agents for up to one year after surgery is the most common practice. Papaverine, phenoxybenzamine and verapamil/ nitroglycerin solution are the most commonly used vasodilator agents used topically to prevent spasm. Studies from Oxford have demonstrated that papaverine is short acting and causes more endothelial damage in RA conduits than phenoxybenzamine [51,52]. We have also shown that phenoxybenzamine is long acting and preferentially prevents adrenergic spasm that may be mediated by the use of inotropic agents in the postoperative period [52,53].

In summary, recent evidence from Possati and associates demonstrating satisfactory long-term RA graft patency, confirms and supersedes the early encouraging findings, and justifies the increasing use of the RA as a conduit for bypass grafting, provided there is due consideration for severity and location of target vessel stenoses. Prospective randomised trials comparing RA to other bypass conduits are currently underway, and will provide strong evidence to determine the use of the RA as a strategy in surgical myocardial revascularisation.

Gastroepiploic artery

Independently described by both Pym [54] and Suma [55] in 1987, the right gastroepiploic artery has also been used as an alternative arterial coronary bypass conduit. It is a muscular artery that can be accessed by extending the median sternotomy incision inferiorly into a limited upper midline laparotomy to expose the greater curvature of the stomach. The right GEA can then be used as an *in situ* graft to the right coronary artery, posterior descending artery or less commonly, to the distal circumflex by passing it through the diaphragm. It can be anastomosed to the left anterior descending artery if passed anterior to the diaphragm. It has also been used as a free graft from the descending aorta [56]. It is not a suitable graft to use if the patient has had previous upper abdominal surgery.

The most recent largest published series of GEA grafts reports clinical and angiographic follow-up in 1000 patients receiving *in situ* GEA grafts, predominantly to the right coronary artery. Angiography revealed early stenosis-free patency rates (within one year of surgery) of 89% and mid-term stenosis-free patency rates of 79% (at 3.1 ± 1.8 years from surgery). In comparison, mid-term angiographic stenosis-free patency rates for left ITA grafts were 93% in the same group of patients [57]. Long-term angiographic follow-up of GEA grafts from Suma and colleagues revealed a cumulative patency rate of 63% at ten years, with concomitant late ITA and saphenous vein graft patency in the same patients found to be 94% and 68% respectively [58]. Hence, despite the initial enthusiasm for this conduit, the poor patency rates compared to the ITA and RA account for the comparatively limited use of the GEA for myocardial revascularisation.

Inferior epigastric artery

The inferior epigastric artery may be harvested via a midline infra-umbilical incision without breaching the peritoneum. The IEA can be identified and then dissected from its origin at the external iliac artery as it passes supero-medially in the anterior abdominal wall, to yield a free graft with a length of between 8cm and 13cm. The IEA is sometimes of small calibre, and therefore, not suitable for direct aortic anastomosis. In these cases the IEA may be anastomosed to the aorta via a cuff or hood of saphenous vein, or to another graft such as a pedicle ITA.

Puig and colleagues first reported the use of the IEA in 1990 [59]. Early postoperative angiography at 8-10 days demonstrated 15 out of 17 patent grafts. Buche and associates then published mid-term angiographic data revealing a 79% perfect patency rate (61 out of 77 IEA grafts) at a mean angiographic follow-up time 15 months [60]. This patency rate is comparable with the reported patency rates of free ITA grafts at 18 months [61]. Despite this, the conduit has not gained in popularity because of the variability in its usable length, with some distal coronary targets beyond its reach and also because of the technical issues surrounding the optimum method of proximal anastomosis.

Total arterial revascularisation

The evidence favouring the use of bilateral internal thoracic arteries as conduits for coronary artery bypass grafting is accumulating. The next logical step is the exclusive use of arterial conduits for myocardial revascularisation. Again, as for bilateral ITAs, there are no large long-term randomised trials comparing total arterial revascularisation with conventional strategies. Furthermore, there are no large observational studies on which to base this strategy.

A retrospective study of 256 patients who underwent total arterial revascularisation using bilateral ITAs and GEA grafts, demonstrated 91% actuarial survival, 97% actuarial freedom from myocardial infarction, and 95% actuarial freedom from re-intervention after a seven year follow-up period. These figures are similar to those of previously published historical cohorts who received up to two arterial grafts. Importantly, the use of total arterial revascularisation resulted in 85% actuarial freedom from angina, a significant increase compared to patients who received a single or even two arterial grafts in other studies [62]. However, comparisons between different patient cohorts should be interpreted with caution due to variations in demographics, extent of disease and exclusion criteria.

Muneretto and colleagues conducted a prospective randomised trial of total arterial revascularisation versus conventional CABG in patients aged over 70, comparing two groups well matched for age, gender, left ventricular function, risk factors for atherosclerosis, and major comorbidity [63]. In-hospital outcome measures (mortality, ventilation time, intensive care stay, major postoperative complications) were similar between the two groups, apart from a greater incidence of limb wound infections in the conventional CABG group (related to saphenous vein harvest) than the total arterial group (no wound complications related to the RA harvest site). Follow-up at 15 months revealed improved angiographic graft patency, and greater freedom from angina and myocardial infarction in the total arterial group. It is encouraging that the benefits of total arterial revascularisation are evident at an early stage, when theoretically most of the benefit is likely to be gained in the longer-term.

The future

Despite the findings of the above well designed study, the expectation that total arterial revascularisation will further improve the prognostic benefit of CABG in the long-term remains to be proven, and is likely to require a long-term randomised trial of total arterial revascularisation versus conventional CABG. However, operative strategies also vary considerably, and the use of different combinations of pedicled, free and composite arterial grafts, as well as choosing the most appropriate target vessels to receive grafts is likely to have a significant impact on outcome. Additional benefits of the use of pedicled and composite arterial grafts, irrespective of improved angiographic patency, is their use in combination with off-pump techniques enabling coronary surgery to be conducted with a no touch aortic technique and thus minimise the risk of macroembolic cerebral injury in patients with severe atherosclerotic disease of the ascending aorta.

Conclusions

Although CABG is the most commonly performed major surgical procedure in the developed world, neither the technique nor the patients are homogeneous. It is therefore difficult to attribute successful or poor outcomes to specific technical aspects (eg. choice of conduit) in isolation. Variations in technique also mean that conducting randomised controlled trials in a multicentre or even multi-surgeon setting present significant challenges. The literature addressing the advantages and disadvantages of different conduits in coronary surgery is therefore littered with retrospective observational studies of angiographic graft patency and clinical outcome. Well designed prospective randomised trials comparing the use of specific conduits to revascularise specific coronary target vessels are in progress, and may address important questions concerning the most suitable conduit to use for revascularisation of a particular coronary target vessel. Evidence is accumulating that off-pump total arterial revascularisation based on composite arterial grafts, reduces the incidence of neurological injury by eliminating all aortic manipulation while obtaining maximal long-term benefits from the potential longevity of arterial conduits.

Recommendations	**Evidence level**
◆ LITA to left anterior descending artery should be performed in all patients undergoing CABG [19,20].	IIb*/B
◆ Bilateral ITA grafting can be safely performed in most CABG patients, and may provide a survival benefit [21, 24, 26].	IIa†/B
◆ RA has better long-term patency compared to GEA and IEA conduits [39, 42, 58, 60].	III/B
◆ RA has not been shown to have improved medium-term patency compared to long saphenous vein or right ITA conduits [44].	Ib/A
◆ Long-term patency of saphenous vein grafts is poor [10-12].	IIb/B
◆ Upper limb veins should only be used if there are no alternative conduits available [13].	III/B

* Despite the lack of randomised controlled trials there is abundant evidence to support this strategy.

† A meta-analysis of seven non-randomised studies is the most compelling evidence to date supporting this strategy.

References

1. Keogh BE, Kinsman R. National Adult Cardiac Surgical Database Report 2002, The Society of Cardiothoracic Surgeons of Great Britain and Ireland; 164-6.
2. Lytle BW, Loop FD, Taylor PC, *et al.* Vein graft disease: the clinical impact of stenoses in saphenous vein bypass grafts to coronary arteries. *J Thorac Cardiovasc Surg* 1992; 103(5): 831-40.
3. Huddleston CB, Stoney WS, Alford WC Jr., *et al.* Internal mammary artery grafts: technical factors influencing patency. *Ann Thorac Surg* 1986; 42(5): 543-9.
4. Paz MA, Lupon J, Bosch X, *et al.* Predictors of early saphenous vein aortocoronary bypass graft occlusion. The GESIC Study Group. *Ann Thorac Surg* 1993; 56(5): 1101-6.
5. Dion R, Glineur D, Derouck D, *et al.* Long-term clinical and angiographic follow-up of sequential internal thoracic artery grafting. *Eur J Cardiothorac Surg* 2000; 17(4): 407-14.
6. Mueller RL, Rosengart TK, Isom OW. The history of surgery for ischemic heart disease. *Ann Thorac Surg* 1997; 63(3): 869-78.
7. Grondin CM, Lesperance J, Bourassa MG, *et al.* Serial angiograpic evaluation in 60 consecutive patients with aorto-coronary artery vein grafts 2 weeks, 1 year, and 3 years after operation. *J Thorac Cardiovasc Surg* 1974; 67(1): 1-6.
8. Sarjeant JM, Rabinovitch M. Understanding and treating vein graft atherosclerosis. *Cardiovasc Pathol* 2002; 11(5): 263-71.
9. Bulkley BH, Hutchins GM. Accelerated "atherosclerosis". A morphologic study of 97 saphenous vein coronary artery bypass grafts. *Circulation* 1977; 55(1): 163-9.
10. FitzGibbon GM, Burton JR, Leach AJ. Coronary bypass graft fate: angiographic grading of 1400 consecutive grafts early after operation and of 1132 after one year. *Circulation* 1978; 57(6): 1070-74.
11. FitzGibbon GM, Leach AJ, Kafka HP, *et al.* Coronary bypass graft fate: long-term angiographic study. *J Am Coll Cardiol* 1991; 17(5): 1075-80.
12. Fitzgibbon GM, Kafka HP, Leach AJ, *et al.* Coronary bypass graft fate and patient outcome: angiographic follow-up of 5,065 grafts related to survival and reoperation in 1,388 patients during 25 years. *J Am Coll Cardiol* 1996; 28(3): 616-26.
13. Stoney WS, Alford WC Jr., Burrus GR, *et al.* The fate of arm veins used for aorta-coronary bypass grafts. *J Thorac Cardiovasc Surg* 1984; 88(4): 522-6.
14. Goldman S, Copeland J, Moritz T, *et al.* Saphenous vein graft patency 1 year after coronary artery bypass surgery and effects of antiplatelet therapy. Results of a Veterans Administration Cooperative Study. *Circulation* 1989; 80(5): 1190-7.
15. The effect of aggressive lowering of low-density lipoprotein cholesterol levels and low-dose anticoagulation on obstructive changes in saphenous-vein coronary-artery bypass grafts. The Post Coronary Artery Bypass Graft Trial Investigators. *N Engl J Med* 1997; 336(3): 153-62.
16. Angell WW, Sywak A. The saphenous vein versus internal mammary artery as a coronary bypass graft. *Circulation* 1977; 56(3 Suppl): II22-5.
17. Lytle BW, Loop FD, Cosgrove DM, *et al.* Long-term (5 to 12 years) serial studies of internal mammary artery and saphenous vein coronary bypass grafts. *J Thorac Cardiovasc Surg* 1985; 89(2): 248-58.
18. Barner HB, Standeven JW, Reese J. Twelve-year experience with internal mammary artery for coronary artery bypass. *J Thorac Cardiovasc Surg* 1985; 90(5): 668-75.
19. Loop FD, Lytle BW, Cosgrove DM, *et al.* Influence of the internal-mammary-artery graft on 10-year survival and other cardiac events. *New Engl J Med* 1986; 314(1): 1-6.
20. Cameron A, Davis KB, Green G, *et al.* Coronary bypass surgery with internal-thoracic-artery grafts – effects on survival over a 15-year period. *N Engl J Med* 1996; 334(4): 216-9.
21. Endo M, Nishida H, Tomizawa Y, *et al.* Benefit of bilateral over single internal mammary artery grafts for multiple coronary artery bypass grafting. *Circulation* 2001; 104(18): 2164-70.
22. Calafiore AM, Contini M, Vitolla G, *et al.* Bilateral internal thoracic artery grafting: long-term clinical and angiographic results of *in situ* versus Y grafts. *J Thorac Cardiovasc Surg* 2000; 120(5): 990-6.
23. Buxton BF, Ruengsakulrach P, Fuller J, *et al.* The right internal thoracic artery graft – benefits of grafting the left coronary system and native vessels with a high-grade stenosis. *Eur J Cardiothorac Surg* 2000; 18(3): 255-61.
24. Lytle BW, Blackstone EH, Loop FD, *et al.* Two internal thoracic artery grafts are better than one. *J Thorac Cardiovasc Surg* 1999; 117(5): 855-72.
25. Endo M, Tomizawa Y, Nishida H. Bilateral versus unilateral internal mammary revascularization in patients with diabetes. *Circulation* 2003; 108(11): 1343-9.
26. Taggart DP, D'Amico R, Altman DG. Effect of arterial revascularisation on survival: a systematic review of studies comparing bilateral and single internal mammary arteries. *Lancet* 2001; 358(9285): 870-5.
27. Loop FD, Lytle BW, Cosgrove DM, *et al.* J. Maxwell Chamberlain memorial paper. Sternal wound complications after isolated coronary artery bypass grafting: early and late mortality, morbidity, and cost of care. *Ann Thorac Surg* 1990; 49(2): 179-86; discussion 186-7.
28. Matsa M, Paz Y, Gurevitch J, *et al.* Bilateral skeletonized internal thoracic artery grafts in patients with diabetes mellitus. *J Thorac Cardiovasc Surg* 2001; 121(4): 668-74.
29. Taggart DP. Effects of a platelet-activating factor antagonist on lung injury and ventilation after cardiac operation. *Ann Thorac Surg* 2001; 71(1): 238-42.
30. Taggart DP. Biochemical assessment of myocardial injury after cardiac surgery: effects of a platelet activating factor antagonist, bilateral internal thoracic artery grafts, and coronary endarterectomy. *J Thorac Cardiovasc Surg* 2000; 120(4): 651-9.
31. Catarino PA, Black E, Taggart DP. Why do UK cardiac surgeons not perform their first choice operation for coronary artery bypass graft? *Heart* 2002; 88(6): 643-4.
32. Carpentier A, Guermonprez JL, Deloche A, *et al.* The aorta-to-coronary radial artery bypass graft. A technique avoiding pathological changes in grafts. *Ann Thorac Surg* 1973; 16(2): 111-21.

33. Geha AS, Krone RJ, McCormick JR, *et al.* Selection of coronary bypass. Anatomic, physiological, and angiographic considerations of vein and mammary artery grafts. *J Thorac Cardiovasc Surg* 1975; 70(3): 414-31.
34. Fisk RL, Brooks CH, Callaghan JC, *et al.* Experience with the radial artery graft for coronary artery bypass. *Ann Thorac Surg* 1976; 21(6): 513-8.
35. Acar C, Jebara VA, Portoghese M, *et al.* Revival of the radial artery for coronary artery bypass grafting. *Ann Thorac Surg* 1992; 54(4): 652-9; discussion 659-60.
36. Kane-ToddHall SM, Taggart DP, Clements-Jewery H, *et al.* Pre-existing vascular disease in the radial artery and other coronary artery bypass conduits. *Eur J Med Res* 1999; 4(1): 11-4.
37. Taggart DP. The radial artery as a conduit for coronary artery bypass grafting. *Heart* 1999; 82(4): 409-10.
38. Tatoulis J, Royse AG, Buxton BF, *et al.* The radial artery in coronary surgery: a 5-year experience – clinical and angiographic results. *Ann Thorac Surg* 2002; 73(1): 143-7; discussion 147-8.
39. Possati G, Gaudino M, Prati F, *et al.* Long-term results of the radial artery used for myocardial revascularization. *Circulation* 2003; 108(11): 1350-4.
40. Acar C, Ramsheyi A, Pagny JY, *et al.* The radial artery for coronary artery bypass grafting: clinical and angiographic results at five years. *J Thorac Cardiovasc Surg* 1998; 116(6): 981-9.
41. Possati G, Gaudino M, Alessandrini F, *et al.* Midterm clinical and angiographic results of radial artery grafts used for myocardial revascularization. *J Thorac Cardiovasc Surg* 1998; 116(6): 1015-21.
42. Iaco AL, Teodori G, Di Giammarco G, *et al.* Radial artery for myocardial revascularization: long-term clinical and angiographic results. *Ann Thorac Surg* 2001; 72(2): 464-8; discussion 468-9.
43. Fremes SE. Multicenter radial artery patency study (RAPS). Study design. *Control Clin Trials* 2000; 21(4): 397-413.
44. Buxton BF, Raman JS, Ruengsakulrach P, *et al.* Radial artery patency and clinical outcomes: five-year interim results of a randomized trial. *J Thorac Cardiovasc Surg* 2003; 125(6): 1363-71.
45. Royse AG, Royse CF, Groves KL, *et al.* Blood flow in composite arterial grafts and effect of native coronary flow. *Ann Thorac Surg* 1999; 68(5): 1619-22.
46. Moran SV, Baeza R, Guarda E, *et al.* Predictors of radial artery patency for coronary bypass operations. *Ann Thorac Surg* 2001; 72(5): 1552-6.
47. Maniar HS, Sundt TM, Barner HB, *et al.* Effect of target stenosis and location on radial artery graft patency. *J Thorac Cardiovasc Surg* 2002; 123(1): 45-52.
48. Chester AH, Marchbank AJ, Borland JA, *et al.* Comparison of the morphologic and vascular reactivity of the proximal and distal radial artery. *Ann Thorac Surg* 1998; 66(6): 1972-6; discussion 1976-7.
49. He GW, Yang CQ, Starr A. Overview of the nature of vasoconstriction in arterial grafts for coronary operations. *Ann Thorac Surg* 1995; 59(3): 676-83.
50. Downing SW, Edmunds LH. Release of vasoactive substances during cardiopulmonary bypass. *Ann Thorac Surg* 1992; 54(6): 1236-43.
51. Dipp MA, Nye PC, Taggart DP. Phenoxybenzamine is more effective and less harmful than papaverine in the prevention of radial artery vasospasm. *Eur J Cardiothorac Surg* 2001; 19(4): 482-6.
52. Mussa S, Guzik TJ, Black E, Dipp MA, Channon KM, Taggart DP. Comparative Efficacy and Duration of Action of Phenoxybenzamine, Verapamil/Nitroglycerin and Papaverine as Topical Antispasmodics for Radial Artery Coronary Artery Bypass Grafting. *J Thorac Cardiovasc Surg.* In press.
53. Taggart DP, Dipp M, Mussa S, *et al.* Phenoxybenzamine prevents spasm in radial artery conduits for coronary artery bypass grafting. *J Thorac Cardiovasc Surg* 2000; 120(4): 815-7.
54. Pym J, Brown PM, Charrette EJ, *et al.* Gastroepiploic-coronary anastomosis. A viable alternative bypass graft. *J Thorac Cardiovasc Surg* 1987; 94(2): 256-9.
55. Suma H, Fukumoto H, Takeuchi A. Coronary artery bypass grafting by utilizing *in situ* right gastroepiploic artery: basic study and clinical application. *Ann Thorac Surg* 1987; 44(4): 394-7.
56. Beretta L, Antonacci C, Santoli C. Gastroepiploic artery free graft for coronary bypass. *Eur J Cardiothorac Surg* 1991; 5(2): 110-1.
57. Hirose H, Amano A, Takanashi S, *et al.* Coronary artery bypass grafting using the gastroepiploic artery in 1,000 patients. *Ann Thorac Surg* 2002; 73(5): 1371-9.
58. Suma H, Isomura T, Horii T, *et al.* Late angiographic result of using the right gastroepiploic artery as a graft. *J Thorac Cardiovasc Surg* 2000; 120(3): 496-8.
59. Puig LB, Ciongolli W, Cividanes GV, *et al.* Inferior epigastric artery as a free graft for myocardial revascularization. *J Thorac Cardiovasc Surg* 1990; 99(2): 251-5.
60. Buche M, Schroeder E, Gurne O, *et al.* Coronary artery bypass grafting with the inferior epigastric artery. Midterm clinical and angiographic results. *J Thorac Cardiovasc Surg* 1995; 109(3): 553-9; discussion 559-60.
61. Loop FD, Lytle BW, Cosgrove DM, *et al.* Free (aorta-coronary) internal mammary artery graft. Late results. *J Thorac Cardiovasc Surg* 1986; 92(5): 827-31.
62. Bergsma TM, Grandjean JG, Voors AA, *et al.* Low recurrence of angina pectoris after coronary artery bypass graft surgery with bilateral internal thoracic and right gastroepiploic arteries. *Circulation* 1998; 97(24): 2402-5.
63. Muneretto C, Bisleri G, Negri A, *et al.* Total arterial myocardial revascularization with composite grafts improves results of coronary surgery in the elderly: a prospective randomized comparison with conventional coronary artery bypass surgery. *Circulation* 2003; 108(10 Suppl 1): II29-33.

Chapter 19

Choice of cardiac valve substitutes

W R Eric Jamieson MD

Professor of Surgery

St. Paul's Hospital, Vancouver, Canada &
Department of Surgery, University of British Columbia, Vancouver, Canada

Introduction

Biological (tissue) and mechanical prostheses have been used for valve replacement surgery for 30 years. There have been extensive advancements over the years, but residual problems still exist with both mechanical and biological prostheses. These extensive developments were introduced to reduce or eliminate deterioration, thromboembolism and anticoagulant-related haemorrhage, as well as to optimise haemodynamic performance.

The continuing problems with mechanical prostheses are thrombus formation from blood stasis and the resultant thromboembolic phenomena despite anticoagulant therapy, which has an inherent risk of haemorrhage. Biological prostheses, both porcine and pericardial bioprostheses are at risk of structural failure over time, with leaflet degeneration and dystrophic calcification occurring either individually or in combination.

The current generations of both biological and mechanical prostheses have been developed to address these complications (Figures 1-33). The present biological valvular prostheses have been developed with tissue preservation techniques to reduce structural failure, together with or without stent designs, contributing to preservation of anatomical characteristics and biomechanical properties of the leaflets. Allografts and autografts have been alternative substitutes for aortic valve and aortic root disease for 40 years, prior to the development of mechanical prostheses and bioprostheses.

The purpose of this chapter is to provide an evidence-based assessment for the use of biological (tissue) and mechanical prostheses. The complications of valvular prostheses, namely - thromboembolism and thrombosis, antithromboembolic-related haemorrhage, structural valve deterioration, non-structural dysfunction and prosthetic valve endocarditis contribute to the evidence-based assessment [1]. The balance is usually related to structural valve deterioration of biological prostheses, and haemorrhage and chronicity of care to prevent thromboembolism and thrombosis with mechanical prostheses. The complications of valvular prostheses contribute to valve-related re-operation, permanent morbidity (neurologic or functional impairment) and mortality. The risk of these valve-related complications in any specific patient is related to life expectancy from comorbidity from concomitant health-related diseases. Careful analysis of valve-related and patient-related factors are of utmost importance, together

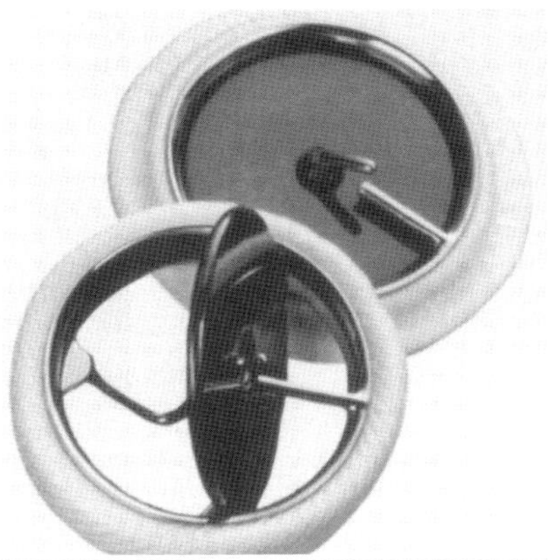

Figure 1. Medtronic Hall.

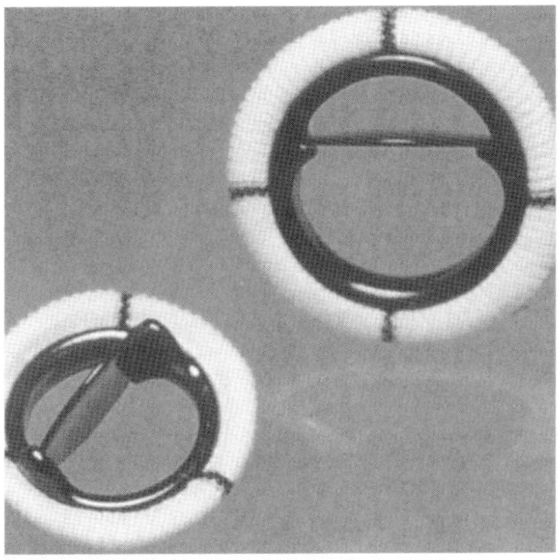

Figure 2. Omnicarbon.

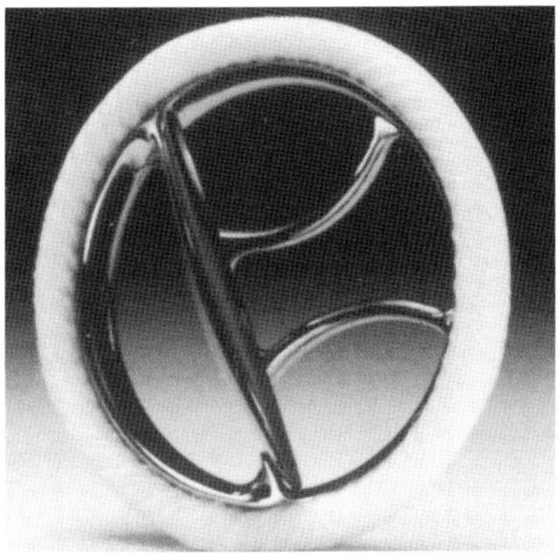

Figure 3. Koehler Ultracor.

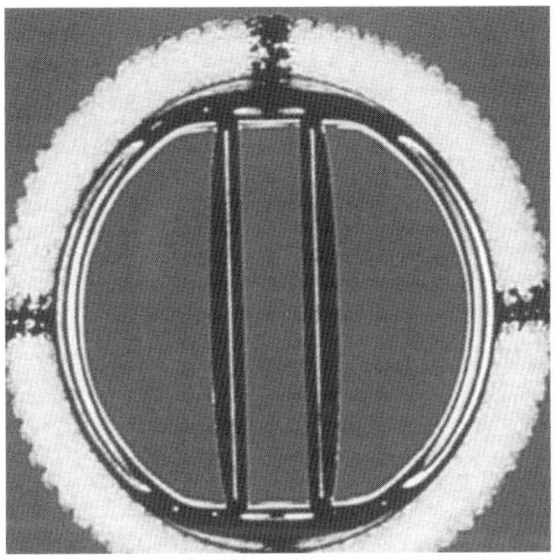

Figure 4. St. Jude Medical Masters (Mitral).

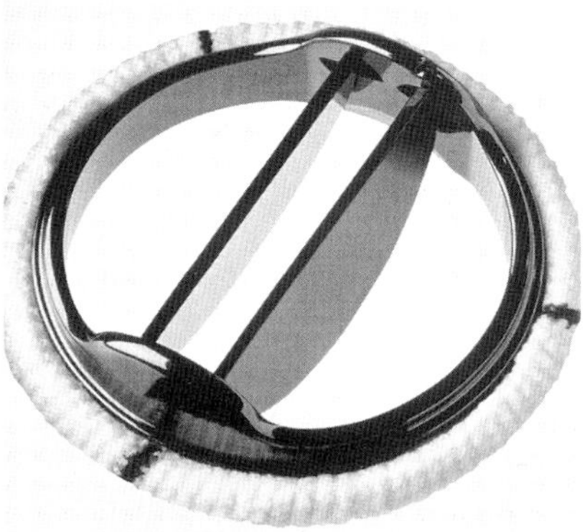

Figure 5. St. Jude Medical Regent (Aortic).

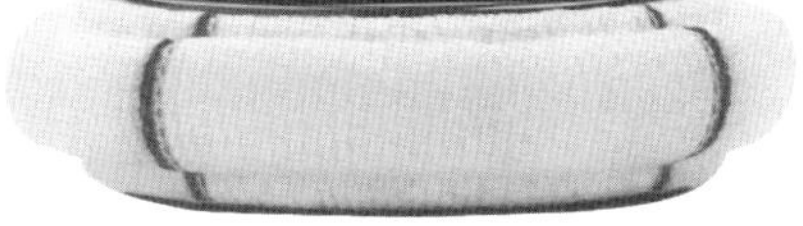

Figure 6. CarboMedics Mitral - Optiform.

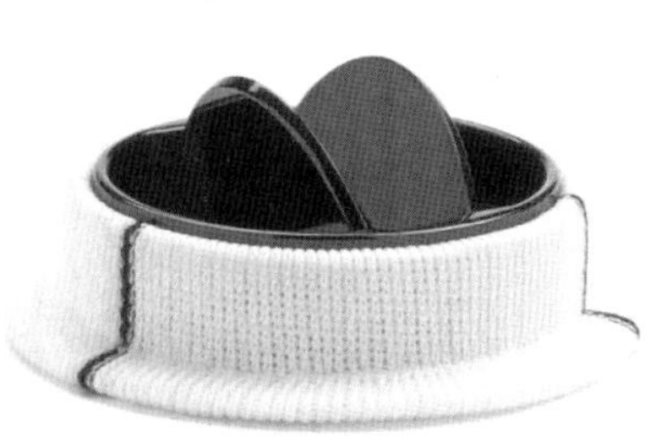

Figure 7. CarboMedics Aortic Top-Hat.

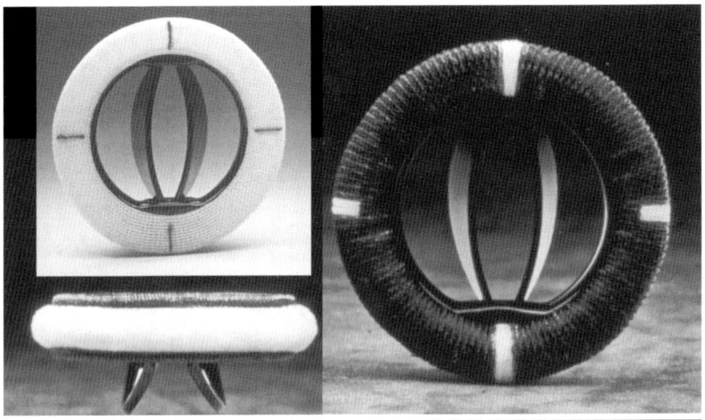

Figure 8. Sorin Bicarbon (Edwards Mira).

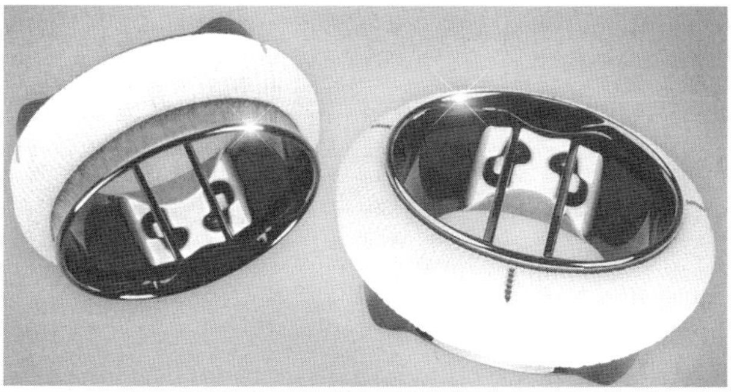

Figure 9. Medical Carbon Research - On-X.

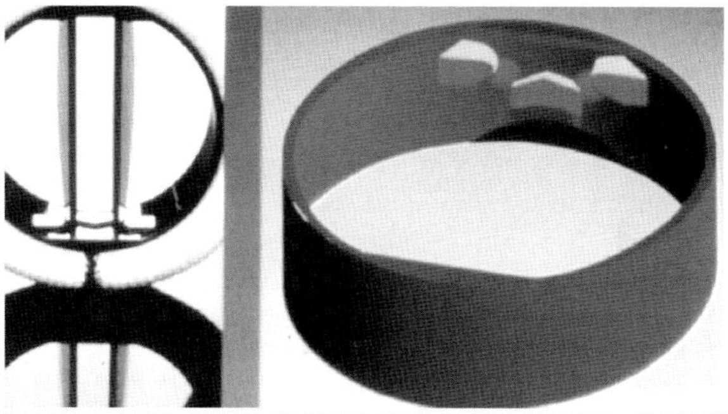

Figure 10. ATS Medical.

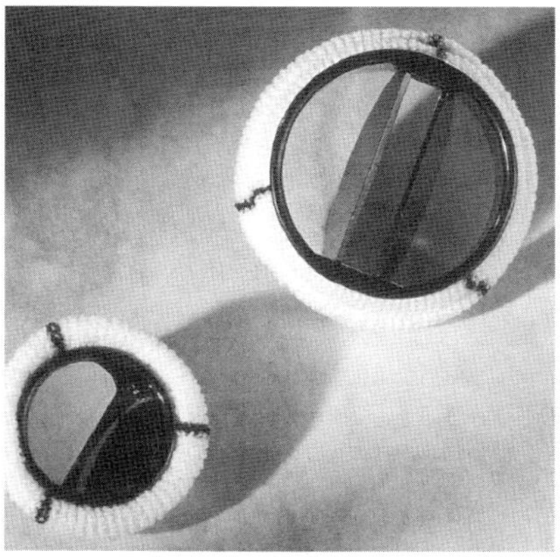

Figure 11. Medtronic Advantage.

with proper indication and optimal timing of surgery, in the selection of appropriate valvular substitutes.

The chapter will deal with current prostheses and the characteristics of these biological and mechanical prostheses to provide an informative understanding for cardiac surgeons and cardiologists. Special attention will be given to the performance or anticipated performance of these prostheses. The valve-related complications and the risk factors of these complications will be provided to support a rational approach for selection of biological and mechanical prostheses with consideration of comorbidity and factors affecting haemodynamic performance.

The current prostheses, the majority available in most parts of the world, are shown in Figures 1-33. These prostheses available for aortic and / or mitral valve replacement are inclusive of monoleaflet and bileaflet mechanical prostheses, allografts, autografts as well as stented and stentless porcine and pericardial bioprostheses. The mechanical prostheses have distinct designs of hinge regions and occluders to control blood stasis and complications. The bioprostheses are formulated with glutaraldehyde-treated porcine leaflet tissue or bovine pericardium designed to minimise mechanical stress and treated with calcium mitigation therapies to minimise calcification.

The Canadian Cardiovascular Society consensus document on *Surgical Management of Valvular Heart Disease* has assessed the evidence for management of valvular lesions and the use of various valvular prostheses [2]. The recommendations have been assigned classes of support and levels of evidence according to the classifications of the American College of Cardiology, the American Heart Association and the Canadian Cardiovascular Society [3, 4].

Class I: Conditions for which there is evidence or general agreement that a given procedure or treatment is useful and effective.

Class II: Conditions for which there is conflicting evidence or a divergence of opinion about the usefulness or efficacy of a procedure or treatment.

IIa: Weight of evidence or opinion is in favour of usefulness and efficacy.

IIb: Usefulness and efficacy is less well established by evidence and opinion.

Class III: Conditions for which there is evidence or general agreement that the procedure or treatment is not useful and in some cases may be harmful.

These recommendations are based on the following levels of evidence:-

Level A: The data were derived from multiple randomised clinical trials.
Level B: The data were derived from single randomised or non-randomised studies.
Level C: The consensus opinion of experts was the primary source of recommendation.

The recommendations for the use of mechanical prostheses and bioprostheses, as detailed in the Canadian Cardiovascular Society consensus document, are presented in Tables 1 and 2 [2].

There are approximately 300,000 valve replacement procedures performed annually worldwide. In the year 2000 the distribution was 64.8% mechanical prostheses (MP) and 35.2% bioprostheses (BP), but changed by 2003 to 54.3% MP and 45.7% BP. In 2003, of the MP replacements

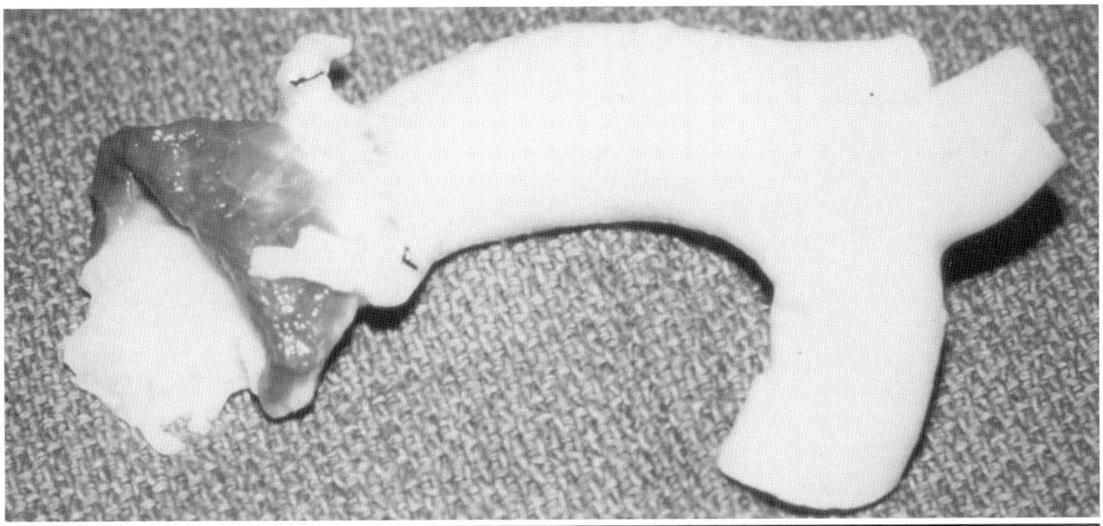

Figure 12. Allograft.

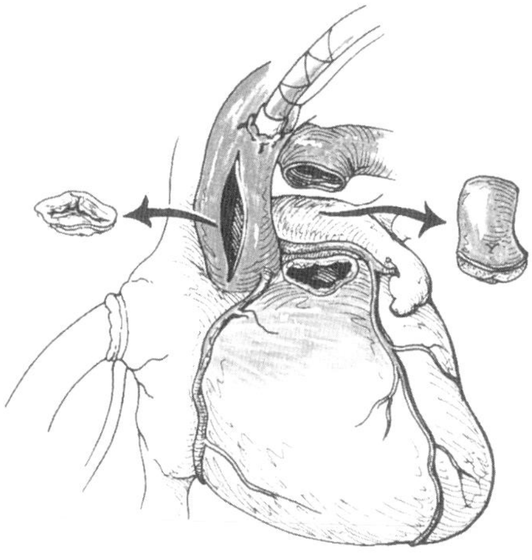

Figure 13. Autograft.

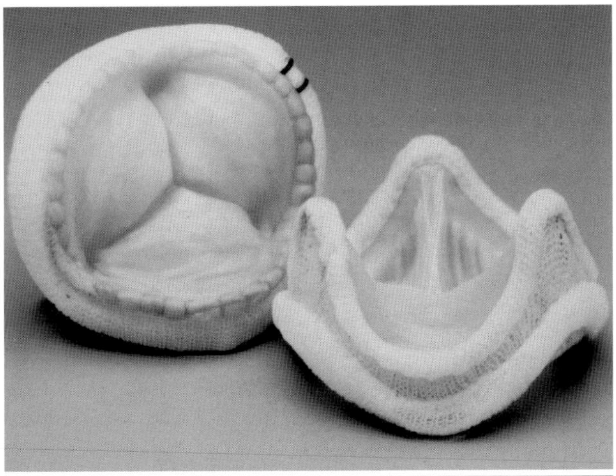

Figure 14. Carpentier-Edwards Supra-Annular.

Table 1. **Recommendations for valve replacement with a mechanical prosthesis.**

	Indication	Class	
1.	Patients with expected long life spans	I	B
2.	Patients with a mechanical prosthetic valve already in place in a different position than the valve to be replaced	I	B
3.	Patients requiring warfarin therapy because of risk factors* for thromboembolism	IIa	C
4.	Patients ≤65 years for aortic valve replacement and ≤70 years for mitral valve replacement†	IIa	C
5.	Valve replacement for thrombosed biological valve	IIb	C
	Contraindication		
6.	Patients in renal failure, on haemodialysis or with hypercalcaemia	III	C
7.	Patients who cannot or will not take warfarin therapy	III	C

* Risk factors: atrial fibrillation, severe left ventricular dysfunction, previous thromboembolism and hypercoagulable condition;
† The age at which patients may be considered for bioprosthetic valves is based on the major reduction in rate of structural valve deterioration after age 65 years for AVR and after age 70 years for MVR, and the increased risk of bleeding in this age group.

Table 2. **Recommendations for valve replacement with a bioprosthesis.**

	Indication	Class	
1.	Patients who cannot or will not take warfarin therapy	I	B
2.	Patients ≥65 years needing aortic valve replacement who do not have risk factors for thromboembolism*	I	B
3.	Patients considered to have possible compliance problem with warfarin therapy	IIa	C
4.	Patients >70 years needing mitral valve replacement who do not have risk factors for thromboembolism*	IIa	C
5.	Valve replacement for thrombosed mechanical valve	IIb	C
6.	Patients <65 years†	IIb	C
7.	Patients in renal failure, on haemodialysis or with hypercalcaemia	IIb	C
	Contraindication		
8.	Adolescent patients who are still growing	III	C

* Risk factors: atrial fibrillation, severe left ventricular dysfunction, previous thromboembolism and hypercoagulable condition;
† The age at which patients should be considered for bioprosthetic valves is based on the major reduction in rate of structural valve deterioration after age 65 years for AVR and after age 70 years for MVR, and the increased risk of bleeding in this age group.

Table 3. Prostheses options for aortic valve replacement according to age range of the patient population.

Age range (years)	Prosthesis type
20 to 40	Pulmonary autograft (no contraindication, i.e. annuloaortic ectasia) Mechanical prosthesis Allograft (if contraindication to autograft or anticoagulation)
41 to 64	Mechanical prosthesis Stentless heterograft prosthesis Stented heterograft prosthesis Pulmonary autograft (to 55 years if good candidate) Allograft
65 and older	Stented heterograft - porcine or pericardial (specifically if large annulus) Stentless heterograft - subcoronary implantation Allograft or stentless porcine root (specifically if small annulus or calcified root) Mechanical prosthesis

18.6% were in North America, 25.3% in Western Europe and 56.2% in the rest of the world; while of BP replacements 54.7% were in North America, 27.4% in Western Europe and 17.9% in the rest of the world.

Since 2000 to 2003 there has been a dramatic increase in bioprostheses in North America from 52.3% to 71.3% and a fall in mechanical prostheses from 48.0% to 28.7%. In Western Europe, the change has been less dramatic; BP increased from 36.0% to 47.7% and MP fell from 64.0% to 52.3%. The proportion of stented and stentless bioprostheses in aortic valve replacement in 2002 in the United States was 92% stented and 8% stentless, while in Western Europe was 91% and 9%, respectively. Between 2000 and 2002 in the United States, stented increased 12%/year and stentless decreased 1%/year, while in Western Europe stented increased 5%/year and stentless decreased 12%/year.

The changes in pattern of practice have been influenced by advanced technologies with bioprostheses, particularly stented bioprostheses without the reporting of the performance of the stentless bioprostheses to the intermediate and long-term (Figures 1-33).

The vast majority of patients having valve replacement surgery are over 50 years of age [5]. The North American experience between 1991 and 1995 inclusive, from the Society of Thoracic Surgeons database revealed 42% of patients were between the ages of 50 and 70 years, and 45% over 70 years of age [6]. During that time in the United States, mechanical prostheses were predominant in aortic valve replacement, as well as mitral valve replacement, when reconstructive procedures are not possible. Since the latter part of the 1990s, there has been a significant resurgence of biological prostheses for aortic valve replacement, but not for mitral valve replacement.

Aortic valve replacement

The prosthesis-type options for aortic valve replacement (AVR) for aortic stenosis or aortic regurgitation by adult age groups are detailed in Table 3 [2]. The choice of prosthesis is a decision made by

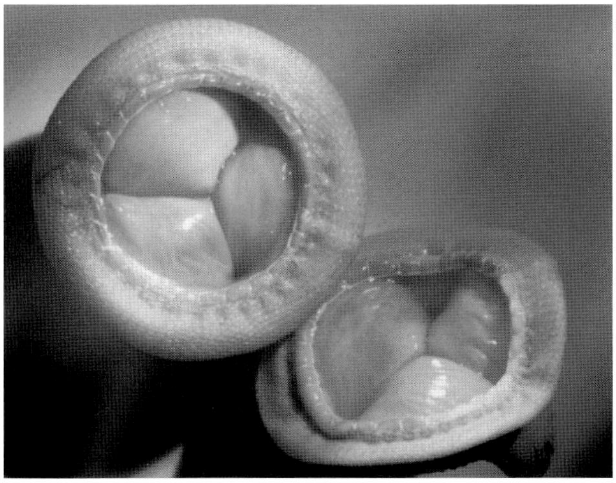

Figure 15. **Hancock II.**

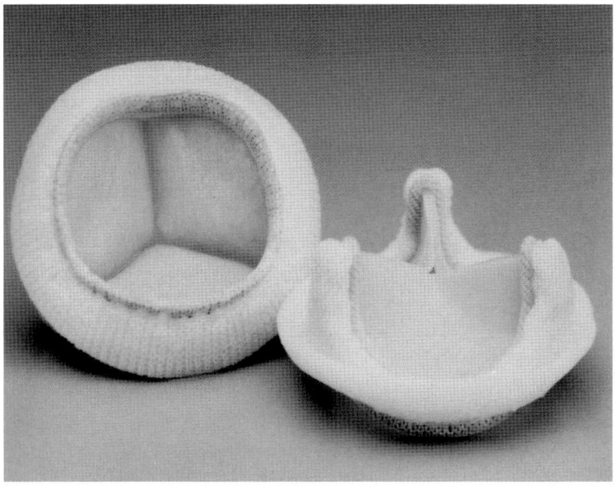

Figure 16. **Carpentier-Edwards PERIMOUNT.**

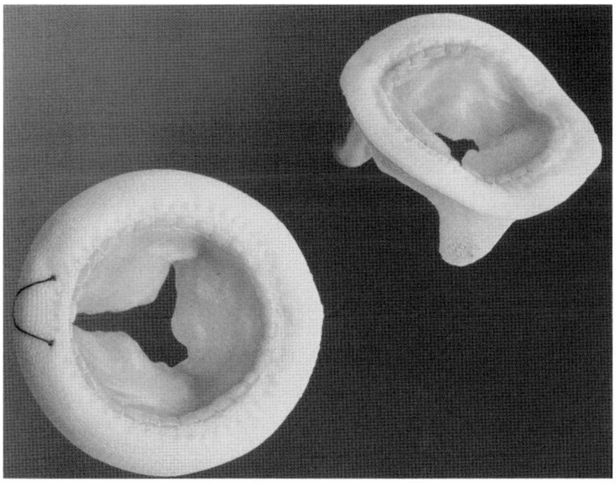

Figure 17. **Medtronic Mosaic.**

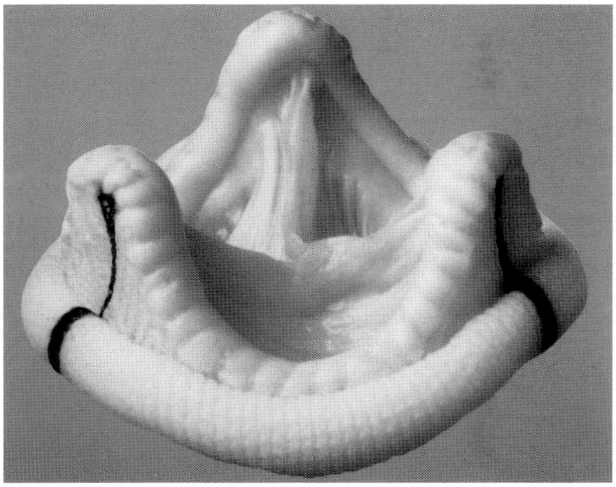

Figure 18. **St. Jude Medical Epic.**

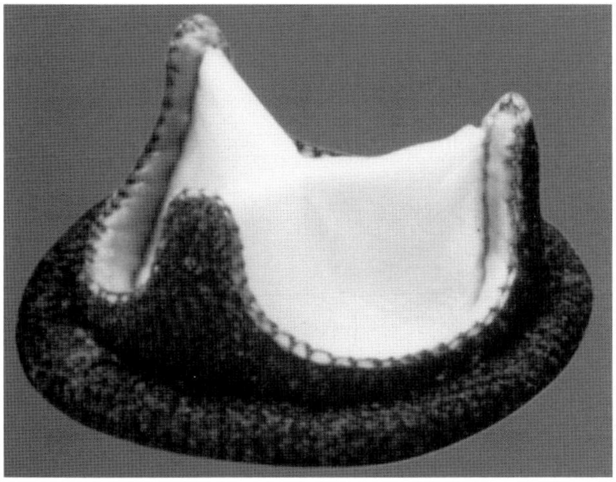

Figure 19. **Sorin Pericarbon "MORE".**

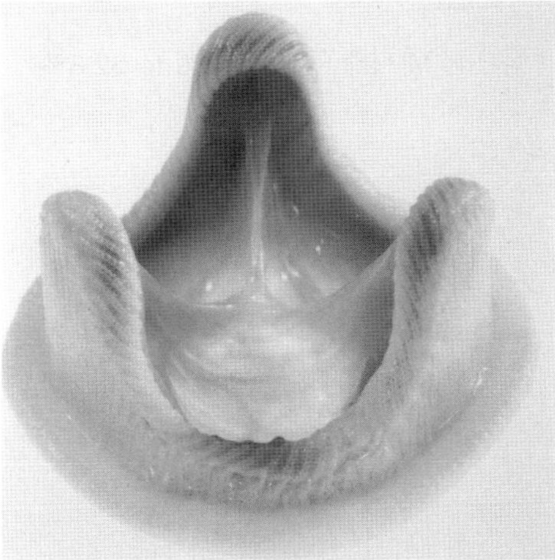

Figure 20. **Koehler Aspire.**

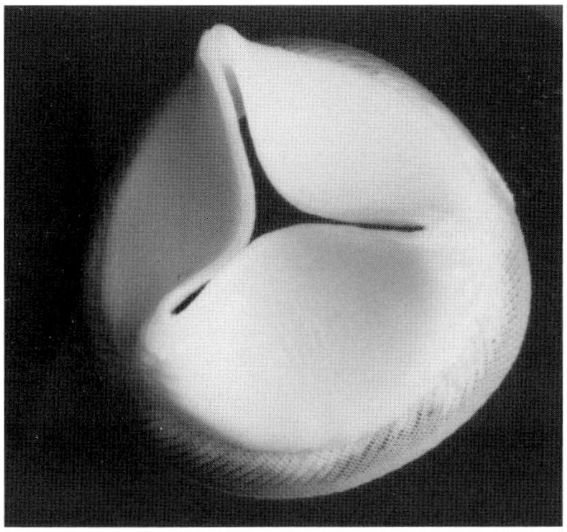

Figure 21. CarboMedics Mitroflow.

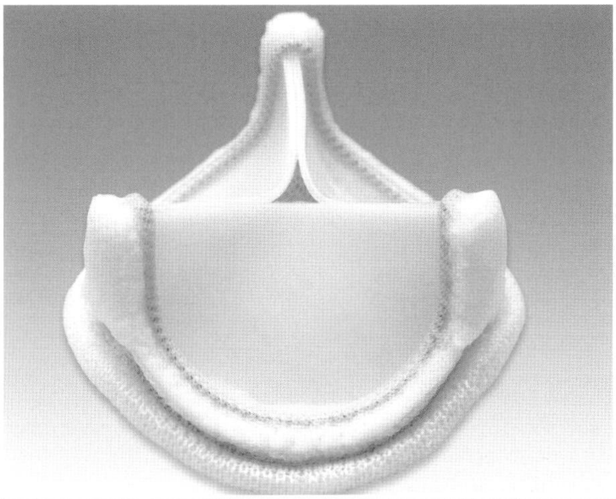

Figure 22. Carpentier-Edwards PERIMOUNT Magna.

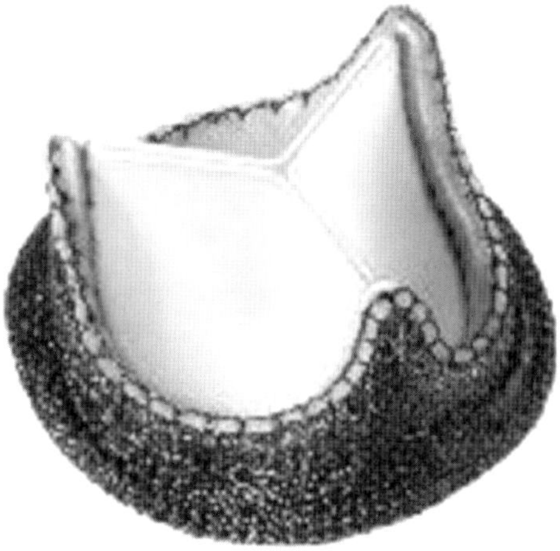

Figure 23. Sorin Soprano.

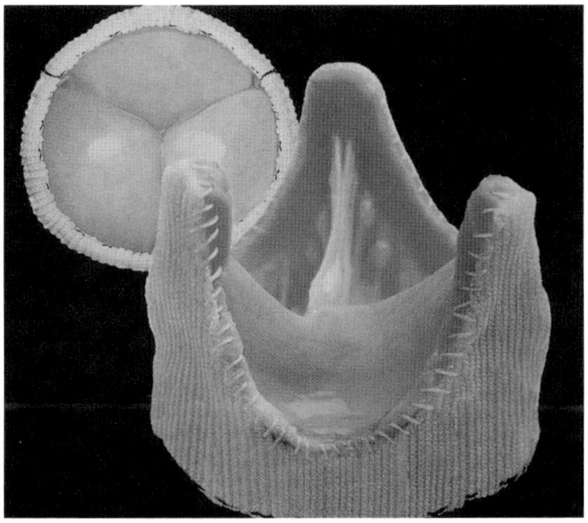

Figure 24. St. Jude Medical Toronto SPV.

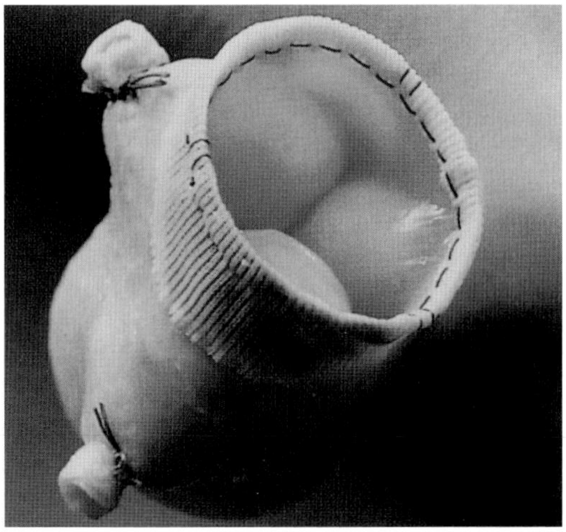

Figure 25. Medtronic Freestyle.

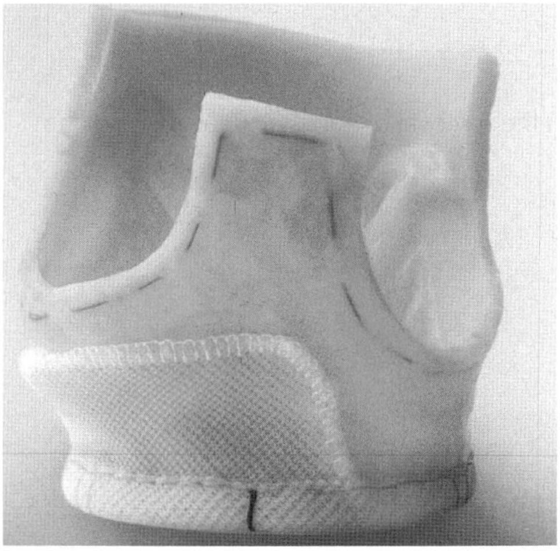

Figure 26. Edwards Prima Plus.

the surgeon and the patient. The patient should be advised of the risks and advantages of the prostheses.

Allografts and autografts

The allograft and autograft were introduced in the 1960s as freehand subcoronary implants for aortic valve disease. The allograft has been used to manage congenital, rheumatic, degenerative and infective disease of the aortic valve and for failed bioprostheses [7]. The major deterrent of the use of allografts is the general limited availability, the shortage of donor organs and priority for heart transplantation over allograft harvesting [8]. Allografts provide excellent haemodynamics with low risk of endocarditis and alleviate the need for anticoagulants. The predominant indications for allografts, in the current era, are children, women in childbearing age and anticoagulant contraindications, and especially in the management of aortic native and prosthetic valve endocarditis [8].

There are limitations to allografts. The predominant limitation is degeneration. Allografts have an age-related limited durability and a lifetime risk of re-operation in younger patients [9]. In children, the re-operation-free survival has been reported at 73% at seven years while in adults the freedom from re-operation is 92% at ten years [7, 10]. The other limitation of allografts is the incidence of significant regurgitation at seven years, greater in the scalloped subcoronary implantation than the cylinder or root techniques [11,12,13]. Early regurgitation can be due to technical issues. To avoid this problem with the freehand scalloped technique with the removal of aortic sinuses, centres do recommend cylinder or root configurations, which both conserve sinuses and the sinotubular junction [11]. The allograft aortic root replacement provides the opportunity for less likelihood of distortion in cases of asymmetry and bicuspid disease, and makes size-matching less critical [14-16].

The consensus in the Canadian document for allografts is class IIb, level B. Because of the limited availability and recognized degeneration with limited long-term durability, the allograft should be used primarily in the management of infective, native and prosthetic endocarditis, especially in cases with destructive annular disease, inclusive of discontinuity, abscesses and fistulas [2]. The general recommendations for allografts have been contributed to by randomised comparisons between allografts and autografts [17, 18].

Autografts are usually reserved for the younger patient and the very active (competitive sports) patient. These patients require ongoing follow-up. The contraindications to the use of autografts must be respected to avoid structural failure. The contradictions are connective tissue disorders (i.e. Marfan's syndrome), immunological disorders, and bicuspid or fenestrated pulmonary valves. The autograft has the advantage of somatic growth and thus, is ideal in the paediatric age group [19]. For autograft aortic root replacement, the pulmonary allograft is used for reconstruction of the RV outflow tract because it is more durable than the aortic allograft [20].

The autograft is safe and reproducible in overall haemodynamic and durability performance in properly selected young adults [17-19, 21]. There have been two documented concerns with the autograft procedure. There is an incidence of late pulmonary allograft stenosis attributed to younger donor age, shorter duration of cryopreservation and smaller homograft size [22,23]. The other concern is late dilatation of the autograft involving the root, sinuses of Valsalva and sinotubular junction [24,25]. Dilatation of the sinotubular junction, and not the sinuses, causes aortic regurgitation [26,27]. The dilatation has been attributed to accompanying pulmonary wall pathology in bicuspid aortic valve morphology and other congenital anomalies. This has been attributed to histological abnormalities of the aortic and pulmonary roots, with common embryogenesis, in conjunction with bicuspid aortic valve disease [28,29]. There is contradictory evidence demonstrating that the abnormalities of the pulmonary artery are the same with bicuspid and tricuspid aortic valves. Root dilatation is relatively common after autograft root replacement, but unrelated to bicuspid aortic valve disease. The latter investigation has demonstrated no correlation between bicuspid aortic valves, degenerative changes of the pulmonary artery and autograft root aneurysm. It is felt that degenerative changes of the pulmonary artery root are negligible and similar in bicuspid and

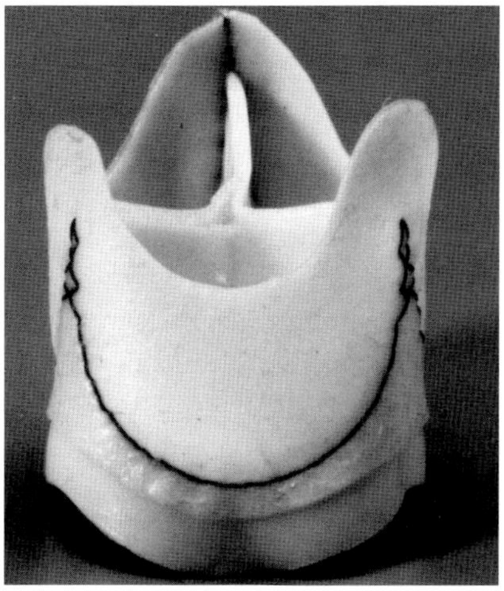

Figure 27. **Sorin Pericarbon Freedom.**

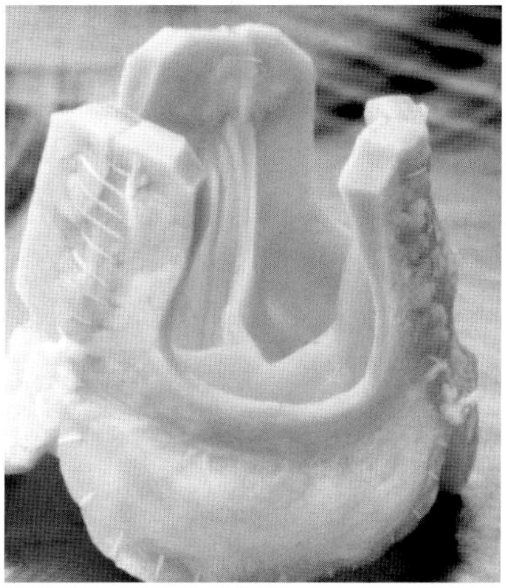

Figure 28. **Cryolife O'Brien.**

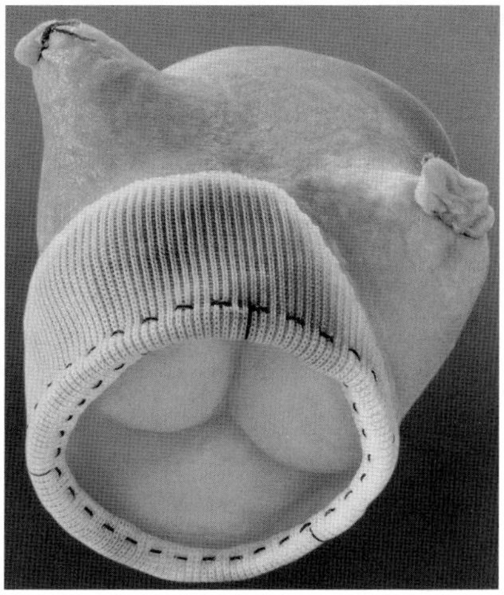

Figure 29. **St. Jude Medical Toronto Duo.**

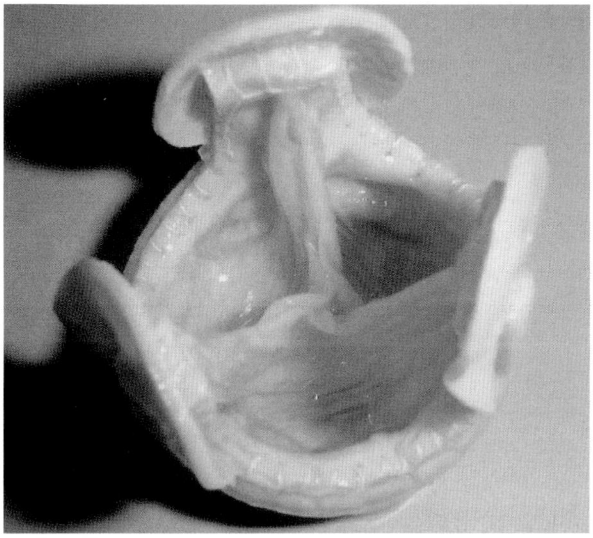

Figure 30. **Shelhigh Supra-Stentless.**

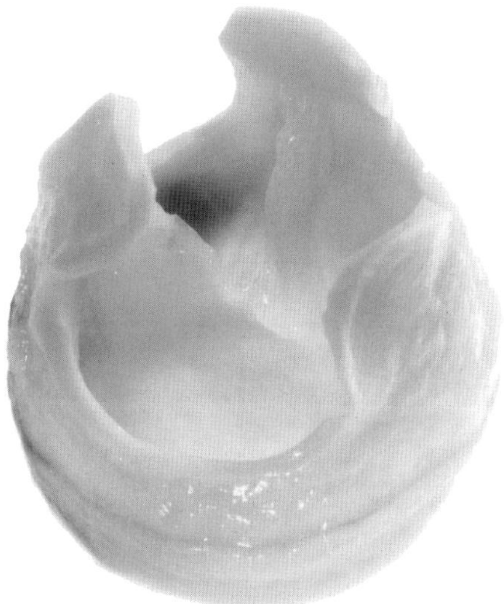

Figure 31. **Koehler Elan and Root Elan.**

tricuspid aortic valves undergoing an autograft procedure. There is consideration that other factors play a role in autograft dilatation.

There are surgical alternatives to deal with this issue, including root inclusion, or buttressing the annulus, coronary artery buttons and sinotubular junction [24]. This technique may be inappropriate in children where somatic growth is desirable. The autograft is contraindicated if the aortic annulus is greater than 30mm.

The autograft has better durability and haemodynamics than the cryopreserved allograft [18]. The trend favouring the autograft over the allograft occurs at eight years of evaluation. Continuing research in the use of autografts is imperative.

The consensus for the use of autografts in the Canadian document for selected patients in the adult population up to 55 years of age (class I-IIa, level B) is based in large part on a randomised trial reported in 2000 evaluating allografts and autografts [17,18]. The

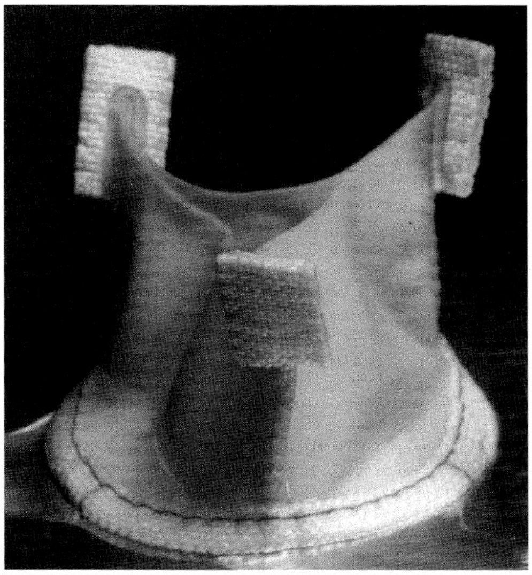

Figure 32. 3F Therapeutics (Aortic).

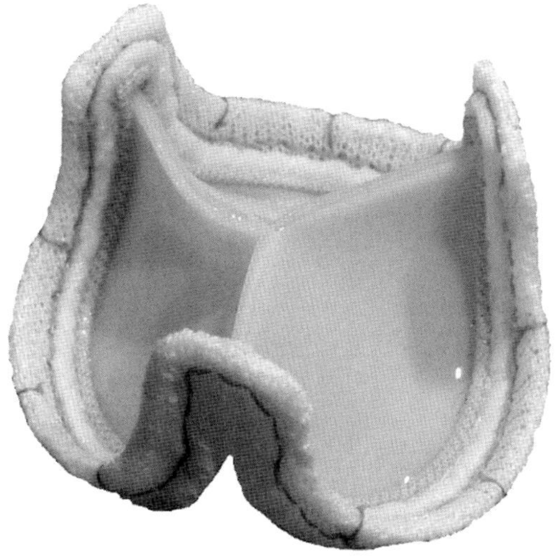

Figure 33. Edwards BioPhysio.

study revealed that, in children, autografts are favoured because of early allograft degeneration. The study also revealed that, in general, autografts had superior durability and haemodynamics. The study failed to identify any significant progressive dilatation of the aortic root. There remains a risk of re-operation of approximately 20% at 20 years inclusive of pulmonary allograft stenosis and complications related specifically to the autograft [21].

Bioprostheses and mechanical prostheses

The majority of aortic valve replacements are performed in patients over 50 years of age. The choice of valvular substitutes is based on results of two randomised trials on obsolete mechanical and heterograft prostheses [30,31], and non-randomised studies of both stand alone prosthesis types and comparative evaluations [32-84]. The choice is made balancing the complications of major thromboembolism, thrombosis and haemorrhage with mechanical prostheses and re-operation for structural valve deterioration of bioprostheses. It is now known that lower-dose anticoagulation and self-monitored anticoagulation can make management with mechanical prostheses safer. Also, re-operation can be performed for structural failure of bioprostheses with low mortality, if patient surveillance can avoid emergent and NYHA class IV circumstances [85, 86].

Fifteen-year outcomes after replacement with a mechanical or bioprosthetic valve are reported by the Veterans Affairs randomised trial [30]. At 15 years, patients undergoing AVR had better survival with a bioprosthetic valve than with a mechanical valve, even though structural valve deterioration was virtually absent with the mechanical valve. Structural valve deterioration was greater with a bioprosthesis for AVR and occurred at a much higher rate in those aged less than 65 years. In patients at least 65 years of age, structural valve deterioration after AVR was not significantly different between the bioprosthesis and the mechanical prosthesis. Re-operation was more common for AVR with the bioprosthesis. Thromboembolism rates were similar with the two valve prostheses, but bleeding was more common with the mechanical prosthesis. All-cause mortality was not different after MVR with mechanical prostheses versus bioprostheses. Structural valve deterioration was greater with bioprostheses for MVR in all age groups but occurred at a much higher rate in those aged less than 65 years. Thromboembolism rates were similar in the two valve prostheses, but bleeding was more common with the mechanical prostheses.

In 2003, the Edinburgh randomised trial reported results to 20 years [31]. The prosthesis type did not influence survival, thromboembolism or endocarditis. Major bleeding was more common with mechanical prostheses. Assessing mortality and re-operation, survival with original prosthesis became different at 8-10 years for MVR and 12-14 years for AVR.

There is sufficient evidence to recommend bioprostheses, porcine or pericardial, for patients at least 65 years of age [34, 42, 51, 54-57, 58, 60, 65, 67]. The evidence pertains to both first and second generation heterograft stented bioprostheses. The actual freedom (cumulative incidence) from structural valve deterioration at 15 years is 87% for 61 to 70 years of age and 96% for greater than 70 years of age; the actuarial freedom is 76% and 82%, respectively [55]. The freedom from structural valve deterioration does not warrant bioprosthesis use in patients below 60 to 65 years of age [55, 56].

The mechanical prostheses currently marketed are free from structural failure [75-78, 80, 84, 87]. The linearized rates of major thromboembolism and haemorrhage in patients less than 65 years of age are both approximately 1.5% per patient year. The literature provides a variation of results dependent on follow-up methodology, adequacy of follow-up, and exclusion or inclusion of events up to 30 days [78]. The rates of thromboembolism and haemorrhage for patients at least 65 years of age are higher [78]. The freedom from major or fatal TE, thrombosis and haemorrhage is 90% at five years for patients less than 65 years of age [78].

Stentless bioprostheses have been shown to have better haemodynamics than stented bioprostheses and mechanical prostheses [88-105]. This is likely related to the ability to implant a larger prosthesis and lack of support structure. The stentless design may increase long-term freedom from structural valve degeneration and potentially improve survival. The potential improvement in survival is considered to be related to completeness of left ventricular mass regression and remodelling. Several studies have revealed that both stented and stentless bioprostheses achieve adequacy of left ventricular mass regression, even though stentless bioprostheses can provide lower transvalvular gradients and better effective orifice area indices [37, 44, 69, 70, 73, 91, 92, 96-100, 103]. It is apparent that mild-to-moderate obstructive phenomena do not influence mass regression and survival.

The use of small size prostheses is controversial. There is evidence of significant residual gradients with valve sizes 19 and 21 with the majority of stented bioprostheses and mechanical prostheses [106-113]. The sewing cuff configurations of small aortic mechanical prostheses, external mounted pericardial bioprosthesis and advanced supra-annular pericardial bioprostheses have been designed to address these issues. The stentless bioprostheses also address this issue.

Haemodynamics-aortic valve substitutes

The optimisation of haemodynamic performance of valvular substitutes in aortic valve replacement has always been recognized as being of extreme importance. The important objective of aortic valve replacement is to minimise postoperative gradients and to optimise the normalization of left ventricular mass and function. The most frequent cause of high postoperative gradients occurs when the effective prosthetic valve area is less than that of the normal human valve. This is known as patient-prosthesis mismatch, even in the presence of normally functioning valve prostheses. Patient-prosthesis mismatch occurs when the size of the prosthesis orifice is too small for the basal surface area of the patient, that is, the relationship of prosthesis size and body size [101, 102]. The effective orifice area (EOA) index, as a measure of patient-prosthesis mismatch, should not be less than $0.85cm^2/m^2$ to avoid significant gradients at rest and exercise [101, 102]. Higher gradients usually occur when the prosthesis size is <21mm. Increased transvalvular gradients occur and cause reduced effective orifice areas and compromise regression of left ventricular mass.

The normally functioning stented bioprostheses are obstructive, by nature, with non-physiological flow patterns and residual pressure gradients. The stentless bioprostheses provide laminar, non-obstructive flow, even though implanted intra-annularly with the prosthesis having a relatively smaller internal diameter for the same label size, not considering the upsizing that is usually achieved.

The importance of optimal haemodynamic performance with low gradients, satisfactory effective orifice areas and normalization of ventricular muscle mass has been extensively evaluated in recent years.

Left ventricular hypertrophy is the physiological response to increased afterload and / or pressure overload. The clinical phenomenon of pressure overload is aortic stenosis, while of increased afterload is systemic hypertension. Aortic valve replacement facilitates left ventricular mass regression and left ventricular remodelling. Left ventricular mass regression is dependent on changes in gradients and changes in effective orifice areas. Left ventricular mass regression commences immediately after aortic valve replacement and is completed by six months. The major factors influencing left ventricular mass are baseline left ventricular mass index and patient-prosthesis mismatch.

The influence of optimal haemodynamics during rest and exercise and consequently, prosthesis type, has been addressed. Stentless bioprostheses have better haemodynamics than stented bioprostheses [88-94]. There is a higher incidence of patient-prosthesis mismatch with stented bioprostheses, and more likely to occur in the small aortic root. There is evidence that left ventricular mass regression may occur even with levels of patient-prostheses mismatch [37, 44, 69, 70, 73, 91, 92, 96-100, 103]. There is some evidence that stentless bioprostheses provide advanced survival over stented bioprostheses. The survival advantage occurs in patients <70 years of age, but not in patients >70 years of age [114]. This may be related to less than adequate regression of left ventricular mass, due to patient-prosthesis mismatch being of lesser significance in patients with more sedentary, less active lifestyles. The issue of durability of stentless porcine bioprostheses compared to stented bioprostheses remains unresolved and is unlikely to be determined until the evaluation period is extended to 10-12 years.

The cardiac surgeon should address the optimisation of haemodynamic performance in aortic valve replacement surgery. The choice of indexed effective orifice area is felt to be the minimal requirement for a given patient, with the knowledge that $0.85cm^2/m^2$ or higher is the optimal value for better haemodynamics.

The Canadian investigators from Laval University have proposed a simple three-step algorithm that can be easily performed in the operating room to prevent patient-prosthesis mismatch [101]. The minimal EOA of valves of patient basal surface area (BSA) to facilitate indexed EOA of three levels ($>0.85cm^2/m^2$, $>0.80cm^2/m^2$, and $>0.75cm^2/m^2$) are delineated. These investigators have determined that the ideal EOA should be $>0.85cm^2/m^2$. The normal *in vitro* and *in vivo* effective orifice areas for the most commonly used prosthetic valves can be made available to surgeons and hospital operating rooms.

The three-step algorithm can easily be performed in the operating room. The steps are as follows:-

1. Calculate the patient's BSA from weight and height using the Dubois equation.
2. Determine the minimal valve EOA required to ensure an indexed EOA of >0.85, >0.80 or $0.75cm^2/m^2$. The choice of EOAI is deemed to be the minimal requirement for a given patient, with the knowledge that $0.85cm^2/m^2$ or higher is the optimal value for better haemodynamics.
3. Select the type and size of prosthesis that has reference values for EOA greater or equal to the minimal EOA value obtained in step 2.

The reference values provided by the manufacturers and /or published by investigators, may be *in vivo* or *in vitro* values. *In vitro* values derived from pre-marketing studies usually overestimate *in vivo* values by 10% to 15%, but otherwise correlate well with *in vivo* values. There is a notable exception, stentless valves *in vitro* values for EOA grossly overestimate *in vivo* values and therefore, cannot be relied upon. The *in vivo* EOA values for bileaflet valves may artifactually be underestimated by Doppler echocardiography, so a value for EOA lower than the reference value does not necessarily mean prosthesis dysfunction [2]. Manufacturers should provide both *in vitro* and *in vivo* values to assist surgeons in minimising patient-prosthesis mismatch.

Mitral valve replacement

The choice of prosthesis is again a decision to be made by the surgeon and the patient, with full knowledge of the advantages and disadvantages of the different types available. The patient must be informed that the valve replacement is only an alternative to valve reconstruction. Bioprostheses have a limited role in MVR because of the increased evidence of structural valve deterioration compared with their use for AVR [55, 60, 76, 79]. Bioprostheses are indicated in patients greater than 70 years of age and for those with comorbidity and anticipated reduced life expectancy. The actual freedom from structural valve deterioration for patients older than 70 years of age at 15 years with bioprostheses is 93% while actuarial freedom is 80%. In the 61- to 70-year age group, these rates are 69% and 26%, respectively [55]. Mechanical prostheses are indicated for patients 70 years of age or older, even though there is significant valve-related morbidity [68,75]. The linearized rate of major thromboembolism, including thrombosis, ranges between 1.5% to 2.5% per patient-year and haemorrhage rates range from 1.5% to 2.0% per patient-year [78, 80, 81].

The outcomes 15 years after valve replacement with a mechanical versus a bioprosthetic valve have been reported by the Veterans Affairs randomised trial [30]. All-cause mortality was not different after MVR with mechanical prostheses versus bioprostheses. Structural valve deterioration was greater with bioprostheses for MVR in all age groups but occurred at a much higher rate in those aged less than 65 years. Thromboembolism rates were similar in the two valve prostheses, but bleeding was more common with the mechanical prostheses.

In 2003, the Edinburgh randomised trial reported results to 20 years [31]. The prosthesis type did not influence survival, thromboembolism or endocarditis. Major bleeding was more common with mechanical prostheses. Assessing mortality and re-operation, survival with the original prosthesis became different at 8-10 years for MVR and 12-14 years for AVR.

The newer generation mechanical prostheses designs with hinge mechanisms to reduce stasis may facilitate control of thromboembolic phenomena with low-dose anticoagulation to reduce the risk of haemorrhage.

The choice of prostheses for multiple replacement surgery must be based on the type of concurrent mitral valve surgery to be performed.

Valve replacement and renal failure

The optimal prosthesis type for valve replacement in patients on chronic renal dialysis is unresolved. In 1998, the ACC/AHA continued to recommend mechanical prostheses [3,4]. The publications since 1998 have overwhelmingly recommended bioprostheses. It was considered that patients on chronic dialysis do not generally survive long enough to experience structural valve deterioration [115-119]. The 2-year survival was only 39% for both bioprostheses and mechanical prostheses, which is poor for both prosthesis types [116]. Mechanical prostheses have been shown to have a 6-fold higher incidence of late bleeding or stroke [115].

Valve replacement - childbearing women

The risk to pregnancy in women with a valve prosthesis is multifactorial [120-121]. The potential problems are related to the hypercoagulable state of pregnancy and increased risk of thromboembolic events, increased haemodynamic volume, risk to the fetus from anticoagulants and the accelerated deterioration of bioprostheses. Normally functioning biological and mechanical prostheses can tolerate the haemodynamic load of the state of pregnancy. Bioprostheses during the childbearing years are subject to accelerated structural deterioration but pregnancy does not advance that deterioration [122-124]. The risk of warfarin embryopathy is 4% to 10% but may be reduced with low-dose warfarin that is acceptable with current generation mechanical prostheses [125]. The hypercoagulable state of pregnancy, on the other hand, increases the risk of prosthesis thrombosis and thromboembolic events. When warfarin is replaced by heparin between the sixth to 12th week of gestation and after the 36th week, there is an increased risk of prosthesis thrombosis and maternal haemorrhage [126]. Warfarin is also associated with an increased risk of spontaneous abortion, prematurity and stillbirth. The livebirth rate is lower with mechanical prostheses than biological prostheses.

The failure of biological prostheses can occur during pregnancy, but pregnancy has not been shown to accelerate failure [122]. Pregnancies in women with biological prostheses require planned conception within a recommended time interval of four to six years after valve implantation, especially for mitral prostheses. The re-operative mortality for elective and urgent re-replacement of failed bioprostheses in the current era is less than 3%.

The optimal type of prosthesis, biological or mechanical, for women considering childbearing has not been fully defined [127-130]. Autografts and heterografts (porcine and bovine pericardial) can be used for AVR and heterografts for MVR, if reconstruction is not feasible [128]. On the other hand, mechanical prostheses can be used at all positions [127, 129, 130].

Tricuspid valve replacement

Tricuspid valve replacement is an uncommon requirement either as an isolated procedure or concomitant with valve replacement in other positions. All substitutes have significant complications, namely, structural valve deterioration of a bioprosthesis or thrombosis of a mechanical prosthesis [131-136]. Endocarditis of the tricuspid valve can be managed with a total or partial mitral allograft [131-134].

Conclusions

The evidence-based assessment for choice of cardiac valve substitutes is primarily class I-II, level B and C (AHA/ACC/CCS) or level Ib-IIa/b-III, grade A and B (based on the grading system used by the National Institute for Clinical Excellence, UK). Autografts are indicated for children with complex congenital left ventricular outflow tract disease and for selected young and middle-aged adults requiring aortic valve replacement. There remains a considerable risk of re-operation during the life expectancy of the patient, either for autograft dysfunction or degeneration of the pulmonary allograft. Due to the risk of degeneration of allografts in aortic valve or aortic root replacement and limited availability, allografts are predominantly used for native and prosthetic valve endocarditis. The use of mechanical prostheses is declining while hinge mechanisms have been improved to reduce blood stasis amenable to lower-dose anticoagulation and the potential of newer antithrombotic agents. Patient-controlled anticoagulation is making anticoagulation management safer. Heterograft bioprostheses have been improved to extend longevity by reducing mechanical stress and providing more effective calcium mitigation management. Age guidelines are arbitrary indications for cardiac valve substitute selection, but comorbid life-compromising disease must always be given considerable attention. The risks of valve-related mortality, permanent morbidity and re-operation must always be given full evaluation by the patient, cardiac surgeon and cardiologist in the selection of a cardiac valve substitute.

Acknowledgement

The author acknowledges and appreciates the support of Kevin Shillitto for the word processing of this manuscript.

Recommendations	Evidence level
◆ Autografts should be considered in the paediatric age group. **AHA / ACC / CCS - IIa/B**	IIa/B
◆ Autografts should be considered for younger, very active patients (maximum 55 years). **AHA / ACC / CCS - IIb/B**	Ib/A
◆ Allografts should be considered in the management of native and prosthetic valve endocarditis. **AHA / ACC / CCS - IIb/B**	III/B
◆ Mechanical prostheses should be considered for AVR below 60-65 years and for MVR below 70 years. **AHA / ACC / CCS - IIa/C, IIa/C**	III/B III/B
◆ Bioprostheses (stented) should be considered for AVR above 60-65 years and for MVR above 70 years who do not have risk factors of thromboembolism. **AHA / ACC / CCS - I/B, I/B**	Ib/A Ib/A
◆ Bioprostheses (stentless) should be considered for active patients 60-70 years to optimise haemodynamic performance. **AHA / ACC / CCS - IIb/B**	IIb/B

References

1. Edmunds LH Jr, Clark RE, Cohn LH, Grunkemeier GL, Miller DC, Weisel RD. Guidelines for reporting morbidity and mortality after cardiac valvular operations. *Ad Hoc* Liaison Committee for Standardizing Definitions of Prosthetic Heart Valve Morbidity of The American Association for Thoracic Surgery and The Society of Thoracic Surgeons. *J Thorac Cardiovasc Surg* 1996; 112(3): 708-11.
2. Jamieson WRE. Primary Panel Members. Canadian Cardiovascular Society. Surgical Management of Valvular Heart Disease. *Can J Cardio* (In Press).
3. Bonow RO, Carabello B, de Leon AC, Edmunds LH Jr, Fedderly BJ, Freed MD, Gaasch WH, McKay CR, Nishimura RA, O'Gara PT, O'Rourke RA, Rahimtoola SH, Ritchie JL, Cheitlin MD, Eagle KA, Gardner TJ, Garson A Jr, Gibbons RJ, Russell RO, Ryan TJ, Smith SC Jr. ACC/AHA Guidelines for the management of patients with valvular heart disease. A report of the American College of Cardiology/American Heart Association Task Force on Practice Guidelines (Committee on Management of Patients with Valvular Heart Disease). *J Am Coll Cardiol* 1998; 32: 1486-588.
4. Bonow RO, Carabello B, de Leon AC, Edmunds LH Jr, Fedderly BJ, Freed MD, Gaasch WH, McKay CR, Nishimura RA, O'Gara PT, O'Rourke RA, Rahimtoola SH, Ritchie JL, Cheitlin MD, Eagle KA, Gardner TJ, Garson A Jr, Gibbons RJ, Russell RO, Ryan TJ, Smith SC Jr. ACC/AHA Guidelines for the management of patients with valvular heart disease. A report of the American College of Cardiology/American Heart Association Task Force on Practice Guidelines (Committee on Management of Patients with Valvular Heart Disease). *J Heart Valve Dis* 1998; 7: 672-707.
5. Jamieson WRE, Edwards FH, Schwartz M, Bero JW, Clark RE, Grover FL. Risk stratification for cardiac valve replacement. National Cardiac Surgery Database. Database Committee of The Society of Thoracic Surgeons. *Ann Thorac Surg* 1999; 67: 943-51.
6. Edwards FH, Peterson ED, Coombs LP, DeLong ER, Jamieson WRE, Shroyer ALW, Grover FL. Prediction of operative mortality after valve replacement surgery. *J Am Coll Cardiol* 2001; 37: 885-92.
7. Doty JR, Salazar JD, Liddicoat JR, Flores JH, Doty DB. Aortic Valve Replacement with Cryopreserved Aortic Allograft: Ten-Year Experience. *J Thorac Cardiovasc Surg* 1998; 115(2): 371-9.
8. Schmid M, Madge M, Geissler HJ, de Vivie ER. Homograft implantation in heart surgery. *Versicherungsmedizin* 1996; 48(2): 46-8.
9. Takkenberg JJ, Eijkemans MJ, van Herwerden LA, Steyerberg EW, Lane MM. Elkins RC. Habbema JD. Bogers AJ. Prognosis after Aortic Root Replacement with Cryopreserved Allografts in Adults. *Ann Thorac Surg* 2003; 75(5): 1482-9.
10. Lupinetti FM, Duncan BW, Lewin M, Dyamenahalli U, Rosenthal GL. Comparison of Autograft and Allograft Aortic Valve Replacement in Children. *J Thorac Cardiovasc Surg* 2003; 126(1): 240-6.
11. Dearani JA, Orszulak TA, Daly RC, Phillips MR, Miller FA, Danielson GK, Schaff HV. Comparison of Techniques for Implantation of Aortic Valve Allografts. *Ann Thorac Surg* 1996; 62(4): 1069-75.
12. Rubay JE, Sluysmans T, Vanoverschelde JL, Buche M, El Khoury G, Dion R, Schoevaerdts JC. Aortic Allograft and Pulmonary Autograft for Aortic Valve Replacement: Mid-Term Results. *Cardiovasc Surg* 1997; 5(5): 533-8.

13. Willems TP, van Herwerden LA, Taams MA, Kleyburg-Linker VE, Roelandt JR, Bos E. Aortic Allograft Implantation Techniques: Pathomorphology and Regurgitant Jet Patterns by Doppler Echocardiographic Studies. *Ann Thorac Surg* 1998; 66(2): 412-6.
14. Lund O, Chandrasekaran V, Grocott-Mason R, Elwidaa H, Mazhar R, Khaghani A, Mitchell A, Ilsley C, Yacoub MH. Primary Aortic Valve Replacement with Allografts over Twenty-Five Years: Valve-Related and Procedure-Related Determinants of Outcome. *J Thorac Cardiovasc Surg* 1999; 117(1): 77-90.
15. Takkenberg JJM, van Herwerden LA, Eijkemans MJ, Bekkers JA, Bogers AJ. Evolution of Allografts Aortic Valve Replacement over 13 Years: Results of 275 Procedures. Eur *J Cardiothorac Surg* 2002; 21(4): 683-91.
16. Takkenberg JJ, Bogers AJ. Allografts for Aortic Valve and Root Replacement: Veni Vidi Vici? *Expert Rev Cardiovasc Ther* 2004; 2(1): 97-105.
17. Carr-White GS, Glennan S, Edwards S, Ferdinand FD, Desouze AC, Pepper JR, Yacoub MH. Pulmonary Autograft Versus Aortic Homograft for Rereplacement of the Aortic Valve: Results from a Subset of a Prospective Randomized Trial. *Circ* 1999; 100(19 Suppl): II103-6.
18. Aklog L, Carr-White GS, Birks EJ, Yacoub MH. Pulmonary autograft versus aortic homograft for aortic valve replacement: interim results from a prospective randomized trial. *J Heart Valve Dis* 2000; 9(2): 176-88.
19. Elkins RC, Knott-Craig CJ, Howell CE. Pulmonary Autografts in Patients with Aortic Annulus Dysplasia. *Ann Thorac Surg* 1996; 61(4): 1141-5.
20. Willems TP, Bogers AJ, Cromme-Dijkhuis AH, Steyerberg EW, van Herwerden LA, Hokken RB, Hess J, Bos E. Allograft Reconstruction of the Right Ventricular Outflow Tract. *Eur J Cardiothorac Surg* 1996; 10(8): 609-14.
21. Kouchoukos NT. Aortic Allografts And Pulmonary Autografts for Replacement of the Aortic Valve and Aortic Root. *Ann Thorac Surg* 1999; 67(6): 1846-8.
22. Schorn K, Yankah AC, Alexi-Meskhishvili V, Weng Y, Lange PE, Hetzer R. Risk Factors for Early Degeneration of Allografts in Pulmonary Circulation. *Eur J Cardiothorac Surg* 1997; 11(1): 62-9.
23. Laforest I, Dumesnil JG, Briand M, Cartier PC, Pibarot P. Hemodynamic Performance at Rest and during Exercise after Aortic Valve Replacement: Comparison of Pulmonary Autografts Versus Aortic Homografts. *Circ* 2002; 106(12 Suppl 1): I57-I62.
24. Dossche KM, de la Riviere AB, Morshuis WJ, Schepens MA, Ernst SM, van den Brand JJ. Aortic root replacement with pulmonary autograft: an invariably competent aortic valve? *Ann Thorac Surg* 1999; 68(4): 1302-7.
25. David TE, Omran A, Ivanov J, Armstrong S, de Sa MP, Sonnenberg B, Webb G. Dilation of the pulmonary autograft after the Ross procedure. *J Thorac Cardiovasc Surg* 2000; 119: 210-20.
26. Elkins RD, Lane MM, McCue C. Pulmonary autograft reoperation: incidence and management. *Ann Thorac Surg* 1996; 62: 450-5.
27. Hokken RB, Bogers AJJC, Taams MA, Schiks-Berghourt MB, van Herwerden LA, Roelandt JR, Bos E. Does the pulmonary autograft in the aortic position in adults increase in diameter? An echocardiographic study. *J Thorac Cardiovasc Surg* 1997; 113: 667-74.
28. Luciani GB, Barozzi L, Tomezzoli A, Casali G, Mazzucco A. Bicuspid aortic valve disease and pulmonary autograft root dilatation after the Ross procedure: a clinicopathologic study. *J Thorac Cardiovasc Surg* 2001; 122: 74-9.
29. Carr-White GS, Afoke A, Birks EJ, Hughes S, O'Halloran A, Glennen S, Edwards S, Eastwood M, Yacoub MH. Aortic Root Characteristics of Human Pulmonary Autografts. *Circ* 2000; 102(19 Suppl 3): III15-21.
30. Hammermeister K, Sethi GK, Henderson WG, Grover FL, Oprian C, Rahimtoola SH. Outcomes 15 years after valve replacement with a mechanical versus a bioprosthetic valve: final report of the Veterans Affairs randomized trial. *J Am Coll Cardiol* 2000 Oct; 36(4): 1152-8.
31. Oxenham H, Bloomfield P, Wheatley DJ, Lee RJ, Cunningham J, Prescott RJ, Miller HC. Twenty year comparison of a Bjork-Shiley mechanical heart valve with porcine bioprostheses. *Heart* 2003; 89: 715-21.
32. Aupart M, Babuty D, Neville P, Fauchier L, Sirinelli A, Marchand M. Influence of age on valve-related events with Carpentier-Edwards pericardial bioprosthesis. *Eur J Cardiothorac Surg* 1997; 11(5): 929-34.
33. Aupart M, Hammami S, Sirinelli A, Dreyfus X, Meurisse Y, Marchand M. Aortic valve replacement using pericardial bioprostheses in patients under the age of 60 years. 10-year experience. *Annales de Chirurgie* 1996; 50(5): 367-373.
34. Aupart MR, Sirinelli AL, Diemont FF, Meurisse YA, Dreyfus XB, Marchand MA. The last generation of pericardial valves in the aortic position: ten-year follow-up in 589 patients. *Ann Thorac Surg* 1996; 61(2): 615-20.
35. Aupart M, Simonnot I, Sirinelli A, Meurisse Y, Babuty D, Marchand M. Pericardial valves in small aortic annuli: ten years' results. *Eur J Cardiothorac Surg* 1996; 10(10): 879-83.
36. Banbury MK, Cosgrove DM 3rd, Thomas JD, Blackstone EH, Rajeswaran J, Okies JE, Frater RM. Hemodynamic stability during 17 years of the Carpentier-Edwards aortic pericardial bioprosthesis. *Ann Thorac Surg* 2002; 73(5): 1460-5.
37. Bortolotti U, Scioti G, Milano A, De Carlo M, Codecasa R, Nardi C, Tartarini G. Performance of 21-mm size perimount aortic bioprosthesis in the elderly. *Ann Thorac Surg* 2000; 69(1): 47-50.
38. Bottio T, Rizzoli G, Gerosa G, Thiene G, Casarotto D. Mid-term follow-up in patients with Biocor porcine bioprostheses. *Cardiovasc Surg* 2002; 10(3): 238-44.
39. Dagenais F, Cartier P, Dumesnil JG, Pibarot P, Lemieux M, Raymond G, Desaulniers D, Perron J, Bauset R, Baillot R, Doyle D. A single center experience with the freestyle bioprosthesis: midterm results at the Quebec Heart Institute. *Sem Thorac Cardiovasc Surg* 2001; 13(4 Suppl 1): 156-62.
40. Danton MH, Sarsam MA, Byrne JG, Campbell NS, Jones JM, Campalani G. Clinical and hemodynamic performance of the Toronto SPV bioprosthesis. *J Heart Valve Dis* 2000; 9(5): 644-52.
41. David TE, Feindel CM, Scully HE, Bos J, Rakowski H. Aortic valve replacement with stentless porcine aortic valves: a ten-year experience. *J Heart Valve Dis* 1998; 7(3): 250-4.
42. David TE, Ivanov J, Armstrong S, Feindel CM, Cohen G. Late results of heart valve replacement with the Hancock II bioprosthesis. *J Thorac Cardiovasc Surg* 2001; 121(2): 268-77.
43. David TE, Ivanov J, Eriksson MJ, Bos J, Feindel CM, Rakowski H. Dilation of the sinotubular junction causes aortic insufficiency after aortic valve replacement with the Toronto SPV bioprosthesis. *J Thorac Cardiovasc Surg* 2001; 122(5): 929-34.

44. Dellgren G, David TE, Raanani E, Armstrong S, Ivanov J, Rakowski H. Late hemodynamic and clinical outcomes of aortic valve replacement with the Carpentier-Edwards Perimount pericardial bioprosthesis. *J Thorac Cardiovasc Surg* 2002; 124(1): 146-54.
45. Dellgren G, Feindel CM, Bos J, Ivanov J, David TE. Aortic valve replacement with the Toronto SPV: long-term clinical and hemodynamic results. *Eur J Cardiothorac Surg* 2002; 21(4): 698-702.
46. Del Rizzo DF, Abdoh A. Clinical and hemodynamic comparison of the Medtronic Freestyle and Toronto SPV stentless valves. *J Cardiac Surg* 1998; 13(5): 398-407.
47. Doty DB, Cafferty A, Cartier P, Huysmans HA, Kon ND, Krause AH, Millar RC, Sintek CF, Westaby S. Aortic valve replacement with Medtronic Freestyle bioprosthesis: 5-year results. *Sem Thorac Cardiovasc Surg* 1999; 11(4 Suppl 1): 35-41.
48. Doty DB, Cafferty A, Kon ND, Huysmans HA, Krause AH Jr, Westaby S. Medtronic Freestyle aortic root bioprosthesis: implant techniques. *J Cardiac Surg* 1998; 13(5): 369-75.
49. Ennker J, Rosendahl U, Ennker IC, Bauer S, Florath I. Risk in elderly patients after stentless versus stented aortic valve surgery. *Asian Cardiovasc Thorac Ann* 2003; 11(1): 37-41.
50. Frater RW, Furlong P, Cosgrove DM, Okies JE, Colburn LQ, Katz AS, Lowe NL, Ryba EA. Long-term durability and patient functional status of the Carpentier-Edwards Perimount pericardial bioprosthesis in the aortic position. *J Heart Valve Dis* 1998; 7(1): 48-53.
51. Hanania G, Michel PL, Montely JM, Warembourg H, Nardi O, Leguerrier A, Agnino A, Despins P, Legault B, Petit H, Bouraindeloup M, Groupe de travail sur les valvulopathies de la Societe francaise de cardiologie. The long-term (15 years) evolution after valvular replacement with mechanical prosthesis or bioprosthesis between the age of 60 and 70 years. *Arch des Mal du Coeur et des Vaiss* 2004; 97(1): 7-14.
52. Hurle A, Meseguer J, Llamas P, Casillas JA. Clinical Experience with the Carpentier-Edwards Supra-Annular Porcine Bioprosthesis Implanted In The Aortic Position. *J Heart Valve Dis* 1998; 7(3): 331-5.
53. Hvass U, O'Brien MF. The stentless Cryolife-O'Brien aortic porcine xenograft: a five-year follow-up. *Ann Thorac Surg* 1998; 66(6 Suppl): S134-8.
54. Jamieson WRE, Aupart MR, Marchand MA, Germann E, Chan F, Miyagishima RT, Neville PH, Janusz MT. Clinical Performance comparison of Carpentier-Edwards SAV porcine and PERIMOUNT pericardial bioprostheses to 15 years in aortic valve replacement. *J Heart Valve Dis* (In Press).
55. Jamieson WRE, Burr LH, Miyagishima RT, Germann E, Anderson WN. Actuarial versus actual freedom from structural valve deterioration with the Carpentier-Edwards porcine bioprostheses. *Can J Cardiol* 1999 Sep; 15(9): 973-8.
56. Jamieson WRE, Burr LH, Miyashima RT, Germann E, MacNab JS, Chan F, Janusz MT, Ling H. Carpentier-Edwards Supra-Annular (SAV) aortic porcine bioprosthesis clinical performance over 20 years. *Eur J Cardiothorac Surg* (In Press).
57. Jamieson WRE, David TE, Feindel CM, Miyagishima RT, Germann E. Performance of the Carpentier-Edwards SAV and Hancock-II porcine bioprostheses in aortic valve replacement. *J Heart Valve Dis* 2002; 11(3): 424-30.
58. Jamieson WRE, Janusz MT, Burr LH, Ling H, Miyagishima RT, Germann E. Carpentier-Edwards supra-annular porcine bioprosthesis: second-generation prosthesis in aortic valve replacement. *Ann Thorac Surg* 2001; 71(5 Suppl): S224-7.
59. Jamieson WRE, MacNab JS, Stanford EA, Abel JG, Cheung A, Fradet GJ, Bur LH, Janusz MT, Germann E. Medtronic Mosaic porcine bioprosthesis investigational centre experience to six years. *J Heart Valve Dis* (In Press).
60. Jamieson WRE, Miyagishima RT, Burr LH, Lichtenstein SV, Fradet GJ, Janusz MT. Carpentier-Edwards porcine bioprostheses: clinical performance assessed by actual analysis. *J Heart Valve Dis* 2000 Jul; 9(4): 530-5.
61. Jamieson WRE, von Lipinski O, Miyashima RT, Burr LH, Janusz MT, Ling H, Fradet GJ, Germann E. Performance of Bioprostheses and Mechanical Prostheses Assessed by composites of valve-related complications at 15 years for mitral valve replacement. *J Thorac Cardiovasc Surg* (In Press).
62. Jamieson WRE, Tyers GF, Janusz MT, Miyagishima RT, Munro AI, Ling H, Burr LH, Tutassaura H. Age as a determinant for selection of porcine bioprostheses for cardiac valve replacement: experience with Carpentier-Edwards standard bioprosthesis. *Can J Cardio* 1991; 7(4): 181-8.
63. Kon ND, Riley RD, Adair SM, Kitzman DW. Cordell AR. Eight-year results of aortic root replacement with the freestyle stentless porcine aortic root bioprosthesis. *Ann Thorac Surg* 2002; 73(6): 1817-21.
64. Logeis Y, Leguerrier A, Rioux C, Chaperon J, Lelong B, Langanay T, Delamber JF, el Issa A, Valla J. The Carpentier-Edwards Porcine Valve in the Supra Annular Aortic Position. Results after 12 Years in a Series of 1108 Patients. *Arch Mal Coeur et des Vais* 1997; 90(6): 887-88.
65. Myken P, Bech-Hanssen O, Phipps B, Caidahl K. Fifteen years follow-up with the St. Jude Medical Biocor porcine bioprosthesis. *J Heart Valve Dis* 2000; 9(3): 415-22.
66. O'Brien MF, Gardner MA, Garlick RB, Davison MB, Thomson HL, Burstow DJ. The Cryolife-O'Brien stentless aortic porcine xenograft valve. *J Cardiac Surg* 1998; 13(5): 376-85.
67. Rizzoli G, Bottio T, Thiene G, Toscano G, Casarotto D, Long-term durability of the Hancock II porcine bioprosthesis. *J Thorac Cardiovasc Surg* 2003; 126(1): 66-74.
68. Sidhu P, O'Kane H, Ali N, Gladstone DJ, Sarsam MA, Campalani G, MacGowan SW. Mechanical or bioprosthetic valves in the elderly: a 20-year comparison. *Ann Thorac Surg* 2001; 71(5 Suppl): S257-60.
69. Thomson DJ, Jamieson WRE, Dumesnil JG, Burgess JJ, Peniston CM, Metras J, Sullivan JA, Parrott JC, Maitland A, Cybulsky IJ. Medtronic Mosaic Porcine Bioprosthesis: Midterm Investigational Trial Results. *Ann Thorac Surg* 2001; 71(5 Suppl): S269-72.
70. Thomson DJ, Jamieson WRE, Dumesnil JG, Metras J, Dewar LRS. Medtronic Mosaic bioprosthesis clinical performance and evaluation of patient-prosthesis mismatch on survival. *Ann Thorac Surg* (In Press).
71. van Nooten GJ, Caes F, Francois K, van Belleghem Y. Toronto stentless aortic valve replacement in elderly patients. *S African Med J* 1996; 86 Suppl 2: C69-73.
72. Van Nooten G, Caes F, Froncois K, Van Belleghem Y, Taeymans Y. Stentless or Stented Aortic Valve Implants in Elderly Patients? *Eur J Cardiothorac Surg* 1999; 15(1): 31-6.
73. Vitale N, Clark SC, Ramsden A, Hasan A, Hilton CJ, Holden MP. Clinical and hemodynamic evaluation of small Perimount aortic valves in patients aged 75 years or older. *Ann Thorac Surg* 2003; 75(1): 35-9.
74. Wendler O, Dzindzibadze V, Langer F, El Dsoki S, Schafers HJ. Aortic valve replacement with a stentless bioprosthesis using the full-root technique. *Thorac Cardiovasc Surg* 2001; 49(6): 361-4.

75. Arom KV, Emery RW, Nicoloff DM, Petersen RJ. Anticoagulant-related complications in elderly patients with St. Jude mechanical valve prostheses. *J Heart Valve Dis* 1996; 5(5): 505-10.
76. Cen YY, Glower DD, Landolfo K, Lowe JE, Davis RD, Wolfe WG, Pieper C, Peterson B. Comparison of survival after mitral valve replacement with biologic and mechanical valves in 1139 patients. *J Thorac Cardiovasc Surg* 2001; 122(3): 569-77.
77. Emery RW, Erickson CA, Arom KV. Northrup WF 3rd, Kersten TE, Von Rueden TJ, Lillehei TJ, Nicoloff DM. Replacement of the aortic valve in patients under 50 years of age: long-term follow-up of the St. Jude Medical prosthesis. *Ann Thorac Surg* 2003; 75(6): 1815-9.
78. Jamieson WRE, Fradet GJ, Miyagishima RT, Henderson C, Brownlee RT, Zhang J, Germann E. CarboMedics mechanical prosthesis: performance at eight years. *J Heart Valve Dis* 2000; 9(5): 678-87.
79. Jamieson WRE, Marchand MA, Pelletier CL, Norton R, Pellerin M, Dubiel TW, Aupart MR, Daenen WJ, Holden MP, David TE, Ryba EA, Anderson WN Jr. Structural valve deterioration in mitral replacement surgery: comparison of Carpentier-Edwards supra-annular porcine and perimount pericardial bioprostheses. *J Thorac Cardiovasc Surg* 1999; 118(2): 297-304.
80. Jamieson WRE, Miyagishima RT, Grunkemeier GL, Germann E, Henderson C, Fradet GJ, Burr LH, Lichtenstein SV. Bileaflet mechanical prostheses performance in mitral position. *Eur J Cardiothorac Surg* 1999; 15(6): 786-94.
81. Jamieson WRE, Miyagishima RT, Tyers GF, Lichenstein SV, Munro AI, Burr LH. Bileaflet mechanical prostheses in mitral and multiple valve replacement surgery: influence of anticoagulant management on performance. *Circ* 1997; 96(9 Suppl): II-134-9.
82. Katircioglu SF, Ulus AT, Yamak B, Ozsoyler I, Birincioglu L, Tasdemir O. Acute mechanical valve thrombosis of the St. Jude medical prosthesis. *J Cardiac Surg* 1999; 14(3): 164-8.
83. Marchand M, Aupart M, Norton R, Goldsmith IR, Pelletier C, Pellerin M, Dubiel T, Daenen W, Casselman F, Holden M, David TE, Ryba EA. Twelve-year experience with Carpentier-Edwards PERIMOUNT pericardial valve in the mitral position: a multicenter study. *J Heart Valve Dis* 1998; 7(3): 292-8.
84. Minakata K, Wu Y, Zerr KJ, Grunkemeier GL, Handy JR Jr, Ahmad A, Starr A, Furnary AP. Clinical evaluation of the carbomedics prosthesis: experience at providence health system in Portland. *J Heart Valve Dis* 2002; 11(6): 844-50.
85. Jamieson WRE, Burr LH, Miyagishima RT, Janusz MT, Fradet GJ, Lichtenstein SV, Ling H. Reoperation for bioprosthetic mitral structural failure: risk assessment. *Circ* 2003; 108 Suppl 1: II98-102.
86. Jamieson WRE, Burr LH, Miyagishima RT, Janusz MT, Fradet GJ, Ling H, Lichtenstein SV. Re-operation for bioprosthetic aortic structural failure - risk assessment. *Eur J Cardiothorac Surg* 2003; 24(6): 873-8.
87. Zellner JL, Kratz JM, Crumbley AJ 3rd, Stroud MR, Bradley SM, Sade RM, Crawford FA Jr. Long-term experience with the St. Jude Medical valve prosthesis. *Ann Thorac Surg* 1999; 68(4): 1210-8.
88. Bach DS, David T, Yacoub M, Pepper J, Goldman B, Wood J, Verrier E, Petracek M, Aldrete V, Rosenbloom M, Azar H, Rakowski H. Hemodynamics and left ventricular mass regression following implantation of the Toronto SPV stentless porcine valve. *Amer J Cardio* 1998; 82(10): 1214-9.
89. Bach DS, Goldman B, Verrier E, Petracek M, Wood J, Goldman S, David T. Toronto SPV Valve Study Group. Impact of small valve size on hemodynamics and left ventricular mass regression with the Toronto SPV stentless aortic bioprosthesis. *J Heart Valve Dis* 2002; 11(2): 236-41.
90. Corbineau H, Lelong B, Langanay T, Verhoye JP, Leguerrier A. Echocardiographic Assessment and Preliminary Clinical Results after Aortic Valve Replacement with the Medtronic Mosaic Bioprosthesis. *J Heart Valve Dis* 2001; 10(2): 171-6.
91. Dellgren G, David TE, Raanani E, Bos J, Ivanov J, Rakowski H. The Toronto SPV: hemodynamic data at 1 and 5 years' postimplantation. *Sem Thoracic Cardiovasc Surg* 1999; 11(4 Suppl 1): 107-13.
92. Eichinger WB, Botzenhardt F, Gunzinger R, Kemkes BM, Bleese N, Sosnowski A, Maiza D, Coto EO, Bauernschmitt R, Lange R. Left ventricular mass regression after aortic valve replacement with the mosaic bioprosthesis. *J Heart Valve Dis* 2002; 11(4): 529-36.
93. Frapier JM, Rouviere P, Razcka F, Aymard T, Albat B, Chaptal PA. Influence of patient-prosthesis mismatch on long-term results after aortic valve replacement with a stented bioprosthesis. *J Heart Valve Dis* 2002; 11(4): 543-51.
94. Fries R, Wendler O, Schieffer H, Schafers HJ. Comparative rest and exercise hemodynamics of 23-mm stentless versus 23-mm stented aortic bioprostheses. *Ann Thorac Surg* 2000; 69(3): 817-22.
95. Gegouskov VA, Eckstein FS, Kipfer B, Berdat PA, Immer FF, Schmidli J, Seiler C, Zobrist C, Carrel TP. The Sorin pericardial bioprosthesis - a stentless aortic valve with very good hemodynamic performance. *Swiss Surg* 2003; 9(5): 247-52.
96. Hurle A, Ibanez A, Meseguer J, Sanchez Paya J, Martinez JG, Gomez Plana J, Llamas P. A comparative study of the follow-up and hemodynamics *in vivo* of 21mm Carpentier-Edwards supra-annular and perimount bioprostheses. *Revista Espanola de Cardiologia.* 2002; 55(7): 733-7.
97. Jamieson WRE, Janusz MT, MacNab J, Henderson C. Hemodynamic Comparison of Second and Third-Generation Stented Bioprostheses in Aortic Valve Replacement. *Ann Thorac Surg* 2001; 71(5 Suppl): S282-4.
98. Jasinski MJ, Hayton J, Kadziola Z, Wos S, Sosnowski AW. Hemodynamic performance after stented vs stentless aortic valve replacement. J Cardiovasc Surg 2002;43(3):313-7.
99. Milano AD, Blanzola C, Mecozzi G, D'Alfonso A, De Carle M, Nardi C, Bortolotti U. Hemodynamic Performance of Stented and Stentless Aortic Bioprostheses. *Ann Thorac Surg* 2001; 72(1): 33-8.
100. Nardi C, Scioti G, Milano AD, De Carlo M, Bortolotti U. Hemodynamic Assessment of The Medtronic Mosaic Bioprosthesis in the Aortic Position. *J Heart Valve Dis* 2001; 10(1): 100-4.
101. Pibarot P, Dumesnil JG. Hemodynamic and clinical impact of prosthesis-patient mismatch in the aortic valve position and its prevention. *J Am Coll Cardiol* 2000; 36: 1131-41.
102. Pibarot P, Dumesnil JG, Leblanc MH, Cartier P, Metras J. Changes in left ventricular mass and function after aortic valve replacement: a comparison between stentless and stented bioprosthetic valves. *J Amer Soc Echo* 1999; 12(11): 981-7.
103. Seitelberger R, Bialy J, Gottardi R, Seebacher G, Moidl R, Mittelbock M, Simon P, Wolner E. Relation between Size of Prosthesis and Valve Gradient: Comparison of Two Aortic Bioprosthesis. *Eur J Cardiothorac Surg* 2004; 25(3): 358-63.

104. Walther T, Falk V, Langebartels G, Kruger M, Schilling L, Diegeler A, Gummert J, Autschbach R, Mohr FW. Regression of left ventricular hypertrophy after stentless versus conventional aortic valve replacement. *Sem Thorac Cardiovasc Surg* 1999; 11(4 Suppl 1): 18-21.
105. Wiseth R, Rossvoll, O, Leavang OW, Skjaerpe T, Hatle L. Two-Dimensional Echocardiography for Prediction of Aortic Valve Prosthesis Size. A Comparative Study of Medtronic-Hall And Carpentier-Edwards Supra-Annular Valves. *Scandinav J Thorac Cardiovasc Surg* 1993; 27(2): 87-92.
106. Bach DS, Sakwa MP, Goldbach M, Petracek MR, Emery RW, Mohr FW. Hemodynamics and early clinical performance of the St. Jude Medical Regent mechanical aortic valve. *Ann Thorac Surg* 2002; 74(6): 2003-9.
107. Bernal JM, Martin-Duran R, Rabasa JM, Revuelta JM. The CarboMedics "Top-Hat" supra-annular prosthesis. *Ann Thorac Surg* 1999; 67(5): 1299-303.
108. Binuani P, Baufreton C, Subayi JB, de Brux JL. The CarboMedics "Top-Hat" aortic valve prosthesis: short-term results. *J Heart Valve Dis* 2000; 9(5): 693-6.
109. Gelsomino S, Morocutti G, Da Col P, Masullo G, Carella R, Guzzi G, Spedicato L, Livi U. Early *in vivo* hemodynamic results after aortic valve replacement with the St Jude Medical Regent mechanical heart valve in patients with pure aortic stenosis. *J Cardiac Surg* 2003; 18(2): 125-32.
110. Gillinov AM, Blackstone EH, Alster JM, Craver JM, Baumgartner WA, Brewster SA, Kleinman LH, Smedira NG. The Carbomedics Top Hat supra-annular aortic valve: a multicenter study. *Ann Thorac Surg* 2003; 75(4): 1175-80.
111. Lundblad R, Hagen OM, Smith G, Kvernebo K. The CarboMedics supra-annular top hat valve improves prosthesis size in the aortic root. *J Heart Valve Dis* 2001; 10(2): 196-201.
112. Strike PC, Edwards TJ, Gardiner D, Livesey SA, Simpson IA. Functional hemodynamic assessment of the 21mm and 23mm CarboMedics Top Hat aortic prosthetic valve. *J Cardiac Surg* 1998; 13(2): 98-103.
113. Sudkamp M, Lercher AJ, Muller-Riemenschneider F, LaRosee K, Tossios P, Mehlhorn U, de Vivie ER. Transvalvular *in vivo* gradients of the new generation bileaflet heart valve prosthesis St. Jude Medical Regent in aortic position. *Thorac Cardiovasc Surg* 2003; 51(3): 126-9.
114. Del Rizzo DF, Abdoh A, Cartier P, Doty D, Westaby S. The effect of prosthetic valve type on survival after aortic valve surgery. *Sem Thorac Cardiovasc Surg* 1999; 11(4 Suppl 1): 1-8.
115. Brinkman WT, Williams WH, Guyton RA, Jones EL, Craver JM. Valve replacement in patients on chronic renal dialysis: implications for valve prosthesis selection. *Ann Thorac Surg* 2002; 74: 37-42.
116. Herzog CA, Ma JZ, Collins AJ. Long-term survival of dialysis patients in the United States with prosthetic heart valves: should ACC/AHA practice guidelines on valve selection be modified? *Circulation* 2002; 105: 1336-41.
117. Kaplon RJ, Cosgrove DM 3rd, Gillinov AM, Lytle BW, Blackstone EH, Smedira NG. Cardiac valve replacement in patients on dialysis: influence of prosthesis on survival. *Ann Thorac Surg* 2000; 70: 438-41.
118. Lucke JC, Samy RN, Atkins BZ, Silvestry SC, Douglas JM Jr, Schwab SJ, Wolfe WG, Glower DD. Results of valve replacement with mechanical and biological prostheses in chronic renal dialysis patients. *Ann Thorac Surg* 1997; 64: 129-33.
119. Chan V, Jamieson WRE, Fleisher AG, Denmark D, Chan F, Germann E. Valve Replacement Surgery in end-stage renal failure - mechanical prostheses versus bioprostheses. *J Thorac Cardiovasc Surg* (In Press).
120. Elkayam UR. Anticoagulation in pregnant women with prosthetic heart valves: a double jeopardy. *J Am Coll Cardiol* 1996; 27: 1704-6.
121. Ginsberg JS, Hirsh J. Use of antithrombotic agents during pregnancy. *Chest* 1998; 114: S524-30.
122. Badduke BR, Jamieson WRE, Miyagishima RT, Munro AI, Gerein AN, MacNab J, Tyers GF. Pregnancy and childbearing in a population with biologic valvular prostheses. *J Thorac Cardiovasc Surg* 1991; 102: 179-86.
123. North RA, Sadler L, Stewart AW, McCowan LM, Kerr AR, White HD. Long-term survival and valve-related complications in young women with cardiac valve replacements. *Circulation* 1999; 99: 2669-76.
124. Jamieson WRE, Miller DC, Akins CW, Munro AI, Glower DD, Moore KA, Henderson C. Pregnancy and bioprostheses: influence on structural valve deterioration. *Ann Thorac Surg* 1995; 60: S282-7.
125. Wong V, Cheng CH, Chan KC. Fetal and neonatal outcome of exposure to anticoagulants during pregnancy. *Am J Med Genet* 1993; 45: 17-21.
126. Salazar E, Izaguirre R, Verdejo J, Mutchinick O. Failure of adjusted doses of subcutaneous heparin to prevent thromboembolic phenomen in pregnant patients with mechanical cardiac valve prostheses. *J Am Coll Cardiol* 1996; 27: 1698-703.
127. Oakley CM. Pregnancy and prosthetic heart valves. *Lancet* 1994; 344: 1643-4.
128. Dore A, Somerville J. Pregnancy in patients with pulmonary autograft valve replacement. *Eur Heart J* 1997; 18: 1659-62.
129. Vural KM, Ozatik MA, Uncu H, Emir M, Yurdagok O, Sener E, Tasdemir O. Pregnancy after mechanical mitral valve replacement. *J Heart Valve Dis* 2003; 12(3): 370-6.
130. Ferraris VA, Klingman RR, Dunn L, Fein S, Eglowstein M, Samelson R. Home heparin therapy used in a pregnant patient with a mechanical heart valve prosthesis. *Ann Thorac Surg* 1994; 58: 1168-70.
131. Kolsi M, Tapia M, Tattevin P, Philip I, Fourchy D, Acar C. Partial tricuspid homograft: a new technique for tricuspid valve repair. Report of a case. *Arch des Mal du Coeur et des Vaiss* 2000; 93(3): 315-8.
132. Mestres CA, Miro JM, Pare JC, Pomar JL. Six-year experience with cryopreserved mitral homografts in the treatment of tricuspid valve endocarditis in HIV-infected drug addicts. *J Heart Valve Dis* 1999; 8(5): 575-7.
133. Miyagishima RT, Brumwell ML, Jamieson WRE, Munt BI. Tricuspid valve replacement using a cryopreserved mitral homograft. Surgical technique and initial results. *J Heart Valve Dis* 2000; 9(6): 805-8.
134. Ramsheyi A, D'Attellis N, Le Lostec Z, Fegueux S, Acar C. Partial mitral homograft for tricuspid valve repair. *Ann Thorac Surg* 1997; 64(5): 1486-8.
135. Rizzoli G, De Perini L, Bottio T, Minutolo G, Thiene G, Casarotto D. Prosthetic replacement of the tricuspid valve: biological or mechanical? *Ann Thorac Surg* 1998; 66(6 Suppl): S62-7.
136. Shapira Y, Nili M, Hirsch R, Vaturi M, Vidne B, Sagie A. Mid-term clinical and echocardiographic follow-up of patients with CarboMedics valves in the tricuspid position. *J Heart Valve Dis* 2000; 9(3): 396-402.

Chapter 20

Interventions on the aortic valve

John R Pepper MA MChir FRCS

Professor of Cardiothoracic Surgery

ROYAL BROMPTON HOSPITAL AND
THE NATIONAL HEART & LUNG INSTITUTE, LONDON, UK

Introduction

In this chapter, aortic valve substitutes will be reviewed as well as conservative approaches to the aortic valve for aortic regurgitation with particular reference to the Marfan's syndrome. Reference will also be made to recent innovatory techniques of percutaneous aortic valvotomy and valve replacement.

Methodology

Searches were made in standard texts, the COCHRANE and PUBMED databases, and from personal reference files.

Indications for surgery

Knowledge of the natural history of aortic stenosis comes from the study of Ross and Braunwald [1]. Once the patient has symptoms of angina, heart failure or syncope, median survival is about two years, so the onset of significant symptoms is the primary indication for an operation with survival being a major consideration as well as symptom relief. Operating on milder degrees of aortic stenosis, in older patients, or coincidentally at the time of coronary artery surgery, is more contentious. Rahimtoola [2] has recently warned against such a policy unless the aortic stenosis is severe, with a valve area equal to or less than $1.0cm^2$ or a subvalvar velocity greater than 4M/sec. The timing of surgery in aortic regurgitation has been the subject of many reviews, but there is general consensus based on echocardiographic dimensions [3,4]. In the absence of symptoms, a left ventricular end diastolic dimension (LVESD) of 55cm or greater is considered an indication for operation.

Results of surgery

The results of valve surgery with regard to survival, complications, valve function, cardiac function and functional class are dependent on patient-related factors, the type of surgery, the type of prosthesis and healthcare-related factors. Ideally, an aortic valve substitute should be non-thrombogenic, it should be durable for the life expectancy of the patient and exhibit satisfactory function with a minimal pressure gradient and allow for complete resolution of abnormal left ventricular function. The clinical performance of valvular substitutes is judged according to the *Guidelines for Reporting Morbidity and Mortality After Cardiac Valvular Operations* [5]. The specific complications associated with cardiac valve prostheses are structural valve degeneration (SVD), non-structural dysfunction, thromboembolism and thrombosis, anticoagulant-related haemorrhage and prosthetic valve endocarditis.

Randomised studies

There have been many reports in the literature documenting the outcome of individual prostheses but few randomised control trials. Two large RCTs have compared patient outcomes with the use of a mechanical valve and a porcine bioprosthetic valve.

The Veterans Affairs Trial

The Department of Veteran Affairs (DVA) trial [6] involved 575 men randomised for the period 1987 to 1992. Three hundred and eighty-four had an aortic valve replacement (AVR) and 181 had a mitral valve replacement (MVR). Follow-up was extended to 18 years with an average follow-up of 15 years. The principal long-term findings were:-

- After AVR, use of a mechanical valve resulted in a lower mortality: 66 +/- 3% v 79 +/- 3% (p=0.02), and a lower re-operation rate (10 +/- 3% v 29 +/- 5% (p=0.004) at 18 years. The difference became apparent after ten years.
- With a bioprosthetic valve, the mortality rate 18 years after MVR (81%) was similar to that of AVR (79%).
- After AVR, 40% of the mortality was related to the valve substitute. After MVR, 44% of the mortality with a mechanical valve and 50% of the mortality with a bioprosthesis was related to the valve substitute.
- There was no structural valve degeneration with the mechanical valve (Bjork-Shiley).
- Primary valve failure occurred mainly in patients less than 65 years old. It began at 5-6 years after MVR and 7-8 years after AVR. The incidence was higher after MVR (44 +/- 8 vs. 23 +/- 5%).
- After ten years of follow-up the incidence and deleterious effects of structural valve degeneration in porcine valves was evident.
- Use of a bioprosthesis resulted in a lower bleeding rate related to less use of anticoagulation.
- There was no significant difference between the two valve types with regard to other valve-related complications, including thromboembolism.

The Edinburgh Heart Valve Trial

A total of 541 men and women were randomised between 1975 and 1979 [7]. Two hundred and eleven had AVR, 261 had MVR and 61 had AVR + MVR. The average follow-up was 12 years. The major findings were:-

- A trend towards an improved survival with a Bjork-Shiley valve (p=0.08).
- Re-operation rates were low and not significant at five years. At 12 years there was a higher re-operation rate with the tissue valve versus the mechanical valve (AVR 22.6 +/- 5.7% v 4.4 +/- 2.1% (p=0.01); MVR 43.1+/- 6% v 9.9 +/- 3.2% (p=0.001). Younger patients were more likely to require re-operation.
- The incidence of thromboembolism and endocarditis were not statistically significantly different.
- The bleeding rate was higher with the mechanical valve versus the tissue valve after AVR (32.6 +/- 6.1% v 9.7 +/- 4.7% (p=0.001), but not after MVR (24.5% v 24.5%).

The bleeding rate in the Edinburgh Heart Valve trial was 2-2.5% per year with the mechanical valve and 0.9-2% per year with a porcine valve. The patients were less heavily anticoagulated and minor bleeding was not recorded for the first five years of follow-up. After MVR, the bleeding rates with a mechanical and porcine valve were not different, probably because many patients with porcine valves needed anticoagulation for other reasons, such as atrial fibrillation. The exact reason for the high bleeding rate in the DVA trial is not clear. In that trial, it was recommended that prothrombin time should be maintained at 2-2.5 times control, which would nowadays be regarded as excessive. Furthermore, some patients with porcine valves were anticoagulated and all bleeding episodes were included because it was not possible to separate bleeding which was due to anticoagulation from that due to other causes.

There has been one randomised controlled trial comparing two mechanical valves, the Starr Edwards and St Jude. At five years there was no difference in thromboembolic event rates or regression of left ventricular mass [20].

Non-randomised studies

The ten and 15-year mortality rates after AVR and MVR are high, of the order of 15-20% [8-18]. The range is large, even with the use of the same type of prosthesis, indicating the overwhelming importance of the patient's risk profile and factors other than the type of valve substitute.

Risk factors for late mortality have included age, left ventricular dysfunction, the presence of heart failure, NYHA functional class III and IV, coronary artery disease, coronary bypass grafting, valve regurgitation, arrhythmias, male gender, pulmonary hypertension and other comorbid conditions, such as lung disease, hypertension, diabetes and renal failure [8,9]. For example, of 842 patients undergoing AVR with the Hancock modified-orifice (MO) porcine valve [10], the 10-year mortality rate was 48 +/- 2%. However, the 10-year mortality rate in those who required concomitant coronary artery surgery (CABG), was 55 +/- 6% versus 39 +/- 3% (p=0.005) in those without CABG.

Not surprisingly, the older the patient at the time of the valve prosthesis implant, the lower is the ten and 20-year survival [10]. Older patients are much more likely to have clinically significantly associated comorbid conditions. Unfortunately, this study provided no information on the patients' condition at base line [10]. Of note, a study of 841 patients undergoing AVR [9] showed that the subgroups with lower survival at ten years were those with renal disease at any age, lung disease in patients older than 60, left ventricular ejection less than 0.40, and coronary artery disease at any age survival.

Do newer valve designs mean better results?

Data from the Mayo Clinic [11] showed that with the Starr-Edwards model 1260 valve, 10-year and 20-year survival after AVR was 60% and 35% respectively. The incidence of thromboembolism was 1.4% per year, although it was higher on exercise. Starr's own data of event rates with the Starr-Edwards valve 1260 model up to 30 years after AVR are good [19]. The 5-year data from a randomised controlled trial reported by Murday and co-workers [20], showed no statistically significant difference in patient outcomes between the St Jude and Starr-Edwards valves, in either the aortic or mitral position. The lesson seems to be that mortality and complication rates in patients with the use of various prosthetic devices followed-up for longer than ten years is required, that most of the variation in outcome is due to patient-related factors, and there are no major differences in patient outcomes among the different valve substitutes.

In the DVA trial, there was not a single instance of mechanical valve failure with the Bjork-Shiley valve up to 18 years of follow-up.

The complications of valve substitutes

To approve a prosthetic heart valve, the Food and Drug Administration (FDA) in the USA [21] requires studies with greater than 800 valve years of follow-up. The incidence of complications should be less than two optimal performance characteristics (OPC) determined by the FDA, which are calculated to allow an alpha error of 5% (p less than 0.05) and a beta error of 20% (p of 80%). A review of mechanical valves [22] comprising 95 published series, 37,253 valves and 187,220 valve years of follow-up and of biological and bioprosthetic valves comprising 70 published series (24,202 valves and 132,519 valve years) of follow-up shows the following:-

- There is no significant difference among the various mechanical valves for thromboembolism or for that matter, among the bioprostheses. This is true for rates of thrombosis, bleeding, endocarditis and paravalvular leak.

- The incidence of thromboembolism is higher in patients with a mitral prosthesis than in those with an aortic prosthesis.
- Bioprostheses are not free of thromboembolic risk, but the risk is lower than with the use of mechanical valves.
- Complication rates with the use of the same type of valve substitute vary widely.
- The risk of structural valve disease with all currently used mechanical valves is negligible.

Patients undergoing implantation with a mechanical valve who are at the lowest risk of thromboembolism are those in sinus rhythm, who have normal left ventricular function and who have not had previous thromboembolism, are non-smokers, do not have thrombus in the left ventricle or left atrium, do not have carotid or coronary disease, do not have diabetes or hypertension and are sero-negative for *Chlamydia pneumoniae*, who had adequate and low anticoagulant variability and do not have a clotting disorder [23,24].

Bleeding

In the randomised trials of anticoagulation and atrial fibrillation, patients' average age ranged from 67-75. The incidence of major bleeding in the placebo group ranged from 0-4.6%, and the incidence of minor bleeding was up to 10.5% per year and there were deaths from bleeding [25,26]. In patients with mechanical valves who were maintained on the same level of anticoagulation at seven years, those greater than age 60 had up to seven times the bleeding rate than those of patients less than 60. In the stroke prevention in atrial fibrillation trial [27], in which the INR was maintained in a range of 2-3, the incidence of bleeding was 1.5% per year, which is what one would expect with AVR in sinus rhythm.

Structural valve disease

The rate of structural valve degeneration (SVD) of bioprostheses is related to:-

- the site of implant - MVR greater than AVR;
- the age of the patient at the time of implant [22]. In patients aged 16-39, at ten years SVD after AVR is 60% and at 16 years is greater than 90%, but in patients over the age of 70 it is less than 15% at 15 years [14]. The rate of SVD is not significantly different with the standard Hancock MO and Carpentier-Edwards porcine valves [28] .

Emerging evidence from non-randomised trials supports the notion of an improved survival in patients with stentless valves owing to its lower valve-related mortality [29]. A case-matched study from Toronto, which compared the Hancock II valve with the Toronto stentless valve showed significant differences in intermediate survival in favour of the stentless valve [30]. At eight years the actuarial survival was 91 +/- 4% for the Toronto stentless valve group and 69 +/- 8% for the Hancock II group (p=0.006); the freedom from cardiac-related death was 95 +/-4% for the Toronto valve and 81 +/- 8% for the Hancock II (p=0.01).

Valve prosthesis patient mismatch

Rahimtoola raised this issue in a report in 1978 [31]. He pointed out that valve prosthesis patient mismatch (VP-PM) occurs when the prosthetic valve area after insertion into the patient is less than that of a normal human valve. The reduced prosthetic valve area is usually mild to moderate in severity and often of no immediate clinical significance. However, occasionally, there can be a severe problem because the patient may be haemodynamically and symptomatically worse after valve replacement.

Pibarot and Dumesnil's review [32] of VP-PM showed that depending on its severity, this may result in higher valve gradients at rest and on exercise, less reduction of left ventricular mass, greater physical limitation, and higher morbidity and mortality. An appropriate sized prosthesis may be important in the peri-operative period in critically ill patients. Connolly and co-workers [33] found that in patients with severe aortic stenosis, mean aortic valve gradient around 30mmHg and heart failure, the only predictor of an operative mortality of 21%, was a small prosthesis size (47% for a bioprosthesis <21mm versus 15% for a valve >23mm diameter, p=0.03).

For long-term outcome, the issue is the effect of prosthetic valve area at 6-12 months after insertion and its relationship to the patient's body size. He *et al* have shown [34] that in patients with a small aortic root who received a prosthetic valve <21mm diameter, the only independent predictor of survival was patient size. In patients with a body surface area >1.7m^2 versus those <1.7m^2, the survival was approximately 10% versus 50% (p=0.014).

The outcome after valve replacement depends on patient-related and other factors and also, on whether the valve substitute produces, mild, moderate or severe VP-PM. One consequence of examining these issues has been a heightened awareness of the importance of left ventricular outflow tract obstruction and the sensitivity of the left ventricle to pressure overload. A range of valves, both mechanical and tissue, have come on to the market designed to be placed in a supra-annular position and to give rise to low transvalvular pressure gradients. Ten-year survival data are not yet available for any of these newer devices.

Homografts and stentless valves

In the early 1960s, Ross and Barrett-Boyes separately introduced the aortic homograft, but in those days only a few skilled surgeons were able to obtain predictable results with a free-sewn valve. Furthermore, the supply of high quality homografts is limited. In 1985, the Toronto stentless porcine valve was introduced as an alternative to stented tissue valves by David [35]. The design of the stentless porcine valve was intended to reduce residual obstruction to trans-aortic flow by maximising the available flow area. Such a feature, it was argued, would permit more complete resolution of left ventricular hypertrophy (LVH), thus improving long-term outcomes and decreasing the incidence of sudden death and congestive heart failure after AVR [34,36,37]. Left ventricular function in the early postoperative period was similar to that of a stented valve in spite of the factor of a longer aortic cross-clamp time required for its implantation [38]. In the medium-term there is an additional increase in effective orifice area (EOA) corresponding to a further reduction of transvalvular pressure gradient, possibly as a result of "ventricular remodelling" [39]. We, and others, have shown rapid resolution of LVH after the use of a homograft or stentless porcine valve in aortic valve stenosis during the first six postoperative months and maintained out to two years [40].

Residual hypertrophy has an important effect on ventricular function and late outcome. In a 22-year follow-up after AVR for aortic stenosis, Lund [41] found that the completeness with which LVH regressed was a dominant mechanism determining overall late outcome. In particular, impaired left ventricular diastolic function at late reinvestigation related to significant residual hypertrophy and was the sole predictor of fatal congestive heart failure irrespective of the initial ejection fraction. Unresolved left ventricular hypertrophy may also result in more frequent and severe ventricular arrhythmias. In 96 patients with aortic valve disease undergoing 24-hour electrocardiographic monitoring, 37% who had severe ventricular arrhythmias (Lown Class III or IV) before AVR proved to have a greater left ventricular mass index and lower ejection fraction than the remaining 63%. Eighteen months after AVR, the incidence of severe ventricular arrhythmia had fallen to 27%; these patients had a significantly lower ejection fraction and larger cavity dimension [42]. Suboptimal left ventricular function after AVR not only increases morbidity and compromises quality of life, but also increases mortality when redo operation becomes necessary [43]. In a retrospective study of 177 patients who underwent repeat AVR using an aortic homograft [44], the early mortality was 5.1% and the actuarial 10-year survival was 71%. Those patients in whom an aortic homograft had been implanted at their first operation had a significantly improved long-term survival compared with those who had received a mechanical valve.

One of the largest and most complete aortic homograft series comes from O'Brien [45] who reported on the relationship between age of the recipient of the homograft and structural degeneration. For cryo-preserved valves, the re-operation rate at 15 years for SVD was 53% for age 1-20 years; 15% for those aged 21 to 40; 19% for those aged 41 to 60, and 16% for those aged over 60 years. In this study, valve preservation techniques (cryo-preservation or storage in antibiotics at 4°C) and implantation technique (full root or subcoronary) had no effect on the overall actuarial 20-year incidence of endocarditis, thromboembolism, SVD or late survival.

The pulmonary autograft

In 1967, Ross introduced the pulmonary autograft (later recognised as the Ross operation) as a possible long-term biological solution for the diseased aortic valve. Although it is a more complex and difficult procedure, the pulmonary autograft has significant advantages, namely, when inserted in children, the valve is able to grow as the child grows [46] and pregnancy may not result in SVD. These authors found that the autograft remained viable and grew in proportion to somatic growth and that the annulus and sinotubular junction increased in size to the normal range. Elkins [46] reported that freedom from re-operation at seven years was 96.5% for autografts in the aortic position or homograft reconstruction of the right ventricular outflow tract. The incidence of thomboembolism is very low as is the incidence of infective endocarditis, 0-1.2% per year. Those with rheumatic heart disease may develop rheumatic valvulitis in the autograft. In 1989, Ross [47] reported 339 cases with an 85% freedom from valve replacement at 20 years. A further report from Gerosa and colleagues [48] in 34 paediatric patients receiving a Ross operation, revealed a 16-year freedom from re-operation of 74% for the left ventricular outflow tract and 80% for the right ventricular outflow tract. The predominant indication for re-operation was bacterial endocarditis. There was no instance of primary structural degeneration of the pulmonary autograft.

The exact role of the pulmonary autograft remains controversial. Its use is confined to a few surgeons in specialist centres, for children or adults under the age of 50.

The bicuspid aortic valve

The bicuspid aortic valve is a common abnormality affecting 1% of the general population. McCusick [49] was among the first to draw attention to an association between bicuspid aortic valves and cystic medial necrosis. It is now well known that a bicuspid aortic valve is found in 10% of acute ascending aortic dissections, but patients with bicuspid aortic valves are not a homogeneous group. They comprise several distinct subgroups including young men with annular dilatation and older men with a normal aortic root. Ideally, surgery needs to be guided by genetic analysis to predict the risk of future dilatation or dissection of the ascending aorta. A recent study from Germany [50] examined tissue from the aortic wall of patients undergoing resection of an ascending aortic aneurysm. Wall segments from patients with bicuspid valves contained more cells bearing markers of apoptosis than tricuspid aortic valve specimens, whereas normal aorta displayed only a few apoptotic cells (p=0.05). The molecular genetics underlying these differences remains to be explored. Meanwhile, the practising surgeon has to rely on serial imaging and surgical judgement.

The standard operation for an ascending aortic aneurysm, which involves the aortic valve and sinuses, is the Bentall operation [51]. In its original form (Classic Bentall), the aortic aneurysmal sac was wrapped around the graft and coronary arteries. Due to a high incidence of false aneurysms between the wrap and the Dacron graft, this has largely been abandoned in favour of a free-standing Dacron graft containing a composite bileaflet mechanical valve with the coronaries implanted as buttons on to the Dacron cylinder (Button Bentall). A third variant of the Bentall procedure was the Cabrol procedure, which has also been largely abandoned. These procedures were carefully reviewed in a retrospective study by Midulla and co-workers [52]. They found in a retrospective review that the overall hospital mortality was 5%. In a univariate analysis, the Cabrol technique was associated with a higher hospital mortality, but this was not confirmed by multivariate analysis. The 5-year actuarial survival for all patients was 79%: Classic Bentall 85%; Button 82%; Cabrol 52%. These authors concluded that the routine procedure is the Button Bentall technique.

Aortic valve repair

The development of aortic valve repair has been gradual and the adoption of techniques has been restricted to only a few enthusiastic surgeons. Indeed, techniques continue to evolve and remain controversial. This stands in marked contrast to mitral valve repair where basic repair techniques have become standardized for the last ten years and are in widespread use.

A significant number of patients develop potentially life-threatening aortic regurgitation secondary to aortic wall disease in the presence of structurally normal aortic leaflets. For example, in aortic root aneurysm the disease process is localized to the wall of the sinuses of Valsalva with complete sparing of the annulus, leaflets and commissures which are initially structurally normal, but can undergo secondary changes if the aortic regurgitation is neglected. In patients with aneurysms of the root, progressive dilatation of the ascending aorta and root result in disappearance of the sinotubular junction and progressive separation of the commissures from each other with resulting failure in coaptation of the leaflets.

These principles apply also to aortic dissection, both acute and chronic. An intimal tear is usually present in the proximal ascending aorta with extension of the dissection both proximally and distally. This results in displacement of one or more commissures, which produces prolapse of one or more leaflets of the aortic valve. An important feature of dissection of the aortic root is that it does not cross the annulus into the left ventricular outflow even when there is rupture into the aorto-atrial space, pericardium or right atrium. All these features render aortic regurgitation due to aortic wall disease, suitable for a valve-conserving operation.

This procedure has also been applied to Marfan's syndrome where the patients are younger and the wish to avoid long-term anticoagulation is strong, particularly for young women who wish to have children. The defect in the fibrillin gene which gives rise to the defective elastin fibres, which is the hallmark of the disease, is widespread affecting both the aortic wall and the valve leaflets. Although this would appear to be a strong theoretical objection, in fact, excellent long-term results have been reported if patients receive their operation before the valve leaflets are too stretched.

The standard against which repair for Marfan's syndrome must be judged, is the report from Johns Hopkins by Gott and colleagues [53] of 455 elective operations with an operative mortality of 1.5% and a 10-year actuarial survival of 75%. These excellent results were achieved by the use of a composite bileaflet mechanical valve and conduit with reimplantation of the coronary arteries. But these patients who have an increased risk of dissection in other parts of their arterial tree, are committed to lifelong anticoagulation with warfarin. A long-term biological solution would be ideal for these patients.

There are no randomised trials of aortic valve repair, so that the evidence to influence our clinical practice comes from case series. One of the largest experiences comes from Yacoub's group [54], who used the remodelling technique exclusively in 82 patients with Marfan's syndrome. They found that by ten years, 17% had required re-operation and an additional 22% had moderate AR at a mean follow-up of 5.5 years. Schafers and colleagues [55] discussed the relative merits of remodelling and reimplantation. In the remodelling operation the proximal suture line attaches the scalloped graft to the base of the aortic sinuses and the commissures. This approach allows tailoring of each individual sinus and a degree of redundancy to mimic the natural sinuses of Valsalva. This should allow more normal leaflet motion and could result in reduced leaflet closing stress and so enhance long-term durability of the valve [56]. In a review of 44 patients with Marfan's syndrome, who underwent aortic root replacement and 61 patients who received a valve-sparing operation, the valve-sparing procedure resulted in a similar survival, but lower rates of valve-related complications than aortic root replacement [57]. Survival at ten years was 87% in the aortic root replacement group and 96% in the aortic valve-sparing group (p=0.3). Freedom from valve-related mortality and morbidity were 65% after root replacement and 100% after the valve-sparing procedure (p=0.02). Unfortunately, within the valve-sparing group there were at least two different operative techniques. While either type of valve-sparing operation is safe, reproducible, and gives reasonable five to 10-year results for selected Marfan patients, the outcomes are not perfect. As Miller [58] points out, by ten years one quarter of Marfan patients who had a valve-sparing procedure had moderate or severe aortic regurgitation. It would appear from deOliviera's report [57] that the actuarial freedom from AR may be lower if the Yacoub technique is used (71% +/- 21% for remodelling versus 96% +/- 4% for reimplantation at eight years), but the numbers are too small to achieve statistical significance.

What we need to know are the 15-year results of valve-sparing versus composite valve replacement in larger numbers of Marfan patients, and a multicentre registry is being established, sponsored by the Marfan Foundation. In the meantime, it would be wise to remain conservative in the application of the valve-sparing procedure to Marfan patients with careful patient selection.

Percutaneous valve replacement

Percutaneous catheter-based systems for the treatment of valvular heart disease have been studied in animal models for several years. The early experience of emergency balloon valvuloplasty in patients with aortic stenosis and cardiogenic shock was not encouraging, as the risks were high and the relief of the gradient only modest [59]. A recent case report from the same team described implantation of a bioprosthetic heart valve in the aortic position in a terminally ill 57-year old man [60]. The calculated valve area increased from 0.6cm^2 to 1.9 immediately and 1.6 to 1.5cm^2 between one and nine weeks. Left ventricular function remained poor with an ejection fraction of 17%. The patient died from non-cardiac complications at 17 weeks postoperatively. This approach remains interesting, but experimental, requiring further device modifications and a clinical trial.

Conclusions

Most of the evidence which guides our clinical practice in aortic valve surgery is of level III status. Randomised trials are expensive, time-consuming and difficult to run, hence it should be no surprise that only two large randomised trials have been reported. The mortality for elective aortic valve replacement is low at 2-3%, but the long-term survival is far from satisfactory and indeed, is similar to that of patients with three vessel coronary artery disease and impaired ventricular function who are on medical treatment. There is much to be done to improve the outlook for our patients who receive an artificial aortic valve. For bioprosthetic valves, there may be improved methods of tissue preservation while for mechanical valves, a safer alternative to warfarin which does not require monitoring, is being actively sought.

Finally, we need to understand much more about the control of left ventricular hypertrophy at the molecular level, since this is the prime abnormality which interventions on the aortic valve are designed to prevent or reverse.

Recommendations	Evidence level
◆ Ten-year survival rates after valve replacement are similar for mechanical and bioprosthetic valves.	Ia/A
◆ Structural valve degeneration is a feature of biological valves and is related to the age of the patient at implant.	IIa/B
◆ Anticoagulant-related bleeding is more common in mechanical compared to bioprosthetic valves.	Ib/A
◆ The incidence of thromboembolism is higher in patients with a mitral prosthesis than with an aortic prosthesis.	IIa/B
◆ Stentless valves in the aortic position offer better haemodynamics than stented valves in the first two years.	IIb/A
◆ The pulmonary autograft is the only valve substitute that may grow with the patient.	IIb/B
◆ Aortic valve repair remains an innovative procedure with excellent results in carefully selected patients in experienced centres.	III/B

References

1. Ross J, Braunwald E. *Circulation* 1968; 38(Suppl 1): 1-6 - 1-7.
2. Eslami M, Rahimtoola SH. Prophylactic aortic valve replacement in older patients for mild aortic stenosis during coronary bypass surgery. *Am J Geriatr Cardiol* 2003; 12: 197-200.
3. ACC/AHA Guidelines for the management of patients with valvular heart disease. Executive Summary. *J Heart Valve Dis* 1998; 7: 672-707.
4. Otto C. Timing of aortic valve surgery. *Heart* 2000; 84: 211-218.
5. Edmunds LH, Clark RE, Cohn LH, *et al.* Guidelines for reporting morbidity and mortality after cardiac valvular operations. *Ann Thorac Surg* 1996; 62: 932-935.
6. Hammermeister KE, Sethi GK, Henderson WC, *et al.* Outcomes 15 years after valve replacement with a mechanical versus bioprosthetic valve: final report of the Veterans Affairs randomized trial. *J Am Coll Cardiol* 2000; 36: 1152-1158.
7. Bloomfield P, Wheatley DJ, Prescott RJ, *et al.* Twelve-year comparison of a Bjork-Shiley mechanical heart valve with porcine bioprosthesis. *N Engl J Med* 1991; 324: 573-579.
8. Butchart EG, Li HH, Payne N, *et al.* Twenty years experience with the Medtronic-Hall valve. *J Thorac Cardiovasc Surg* 2001; 121: 1090-1100.
9. Peterseim DS, Chen Y-Y, Cheruvu S. Long-term outcome after biological versus mechanical aortic valve replacement in 841 patients. *J Thorac Cardiovasc Surg* 1999; 117: 890-897.
10. Grunkemeier GL, Li HH, Starr A. Heart valve replacement: a statistical review of 35 years results. *J Heart Valve Dis* 1999; 8: 466-471.
11. Orszulak TA, Schaff HV, Puga FJ. Event status of the Starr-Edwards aortic valve to 20 years: a benchmark for comparison. *Ann Thorac Surg* 1997; 63: 620-626.
12. Lindblom D. Long-term clinical results after aortic valve replacement with the Bjork-Shiley prosthesis. *J Thorac Cardiovasc Surg* 1988; 95: 658-667.
13. Lund O, Nielson SL, Arildsen H, *et al.* Standard aortic St. Jude valve at 18 years: performance profile and determinants of outcome. *Ann Thorac Surg* 2000; 69: 1459-1465.
14. Yun KL, Miller DC, Moore KA. Durability of the Hancock MO bioprosthesis compared with the standard aortic valve bioprosthesis. *Ann Thorac Surg* 1995; S221-S228.
15. Jamieson WRE, Burr LH, Munro AI, *et al.* Carpentier-Edwards supra-annular porcine bioprosthesis: clinical performance to twelve years. *Ann Thorac Surg* 1995; 60: S235-S240.
16. Cohn LH, Collins JJ, Rizzo RJ, *et al.* Twenty-year follow-up of the Hancock modified orifice porcine aortic valve. *Ann Thorac Surg* 1998; 66: S30-S34.
17. Frater RWM, Furlong P, Cosgrove DM. Long-term durability and patient functional status of the Carpentier-Edwards Perimount pericardial bioprosthesis in the aortic position. *J Heart Valve Dis* 1998; 7: 48-53.
18. David TE, Ivanor J, Armstrong S, *et al.* Late results of heart valve replacement with the Hancock II bioprosthesis. *J Thorac Cardiovasc Surg* 2001; 121: 268-278.
19. Rahimtoola SH, Frye RL. Valvular heart disease. *Circulation* 2000; 102(Suppl.IV): IV24 - IV33.
20. Murday A, Hochstitzky A, Mansfield J, *et al.* A prospective randomized trial of St. Jude versus Starr-Edwards aortic and mitral valve prostheses. *Ann Thorac Surg* 2003; 76: 66-74.
21. Johnson DM, Sapirstein W. FDA's requirements for *in vivo* performance data for prosthetic heart valves. *J Heart Valve Dis* 1994; 3: 350-355.
22. Grunkemeier GL, Li H-H, Naftel DC, *et al.* Long-term performance of heart valve-prostheses. *Curr Probl Cardiol* 2000; 25: 73-86.
23. Bonow RO, Carabello B, deLeon AC. ACC/AHA guidelines for the management of patients with valvular heart disease. *J Am Coll Cardiol* 1998; 32: 1486-1588.
24. Butchart EG, Payne N, Li H-H *et al.* Better anticoagulation control improves survival after valve replacement. *J Thorac Cardiovasc Surg* 2002; 123: 715-723.
25. Ezekowitz MD, Bridgers SL, Jame KE. Warfarin in the prevention of stroke associated with non-rheumatic atrial fibrillation. *N Engl J Med* 1992; 327: 1406-1412.
26. EAFT Study Group. Secondary prevention in non-rheumatic atrial fibrillation after transient ischaemic attack or minor stroke. *Lancet* 1993; 342: 1255-1262.
27. Stroke Prevention in Atrial Fibrillation Investigators. Adjusted-dose warfarin versus low-intensity, fixed warfarin plus aspirin for high-risk patients with atrial fibrillation: Stroke Prevention in Atrial Fibrillation III randomized clinical trial. *Lancet* 1996; 348: 633-638.
28. Grunkemeier GL, Bodnar E. Comparative assessment of bioprosthesis durability in the aortic position. *J Heart Valve Dis* 1995; 4: 49-55.
29. Westaby S, Horton M, Jin XY, *et al.* Survival advantage of stentless aortic bioprosthesis. *Ann Thorac Surg* 2000; 70: 785-790.
30. David TE, Puschmann R, Ivanov J, *et al.* Aortic valve replacement with stentless and stented porcine valves: a case-match study. *J Thorac Cardiovasc Surg* 1998; 116: 236-241.
31. Ramhimtoola SH. The problem of valve prosthesis-patient mismatch. *Circulation* 1978; 58: 20-24.
32. Pibarot P, Dumesnil JG. Hemodynamic and clinical impact of prosthesis-patient mismatch in the aortic valve position and its prevention. *J Am Coll Cardiol* 2000; 36: 1131-1141.
33. Connolly HM, Oh JK, Schaff HV. Severe aortic stenosis with low transvalvular gradient and severe left ventricular dysfunction: result of aortic valve replacement in 52 patients. *Circulation* 2000; 101: 1940-1946.
34. He GW, Grunkemeier GL, Gately HL, *et al.* Up to thirty-year survival after aortic valve replacement in the small aortic root. *Ann Thorac Surg* 1995; 59: 1056-1062.
35. David TE, Pollick C, Bos J. Aortic valve replacement with stentless porcine aortic bioprosthesis. *J Thorac Cardiovasc Surg* 1990; 99: 113-118.

36. Lund O, Pilegaard HK, Magnussen K, *et al.* Long-term prosthesis-related and sudden cardiac-related complications after aortic valve replacement for aortic stenosis. *Ann Thorac Surg* 1990; 50: 396-406.
37. Lytle BW, Cosgrove DM, Taylor PC, *et al.* Primary isolated aortic valve replacement: early and late results *J Thorac Cardiovasc Surg* 1989; 97: 675-694.
38. Jin XY, Gibson DG, Yacoub MH, *et al.* Perioperative assessment of aortic homograft, Toronto stentless valve and stented valve in the aortic position. *Ann Thorac Surg* 1995; 60: S395-S401.
39. Walther T, Falk V, Autschenbach R, *et al.* Haemodynamic assessment of the stentless Toronto SPV bioprosthesis by echocardiography. *J Heart Valve Dis* 1994; 3: 657-665.
40. Jin XY, Zhong MZ, Gibson DG, *et al.* Effect of valve substitutes on changes in left ventricular function and hypertrophy after aortic valve replacement. *Ann Thorac Surg* 1996; 62: 683-690.
41. Lund O. Valve replacement for aortic stenosis: the curative potential of early operation. *Scand J Thorac Cardiovasc Surg* 1993; 40 (Suppl): 1-137.
42. Michel PL, Mandagout O, Vahanian A, *et al.* Ventricular arrhythmias in aortic valve disease before and after aortic valve replacement. *Acta Cardiol* 1992; 47: 145-156.
43. Bortolotti U, Milano A, Mossuto E, *et al.* The risk of reoperation in patients with bioprosthetic valves. *J Card Surg* 1991; 6(Suppl 4): 638-643.
44. Albertucci M, Wong K, Petrou M, *et al.* The use of unstented homograft valves for aortic valve reoperations: review of a twenty-three-year experience. *J Thorac Cardiovasc Surg* 1994; 107: 152-161.
45. O'Brien MF, Hancock S, Stafford EG. The homograft aortic valve: a 29-year, 99.3% follow-up of 1,022 valve replacements. *J Heart Valve Dis* 2001; 10: 334-344.
46. Elkins RC, Knott-Craig CJ, Ward KE. Pulmonary autograft in children: realized growth potential. *Ann Thorac Surg* 1994; 57: 1387-1392.
47. Ross D. The versatile homograft and autograft valve. *Ann Thorac Surg* 1989; 48: S69-S71.
48. Gerosa G, McKay R, Ross DN. Replacement of the aortic valve with a pulmonary autograft in children. *Ann Thorac Surg* 1991; 51: 424-429.
49. McCusick VA. An association between aortic valve disease and cystic medial necrosis. *Circulation* 1956; 46: 188-190.
50. Schmid FX, Bielenberg K, Schneider A, *et al.* Ascending aortic aneurysm associated with bicuspid and tricuspid aortic valve: involvement and clinical relevance of smooth muscle cell apoptosis and expression of cell death-initiating proteins. *Eur J Cardiothorac Surg* 2003; 23: 537-543.
51. Bentall H, DeBono A. A technique for complete replacement of the ascending aorta. *Thorax* 1968; 23: 338-339.
52. Midulla PS, Ergin MA, Galla J, *et al.* Three faces of the Bentall procedure. *J Card Surg* 1994; 9: 466-481.
53. Gott VI, Greene PS, Alejo DE, *et al.* Replacement of the aortic root in patients with Marfan's syndrome. *N Engl J Med* 1999; 340: 1307-1313.
54. Birks EJ, Webb C, Child A, *et al.* Early and long-term results of a valve-sparing operation for Marfan syndrome. *Circulation* 1999; 100 (Suppl II): II-29 - II-35.
55. Schafers H-J, Fries R, Langer F, *et al.* Valve-preserving replacement of the ascending aorta: remodelling versus reimplantation. *J Thorac Cardiovasc Surg* 1998; 116: 990-996.
56. Leyh RG, Schmidtke C, Sievers H-H, *et al.* Opening and closing characteristics of the aortic valve after different types of valve-preserving surgery. *Circulation* 1999; 100: 2153-2160.
57. DeOliveira NC, David TE, Ivanov J, *et al.* Results of surgery for aortic root aneurysm in patients with Marfan syndrome. *J Thorac Cardiovasc Surg* 2003; 125: 789-796.
58. Miller DC. Valve-sparing aortic root replacement in patients with the Marfan syndrome. *J Thorac Cardiovasc Surg* 2003; 125: 773-778.
59. Cribier A, Remadi F, Koning R. Emergency balloon valvuloplasty as initial treatment of patients with aortic stenosis and cardiogenic shock. *N Engl J Med* 1992; 323: 646.
60. Cribier A, Eltchaninoff H, Bash A, *et al.* Percutaneous transcatheter implantation of an aortic valve prosthesis for calcific aortic stenosis. *Circulation* 2002; 106: 3006-3008.

Chapter 21

Surgery for mitral regurgitation

Richard C Daly MD
Consultant in Cardiac Surgery &
Director of Cardiac and Pulmonary Transplantation

Mayo Clinic, Rochester, MN, USA

Introduction

The pathology and mechanism of mitral regurgitation has changed considerably over time. "Floppy" or myxomatous mitral valve disease has now become the predominant pathology in the western world (Figure 1) [1] although rheumatic disease remains an important cause worldwide. The leaflet prolapse and chordal rupture associated with this disease is more amenable to repair than inflammatory (primarily rheumatic) disease. As a result of the changing pathology much of the debate around surgical treatment of mitral regurgitation revolves around the relative merits of repair versus replacement and the timing of surgery.

The timing and indications for surgical intervention on the mitral valve have evolved with:-

- better understanding of the natural history of mitral insufficiency and the benefits of surgical treatment;
- the ability to predict whether mitral disease is repairable;
- the development of reliable techniques to repair mitral insufficiency; and
- improving techniques and outcome with reparative valve surgery.

Ultimately, the likelihood that mitral insufficiency can be repaired depends on the pathology and mechanism of the mitral regurgitation, as well as the experience and training of the surgeon.

Natural history of mitral insufficiency

Mitral regurgitation (MR) is not a benign condition. The volume overload that results from MR clearly causes progressive deterioration in left ventricular function and the effects can be irreversible even in the asymptomatic patient.

Widely disparate estimates of long-term survival have been reported [2]. Data from the Mayo Clinic indicate that only 57% of patients with flail mitral leaflets will survive ten years, which is significantly reduced from expected survival (Figure 2) [3].

Furthermore, asymptomatic patients with severe MR due to flail leaflets will become symptomatic at a rate of 10.3% per year. This is associated with an annual mortality of 6.3%, and sudden death at a rate of 1.8% per year [3,4].

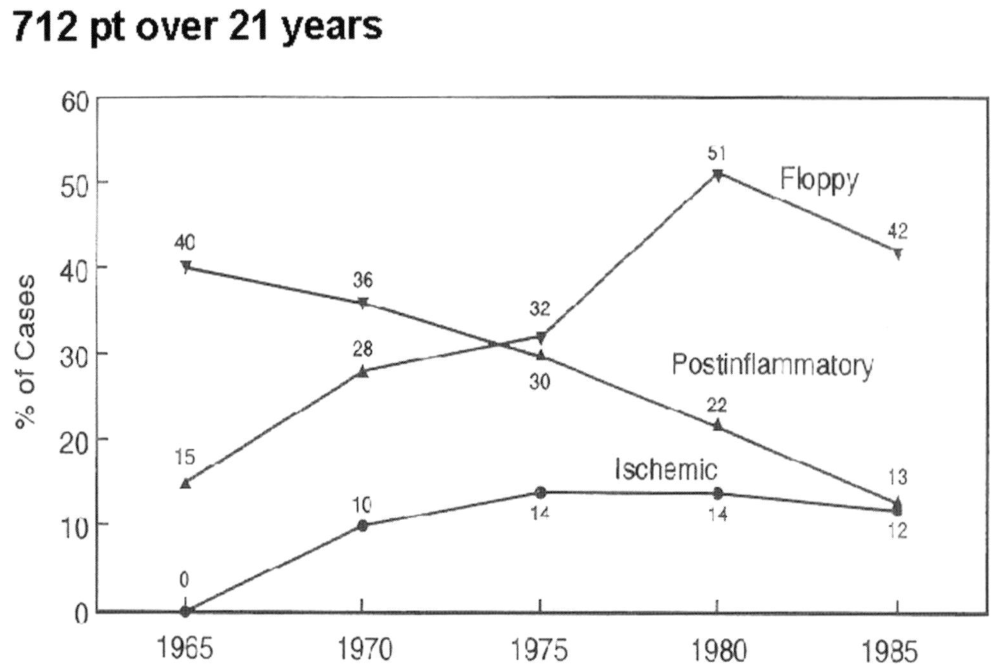

Figure 1. The pathology and mechanism of mitral regurgitation in patients undergoing surgery at the Mayo Clinic has changed considerably over time [1].

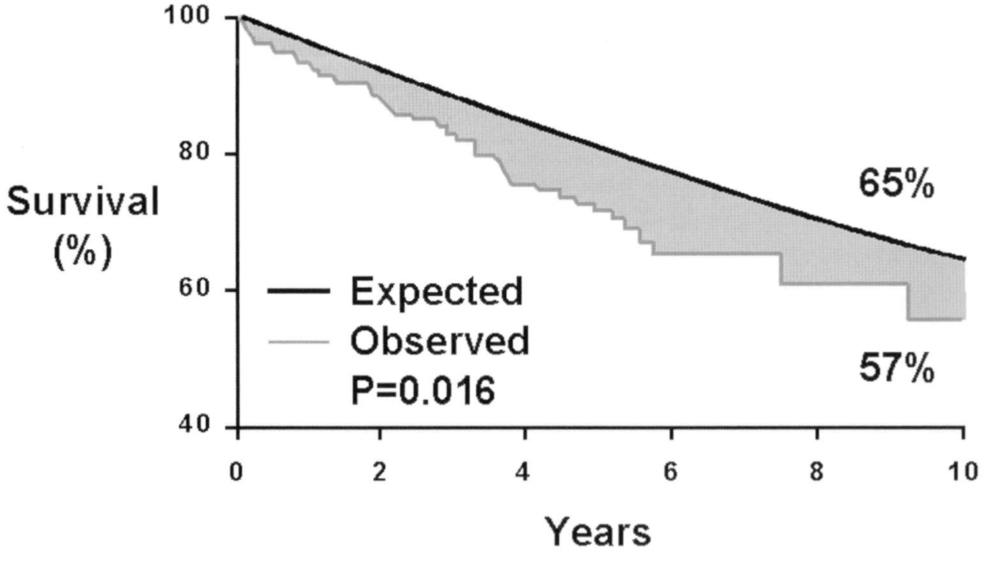

Figure 2. Survival with severe mitral regurgitation due to flail mitral leaflets is significantly reduced from expected survival [3].

These rates are increased in patients with symptoms or reduced ejection fraction.

More specifically, predictors of poor outcome include severe symptoms [3], reduced ejection fraction [3], pulmonary hypertension, and increased LV end-diastolic volume [5]. Patients with class I or II symptoms have a yearly mortality of 4.1%, but once a patient develops NYHA class III or IV symptoms, even if transient, the yearly mortality rises to 34% [3].

MR can also result in increased morbidity over time. Among patients who are asymptomatic, 10% per year will develop symptoms, and symptoms develop more rapidly with atrial fibrillation [8]. In patients with flail leaflets followed for ten years, 30% will develop atrial fibrillation and 63% will develop heart failure [3].

Timing of surgery

The LV volume overload due to MR is corrected by surgery, but underlying LV dysfunction is not reversible. Late survival is reduced if LV dysfunction is allowed to develop pre-operatively. Figure 3 shows that late survival after repair of MR is reduced once pre-operative LV ejection fraction falls below 60%, and survival falls further if pre-operative LV ejection fraction is below 50% [3,9].

More severe pre-operative symptoms correlate with a lower postoperative ejection fraction and a higher incidence of late congestive heart failure [7]. Persistent LV dysfunction is the major cause of late mortality after surgery [7]. Among patients with preserved LV function, late survival is similar to expected survival if MR is corrected prior to development of advanced symptoms (Figure 4) [3].

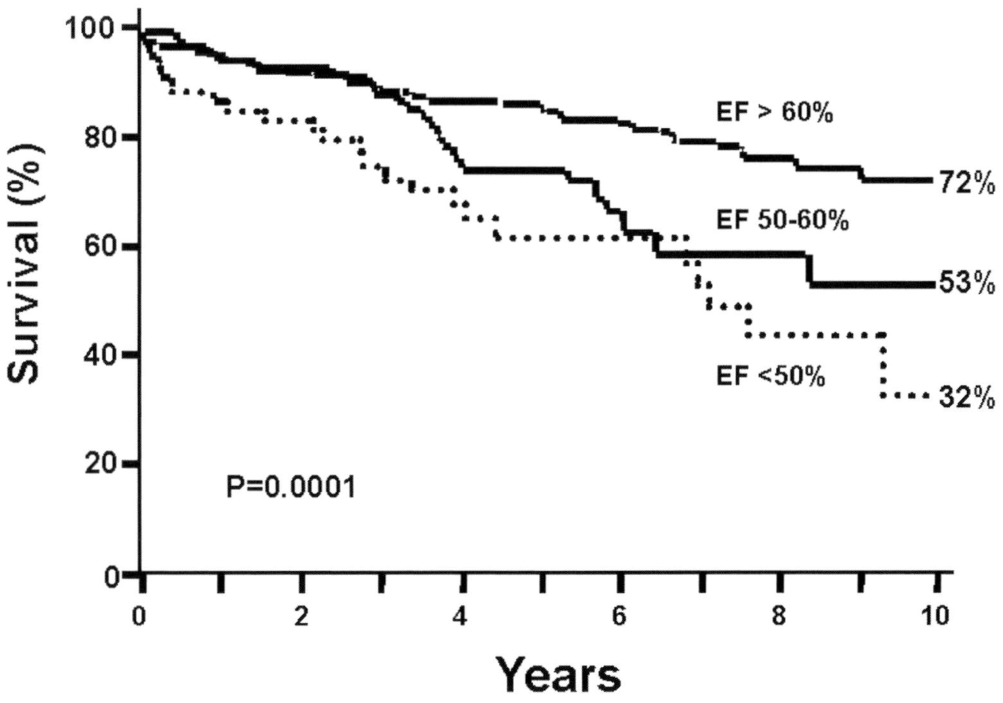

Figure 3. Late survival after repair of MR is dependent on pre-operative LV ejection fraction [3].

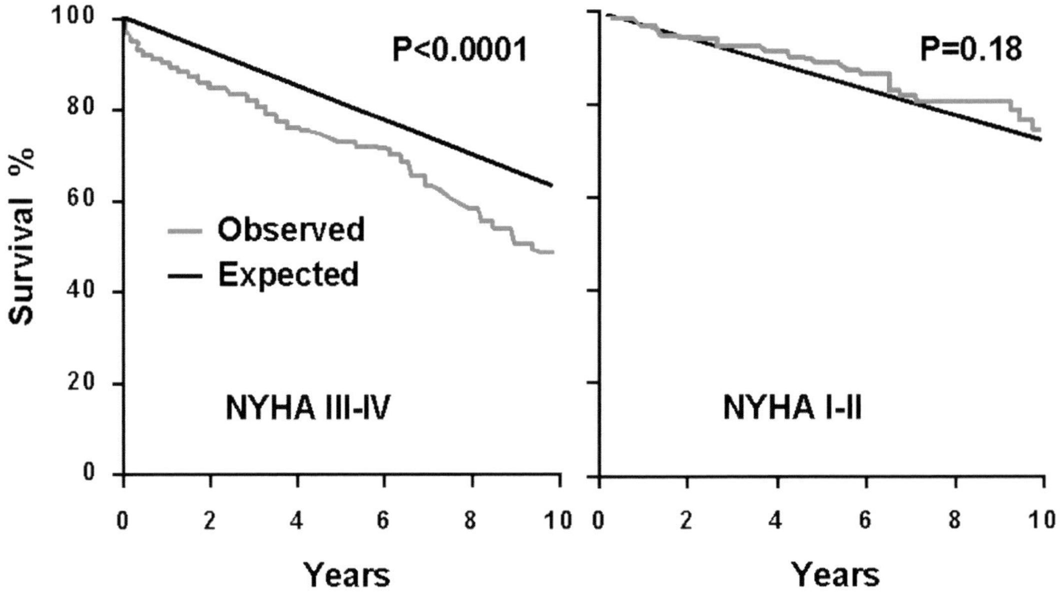

Figure 4. **Among patients with preserved LV function, late survival is similar to expected survival if MR is corrected [3].**

Myxomatous mitral valve disease is the most common aetiology of MR in patients requiring surgery. The vast majority of these valves are repairable and this is generally predictable from the pre-operative echocardiogram. Prolapse or flail segments of the posterior leaflet is present in about two thirds of patients with myxomatous disease, isolated anterior leaflet prolapse in 10% and bileaflet prolapse in about 20% [11].

The operative mortality for surgical correction, especially with valve replacement has been high in the past and led to a conservative approach to MR for many years. Operative mortality for ischaemic MR remains high enough that surgery is generally not recommended for asymptomatic patients. Operative mortality for the surgical repair of organic MR at the Mayo Clinic has been low. In a review of 898 patients undergoing mitral valve repair from 1994 to 1998, overall mortality was 1.2%. However, mortality was zero for patients who were class I or II pre-operatively. Among patients of all functional classes less than 75 years old, mortality was 0.4% and was zero in about 450 patients in the last three years of the review [10].

Techniques for mitral valve repair

Inspection of the valve

Repair is not possible without a good understanding of the mechanism of MR in each case. We expose the MV through an incision parallel to the interatrial groove. In some cases with small left atria, or rightward displacement of the heart, alternate approaches may be necessary (eg. trans-septal, T-incisions in the right atrium and septum, dome of the left atrium, division of the superior vena cava) [12-19]. The annulus, leaflets, chordae and papillary muscles are carefully inspected. If the cause of the MR is not apparent, saline is injected into the LV with a bulb syringe. The same maneuver is used to test the repair at the end of the procedure [10].

Repair of the valve

Severe MR resulting from chordal elongation (resulting in leaflet prolapse) or chordal rupture (resulting in flail segment of leaflets) can be repaired by plicating or resecting the involved portion of the posterior leaflet. The anterior leaflet requires a more complex approach.

Plication of flail segments of the posterior leaflet was described by McGoon in 1960 [20]. Leaflet resection is necessary when large sections of the posterior leaflet prolapse or are flail. Quandrangular resection, or removal of a rectangular segment of the posterior leaflet has been advocated by some authors [21]. We prefer a triangular resection of the posterior leaflet. The triangular technique results in no resected tissue at the annular portion of the leaflet and is easily reconstructed by approximating the cut edges with a simple running suture from the annulus to the coapting edge. We use two layers of 4-0 polypropylene.

Resection of a significant portion of the anterior leaflet is not usually possible. The anterior leaflet is positioned between the fibrous trigones of the heart, and excess tension in the repair or excessive reduction in the area of the leaflet will result if much of the leaflet is excised. Occasionally, resection of a small portion of the anterior leaflet is possible, and a triangular approach is used. Larger areas of prolapse involving the anterior leaflet require chordal repair techniques.

Leaflet perforation (usually from infective endocarditis) can be repaired with an autologous pericardial patch.

Prolapse or flail segments of the anterior leaflet generally cannot be excised and elimination of the MR requires re-supporting the leaflet. This is also required on occasion for the posterior leaflet when a very large portion of this leaflet has prolapsed or is flail. Chordal repair methods include chordal shortening, chordal transfer and artificial chordal implantation.

Chordal shortening involves retracting a portion of the chord into an incision made in the papillary muscle [22]. The chord is pulled into the papillary muscle incision and secured with a suture. In our opinion, this technique has the disadvantage of relying on a chord that is often thin and tenuous. Also, the suture securing the chord into the papillary muscle may erode the chord.

Cordal transposition has been described [22,23]. This technique involves moving a small segment of posterior leaflet with normal supporting chordae to the leaflet area needing support, usually to an area of the anterior leaflet. The defect in the posterior leaflet is repaired primarily. It is sometimes possible to use secondary chordae (not on the coapting edge) from the posterior leaflet when a large segment of the posterior leaflet prolapses or is flail. These secondary chordae, which are adjacent to the resected segment of the posterior leaflet, are moved (with a small portion of leaflet tissue) to the coapting edge where the leaflet has been repaired. This reduces the size of the resected portion of the posterior leaflet and is useful if there is prolapse of an entire, large middle scallop. The advantage of chordal transposition is that chordal length does not have to be adjusted by the surgeon; a chord of normal length for the valve is used.

Artificial chordae can be constructed from a PTFE suture [11, 24]. A 4-0 PTFE suture is passed through the fibrotic area at the head of a papillary muscle in a mattress fashion. Felt pledgets have been described for supporting the suture at the papillary muscle, but are probably not necessary if the suture is placed through the fibrotic head of the muscle and not through the soft body of the papillary muscle. The suture is not usually tied on the papillary muscle; if it is tied, an "air knot" should be used to avoid the possibility of strangling the blood supply to the tip of the muscle. The two ends of the suture are then each passed twice through the coapting edge of the region of the leaflet to be supported. Passing the suture through the leaflet twice provides resistance to slippage while the length of the artificial chord is tested. The chord length is tested by filling the LV with saline from a bulb syringe, and can be re-adjusted until the length is correct and the leaflet is held just at the plane of the annulus. The knot is tied, taking care not to allow the knot to slip and over shorten the chord (again, the resistance provided by passing the sutures through the leaflet twice assists with this knot). The common tendency is to make the artificial chords too short.

Annuloplasty is routinely performed with leaflet repair to correct the annular dilatation associated with severe MR, and to support the repair.

Annuloplasty

The volume overload of severe MR eventually results in LV and annular dilatation. The mitral annulus adjacent to the anterior leaflet lies between the fibrous trigones of the heart and is part of the fibrous continuity between the mitral and aortic valves. This anterior portion of the annulus is not prone to stretching or dilatation. The annulus adjacent to the posterior leaflet lies along the wall of the LV and can become dilated. Dilatation of the posterior mitral annulus may be isolated and related to the nature of the underlying connective tissue that results in myxomatous changes in the mitral leaflets, or related to dilatation of the LV. Ventricular dilatation as a result of ischaemic disease, dilated cardiomyopathy, the volume overload of severe MR or other aetiologies may all cause annular dilatation.

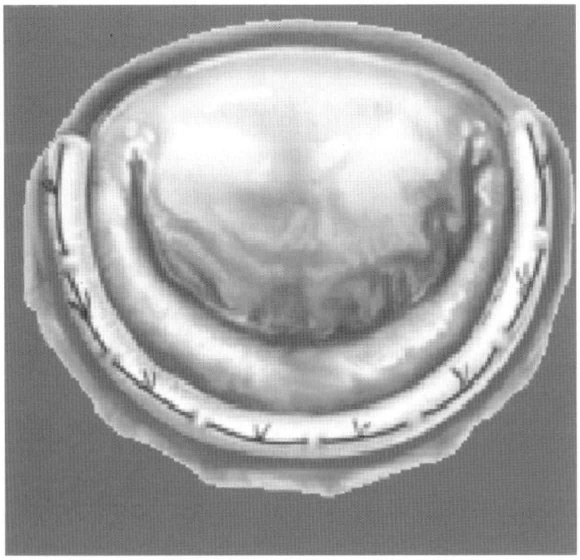

Figure 5. Posterior mitral annuloplasty with an unmeasured partial ring. The ring is anchored in the fibrous trigones above each commissure. The anterior annulus is fixed in size and is 30 to 35% of the total annular circumference. The posterior annulus is 65 to 70% of the circumference. The "partial ring" or band measures 6.3cm [29].

When annular dilatation is sufficient to interfere with leaflet coaptation the MR ensues even with normal leaflets and existing MR from other causes becomes worse.

Annuloplasty is an important component of every mitral repair. Annuloplasty reduces the size of the mitral annulus and improves leaflet coaptation. It also compensates for the decrease in leaflet area following resection. Improved leaflet coaptation reduces the strain on leaflet repairs. MR due to isolated annular dilatation and some cases of anterior leaflet prolapse are adequately treated with annuloplasty alone.

Early annuloplasty techniques such as the Kay and Reed procedures involved plication of the annulus at the commissures [25,26]. In 1971, Carpentier described symmetric reduction of the annulus using a measured, rigid annuloplasty ring which spread out the suture tension evenly along the posterior annulus [22]. Subsequently, Duran described a flexible ring that allows dynamic movement of the annulus through the cardiac cycle [27,28].

Orszulak and Schaff at the Mayo Clinic, and others elsewhere, modified the annuloplasty ring concept further by using a partial ring or band that reduces only the size of the posterior annulus [29]. This has several theoretical and practical advantages. First, sutures are only placed in the posterior annulus, so exposure of the anterior annulus is not necessary. Second, the risk of suture injury to the anterior leaflet, aortic valve and conduction tissue is reduced. Third, a single, standard partial ring size is suitable for most patients, which eliminates the need to measure the size of the annulus. Use of a posterior partial ring has reduced cross-clamp and cardiopulmonary bypass time by 25% compared to a complete ring in our practice [29].

We have used a standard 6.3cm band as an "unmeasured" partial ring in most patients (Figure 5).

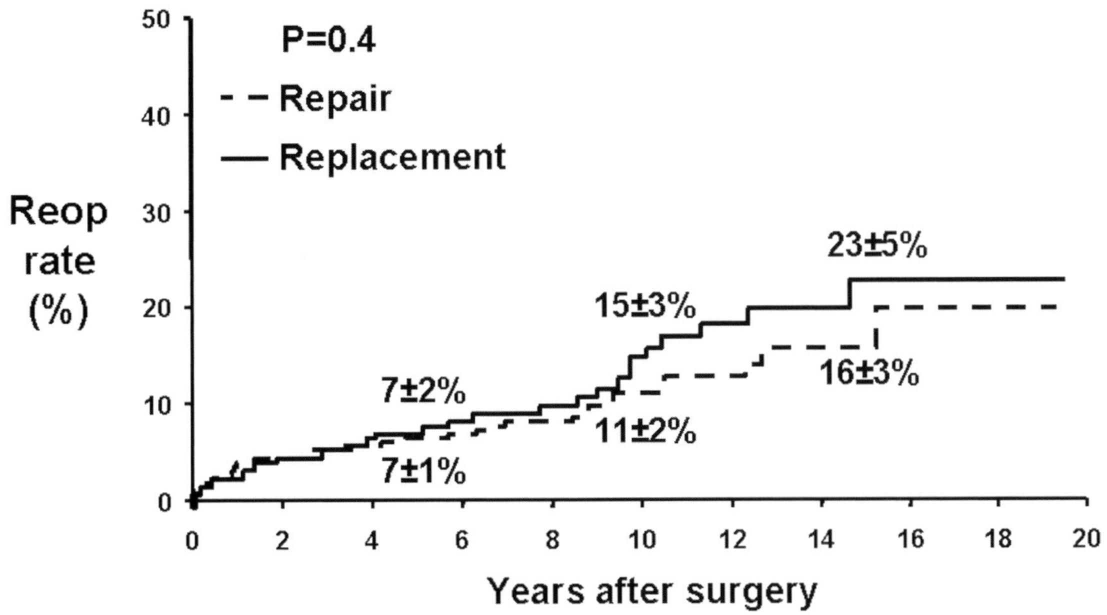

Figure 6. Rate of re-operation is not different for mitral repair and replacement [30].

The geometric justification for this size are:-

- The normal mitral annulus is about 10cm in diameter.
- The anterior annulus is fixed in size.
- The anterior annulus is 30 to 35% of the total annular circumference and the posterior annulus is 65 to 70%.
- Small differences in the size of a partial ring used to reduce the posterior annulus will have a minimal effect on the final valve orifice area. Reduction in MR, valve area, and gradients are similar between complete ring, partial ring and commissural plication techniques [29].

Annuloplasty with a partial ring is performed by placing permanent, braided horizontal mattress sutures along the posterior annulus and then through the partial ring. The sutures on each end are anchored in the fibrous trigones. The fibrous trigones are located just anterior to the lateral and medial commissures, and are usually identifiable by a dimple in the annulus. The partial ring is lowered to the annulus and the sutures are tied just tight enough to avoid kinking of the partial ring.

Results

Operative mortality is low for mitral repair. In 898 patients at our institution, overall mortality was 1.2%. Mortality was zero in all patients in functional class I or II, and was also zero in patients less than 75 years old in all functional classes [10]. Compared to mitral valve replacement, mitral valve repair has a lower operative mortality, improved long-term survival, improved late ventricular function, and lower rates of thrombo-emboli, anticoagulant-related complications and endocarditis [2].

In terms of durability, there was no statistically significant difference in rate of re-operation between mitral repair and replacement [10, 30] (Figure 6). In a review of 917 patients operated on at the Mayo Clinic from 1980 to 1995, isolated posterior leaflet repair has a very low re-operation rate of 11% at 15 years

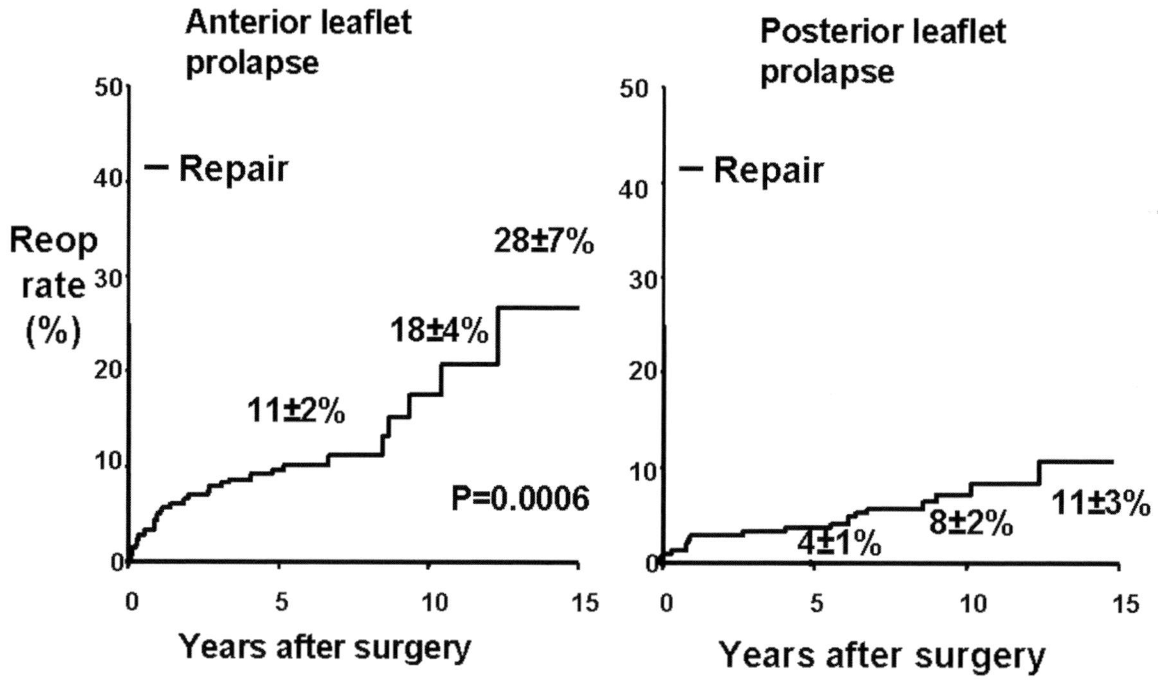

Figure 7. In a review of 917 patients operated on at the Mayo Clinic, posterior leaflet repair has a lower re-operation rate than that for anterior leaflet repair (p=0.0006) [30].

and is significantly lower (p=0.0006) than that for anterior leaflet repair, 28% at 15 years [30] (Figure 7). These rates compare favourably to the rate of re-operation for mitral valve replacement, which has a 15-year re-operation rate of 21% and 24%, respectively, for posterior and anterior leaflet prolapse at the time of valve replacement [30]. Although patients with mechanical prostheses underwent fewer instances of re-operation than did those with bioprostheses (p=0.002), they had re-operation rates similar to those with repair (at ten years, 9% vs 11%).

The presence of residual, intra-operative mild, or mild to moderate MR by transoesophageal echocardiography after mitral valve repair, is associated with a higher incidence of late re-operation when compared to no residual MR. In 669 patients reviewed, 122 had residual MR after repair (mild or mild to moderate). The re-operation rates at five, ten and 15 years were 14%, 18% and 21%, respectively, with residual MR, and 5%, 9% and 14%, respectively, with no residual MR [30].

We reviewed the outcome of anterior leaflet repair in 334 patients with anterior or bileaflet prolapse undergoing mitral valve repair from 1988 to 1996. One third were repaired with annuloplasty alone. Chordal shortening was performed in 46 patients and artificial chordae were placed in 75 patients. The remaining patients had anterior leaflet plication or other procedures. Chordal replacement had a significantly lower incidence of re-operation at mean follow-up of 3.5 years compared to chordal shortening (1.4% vs 14.8%, p=0.025) [11]. Others have had similar results [23, 24] (Table 1).

Postoperative LV dysfunction is associated with poorer survival [6]. Postoperative congestive heart failure is associated with a 5-fold increase in late mortality [7].

Table 1. Incidence of re-operation after surgical repair of mitral regurgitation with anterior leaflet prolapse.

	Follow-up (years)	Chordal shortening	Chordal transfer	Chordal replacement
Mayo Clinic (11)	3.5	14.8%	-	1.4%
Cleveland Clinic (23)	5	26%	4%	-
Toronto (24)	5	-	-	4%

Mitral valve replacement and the subvalvular apparatus

While this chapter has focused on repair of the mitral valve, replacement is necessary in many situations. A point to emphasize at the time of mitral valve replacement (MVR) is the importance of preservation of the chordae tendonae and their attachments to the papillary muscles. In 1964, Lillehei reported a reduction in operative mortality for MVR from 37% to 14% when the chordae tendonae and papillary muscle attachments to the posterior leaflet were preserved [31]. In a non-randomised comparison of 68 patients who had mitral valve repair, MVR with complete chordal preservation, and conventional MVR, the chordal preservation and repair groups had improved ventricular size and ejection fraction both early and late [32]. In a randomised, prospective trial of 100 patients undergoing MVR with or without posterior chordal preservation, the group with preserved posterior chordae had lower LV volume, improved exercise tolerance, fewer thromboemboli, and improved late survival (92% vs 80% at six years) [33].

Preservation of the posterior leaflet and attached chordae is generally straightforward. The leaflet is plicated between the annulus and the sewing ring of the prosthesis with the valve sutures. Preservation of the anterior leaflet may be more problematic, especially if the anterior leaflet is thickened or calcified. Rheumatic and other inflammatory processes may result in severe leaflet thickening as well as subvalvular disease, and resection of the anterior leaflet may be unavoidable. In some cases, resection of the midportion of one or both leaflets, with preservation of the chordal attachments at the lateral aspect of the leaflet(s) will be possible. When chordal preservation is not feasible placement of artificial chordae to suspend the papillary muscles and support the LV has been described [34].

Mitral valve replacement with homografts has been studied and performed clinically to limited extent. This technique allows support of the LV by the homograft tissue. However, technical issues, size matching, and preservation are persistent challenges [35, 36].

Conclusions

Understanding of the natural history of mitral insufficiency has improved as success with valve repair has evolved. Untreated patients with severe MR due to flail leaflets have significant morbidity and mortality over time even with minimal symptoms. Delaying surgical intervention until the development of severe symptoms, atrial fibrillation, or reduced LV function only results in a high incidence of late complications and poor late survival. Mitral valve repair has a low operative mortality and good durability. Techniques are available to repair anterior and posterior leaflet prolapse. We have simplified annuloplasty to a single, unmeasured, posterior, partial ring.

Early surgical repair of severe MR, even in asymptomatic patients is appropriate if the following conditions exist [10]:-

- Low predicted operative risk.
- Echocardiographic demonstration of a "repairable" valve.
- Severe MR with criteria:
  - Regurgitant volume ≥60ml/beat.
  - Regurgitant fraction ≥50%.
  - Effective regurgitant orifice ≥40mm^2.
- Availability of intra-operative echocardiography performed by an experienced physician.

Late outcome is less favourable when symptoms and signs of LV dysfunction develop; however, surgical outcome remains superior to medical management in these patients.

Thus, delaying intervention until the development of severe symptoms, reduced LV function or atrial fibrillation places the patient at high risk of mortality and morbidity as well as higher peri-operative risk. Furthermore, even with surgery, late survival is reduced.

Traditional indications for surgery had been based on the patients' symptoms. Understanding the natural history as well as the influence of surgical repair on MR has led to recommendation for early surgery provided operative mortality is low and repair is likely.

Thus, early surgery for organic MR is strongly recommended, and should be offered to asymptomatic patients with minimal comorbid conditions. Reparability can generally be predicted pre-operatively. Operative mortality is very low, progressive LV dysfunction and congestive heart failure are prevented, and late survival is improved and is similar to expected survival.

Recommendations	Evidence level
• Early repair of mitral regurgitation prior to symptoms, deterioration in LV function or the onset of atrial fibrillation reduces operative risk and improves long-term survival following surgery.	III/B
• Annuloplasty is an important component of surgical repair of mitral regurgitation. In many cases of anterior leaflet prolapse, anterior annuloplasty is sufficient to eliminate the mitral regurgitation.	III/B
• Chordal transposition and chordal replacement have superior long-term durability compared to chordal shortening.	III/B
• Operative mortality for surgical repair of mitral regurgitation is low and is near zero for patients with funcitonal class I or II, or in patients less than 75 years old without significant comorbidity.	III/B
• Compared to mitral valve replacement, mitral valve repair has a lower operative mortality, improved long-term survival, improved late ventricular function, and lower rates of thromboemboli, anticoagulant-related complications, and endocarditis.	III/B
• Late re-operation rates after surgical repair of mitral regurgitation is lower following repair of posterior leaflet prolapse rather than anterior leaflet, and is comparable to that following mitral valve replacement.	III/B
• Preservation of the subvalvular apparatus at the time of mitral valve replacement reduces late morbidity and improves long-term survival.	Ib/A

References

1. Olson LJ, Subramanian R, Ackermann DM, Orszulak TA, Edwards WD. Surgical pathology of the mitral valve: a study of 712 cases spanning 21 years. *Mayo Clin Proc* 1987; 62: 22-34.
2. Enriquez-Sarano M, Orszulak TA, Schaff HV, Abel MD, Tajik AJ, Frye RL. Mitral regurgitation: a new clinical perspective. *Mayo Clin Proc* 1997; 72(11): 1034-1043.
3. Ling LH, Enriquez-Sarano M, Seward JB, Tajik AJ, Schaff HV, Bailey KR, *et al.* Clinical outcome of mitral regurgitation due to flail leaflet. *N Engl J Med* 1996; 335: 1417-1423.
4. Grigioni F, Sarano ME, Ling HL, Bailey KR, Tajik AJ. Sudden death in mitral regurgitation due to flail leaflets: when is it unexpected? *European Heart Journal* 1999 Aug; 20 (ABSTR. Suppl): 599.
5. Hammermeister K, Fisher L, Kennedy W, *et al.* Prediction of late survival in patients with mitral valve disease from clinical, hemodynamic and quantitative angiographic variables. *Circulation* 1978; 57: 341-349.
6. Enriquez-Sarano M, Tajik AJ, Schaff HV, Orszulak TA, McGoon MD, Bailey KR, *et al.* Echocardiographic prediction of left ventricular function after correction of mitral regurgitation: results and clinical implications. *J Am Coll Cardiol* 1994; 24: 1536-1543.
7. Enriquez-Sarano M, Schaff HV, Orszulak TA, Bailey KR, Tajik AJ, Frye RL. Congestive heart failure after surgical correction of mitral regurgitation: a long-term study. *Circulation* 1995; 92: 2496-2503.
8. Rosen SE, Borer JS, Hochreiter C, Supino P, Roman MJ, Devereux RB, *et al.* Natural history of the asymptomatic/minimally symptomatic patient with severe mitral regurgitation secondary to mitral valve prolapse and normal right and left ventricular performance. *Am J Cardiol* 1994; 74: 374-380.
9. Enriquez-Sarano M, Tajik AJ, Schaff HV, Orszulak TA, Bailey KR, Frye RL. Echocardiographic prediction of survival after surgical correction of organic mitral regurgitation. *Circulation* 1994; 90: 830-837.
10. Secombe, JF, Schaff HV. Mitral Valve Repair: Current Techniques and indications. In: *Advanced Therapy in Cardiac Surgery.* Franco KL, Verrire ED, Eds. BC Decker Inc., Hamilton, 1999; 220-231.
11. Phillips MR, Daly RC, Schaff HV, Dearani JA, Mullany CJ, Orszulak TA. Repair of anterior leaflet mitral valve prolapse: chordal replacement versus chordal shortening. *Ann of Thorac Surg* 2000; 69(1): 25-9.
12. Balasundaram SG, Duran C. Surgical approaches to the mitral valve. *J Cardiac Surg* 1990; 5: 163-9.
13. Brawley RK. Improved exposure of the mitral valve in patients with a small left atrium. *Ann Thorac Surg* 1980; 29: 179-81.
14. Meyer Bw Verska JJ, Lindesmith GG, Jones JC. Open repair of mitral valve lesions - the superior approach. *Ann Thorac Surg* 1965; 1: 453-7.
15. Selle JG. Temporary division of the superior vena cava for exceptional mitral valve exposure. *J Thorac Cardiovasc Surg* 1984; 88: 302-4.
16. Bowman FO Jr, Malm JR. The transeptal approach to the mitral valve. *Arch Surg* 1965; 90: 329-31.
17. Dubost C, Guilmet D, Parades B, Pedeferri G. Nouvelle Technique d'ouverture de l'oritellette gauche en chirugie a couer ouvert: l'abord bi-auriculaire transeptal. *Presse Med* 1996; 74: 1607-10.
18. Guiraudon GM, Ofiesh JG, Kaushik R. Extended vertical transatrial septal approach to the mitral valve. *Ann Thorac Surg* 1991; 52: 1058-62.
19. Couetil PA, Ramsheyi A, Tolan MJ, *et al.* Biatrial inferior transeptal approach to the mitral valve. *Ann Thorac Surg* 1995; 60: 1432-3.
20. McGoon DC. Repair of mitral insufficiency due to ruptured chordae tendineae. *J Thorac Cardiovasc Surg* 1960; 39: 357-362.
21. Carpentier A. Cardiac valve surgery - The "French correction." *J Thorac Cardiovasc Surg* 1983; 86: 323-37.
22. Carpentier A, Deloche A, Dauptain J, Soyer R, Blondeau P, Piwnica A, *et al.* A new reconstructive operation for correction of mitral and tricuspid insufficiency. *J Thorac Cardiovasc Surg* 1971; 61: 1-13.
23. Smedira N, Selman R, Cosgrove D, *et al.* Repair of anterior leaflet prolapse. *J Thorac Cardiovasc Surg* 1996; 112: 287-291.
24. David TE, Omran A, Armstrong S, *et al.* Long-term results of mitral valve repair for myxomatous disease with and without chordal replacement with expanded polytetrafluoroethylene sutures. *J Thorac Cardiovasc Surg* 1998; 115: 1279-85.
25. Kay JH, Egerton WS, Zubiate P. The surgical treatment of mitral insufficiency with the use of the heart-lung machine. *Surgery* 1961; 50: 67.
26. Reed GE, Tice DA, Clauss RH. Asymmetric exaggerated mitral annuloplasty: repair of mitral insufficiency. *J Thorac Cardiovasc Surg* 1965; 49: 752.
27. Duran CM, Pomar JL, Cucchiara G. A flexible ring for atrioventricular heart valve reconstruction. *J Cardiovasc Surg* 1978; 19: 417-20.
28. Duran C, Ubago JL. Cinical and hemodynamic performance of a totally flexible prosthetic ring for atrioventricular valve reconstruction. *Ann Thorac Surg* 1976; 22: 458-63.
29. Odell JA, Schaff HV, Orszulak TA. Early results of a simplified method of mitral valve annuloplasty. *Circulation* 1995 Nov 1; 92(9 Suppl): II150-4.
30. Mohty D, Orszulak TA, Schaff HV, Avierinos JF, Tajik JA, Enriquez-Sarano M. Very long-term survival and durability of mitral valve repair for mitral valve prolapse. *Circulation* 2001 Sep 18; 104(12 Suppl): I-1-I-7
31. Lillehei CW, Levy MJ, Bonnabeau RC. Mitral valve replacement with preservation of the papillary muscles and chordae tendonae. *J Thorac Cardiovasc Surg* 1964; 47: 532-543.
32. Okita Y, Miki S, Ueda Y, Tahata T, Sakai T, Matsuyama K. Comparative evaluation of left ventricular performance after mitral valve repair or valve replacement with or without chordal preservation. *J Heart Valve Dis* 1993; 2: 159-166.

33. Horstkotte D, Schulte HD, Bircks W, Strauer BE. The effect of chordal preservation on late outcome after mitral valve replacement: a randomized study. *J Heart Valve Dis* 1993; 2: 150-158.
34. Reardon MJ, David TE. Mitral valve replacement with preservation of the subvalvular apparatus. *Curr Opin Cardiol* 1998; 14: 104-110.
35. Acar C, Farge A, Ramsheyi A, *et al.* Mitral valve replacement using a cryopreserved mitral homograft. *Ann Thorac Surg* 1994; 57: 746-748.
36. Duran CMG. Editorial: mitral valve allografts. An opportunity. *J Heart Valve Dis* 1995; 4: 29-30.

Chapter 22

Anticoagulation in cardiac disease

Kiat T Tan MRCP
Research Fellow, Cardiovascular Medicine
Gregory YH Lip MD FRCP
Professor of Cardiovascular Medicine

HAEMOSTASIS, THROMBOSIS AND VASCULAR BIOLOGY UNIT,
UNIVERSITY DEPARTMENT OF MEDICINE, CITY HOSPITAL, BIRMINGHAM, UK

Introduction

One of the greatest developments in cardiovascular medicine in the past century has been the discovery of antithrombotic agents. The use of the various antiplatelet agents, anticoagulants, and thrombolytic agents have saved millions of lives each year and improved the quality of life of many others.

Unfortunately, as many of these drugs were discovered before the advent of randomised controlled trials (RCT), evidence is often lacking for the use of many of these agents in adult practice, at least until recently. Indications for anticoagulation in childhood are even less clear, with virtually no RCT data on this controversial topic.

Currently, most of our guidance for the anticoagulation of patients with cardiac disease is derived from guidelines published by the American College of Cardiologists (ACC), the American Heart Association (AHA), the European Society of Cardiologists (ESC), and the American College of Chest Physicians (ACCP).

Methodology

We combined a manual search of the literature mentioned above with a Medline search using the following search terms: "anticoagulation"; "warfarin"; "heparin"; and "atrial fibrillation", and the following terms for pathology "mitral valve", "pulmonary hypertension"; "prosthetic valve"; "percutaneous coronary intervention", etc. We then combined the search terms for anticoagulation with that of pathology, eg. ("anticoagulation" or "warfarin" or "heparin") and mitral valve.

Indications for anticoagulation in cardiac disease

The various cardiac conditions for which anticoagulation has been used are summarized in alphabetical order in Table 1. Some of these conditions will be discussed in further detail in this chapter.

Table 1. Cardiac indications for anticoagulation.

Condition	Drug used	Comments
Atrial fibrillation	Warfarin	Effective in reducing thromboembolic events
Coronary heart disease (acute)	(1) Heparin* (2) Hirudin ** (3) Fondaparinux***	* Major benefits on mortality and morbidity ** Benefits on mortality and morbidity *** May be effective in acute coronary syndrome Further data awaited
Coronary angioplasty/ stenting	Heparin	Shown to improve procedural outcome
Coronary artery bypass grafting (vein grafts)	Warfarin	Benefits unclear
Infective endocarditis - associated thromboembolism	Warfarin and heparin	May be beneficial BUT substantial risk of intracranial haemorrhage
Mitral annular calcification	Warfarin	Beneficial in those with documented arterial thromboembolism and/or atrial fibrillation
Mitral regurgitation (non-rheumatic)	Warfarin	Beneficial in those with documented arterial thromboembolism and/or atrial fibrillation
Mitral regurgitation (rheumatic)	Warfarin	(1) Beneficial in those with documented arterial thromboembolism and/or atrial fibrillation (2) Probably beneficial in those with other associated risk factors for thromboembolism (eg. the elderly, atrial size (>5.5cm), and severe lesion)
Mitral stenosis	Warfarin	As per rheumatic mitral regurgitation BUT possible increased risk of haemorrhage (eg. haemoptysis)
Mitral valve prolapse	Warfarin	Beneficial in patients with MVP who have documented arterial thromboembolism and/or atrial fibrillation
Mural thrombus (post-myocardial infarction)	(1) Heparin* (2) Warfarin**	* Reduces incidence of LV thrombus in patients post-MI ** Possibly beneficial in treatment of post-MI mural thrombus (good data lacking)
Patent foramina ovale	Warfarin	Indicated if thromboembolic events occur
Prosthetic heart valves (bioprosthetic)	Warfarin and heparin	Patients should be anticoagulated with warfarin for the first three months post-valve insertion Heparin cover should be used until INR reaches target range
Prosthetic heart valves (mechanical)	Heparin and warfarin	All patients should be anticoagulated with warfarin for life Heparin cover should be used until INR reaches target range. Patients with other risk factors (eg. AF) may require life-long anticoagulation
Pulmonary hypertension (primary)	Warfarin	May improve survival

Table 2. **Practical guidelines for antithrombotic therapy in non-valvar atrial fibrillation.**

Assess risk, and reassess regularly

High risk (annual risk of cerebrovascular accident = 8-12%)

- All patients with previous transient ischaemic attack or cerebrovascular accident
- All patients aged ≥75 with diabetes or hypertension
- All patients with clinical evidence of valve disease, heart failure, thyroid disease, and impaired left ventricular function on echocardiography *

Treatment - Give warfarin (target INR 2-3) if no contraindications and possible in practice.

Moderate risk (annual risk of cerebrovascular accident = 4%)

- All patients <65 with clinical risk factors: diabetes, hypertension, peripheral vascular disease, ischaemic heart disease
- All patients >65 not in high risk group

Treatment - Either warfarin (INR 2-3) or aspirin 75-300mg daily. In view of insufficient clear cut evidence, treatment may be decided on individual cases. Referral and echocardiography may help.

Low risk (annual risk = 1%)

- All patients aged <65 with no history of embolism, hypertension, diabetes, or other clinical risk factors

Treatment - Give aspirin 75-300mg daily.

* Echocardiogram not needed for routine risk assessment but refines clinical risk stratification in case of moderate or severe left ventricular dysfunction and valve disease. A large atrium *per se* is not an independent risk factor on multivariate analysis.

Atrial fibrillation

Atrial fibrillation (AF) is the commonest cardiac arrhythmia encountered in clinical practice. The joint ACC/AHA/ESC guidelines have classified AF into:-

- paroxysmal, defined as self-terminating episodes of AF;
- persistent, when the arrhythmia is sustained and potentially cardioverted to sinus rhythm; and
- permanent, where cardioversion is inappropriate or has failed and the objective of management is rate control [1].

The presence of AF is associated with a substantial increase in the risk of thromboembolism (particularly strokes). The incidence of thromboembolic stroke in all patients with atrial fibrillation who are not on anticoagulation is around 5%[1,2]. However, this figure masks the fact that there is a wide variation in stroke incidence in the various sub-populations of patients with atrial fibrillation, a fact which highlights the need for appropriate risk-stratification techniques to detect those at risk.

Independent risk factor predictors for stroke in patients with atrial fibrillation include increasing age, hypertension, diabetes, heart failure, associated structural heart disease (eg. valvular heart disease), and thyroxicosis. Based on mainly clinical criteria, risk stratification is possible for AF and forms the basis of a practical guideline for the management for the provision of thromboprophylaxis in this condition (Table 2), and the evidence is summarised further below.

Anticoagulation for AF

Antithrombotic therapy should be considered for virtually all patients with AF, in the absence of any contraindicatory factors. The only exception to this rule is in the patient who has lone AF, defined as an AF with no other risk factors for a thromboembolic event, and is less than 65 years of age. However, it should be borne in mind that nearly all patients with "lone AF" will eventually need to be considered for antithrombotic therapy at some stage, due to increasing age and the development of associated comorbidities.

Anticoagulation is the treatment of choice for the prevention of stroke in moderate to high-risk patients with AF, with a stroke risk reduction of 62% (95% CI 48%-78%) with warfarin use compared to controls. This is in marked contrast to a risk reduction of 22% (95% CI 2%-33%) seen with aspirin compared to controls [3]. The reason behind the superiority of warfarin lies in the fact that thrombi formed in the low-pressure systems are often composed of fibrin and trapped erythrocytes ("red thrombi"), rather than platelets ("white thrombi") [4]. The evidence-based guidelines for anticoagulation in AF are summarised below (modified from the ACC / AHA / ESC / ACCP guidelines)[1]. References are given for recommendations which differ from the guidelines due to the availability of new trial data.

(a) Indications for antithrombotic therapy

- Anticoagulation using warfarin should be considered for all patients with AF, with the sole exception of patients with lone AF. The target international normalised ratio (INR) should be between two to three for the optimal prevention of stroke, and the need for anticoagulation should be reviewed at regular intervals (Ia/A).
- Administration of a daily dose of 300mg of aspirin should be considered for those for whom anticoagulation is unsuitable (Ia/A).
- Combination therapy with aspirin and fixed-dose warfarin should NOT be used (Ia/A).
- Patients with lone AF can either be left untreated or given low-dose aspirin (IV/C).

(b) Interruption of anticoagulation for surgical procedures

- Stop warfarin for up to one week without giving alternative anticoagulation (eg. unfractionated heparin [UFH] or low molecular weight heparin [LMWH]) (IV/C).
- Stop warfarin for up to one week with heparin cover (either unfractionated or low molecular weight) (IV/C).

(c) Cardioversion and anticoagulation

- All patients with recurrent/persistent AF and risk factors for thromboembolism should be given a choice either of lifelong rate control and anticoagulation, or cardioversion with anticoagulation for three to four weeks before and after the procedure, as there is no difference in outcome (Ib/A) [5,6].
- If cardioversion is the preferred option for the restoration of sinus rhythm in patients with AF lasting more than 48 hours, the patient should be anticoagulated for three to four weeks before and after cardioversion, with a target INR of 2-3 (IIa/B).
- If the decision is made to opt for immediate cardioversion of a patient in AF accompanied by symptoms of haemodynamic instability, heparin should be administered by an initial bolus followed by a continuous infusion, to achieve an activated partial thromboplastin time ratio (APTTR) of 1.5-2.0. The patient should also be anticoagulated for four weeks post-cardioversion (INR 2-3). Heparin cover should be maintained until the target INR has been achieved (IV/C).
- If no thrombus is seen on transoesophageal echocardiography, the patient may be cardioverted without prior oral anticoagulation. However, the patient will still need to be started on intravenous heparin (APTTR of 1.5-2), with subsequent oral anticoagulation (INR 2-3) for four weeks post-cardioversion (Ib/A) [7].
- Patients with AF lasting less than 48 hours may be cardioverted without prior anticoagulation. Anticoagulation post-cardioversion is optional, depending on risk (IV/C).

Coronary heart disease (acute)

Anticoagulation for acute coronary heart disease

Anticoagulation has long been established as standard therapy for the treatment of the acute coronary syndromes, having been shown to have a beneficial effect on morbidity and mortality [8-10]. Again, recommendations which differ from the AHA or ESC guidelines are referenced.

(a) Non-ST elevation acute coronary syndromes (NSTACS)

- Patients admitted with non-ST elevation syndromes should be treated with either intravenous heparin (to maintain APTTR between 1.5-2) or low molecular weight heparin, in combination with antiplatelet agents until the patient has been asymptomatic for 48 hours (Ia/A).
- There is general agreement that LMWH may be better than UFH in the treatment of NSTACS (Ib/A).
- Heparin (either unfractionated or LMW) may be safely administered with GPIIb/IIIa antagonists in patients being considered for percutaneous coronary intervenion (PCI) (IIa/B).
- The direct thrombin inhibitor, hirudin, can be used if the patient has heparin-induced thrombocytopenia (Ia/A).

(b) ST elevation myocardial infarction (STEMI)

- Intravenous unfractionated heparin should be given together with selective thrombolytic agents (eg. alteplase, tenecteplase), to achieve an APTTR of 1.5-2 for 48 hours in uncomplicated cases (Ib/A).
- Low molecular weight heparin, administered either intravenously or subcutaneously, may be a suitable alternative to unfractionated heparin for the above purpose [11,12] (Ib/A).
- Heparin is not indicated in patients receiving non-selective thrombolytic agents, but its use should be considered for those at high risk of developing thromboembolic events (eg. large anterior MI, AF, mural thrombus) (Ib/A).
- Close monitoring of APPTR is required if UFH is used (IV/C).

(c) Mural thrombus

- Patients with mural thrombus should be treated initially with intravenous UFH (APTTR 1.5-2) (or subcutaneous LMWH) and commenced on warfarin. Heparin can be discontinued after the INR of 2-3 has been achieved (IV/C).
- The recommendation above is also true in the presence of a left ventricular aneurysm, although there is some controversy over this (IV/C).

Percutaneous coronary intervention

One of the greatest achievements in cardiology has been the development of percutaneous coronary intervention (PCI) to dilate both the acutely or chronically narrowed coronary artery. However, the presence of the various thrombogenic components of the PCI system and the injury to the vessel wall caused by the procedure itself (eg. angioplasty/stent deployment, atherectomy) results in the activation of platelets and the activation of the coagulation cascade. Indeed, the use of coronary stents can be associated with thrombotic rates of up to 10%, if the appropriate antithrombotic agents were not used, as observed in the early years of stent use. Therefore, the use of anticoagulants and antiplatelet agents is crucial to the success of PCI.

(a) PCI for chronic coronary heart disease

- Use of unfractionated heparin is indicated just prior to stent deployment, to achieve an activated clotting time (ACT) of 250 to 300s (HemoTec) or 300 to 350s (Hemochron) (IIb/B).
- Heparin should not be used routinely post-PCI due to excess local complications (IIb/B).
- The sheath should be removed as soon as the ACT falls to 150-180s in routine cases (IIb/B).

(b) PCI for acute coronary heart disease

- Heparin (LMWH and UFH) may be combined with GPIIb/IIIa inhibitors in patients (Ib/A).

(c) Anticoagulation to prevent stent restenosis

- There is no indication for anticoagulation for this purpose (Ib/A).

Warfarin use in coronary artery bypass grafting (CABG)

- Warfarin may be used in place of aspirin in patients in whom oral anticoagulants are simultaneously required (eg. atrial fibrillation) (III/B).

Mitral valve disease

Abnormalities of the mitral valve are the commonest form of valvular disease in adults. Thromboembolism can be a major problem and many patients with certain forms of mitral valve disease need to be adequately anticoagulated.

(a) Rheumatic mitral valve disease

Patients with rheumatic mitral valve disease have a much higher risk of developing a thromboembolic event than patients with other forms of valvular heart disease. The risk of developing an embolic event increases with age, the presence of AF, the presence of left atrial thrombus, and the presence of significant aortic regurgitation [13,14]. The guidelines below are modified from those of the ACC / AHA / ACCP [15].

(b) Mitral stenosis (MS) and mitral regurgitation (MR)

- Patients with AF should be anticoagulated with warfarin (INR of 2-3) (III/B).
- All patients with a prior embolic event should be considered for anticoagulation (INR 2-3) (III/B).
- Patients should be considered for anticoagulation if they have severe mitral stenosis and a left atrial dimension of more than 50mm, although this recommendation remains controversial (IV/C).
- There are no indications to anticoagulate the patient with uncomplicated MS and/or MR (III/C).

(c) Mitral valve prolapse (MVP)

- Patients with MVP who experience unexplained TIAs should be considered for long-term aspirin therapy (III/B).
- Patients under the age of 65 with AF, MVP, and no other risk factors could be treated with aspirin (III/B).
- Patients over the age of 65 with AF, MVP, and any risk factor (eg. hypertension, heart failure) should be anticoagulated (III/B).
- Patients should be anticoagulated after a stroke (III/B).
- Patients should be anticoagulated if TIAs occur despite aspirin therapy (IV/C).

(d) Non-rheumatic MR and mitral annulus calcification (MAC)

- Patients with MAC complicated by systemic embolism, not documented to be calcific embolism, should be anticoagulated with warfarin (IV/C).
- Patients with MAC and AF should be anticoagulated (III/B).
- Patients with MR and AF or previous history of embolism should be anticoagulated (III/B).

Infective endocarditis (IE)

Anticoagulation therapy in the presence of an infected heart valve is controversial. Although symptomatic thromboembolism is a frequent occurrence with IE, cerebral haemorrhage due to septic emboli can also occur.

Evidence for (or against) the use of anticoagulation in IE is lacking and most of the current recommendations are based on expert opinions of the ACC/ AHA/ ACCP/ ESC [15,16].

(a) The infected prosthetic valve

- Patients who are already on warfarin should be switched to heparin, as urgent surgery may be required (IV/C).
- If neurological symptoms develop whilst on anticoagulation, anticoagulation should be discontinued until an intracranial haemorrhage can be ruled out (IV/C).

(b) Thromboembolism in IE

- The indications for use of anticoagulants in native valve or bioprosthetic valve IE is uncertain [16]. The ACCP recommends basing any therapeutic decisions on the presence of comorbidities, echocardiographic features, and the success of antibiotic therapy [16] (IV/C).

Prosthetic heart valves

These recommendations are based on the ACCP/ ACC/ AHA guidelines [15,17]. The ESC guidelines are slightly different [18].

(a) Mechanical heart valves

- Every patient should be anticoagulated for life (Ib/A).
- The INR can be maintained between 2-3 in patients who had aortic valve replacement with bileaflet valves (eg. St Jude, Carbomedics) or the Medtronic-Hall valve AND there are no other risk factors for thromboembolism (Ib/A).
- An INR of 2.5-3.5 should be maintained for patients who had aortic valve replacement with the Starr-Edwards valve (Ib/A).
- Patients with a mechanical aortic valve AND at least one other risk factor for thromboembolism should have an INR of between 2.5-3.5 (III/B).
- All patients with mitral valve prostheses (Ib/A).

(b) Bioprosthetic valves

- Every patient should be anticoagulated for the first three months after valve replacement (IIb/B).
- Lifetime anticoagulation should be considered for those with at least one other risk factor for thromboembolism. The INR should be between 2-3 and 2.5-3.5 for those with aortic valve replacement (AVR) and mitral valve replacement (MVR) respectively (III/B).
- The use of aspirin should be considered to prevent thromboembolic events in patients with a bioprosthetic valve who do not have any other risk factors (IV/C).

(c) Thromboembolism despite adequate anti-coagulation

- Warfarin, INR 2-3. The warfarin dose may need to be increased to 2.5-3.5 (IV/C).
- Warfarin, INR 2.5-3.5. The warfarin dose may need to be increased to 3.5-4.5 (IV/C).
- If the higher dose of warfarin does not achieve the desired effect, the addition of aspirin should be considered (IV/C)

Pulmonary hypertension (primary)

- Anticoagulation with warfarin should be considered in patients with primary pulmonary hypertension [19] (III/B).

Conclusions

Antithrombotic therapy in patients with cardiac disease is a rapidly expanding field. The recent introduction of two novel anticoagulants, fondaparinux and ximelagatran, provides much needed stimuli for research into this field. At present, the direct thrombin inhibitor fondaparinux is being assessed for use as an alternative to heparin in the treatment of the acute coronary syndromes [20]. For example, data from the PENTALYSE study suggests that fondaparinux may even be superior to unfractionated heparin in the treatment of STEMI [21]. However, this finding will need to be confirmed by larger studies.

There is no doubt that the guidance on anticoagulation in patients with cardiac disease will become more evidence-based and the benefits (or lack thereof) of anticoagulation in the various disease groups will become clearer.

Recommendations	Evidence level
There is current sound evidence for anticoagulation for the following:-	
◆ AF (with the exception of lone AF).	Ia/A
◆ Acute coronary syndromes.	Ia/A
◆ Percutaneous coronary intervention.	Ia/A
◆ Prosthetic mechanical heart valve.	Ia/A
There is evidence needed for the following:-	
◆ Infective endocarditis-associated thromboembolism.	IV/C
◆ Thromboembolism from prosthetic heart valves despite adequate anticoagulation.	IV/C
◆ The optimal regime for anticoagulation in the infected prosthetic valve.	IV/C
◆ The role of the new anticoagulants in cardiac disease.	IV/C

References

1. Committee to Develop Guidelines For The Management of Patients With Atrial Fibrillation. ACC/AHA/ESC Guidelines for the management of patients with atrial fibrillation: Executive Summary. *J Am Coll Cardiol* 2001; 38: 1231-65.
2. Atrial Fibrillation Investigators. Risk factors for stroke and efficacy of antithrombotic therapy in atrial fibrillation. Analysis of pooled data from five randomized controlled trials. *Arch Intern Med* 1994; 154: 1449-57.
3. Hart RG, Benavente O, McBride R, Pearce LA. Antithrombotic therapy to prevent stroke in patients with atrial fibrillation: a meta-analysis. *Ann Intern Med* 1999; 131: 492-501.
4. Kamath S, Blann AD, Lip GY. Platelets and atrial fibrillation. *Eur Heart J* 2001; 22: 2233-42.
5. Carlsson J, Miketic S, Windeler J, *et al.* Randomized trial of rate-control versus rhythm-control in persistent atrial fibrillation: the Strategies of Treatment of Atrial Fibrillation (STAF) study. *J Am Coll Cardiol* 2003; 41: 1690-6.
6. Atrial Fibrillation Follow-up Investigation of Rhythm Management (AFFIRM) Investigators. A comparison of rate control and rhythm control in patients with atrial fibrillation. *N Engl J Med* 2002; 347: 1825-33.
7. Klein AL, Grimm RA, Murray RD, *et al.* Use of transesophageal echocardiography to guide cardioversion in patients with atrial fibrillation. *N Engl J Med* 2001; 344: 1411-20.
8. Committee on the Management of Patients With Unstable Angina. ACC/AHA 2002 guideline update for the management of patients with unstable angina and non-ST-segment elevation myocardial infarction - summary article: a report of the American College of Cardiology/American Heart Association task force on practice guidelines. *J Am Coll Cardiol* 2002; 40: 1366-74.
9. Committee on the Management of Patients With Unstable Angina. ACC/AHA Guidelines for the management of patients with unstable angina and non-ST elevation myocardial infarction. *J Am Coll Cardiol* 2000; 36: 970-1062.
10. The Task Force on the Management of Acute Myocardial Infarction of the European Society of Cardiology. Management of acute myocardial infarction in patients presenting with ST-segment elevation. *Eur Heart J* 2003; 24: 28-66.
11. ASSENT-3 Investigators. Efficacy and safety of tenecteplase in combination with enoxaparin, abciximab, or unfractionated heparin: the ASSENT-3 randomised trial in acute myocardial infarction. *Lancet* 2001; 358: 605-13.
12. Wallentin L, Bergstrand L, Dellborg M, *et al.* Low molecular weight heparin (dalteparin) compared to unfractionated heparin as an adjunct to rt-PA (alteplase) for improvement of coronary artery patency in acute myocardial infarction - the ASSENT Plus study. *Eur Heart J* 2003; 24: 897-908.
13. Cassella K, Abelmann WH, Ellis LB. Patients with mitral stenosis and systemic emboli. *Arch Intern Med* 2003; 114: 773.
14. Chiang CW, Lo SK, Ko YS, *et al.* Predictors of systemic embolism in patients with mitral stenosis: a prospective study. *Ann Intern Med* 1998; 128: 885-9.
15. Committee on Management of Patients with Valvular Heart Disease. Guidelines for the management of patients with valvular heart disease: executive summary. A report of the American College of Cardiology/American Heart Association Task Force on Practice Guidelines. *Circulation* 1998; 98: 1949-84.

16. Salem DN, Daudelin DH, Levine HJ, *et al.* Antithrombotic therapy in valvular heart disease. *Chest* 2001; 119: 207S-19S.
17. Stein PD, Alpert JS, Bussey HI, *et al.* Antithrombotic Therapy in Patients With Mechanical and Biological Prosthetic Heart Valves. *Chest* 2001; 119: 220S-7S.
18. Gohlke-Barwolf C, Acar J, Oakley C, *et al.* Guidelines for prevention of thromboembolic events in valvular heart disease. Study Group of the Working Group on Valvular Heart Disease of the European Society of Cardiology. *Eur Heart J* 1995; 16: 1320-30.
19. Fuster V, Steele PM, Edwards WD, *et al.* Primary pulmonary hypertension: natural history and the importance of thrombosis. *Circulation* 1984; 70: 580-7.
20. Tan KT, Makin A, Lip GYH. Factor X inhibitors. *Expert Opin Investig Drugs* 2003; 12: 799-804.
21. Coussement PK, Bassand JP, Convens C, *et al.* A synthetic factor Xa inhibitor as an adjunct to fibrinolysis in acute myocardial infarction. *Eur Heart J* 2001; 22: 2726-31.

Chapter 23

Interventions for thoracic aortic disease

Aaron M Ranasinghe MRCS
Specialist Registrar, Cardiothoracic Surgery
Robert S Bonser FRCP FRCS FESC
Consultant Cardiothoracic Surgeon

QUEEN ELIZABETH HOSPITAL, UNIVERSITY HOSPITAL BIRMINGHAM NHS TRUST, BIRMINGHAM, UK

Introduction

Patients with untreated chronic thoracic aortic aneurysms or chronic dissection have a 5-year survival between 13-39% [1-3] (Figure 1). The predominant cause of death in these patients is rupture.

There are no randomised controlled trials of intervention versus medical therapy for pathologies of the thoracic aorta. The current levels of evidence available for surgical intervention in pathologies of the thoracic aorta are levels III and IV.

Repair of thoracic aneurysms remains a formidable undertaking, despite advances in surgical technique and peri-operative management, and surgery carries a significant hazard of mortality and permanent neurological deficit for patients undergoing surgical repair. The risks of these complications must be carefully weighed against the risk of rupture with conservative management, which occurs in approximately 40% of unoperated cases and is almost universally fatal [3]. Recent database reports together with retrospective cohort studies provide us with the best available evidence for management of thoracic aortic disease.

Methodology

A systematic review of the literature on thoracic aortic aneurysms was performed. This was carried out by a search of databases that included Pubmed, Ovid Medline, National Electronic Library for Health and the Cochrane Library between 1966 and 2004. The bibliographies of all relevant articles and reviews as well as the authors' personal files were also searched. This chapter considers thoracic aneurysmal disease and dissection, as well as trauma and coarctation in adults.

Dissection

An aortic dissection occurs when there is splitting of the tunica media with extraluminal blood in the aortic wall. There are two widely used classification systems for aortic dissections: the DeBakey and Stanford classifications [4,5]. The Stanford classification is based on the presence (type A) or absence (type B) of dissection in the ascending aorta regardless of the site of initial aortic intimal tear. Dissections of the aorta are arbitrarily defined as acute if their onset is less than two weeks and chronic if longer. Risk factors for aortic dissection are listed in Table 1. Actuarial

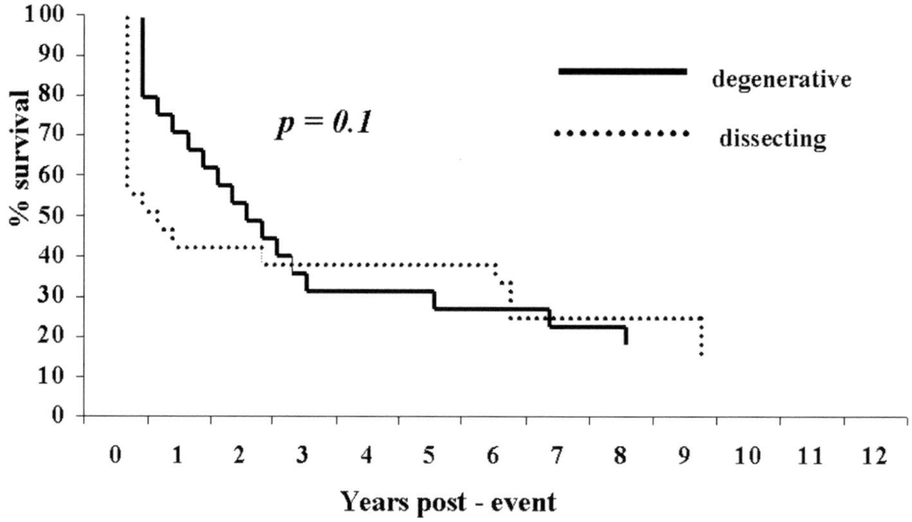

Figure 1. **Kaplan Meier survival curve of non-operated dissecting versus degenerative aneurysms. Adapted from Perko** *et al* [3]. ***Reprinted with permission from the Society of Thoracic Surgeons.***

Table 1. **Risk factors for aortic dissection. Adapted from Nienaber and Eagle** [7]. ***Reprinted with permission from Lippincott, Williams and Wilkins.***

- Long standing hypertension
  Smoking, dyslipidaemia
- Connective tissue disorders
  Marfan's syndrome
- Vasculitides
  Giant cell arteritis, Bechet's disease, syphilis
- Deceleration trauma
  Motor vehicle accident
- Iatrogenic
  Catheter interventions, cannulation sites, aortic clamping, aortic wall fragility

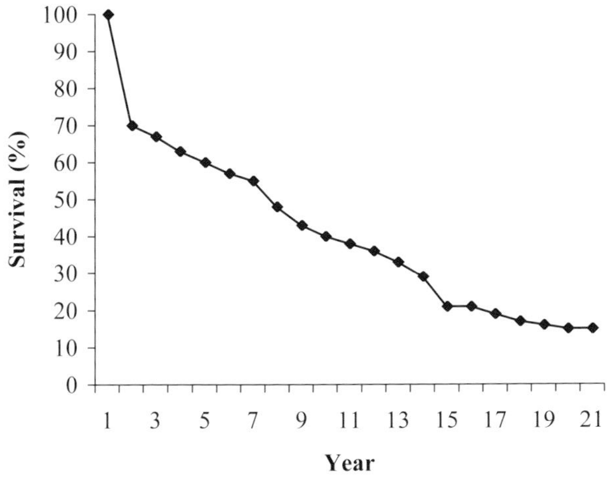

Figure 2. **Plot of actuarial late survival estimates for all patients with aortic dissection. Adapted from Fann,** *et al* [6]. ***Reprinted with permission from Lippincott, Williams and Wilkins.***

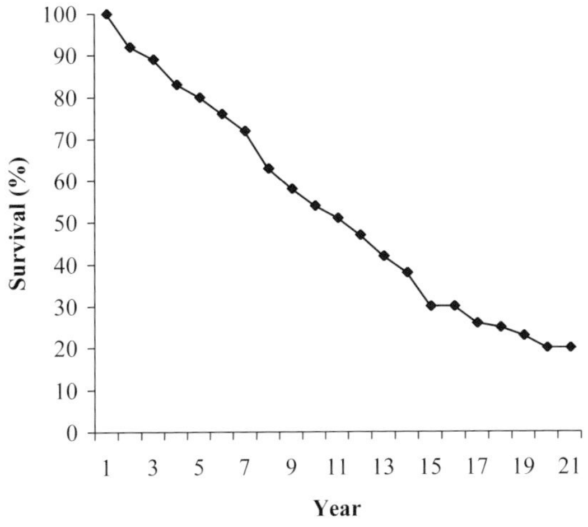

Figure 3. **Plot for all actuarial late survival estimates for all discharged patients with aortic dissection. Adapted from Fann** *et al* [6]. ***Reprinted with permission from Lippincott, Williams and Wilkins.***

survival rates for all patients presenting to hospital with acute aortic dissection are 69%, 57%, 39% and 23% at one, five, ten and 15 years. These figures rise to 92%, 76%, 52% and 30% at the same time-points for patients who survive to discharge. Late deaths are related, in 15% of cases, to complications or extension of the dissection [6] (Figures 2 and 3).

Type A dissection

Natural history

Untreated acute type A dissections carries a mortality rate of 20% by 24 hours post-presentation, 30% by 48 hours, 40% by day seven and 50% at one month with medical management alone [7] (Figure 4). Few patients survive more than one year after the initial event without operative intervention [3] (Figure 5). Mortality in non-operated patients is mainly attributed to rupture with cardiac tamponade as well as bleeding, malperfusion phenomena and intractable heart failure due to severe aortic valve incompetence. In contrast, the most common causes of mortality in patients undergoing surgical intervention are cardiac failure, intra-operative haemorrhage, multiple organ failure and major neurological injury (95% of post-operative deaths) [8].

Intervention

The aim of surgical treatment in this group of patients is to prevent rupture, protect the coronary arteries and other main aortic branch vessels from malperfusion and to restore competence to the aortic valve. Surgery is performed according to the following principles:-

- Resection and replacement of the aortic tear site.
- Repair/replacement of aortic sinus segments with false lumen obliteration to prevent coronary malperfusion and late aortic root complications.
- Resuspension/replacement of the aortic valve.
- Obliteration of the false lumen at the distal anastomosis and re-establishing primary flow into the true lumen.

Despite advances in surgical technology, mortality rates for acute type A dissection repair remain high. Nearly one in three patients dies, even in centres that

Chapter 23

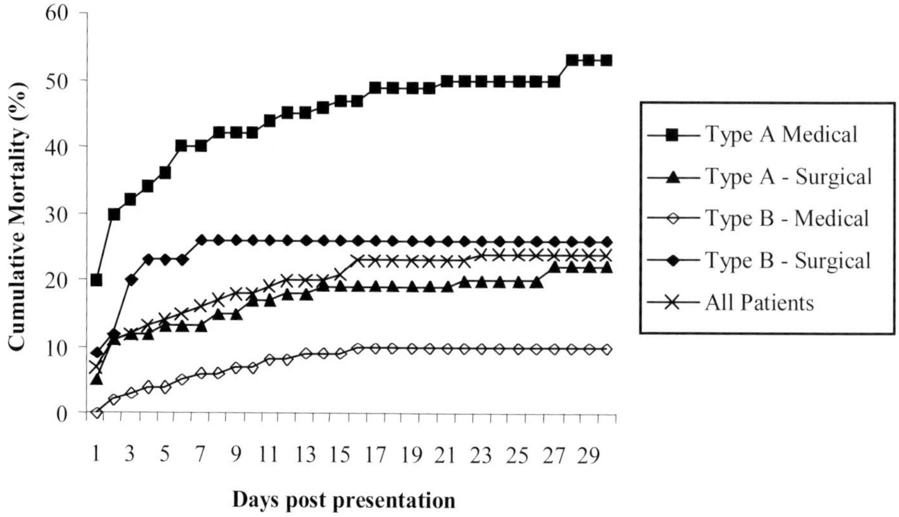

Figure 4. 30-day mortality by dissection type and intervention. Adapted from Nienaber and Eagle [7]. *Reprinted with permission from Lippincott, Williams and Wilkins.*

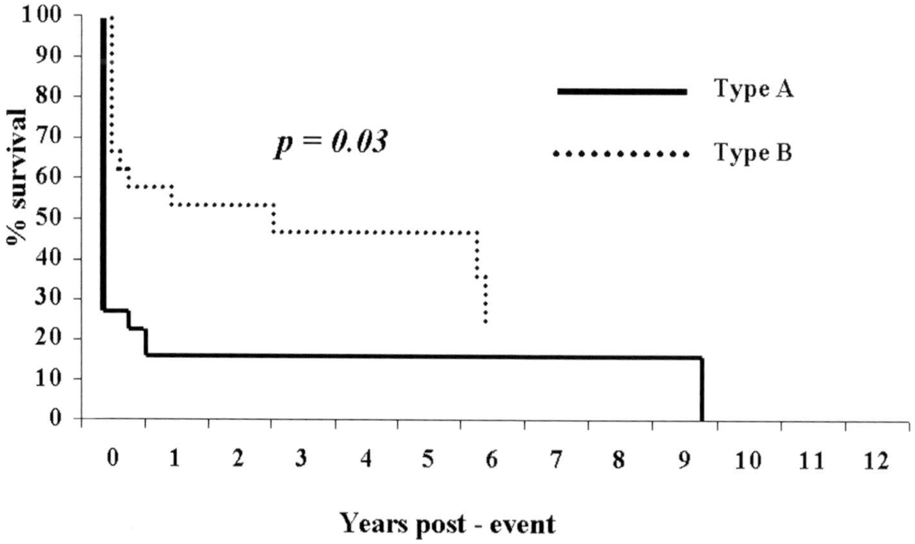

Figure 5. Kaplan Meier survival curve of non-operated type A and type B dissections. Perko *et al* [3]. *Reprinted with permission from the Society of Thoracic Surgeons.*

Table 2. Factors associated with prediction of in-hospital mortality in acute type A dissection [1]. On presentation [2]. Adapted from Mehta *et al* [87]. *Reprinted with permission from Lippincott, Williams and Wilkins.*

- Age >70 years.
- Female.
- Abrupt onset pain [1].
- Abnormal ECG [1].
- Any pulse deficit [1].
- Renal failure [2].
- Hypotension/shock/tamponade.
- No prior history of hypertension.

have extensive experience in the treatment of this condition. Mortality rates quoted in the literature for intervention in acute type A dissections range from 9% to 50%, with typical figures of 15-25% [6,9-15]. For patients greater than 70 years the risk of in-hospital mortality is significantly higher that of younger patients (43% vs. 28%) [16]. Patients less than 40 years of age are more likely to have Marfan's, bicuspid aortic valve and larger aortic dimensions at time of presentation [17]. Overall, five and 10-year survival for patients undergoing immediate surgical treatment of acute type A dissection are 71% and 54% respectively. For those patients that survive the operation the figures are 84% and 64% [15], thus, early mortality remains high, but good long-term survival is achieved in patients who leave hospital. There are a number of clinical variables that are predictors for in-hospital mortality (Table 2), which primarily relate to the presence of advanced age, rupture or pre-operative malperfusion.

Recent studies have suggested progressive improvements in surgical outcomes for patients with acute type A aortic dissection [18]. These improvements in outcome are based upon improvements in both surgical and perfusion strategies and include earlier non-invasive diagnosis, hypothermic circulatory arrest to facilitate an open distal aortic anastomosis [19], the use of biological glues [11], prevention of organ malperfusion with antegrade arterial perfusion [12] and improvements in neuroprotection.

The extent of dissection is an important consideration. If the dissection extends into the aortic arch or descending aorta then it may not be possible to resect the entire intimal flap, and current surgical treatment fails to eliminate a patent distal false lumen in 70% of cases. Attempts to resect the entire intimal flap when it extends into the descending thoracic aorta, leads to a sharp rise in mortality, 14% in the ascending aorta or proximal arch only vs. 43% including the descending aorta [15]. However, on occasion, aortic arch involvement may be dealt with at the same time as the ascending aorta without excessively increasing mortality. However, this appears to depend upon the availability of specialist expertise in centres performing significant volumes of aortic arch surgery [20].

Patients with type A dissection are at risk of both permanent and temporary neurological dysfunction postoperatively, and if brain injury occurs this is a major risk factor for early death [8,21]. Transient neurological dysfunction occurs in 11.8-32% of patients and the main risk factors for this are advancing age (greater than 60 years) and coronary artery disease. Permanent neurological dysfunction can occur in between 10-12.9% of patients [10,15,22].

Aortic incompetence, due to commissural disruption and leaflet prolapse is a common complication in acute type A dissection. Opinion is divided as to whether these patients should undergo prosthetic aortic valve replacement, adhesive reconstruction of the aortic root or valve sparing root replacement. It is generally accepted that for patients with aortic root dilatation, Marfan's and abnormalities of the aortic valve, that an aggressive surgical approach with total aortic root replacement should be undertaken. Patients without or with only mild aortic incompetence can be treated with surgical conservatism, i.e. preservation of the native valve. In these cases there is a freedom from re-operation at five and ten years post initial surgery of 93% and 80% respectively. Patients with moderate to severe aortic incompetence treated in this manner have a freedom from re-operation at five and ten years post initial surgery of 80% and 40% respectively [23]. Re-operation is predominantly required in patients with progressive aneurysmal aortic root dilatation who require total root replacement. More extensive operation in terms of composite aortic root replacement or valve-sparing reconstruction may be

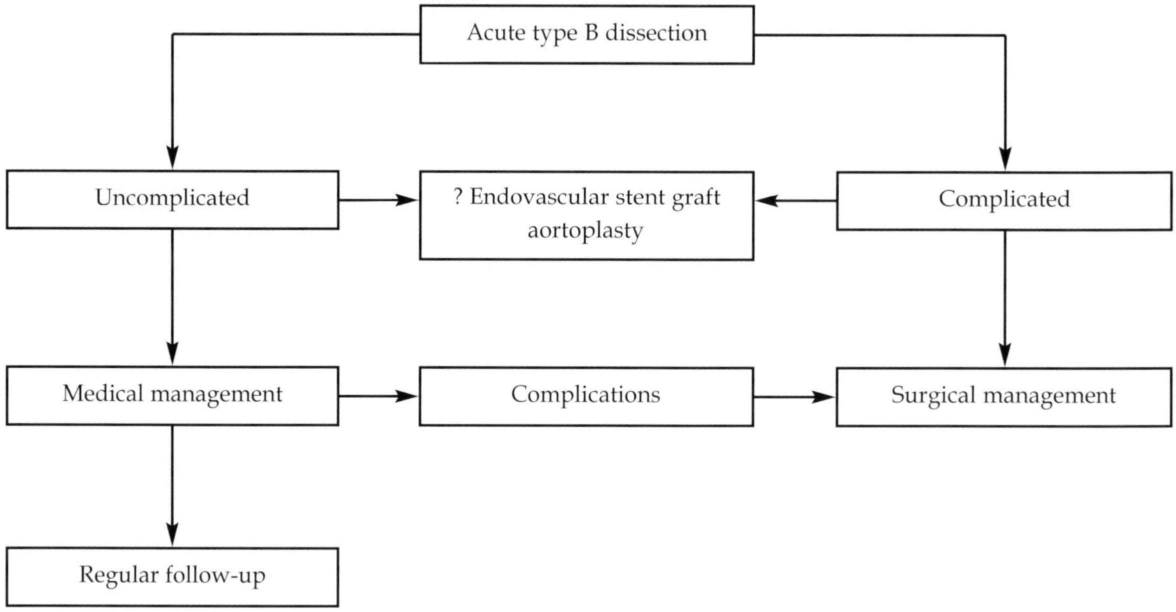

Figure 6. **"Complication-specific" management of acute type B dissection.**

more appropriate for those patients with moderate to severe aortic regurgitation. However, this adds the hazards of long-term anticoagulation and other risks associated with prosthetic aortic valve replacement. These risks need to be weighed against the finding that 61% of patients presenting with severe aortic incompetence who have undergone valve repair are free from significant aortic incompetence and 74% are free from re-operation at five years.

There is ongoing debate regarding the employment of methods of cerebral perfusion (retrograde or antegrade) in patients with acute type A dissection. Rates of neurological complications appear higher in patients who do not undergo some form of cerebral perfusion during surgery (36.4% vs. 12.2%) [10]. Most reported series are retrospective analyses comparing non-contemporary series. Although both retrograde and antegrade cerebral perfusion techniques have produced comparable results, the use of a relatively short period of hypothermic circulatory arrest (HCA) to construct an open distal anastomosis remains the primary neuroprotective strategy. Neurological injury rates are similar whether the adjunctive technique used is retrograde or antegrade cerebral perfusion. Use of antegrade cerebral perfusion in acute type A dissection can produce acceptable results, with in-hospital mortality of 19.7% and permanent and temporary neurological dysfunction rates of 7% and 11.2% respectively [24].

In the absence of any randomised studies, the outcome data for information in acute type A dissection provides irrefutable evidence of an overwhelming benefit versus the natural history of the disease process.

Type B dissection

Natural history

The majority of patients that present with acute type B dissection are uncomplicated and can be treated initially by medical intervention [25]. Patients with dissections of the descending aorta fare better with initial conservative management than those involving the ascending aorta (Figures 4 and 5). A "complication-specific" line of management is usually employed in patients with acute descending aortic dissection (Figure 6). For uncomplicated cases medical management in the form of antihypertensive and cardiac output suppressive therapy is the first line of treatment.

For uncomplicated cases of acute type B dissection, medical therapy can be employed with excellent early survival rates (90%) [26] (Figure 4). Medical therapy is directed towards control of hypertension and "anti-impulse" therapy (controlling forceful ejection from the heart). This is brought about in both the early and late stages by the use of first intravenous and then oral beta blocker therapy, or other suitable antihypertensive agents, if beta blockers are contraindicated. Prescription and tolerance of beta blocker therapy leads to a reduction in the rate of late complication in type B dissections [27]. Patients should have a repeat CT scan prior to discharge to note the maximal aortic diameter. Once discharged, these patients should be managed in an aggressive fashion in the out-patient department with regular follow-up CT scanning at 6-monthly intervals to detect expansion [28].

For cases with complications such as rupture, occlusion of major branch vessels, extension and rapid enlargement, surgical management is the usual line of treatment. Patients that fail to respond to conservative medical therapy or develop complications such as uncontrolled hypertension and pain, rapid enlargement or rupture, should be considered for surgical therapy. On presentation, this group of patients are typically male, in their mid-60s, hypertensive with sudden onset of chest or back pain [26].

Surgical intervention

Although early operative mortality for acute type B dissection has fallen from 57% (1963-1969) to 27% (1990-1999) [29], it is still prohibitively high in comparison to conservative medical therapy in uncomplicated cases and carries with it a significant risk of paraplegia/paraparesis of 24% [30]. For this reason surgery for acute type B dissections is limited to the prevention of life-threatening complications such as rupture, rapid expansion and intractable pain.

The prognosis for patients with acute type B dissections is determined primarily by presentation and patient-related risk factors that are not readily modifiable. These include shock, visceral malperfusion and extension into the aortic arch, aortic diameter greater than 6cm, lack of chest/back pain, rupture, stroke, previous sternotomy, coronary artery disease, chronic obstructive pulmonary disease and female sex [26,29,31]. There is disagreement as to whether the presence of a persistent patent false lumen is associated with an increased risk of death [26].

Surgery for the acutely dissected descending aorta is complicated by two major problems: bleeding and paraplegia. The acutely dissected descending aorta is extremely friable and holds sutures poorly. Major haemostatic problems may be encountered even with the application of new techniques such as the use of aprotinin, non-porous grafts, glue, suture line reinforcement and autologous blood [32]. Of all deaths post-surgery for acute descending dissection, 35% are due to bleeding from the anastomosis or aorta itself [33]. Paraplegia rates are much higher for this acute group of patients when compared with those with chronic descending aortic aneurysms. Patients with chronic aneurysms collateralise intercostal vessels, but this process does not have time to occur in acute type B dissection and consequently, during operation, transient or permanent interruption of the intercostal blood supply is more likely to result in paraplegia/paraparesis.

For chronic type B dissections management should be as for aneurysms of the descending aorta (discussed later). Continued expansion of the aorta is the main problem in these patients with the consequent risk of rupture.

On the basis of these data, current evidence supports medical therapy for uncomplicated type B dissections. The high mortality in complicated patients leads to an obvious need for intervention. Both surgical repair and stent aortoplasty (*vide infra*) carry significant risk, but are likely to improve survival in this compromised group.

Thoracic and thoracoabdominal aortic aneurysms

Natural history

Five-year survival rates for non-operated thoracic (TAA) and thoracoabdominal aortic aneurysms (TAAA) are quoted at 39% and 23% respectively. The main cause of death is rupture [3,34]. Elective repair of these aneurysms in selected patients has a superior outcome to emergency intervention for rupture [35]. However, elective operation requires careful assessment of the balance of risk of rupture versus operative risk (mortality and permanent neurological deficit). Mortality for ascending aortic aneurysms is quoted between 2.5-12.8% and for TAA and TAAA between 8-31% [36-38], while stroke risk for ascending and descending aneurysms are typically quoted at 8% and 5% respectively, with a further 4.5-8% risk of paraplegia for operations that involve the descending thoracic aorta [36,38,39]. Figures in the UK are shown in Table 3. These figures are all increased in patients undergoing emergency intervention with operative mortality quoted as high as 57% [40,41].

The presumed natural progression of thoracic aneurysm disease is expansion, rupture and death, and the larger the aneurysm, the greater the risk of rupture and death. Over 80% of thoracic aneurysms detected at post-mortem have ruptured and follow-up series of large unoperated aneurysms have a dismal prognosis (<20% 5-year survival) [3,42]. The very factors that influence expansion rate and risk of rupture also increase the risk of surgery, eg. age, chronic obstructive pulmonary disease (COPD). Therefore, management of these patients is a careful balance between weighing the risk of rupture against the complications associated with operative intervention.

There are a small number of patients who survive the initial event and may be referred to specialist centres for treatment [43]. For these patients operative mortality is high between 10% and 57% [43-46]. It is therefore important to identify patients who are at an increased risk of rupture, so that elective surgery (with a lower mortality and morbidity) can be considered.

The rate of aneurysm expansion determines the rupture risks of the aneurysm [47]. Maximal cross-sectional diameter is strongly associated with increased rate of expansion. While overall median expansion rates for thoracic aneurysms are between 1-4.3mm/year [36,48,49], expansion rates increase exponentially with incremental increases in aortic diameter. Aneurysms with a greater than 50mm maximal cross-sectional diameter expand at a far greater rate than those less than 50mm in diameter, (7.9mm/year in comparison to 1.7mm/year respectively) [49]. Several formulae are available for calculating expansion rates of thoracic aneurysms and the fundamental component of the formulae is the initial aortic diameter [35,48-50].

Table 3. Number and associated mortality of aortic procedures performed within the United Kingdom for 2000-2001 [37].

Aortic procedure	Number cases	Mortality (%)
Ascending aorta and valve	94	12.8
Ascending aorta without valve	191	19.9
Ascending aorta, valve and coronary root	247	14.6
Aortic arch	43	27.9
Descending aorta	76	31.5
Ruptured thoracic aorta	9	11.1

Other factors that have been shown to impact on expansion rate are smoking, age, hypertension, COPD and non-use of ß-blockers.

As aneurysm size increases so does the probability of rupture. This correlates to the law of LaPlace that relates the pressure (P) on a cylinder to its wall thickness (t), wall tension (T) and radius (r) by the equation:-

$$P = (2txT)/r$$

Thus, at a given pressure, any increase in dimension with associated wall thinning leads to an increase in wall tension until rupture occurs.

The risk of rupture is 25 times greater in patients with 60mm or greater aneurysms when compared to those of 40-49mm. Even aneurysms within the 50-59mm range are associated with 11 times the risk of rupture when compared to those in the 40-49mm range [51]. For every 10mm increase in maximal aortic diameter the risk of rupture increases by a factor of 1.9 [52]. For aneurysms less than 50mm in diameter the yearly rate for risk of rupture is close to zero. This rupture rate rises to 1.7% and 3.6% per year for aneurysms between 50mm and 59mm and those greater than 60mm respectively [51] (Table 4).

Table 4. Complications based on aortic size. Adapted from Elefteriades *et al* [36]. *Reprinted with permission from the Society of Thoracic Surgeons.*

	Aortic size			
Yearly risk of	>3.5cm	>4cm	>5cm	>6cm
Rupture	0.0%	0.3%	1.7%	3.6%
Dissection	2.2%	1.5%	2.5%	3.7%
Death	5.9%	4.6%	4.8%	10.8%
Any of the above	7.2%	5.3%	6.5%	14.1%

There is a steady increase in the risk of rupture with age [53]. Smoking increases the risk of rupture by 6.5 times independently of COPD [54] and the presence of COPD increases the risk of rupture by a factor of 3.6 [52,55].

Untreated hypertension may also be a risk factor for rupture. Non-prescription or intolerance of ß-blockers is also a factor, but this may be due to an existing phenomena in COPD patients [34]. It would therefore seem appropriate that patients who are hypertensive should receive appropriate medical therapy to control their hypertension.

Non-specific pain in the presence of aneurysmal disease is also of prognostic significance. In a study of non-operated aneurysms [52], the presence of vague or uncharacteristic pain emerged as an independent risk factor for rupture in patients with non-dissecting aneurysms.

Thus, it is possible to identify patients with a high risk of rupture and compare their anticipated outcomes with those achieved by intervention.

Surgical intervention

Surgical intervention for patients with TAA and TAAA should be offered at a time when the combined centre-specific risk of operative mortality and permanent neurological deficit is less than or equal to the risk of rupture. Many patients are inoperable as the expected mortality from elective surgery may be prohibitively high. The factors discussed above that influence the risk of rupture can all be considered in a formula that calculates the risk of rupture [52,56] (Figures 7 and 8). The main factor that determines the need for

$$\ln \lambda = -21.055 + 0.093\,(\text{age}) + 0.841\,(\text{pain}) + 1.282\,(\text{COPD}) + 0.643\,(\text{descending diameter, cm}) + 0.405\,(\text{abdominal diameter, cm})$$

Pain and COPD are 1 if present and 0 if absent.

Probability of rupture within 1 year = $1 - e^{-\lambda(365)}$

Figure 7. **Equation to estimate the rate of rupture (λ) after CT scan [52,56].**

Chapter 23

a. 50-year- old

b. 60-year- old

c. 70-year- old

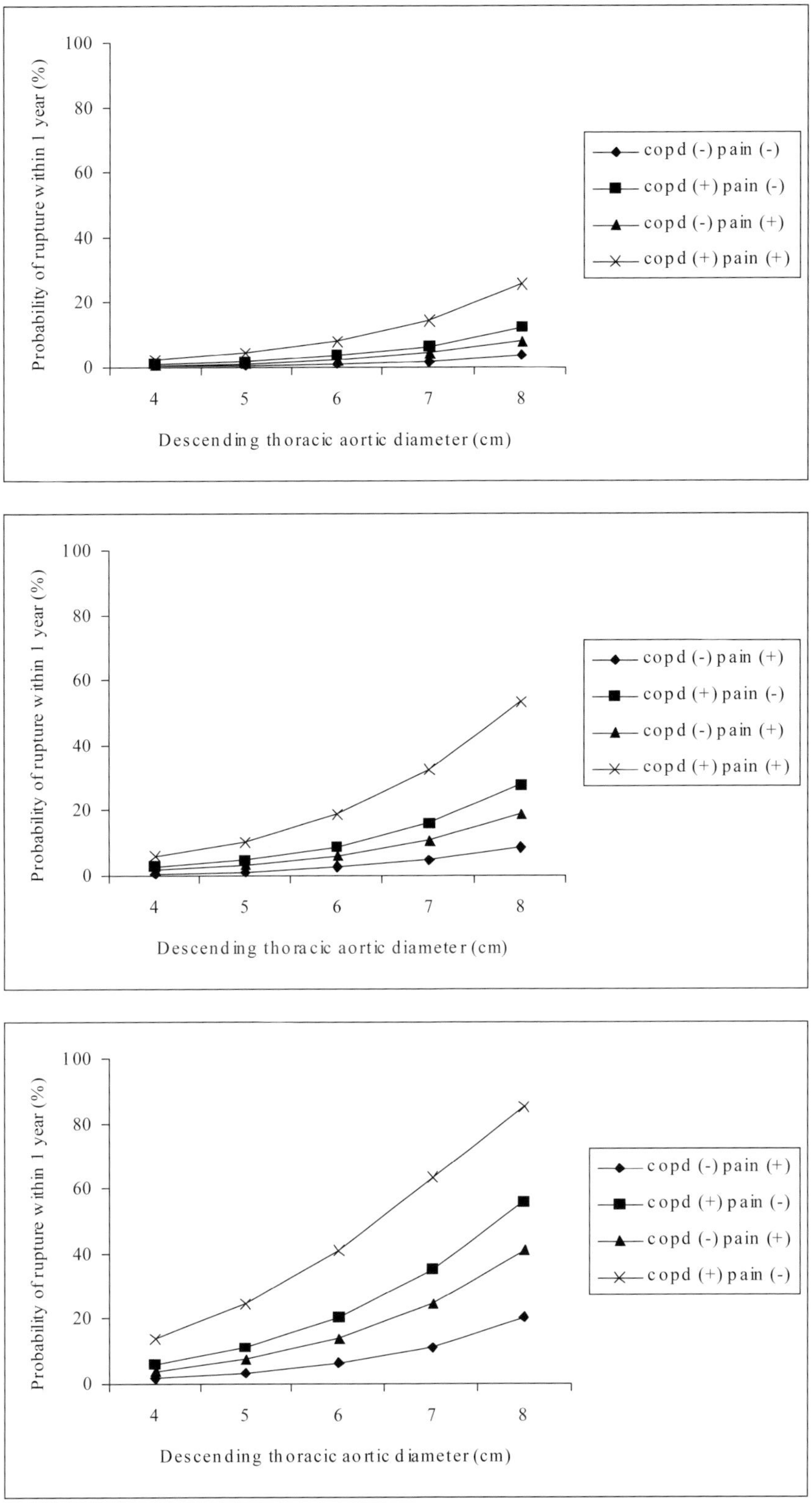

Figure 8. **Diagrams to show calculated risks of rupture for various age groups of patients with increasing descending thoracic aortic diameter and varying comorbidities [52]. Abdominal aortic diameter is constant at 5cm.**

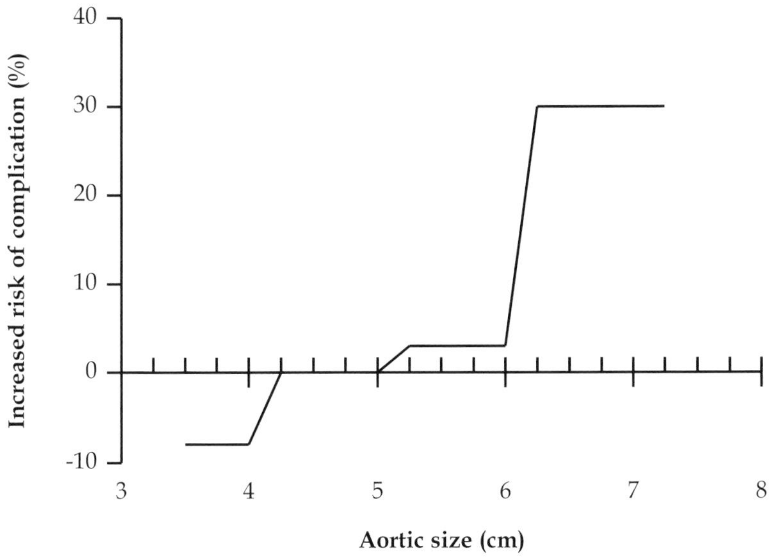

Figure 9. **Influence of ascending aortic size on cumulative, lifetime incidence of natural complications of aortic aneurysm [36].** ***Reprinted with permission from the Society of Thoracic Surgeons.***

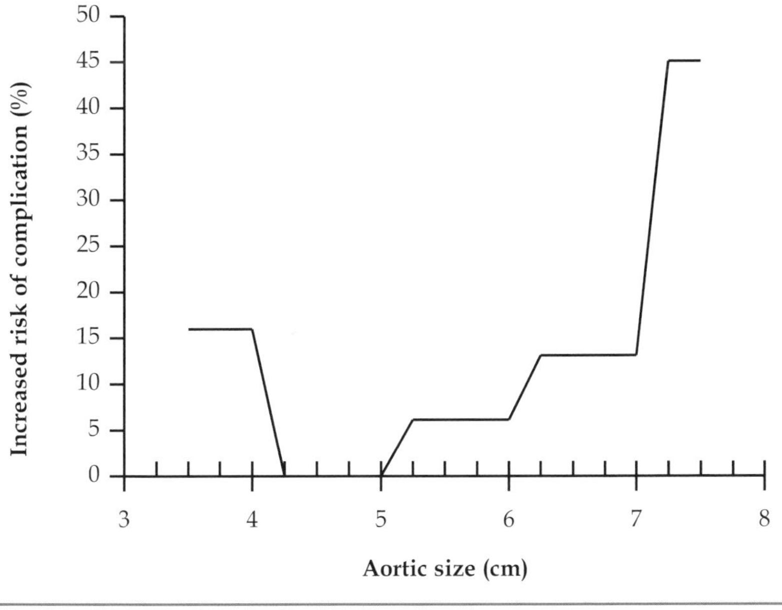

Figure 10. **Influence of descending aortic size on cumulative, lifetime incidence of natural complications of aortic aneurysm [36].** ***Reprinted with permission from the Society of Thoracic Surgeons.***

operative intervention is size. Recommendations for intervention based on the expected rate of complication (Table 4, Fgures 9 and 10) are 5.5cm and 6.5cm for asymptomatic patients in the ascending and descending aorta respectively [36].

Surgical repair of thoracoabdominal aortic aneurysms (TAAA) is a technically challenging procedure with significant mortality and morbidity (particularly the devastating complication of

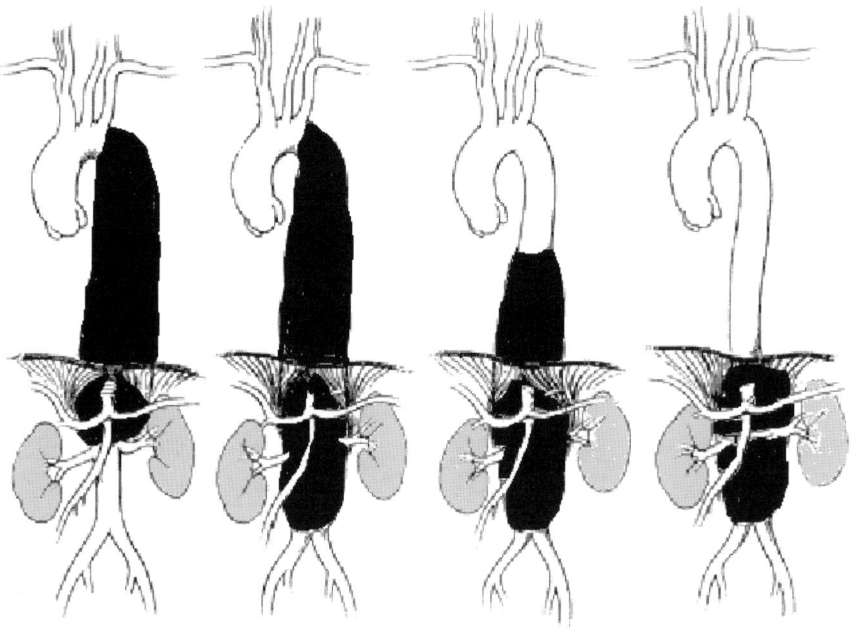

Figure 11. **Crawford classification of thoracoabdominal aneurysms [43].** *Reprinted with permission from John Wiley & Sons Ltd on behalf of the BJSS Ltd.*

paraplegia/paraparesis). They are classically classified under the Crawford system (Figure 11).

- Extent I - Proximal descending aorta to upper abdominal aorta.
- Extent II - Proximal descending aorta to below the origin of the renal arteries.
- Extent III - Distal half of descending aorta extending into the abdomen.
- Extent IV - Most of/entire abdominal aorta.

Extent II TAAA which typically involve the entire thoracoabdominal aortic segment carry the greatest risk of mortality and paraplegia [57] compared with the other extents (Table 5). Five-year survival rates for extents I-IV TAAA are 80.4%, 68.7%, 69.4% and 65.3% respectively [58]. In an attempt to minimise major morbidity from repair of TAAAs there are a number of strategies available (Table 6) [58]. Cross-clamping of the proximal aorta leads to distal hypoperfusion with spinal cord ischaemia and increased cerebrospinal

Table 5. **Results of TAAA repair in large series of patients (n=1773). Note the increased mortality and paraplegia rates for type II aneurysms. Adapted from Coselli** *et al* **[58].** *Reprinted with permission from the Society of Thoracic Surgeons.*

Extent	No. patients (%)	30-day mortality (%)	Paraplegia rate (%)
I	32.7	5.5	3.7
II	32.3	7.5	7.8
III	16.4	4.8	2.8
IV	18.6	3.6	2.1
Total	100	5.7	4.5

Table 6. Strategies for spinal cord, visceral and renal protection during TAAA repair. Adapted from Coselli *et al* [58]. *Reprinted with permission from the Society of Thoracic Surgeons.*

All Extents

- Permissive mild hypothermia
- Moderate heparinisation
- Perfusion of renal arteries with crystalloid
- Aggressive reattachment of segmental arteries, especially between T8 and L1

Extent I and II

- CSF drainage
- Left heart bypass during proximal anastomosis
- Selective perfusion of celiac axis and superior mesenteric artery during intercostal and visceral / renal anastomosis

fluid (CSF) pressure. Adjuncts for spinal cord protection include distal aortic perfusion, CSF drainage and aggressive reattachment of critical intercostal arteries. The use of distal perfusion techniques leads to an increase in spinal artery perfusion. CSF drainage may further improve spinal cord perfusion and has been shown in a randomised study to decrease the incidence of paraplegia/ paraparesis in surgery for extent I and II TAAAs (12.2% vs. 2.7%, an 80% reduction in the relative risk of postoperative deficit) [59]. Other non-randomised studies have also shown benefit in the reduction of this devastating complication [60]. Alternative techniques that have met with similarly low neurological injury rates include reconstruction of the TAAA with profound hypothermia and circulatory arrest [61,62].

Ten-year survival rates for TAA and TAAA repair approximate 40% [63]. On the basis of the observed natural history, there is good evidence that intervention in selected patients with high rupture risk improves survival.

Marfan's syndrome

Marfan's syndrome is an autosomal dominant inherited connective tissue disorder with a deficiency in the glycoprotein fibrillin. This leads to an alteration in the deposition of elastin within the aortic wall and consequently, these patients are more likely to develop aneurysms of the elastic arteries [64]. Dilatation of the aortic root is present in up to 80% of these patients by their twenties. These patients also have a greater maximal aortic diameter than age and sex-matched controls without Marfan's [65]. Marfan's patients have a reduced life expectancy with 90% of deaths being due to aortic rupture [66]. Advances in medical and surgical therapy has led to a greater than 25% increase in life expectancy [67]; reasons for this may include greater awareness of the condition (so that patients with less clinically severe disease may be being diagnosed), earlier surgical interventions, improvements in surgical techniques and use of ß-blockers to slow the rate of aortic dilatation [68]. Patients with Marfan's may have aneurysms at more than one site in the aorta. The most common site is the aortic root and ascending aorta, followed by the descending thoracic aorta. The majority of patients who undergo surgery with Marfan's will develop further aneurysmal disease or dissection at secondary sites and it is not uncommon for this group to undergo additional procedures. Variables which predict the requirement of subsequent surgery are acute or chronic dissection at the time of the primary surgical intervention, uncontrolled hypertension after the initial surgery and smoking [69]. It is recommended that Marfan's patients undergo repair of thoracic aneurysms at lower limits than the general population

Table 7. Anatomical considerations for use of endovascular stent grafts in the thoracic aorta [76].

- A "landing zone" of normal aorta 1.5cm distal to the left subclavian artery (or left common carotid if the subclavian is sacrificed) and proximal to the coeliac axis
- Greater success for "straighter" segments of aorta
- Access through femoral or iliac arteries with vessels of greater than 7mm diameter

Table 8. Description of types of endoleak [76].

- Type I - leak at anastomotic junction of aorta and stent graft
- Type II - back bleeding vessels within the aneurysm sac
- Type III - Stent graft junctions (treated with further stent graft insertion)
- Type IV - Leak though stent graft fabric

because of the increased risk of dissection in these patients at relatively smaller sizes [36].

Many surgeons believe that aortic valve-sparing procedures should not be performed when operating on Marfan's patients with aortic root aneurysms. The standard treatment for Marfan's patients with aortic root aneurysm is composite replacement of the aortic valve and ascending aorta. However, in expert centres good clinical outcomes have been obtained in treating these patients with aortic valve-sparing procedures. The size of the aneurysm determines the feasibility of the valve-sparing procedure and valve-sparing surgery is recommended for patients with Marfan's who have echocardiographically normal aortic valve cusps once the aortic root reaches 5cm [70].

Endovascular stent grafts

Endovascular stent graft aortoplasty (ESGA) is a novel technique and its efficacy remains under evaluation. In centres experienced with their use they have been used in up to 65% of cases of dissection or aneurysm including rupture [71-74]. They have been used in aneurysms of the abdominal aorta since 1991 [75] and shortly afterwards in thoracic aortic aneurysms. However, as with many other interventions in thoracic aortic pathology, there is a paucity of evidence regarding their use and there are currently no randomised studies available with long-term data for the use of ESGA in pathologies of the aorta.

The principle of ESGA is to achieve exclusion of the diseased portion of the aorta and suppress pressure stress within these areas. As they are a less invasive option, it is hoped that their use may be of particular benefit in those patients with multiple comorbidities in whom surgery carries excessively high morbidity and mortality. ESGA has been used in the treatment of thoracic aneurysms and type B dissections with primary successful stent deployment of around 90% [74]. However, aneurysm exclusion without primary endoleak is achieved in 70-80%. Successful use of ESGA implies exclusion of thoracic intimal tears or the aneurysm sac without further leak.

There are a number of anatomical considerations that must be taken into account for successful deployment of ESGA (Table 7) [76]. The efficacy of ESGA is limited by the complication of early and late endoleak (Table 8) which allow for continued pressurisation of the aneurysm sac. Their exact incidence is unknown, but may be as high as 30% and will become apparent as long-term studies become available [76].

There are a number of small series available within the literature for the use of ESGA; some of these are summarised in Table 9. The overall long-term survival data published from the Stanford group [73] were considerably lower than that expected for an age and sex-matched population. However, 60% of their ESGA patient population were judged to be unsuitable for open surgical repair due to comorbidities. Life expectancy for this group was

Table 9. Comparison of studies involving endovascular stent grafts for aortic pathologies. 1) Success rate for uncomplicated type B and chronic type B 100%; 2) in-hospital mortality for acute type B with complication 6.3%, no mortality in acute type B without complication and chronic dissection; 3) primary success rate, secondary success rate defined as complete exclusion of aneurysm after second intervention (84%); 4) also a cerebrovascular accident rate of 7%.

Study	Number of patients	Aortic pathology included	Success rate	Conversion to surgery	In-hospital survival	Long-term survival	Paraplegia	Endoleak
Ehrlich 1998 [88]	10	Aneurysm and chronic dissection	80%	Nil	90%	Not available	0	20%
Buffolo 2002 [74]	191	Aneurysm, type B dissection and trauma	91.1%	3.1%	89.6%	87.4% at 70 months	0	Not available
Shimono 2002 [89]	37	Acute and chronic type B dissection	94.4%[1]	Nil	97.3%[2]	97.3% at 2 years	0	13.5%
Doss 2003 [71]	26	Acute rupture	Not available	Not available	96.2%	Not available	0	7.7%
Demers 2004 [73]	103	Descending thoracic aneurysms	73%[3]	0.97%	91%	1 yr 82% 5 yr 49% 8 yr 27%	3%[4]	21.4%

considerably less than those who were deemed to be operable (31% 5-year vs. 78% 5-year survival respectively) (Figure 12) due mainly to death from co-existing medical conditions and this raises the important point of whether endovascular treatment should be offered to this group who are likely to die from their comorbidities rather than aortic rupture.

In type B dissection, long-term data are also required as there is a high incidence of persistently patent false lumen and increasing dimensions of the distal aorta. These factors argue against the use of ESGA in uncomplicated type B dissection. For these reasons it is of great importance that patients who undergo ESGA placement should receive serial radiological imaging to monitor the potential long-term complications that may ensue.

The current evidence for use of ESGA is limited and further studies and long-term follow-up data are required.

Trauma

Thoracic aortic injury occurs in 10-30% of fatally injured adult blunt trauma victims [77]. Survival is rare, with 85% of patients failing to reach hospital alive. Management of traumatic aortic rupture is controversial with conventional wisdom stating that urgent operative intervention should be performed. However, it has been noted that in selected groups of patients, delay in operative intervention can be performed with satisfactory morbidity and mortality [78-80]. The majority of patients with this type of injury are

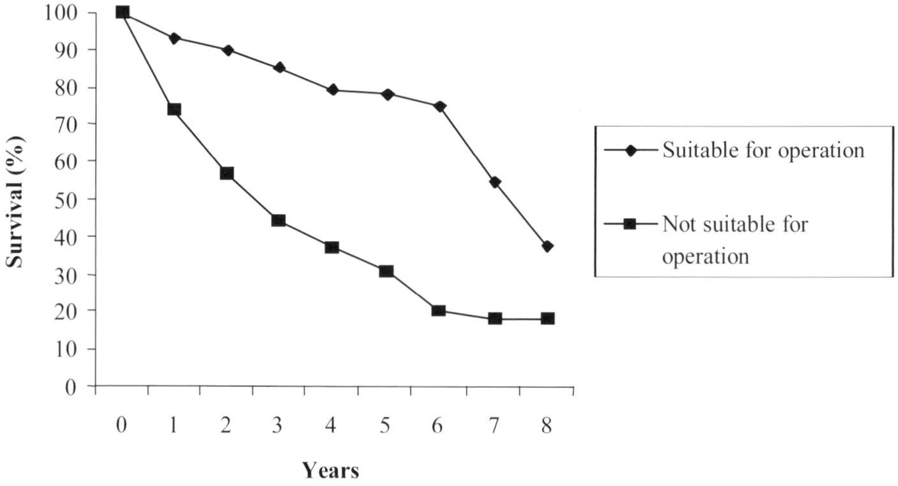

Figure 12. Actuarial survival for patients with descending thoracic aneurysms treated by endovascular stent grafting according to whether or not the patient was judged to be a suitable surgical candidate. Adapted from Demers [73]. *Reprinted with permission from the American Association for Thoracic Surgery.*

involved in motor vehicle accidents with deceleration injuries, most of which occur at the level of the aortic isthmus. Risk factors for death in this population in one retrospective study include higher injury severity scores, lower Glasgow Coma Scale, higher age and earlier surgical intervention [81]. In this series, a mortality rate of 38% was found for immediate repair (less than 24 hours, mean seven hours) and 10% for late repair (greater than 24 hours, mean 66 days). Mortality rates elsewhere in the literature are quoted at 10-14.3% for urgent surgical intervention and 0-10% for delayed intervention [78,81,82]. Delay in surgical intervention allows for diagnosis and treatment of other life-threatening conditions, which are responsible for a large proportion of mortality in this group. Delayed management relies on the same principles as that of medical management for acute type B dissection, with adequate blood pressure control using ß-blocker therapy and anti-impulse therapy. Historical controls treated urgently may not have benefited from sophisticated improvements in surgical and peri-operative management. Management of this area of aortic pathology is likely to remain controversial as it is impossible to perform a randomised controlled trial in this group and in many studies the numbers of patients involved are small.

Coarctation of the aorta in adults

Coarctation of the aorta is characterised by congenital stenosis of a site in the descending thoracic, distal arch or abdominal aorta with a pressure gradient across the stenosis. Diagnosis of untreated coarctation is now rare in the adult population and more frequently, adults are seen with late complications that include aneurysm formation, restenosis, inadequate graft size or graft infection.

If untreated, 90% of patients die before the age of 50. This is generally due to cardiac causes and problems related to hypertension such as stroke. Rupture from either proximal dissection or a post-stenotic aneurysm may also occur [83].

Options for treatment of coarctation in adults include surgical intervention, balloon angioplasty and the use of stent grafts to the stenotic segment.

Surgical repair of coarctation may be performed by patch repair, coarctectomy or prosthetic graft replacement, and is indicated when the gradient across the coarctation is greater than or equal to 30mmHg. Outcome following coarctation repair is generally good. Patients should undergo regular follow-up to detect the most important complication of repair, which is late aneurysm formation at the site of repair and recoarctation. Management of systemic hypertension requires lifelong monitoring. One of the benefits conferred by surgery for this group of patients is normalisation of blood pressure. Persistent systemic hypertension following repair occurs in between 5.4-9% of patients and is associated with expansion, rupture and death [84,85]. Aneurysm formation is more common in patients who undergo synthetic patch repair vs. coarctectomy vs. prosthetic graft replacement [84]. Surgical repair carries with it a risk of mortality and paraplegia in adults and comparable results are now being obtained with balloon angioplasty.

The indications for stent implantation are not clearly defined. Possible indications include long segment and tortuous coarctation, and recurrent coarctation after surgical repair. Recoarctation is rare in adult and adolescent patients with discrete coarctation treated by balloon angioplasty. Compared with surgery, balloon angioplasty offers fewer burdens to the patient, with a short in-hospital stay varying from one to two days. This also applies to the financial costs of the angioplasty that are relatively low. Long-term results for balloon angioplasty treatment of coarctation are now available and are favourable when compared to surgical results with a reintervention rate of 7.5% and late aneurysm formation rate of 7.5% also [86].

Conclusions

There are no randomised controlled trials considering surgical intervention in thoracic aortic disease. The evidence for intervention is based upon a comparison of anticipated natural history versus reported long-term outcomes following repair. Natural history prediction is becoming increasingly refined (at least for populations, if not individuals) and this allows an analysis of the risks and potential benefits of intervention. The surgical results in thoracic aortic surgery are variable and it is important that local institutional outcomes are compared with natural history rupture risk estimates, when recommending intervention.

Recommendations	Evidence level
◆ Surgical management of acute type A dissection confers an overwhelming benefit compared with the natural history of the disease.	III/B
◆ A "complication-specific" line of management for acute type B dissection should be employed.	III/B
◆ Medical therapy with regular follow-up is the current treatment of choice for "uncomplicated" type B dissection.	III/B
◆ Surgical therapy is the current treatment of choice for "complicated" type B dissection.	IV/C
◆ Surgical intervention for thoracic aneurysm disease still carries a significant risk of mortality and permanent neurological deficit.	III/B
◆ Intervention in patients with a high risk of rupture improves survival.	III/B
◆ The current evidence for the use of endovascular stent grafts is limited and so further studies are required.	III/B

References

1. Bickerstaff LK, Pairolero PC, Hollier LH, Melton LJ, Van Peenen HJ, Cherry KJ, *et al.* Thoracic aortic aneurysms: a population-based study. *Surgery* 1982; 92(6): 1103-8.
2. Pressler V, McNamara JJ. Aneurysm of the thoracic aorta. Review of 260 cases. *J Thorac Cardiovasc Surg* 1985; 89(1): 50-54.
3. Perko MJ, Norgaard M, Herzog TM, Olsen PS, Schroeder TV, Pettersson G. Unoperated aortic aneurysm: a survey of 170 patients. *Ann Thorac Surg* 1995; 59(5): 1204-9.
4. DeBakey ME, Beall AC Jr, Cooley DF, Crawford ES, Morris GC Jr, Garrett HE, *et al.* Dissecting aneurysms of the aorta. *Surg Clin North Am* 1966 Aug; 46(4): 1045-55.
5. Daily PO, Trueblood HW, Stinson EB, Wuerflein RD, Shumway NE. Management of acute aortic dissections. *Ann Thorac Surg* 1970; 10(3): 237-247.
6. Fann JI, Smith JA, Miller DC, Mitchell RS, Moore KA, Grunkemeier G, *et al.* Surgical Management of Aortic Dissection During a 30-Year Period. *Circulation* 1995; 92(9): 113-121.
7. Nienaber CA, Eagle KA. Aortic Dissection: New Frontiers in Diagnosis and Management: Part I: From Etiology to Diagnostic Strategies. *Circulation* 2003; 108(5): 628-635.
8. Van Arsdell GSM, David TEM, Butany JM. Autopsies in Acute Type A Aortic Dissection: Surgical Implications. *Circulation* 1998; 98(19S): 299II-302II.
9. Long SM, Tribble CG, Raymond DP, Fiser SM, Kaza AK, Kern JA, *et al.* Preoperative shock determines outcome for acute type A aortic dissection. *Ann Thorac Surg* 2003; 75(2): 520-524.
10. Sinatra R, Melina G, Pulitani I, Fiorani B, Ruvolo G, Marino B. Emergency operation for acute type A aortic dissection: neurologic complications and early mortality. *Ann Thorac Surg* 2001; 71(1): 33-38.
11. Bachet J, Goudot B, Dreyfus GD, Brodaty D, Dubois C, Delentdecker P, *et al.* Surgery for acute type A aortic dissection: the Hopital Foch experience (1977-1998). *Ann Thorac Surg* 1999; 67(6): 2006-2009.
12. David TE, Armstrong S, Ivanov J, Barnard S. Surgery for acute type A aortic dissection. *Ann Thorac Surg* 1999; 67(6): 1999-2001.
13. Lansman SL, McCullough JN, Nguyen KH, Spielvogel D, Klein JJ, Galla JD, *et al.* Subtypes of acute aortic dissection. *Ann Thorac Surg* 1999; 67(6): 1975-1978.
14. Kazui T, Washiyama N, Bashar AHM, Terada H, Suzuki T, Ohkura K, *et al.* Surgical outcome of acute type A aortic dissection: analysis of risk factors. *Ann Thorac Surg* 2002; 74(1): 75-81.
15. Ehrlich MP, Ergin MA, McCullough JN, Lansman SL, Galla JD, Bodian CA, *et al.* Results of Immediate Surgical Treatment of All Acute Type A Dissections. *Circulation* 2000; 102(90003): 248III-252.
16. Mehta RH, O'Gara PT, Bossone E, Nienaber CA, Myrmel T, Cooper JV, *et al.* Acute type A aortic dissection in the elderly: clinical characteristics, management, and outcomes in the current era. *J Amer Coll Cardiol* 2002; 40(4): 685-692.
17. Januzzi JL, Isselbacher EM, Fattori R, Cooper JV, Smith DE, Fang J, *et al.* Characterizing the young patient with aortic dissection: results from the international registry of aortic dissection (IRAD)*1. *J Amer Coll Cardiol* 2004; 43(4): 665-669.
18. Bavaria JE, Brinster DR, Gorman RC, Woo YJ, Gleason T, Pochettino A. Advances in the treatment of acute type A dissection: an integrated approach. *Ann Thorac Surg* 2002; 74(5): S1848-S1852.
19. Livesay JJ, Cooley DA, Duncan JM, Ott DA, Walker WE, Reul GJ. Open aortic anastomosis: improved results in the treatment of aneurysms of the aortic arch. *Circulation* 1982; 66(2:Pt 2): t-7.
20. Urbanski PP, Siebel A, Zacher M, Hacker RW. Is extended aortic replacement in acute type A dissection justifiable? *Ann Thorac Surg* 2003; 75(2): 525-529.
21. Wong CH, Bonser RS. Does retrograde cerebral perfusion affect risk factors for stroke and mortality after hypothermic circulatory arrest? *Ann Thorac Surg* 1999; 67(6): 1900-1903.
22. Ehrlich MP, Schillinger M, Grabenwoger M, Kocher A, Tschernko EM, Simon P, *et al.* Predictors of Adverse Outcome and Transient Neurological Dysfuntion Following Surgical Treatment of Acute Type A Dissections. *Circulation* 2003; 108(90101):318II-323.
23. Pessotto R, Santini F, Pugliese P, Montalbano G, Luciani GB, Faggian G, *et al.* Preservation of the aortic valve in acute type A dissection complicated by aortic regurgitation. *Ann Thorac Surg* 1999; 67(6): 2010-2013.
24. Di Eusanio M, Tan ME, Schepens MAAM, Dossche KM, Di Bartolomeo R, Pierangeli A, *et al.* Surgery for acute type A dissection using antegrade selective cerebral perfusion: experience with 122 patients. *Ann Thorac Surg* 2003; 75(2): 514-519.
25. Hagan PG, Nienaber CA, Isselbacher EM, Bruckman D, Karavite DJ, Russman PL, *et al.* The International Registry of Acute Aortic Dissection (IRAD): New Insights Into an Old Disease. *JAMA* 2000; 283(7): 897-903.
26. Suzuki T, Mehta RH, Ince H, Nagai R, Sakomura Y, Weber F, *et al.* Clinical Profiles and Outcomes of Acute Type B Aortic Dissection in the Current Era: Lessons From the International Registry of Aortic Dissection (IRAD). *Circulation* 2003; 108(90101): 312II-31317.
27. Genoni M, Paul M, Jenni R, Graves K, Seifert B, Turina M. Chronic beta-blocker therapy improves outcome and reduces treatment costs in chronic type B aortic dissection. *Eur J Cardiothorac Surg* 2001; 19(5): 606-10.
28. Hata M, Shiono M, Inoue T, Sezai A, Niino T, Negishi N, *et al.* Optimal treatment of type B acute aortic dissection: long-term medical follow-up results. *Ann Thorac Surg* 2003; 75(6): 1781-1784.
29. Umana JP, Miller DC, Mitchell RS. What is the best treatment for patients with acute type B aortic dissections - medical, surgical, or endovascular stent-grafting? *Ann Thorac Surg* 2002; 74(5): S1840-S1843.
30. Svensson LG, Crawford ES, Hess KR, Coselli JS, Safi HJ. Dissection of the aorta and dissecting aortic aneurysms. Improving early and long-term surgical results. *Circulation* 1990; 82(5 Suppl): 24-38.
31. Umana J, Lai D, Mitchell R, Moore K, Rodriguez F, Robbins R *et al.* Is medical therapy still the optimal treatment strategy for patients with acute type B aortic dissections? *J Thorac Cardiovasc Surg* 2002; 124(5): 896-910.

32. Svensson LG. How to obtain hemostasis after aortic surgery. *Ann Thorac Surg* 1999; 67(6): 1981-1982.
33. Miller DC, Mitchell RS, Oyer PE, Stinson EB, Jamieson SW, Shumway NE. Independent determinants of operative mortality for patients with aortic dissections. *Circulation* 1984; 70(3:Pt 2): t-64.
34. Bonser RS, Pagano D, Lewis ME, Rooney SJ, Guest P, Davies P, *et al.* Clinical and patho-anatomical factors affecting expansion of thoracic aortic aneurysms. *Heart* 2000; 84(3): 277-283.
35. Coady MA, Rizzo JA, Hammond GL, Mandapati D, Darr U, Kopf GS, *et al.* What is the appropriate size criterion for resection of thoracic aortic aneurysms? *J Thorac Cardiovasc Surg* 1997; 113(3):476-91.
36. Elefteriades JA. Natural history of thoracic aortic aneurysms: indications for surgery, and surgical versus nonsurgical risks. *Ann Thorac Surg* 2002; 74(5): S1877-S1880.
37. The Society of Cardiothoracic Surgeons of Great Britain and Ireland. National Adult Cardiac Surgical Database Report 2000-2001. October 2002 ed. Dendrite Clinical Systems Ltd, 2002.
38. LeMaire SA, Miller III, Conklin LD, Schmittling ZC, Coselli JS. Estimating group mortality and paraplegia rates after thoracoabdominal aortic aneurysm repair. *Ann Thorac Surg* 2003; 75(2): 508-513.
39. Coselli JS, LeMaire SA, Miller CC3, Schmittling ZC, Koksoy C, Pagan J, *et al.* Mortality and paraplegia after thoracoabdominal aortic aneurysm repair: a risk factor analysis. *Ann Thorac Surg* 2000; 69(2): 409-14.
40. Clouse WD, Hallett JW, Jr., Schaff HV, Gayari MM, Ilstrup DM, Melton LJ3. Improved prognosis of thoracic aortic aneurysms: a population-based study. *JAMA* 1998; 280(22): 1926-9.
41. LeMaire SA, Rice DC, Schmittling ZC, Coselli JS. Emergency surgery for thoracoabdominal aortic aneurysms with acute presentation. *J Vasc Surg* 2002; 35(6):1171-8.
42. Cambria RA, Gloviczki P, Stanson AW, Cherry KJ, Jr., Bower TC, Hallett JW, Jr. *et al.* Outcome and expansion rate of 57 thoracoabdominal aortic aneurysms managed nonoperatively. *Am J Surg* 1995; 170(2): 213-7.
43. Lewis ME, Ranasinghe AM, Revell MP, Bonser RS. Surgical repair of ruptured thoracic and thoracoabdominal aortic aneurysms. *Br J Surg* 2002; 89(4): 442-5.
44. Mastroroberto P, Chello M. Emergency thoracoabdominal aortic aneurysm repair: clinical outcome. *J Thorac Cardiovasc Surg* 1999; 118(3):477-81.
45. von Segesser LK, Genoni M, Kunzli A, Lachat M, Niederhauser U, Vogt P, *et al.* Surgery for ruptured thoracic and thoraco-abdominal aortic aneurysms. *Eur J Cardiothorac Surg* 1996; 10(11): 996-1001.
46. Bradbury AW, Bulstrode NW, Gilling-Smith G, Stansby G, Mansfield AO, Wolfe JH. Repair of ruptured thoracoabdominal aortic aneurysm is worthwhile in selected cases. *Eur J Vasc Endovasc Surg* 1999; 17(2): 160-165.
47. Lobato AC, Puech-Leao P. Predictive factors for rupture of thoracoabdominal aortic aneurysm. *J Vasc Surg* 1998; 27(3): 446-453.
48. Shimada I, Rooney SJ, Pagano D, Farneti PA, Davies P, Guest PJ, *et al.* Prediction of thoracic aortic aneurysm expansion: Validation of formulae describing growth. *Ann Thorac Surg* 1999; 67(6): 1968-1970.
49. Dapunt OE, Galla JD, Sadeghi AM, Lansman SL, Mezrow CK, de Asla RA, *et al.* The natural history of thoracic aortic aneurysms. *J Thorac Cardiovasc Surg* 1994; 107(5): 1323-32.
50. Hirose Y, Hamada S, Takamiya M. Predicting the growth of aortic aneurysms: a comparison of linear vs exponential models. *Angiology* 1995; 46(5): 413-9.
51. Davies RR, Goldstein LJ, Coady MA, Tittle SL, Rizzo JA, Kopf GS, *et al.* Yearly rupture or dissection rates for thoracic aortic aneurysms: simple prediction based on size. *Ann Thorac Surg* 2002; 73(1): 17-27.
52. Juvonen T, Ergin MA, Galla JD, Lansman SL, Nguyen KH, McCullough JN, *et al.* Prospective study of the natural history of thoracic aortic aneurysms.[erratum appears in *Ann Thorac Surg* 1997; 64(2): 594]. *Ann Thorac Surg* 1997; 63(6): 1533-1545.
53. Johansson G, Markstrom U, Swedenborg J. Ruptured thoracic aortic aneurysms: a study of incidence and mortality rates. *J Vasc Surg* 1995; 21(6): 985-988.
54. Strachan DP. Predictors of death from aortic aneurysm among middle-aged men: the Whitehall study. *Br J Surg* 1991; 78(4): 401-4.
55. Juvonen T, Ergin MA, Galla JD, Lansman SL, McCullough JN, Nguyen K, *et al.* Risk factors for rupture of chronic type B dissections. *J Thorac Cardiovasc Surg* 1999; 117(4): 776-786.
56. Griepp RB, Ergin MA, Galla JD, Lansman SL, McCullough JN, Nguyen KH, *et al.* Natural history of descending thoracic and thoracoabdominal aneurysms. *Ann Thorac Surg* 1999; 67(6): 1927-30.
57. Coselli JS, LeMaire SA, Conklin LD, Koksoy C, Schmittling ZC. Morbidity and mortality after extent II thoracoabdominal aortic aneurysm repair. *Ann Thorac Surg* 2002; 73(4): 1107-15.
58. Coselli JS, Conklin LD, LeMaire SA. Thoracoabdominal aortic aneurysm repair: review and update of current strategies. *Ann Thorac Surg* 2002; 74(5): S1881-S1884.
59. Coselli JS, LeMaire SA, Koksoy C, Schmittling ZC, Curling PE. Cerebrospinal fluid drainage reduces paraplegia after thoracoabdominal aortic aneurysm repair: results of a randomized clinical trial. *Ann Thorac Surg* 2002; 35(4): 631-639.
60. Khan SN, Stansby G. Cerebrospinal fluid drainage for thoracic and thoracoabdominal aortic aneurysm surgery (Cochrane review). *The Cochrane Library*, Issue 2, 2004. John Wiley & Sons, Ltd, Chichester, UK, 2003.
61. Kouchoukos NT, Rokkas CK. Hypothermic cardiopulmonary bypass for spinal cord protection: rationale and clinical results. *Ann Thorac Surg* 1999; 67(6): 1940-1942.
62. Kouchoukos NT, Masetti P, Rokkas CK, Murphy SF. Hypothermic cardiopulmonary bypass and circulatory arrest for operations on the descending thoracic and thoracoabdominal aorta. *Ann Thorac Surg* 2002; 74(5): S1885-S1887.
63. Svensson LG, Crawford ES, Hess KR, Coselli JS, Safi HJ. Variables predictive of outcome in 832 patients undergoing repairs of the descending thoracic aorta. *Chest* 1993; 104(4): 1248-1253.
64. Marsalese DL, Moodie DS, Vacante M, Lytle BW, Gill CC, Sterba R, *et al.* Marfan's syndrome: natural history and long-term follow-up of cardiovascular involvement. *J Am Coll Cardiol* 1989; 14(2): 422-8.

65. Hwa J, Richards JG, Huang H, McKay D, Pressley L, Hughes CF, *et al.* The natural history of aortic dilatation in Marfan syndrome. *Med J Aust* 1993; 158(8): 558-62.
66. Murdoch JL, Walker BA, Halpern BL, Kuzma JW, McKusick VA. Life expectancy and causes of death in the Marfan syndrome. *N Engl J Med* 1972; 286(15): 804-808.
67. Silverman DI, Burton KJ, Gray J, Bosner MS, Kouchoukos NT, Roman MJ, *et al.* Life expectancy in the Marfan syndrome. *Am J Cardiol* 1995; 75(2): 157-160.
68. Shores J, Berger KR, Murphy EA, Pyeritz RE. Progression of aortic dilatation and the benefit of long-term beta-adrenergic blockade in Marfan's syndrome. *N Engl J Med* 1994; 330(19): 1335-41.
69. Finkbohner R, Johnston D, Crawford ES, Coselli J, Milewicz DM. Marfan Syndrome: long-term survival and complications after aortic aneurysm repair. *Circulation* 1995; 91(3): 728-733.
70. Tambeur L, David TE, Armstrong S, Ivanov J, Webb G. Results of surgery for aortic root aneurysm in patients with the Marfan syndrome. *Eur J Cardiothorac Surg* 2000; 17(4): 415-419.
71. Doss M, Balzer J, Martens S, Wood JP, Wimmer-Greinecker G, Fieguth HG, *et al.* Surgical versus endovascular treatment of acute thoracic aortic rupture: a single-center experience. *Ann Thorac Surg* 2003; 76(5): 1465-1470.
72. Hutschala D, Fleck T, Czerny M, Ehrlich M, Schoder M, Lammer J, *et al.* Endoluminal stent-graft placement in patients with acute aortic dissection type B. *Eur J Cardiothorac Surg* 2002; 21(6): 964-9.
73. Demers P, Miller D, Mitchell R, Kee S, Sze D, Razavi M, *et al.* Midterm results of endovascular repair of descending thoracic aortic aneurysms with first-generation stent grafts. *J Thorac Cardiovasc Surg* 2004; 127(3):664-673.
74. Buffolo E, da Fonseca JHP, de Souza JAM, Alves CMR. Revolutionary treatment of aneurysms and dissections of descending aorta: the endovascular approach. *Ann Thorac Surg* 2002; 74(5): S1815-S1817.
75. Parodi JC, Palmaz JC, Barone HD. Transfemoral intraluminal graft implantation for abdominal aortic aneurysms. *Ann Vasc Surg* 1991; 5(6): 491-499.
76. Mitchell RS. Stent grafts for the thoracic aorta: a new paradigm? *Ann Thorac Surg* 2002; 74(5): S1818-S1820.
77. Smith RS, Chang FC. Traumatic rupture of the aorta: Still a lethal injury*1. *Am J Surg* 1986; 152(6): 660-663.
78. Galli R, Pacini D, Bartolomeo R, Fattori R, Turinetto B, Grillone G, *et al.* Surgical Indications and Timing of Repair of Traumatic Ruptures of the Thoracic Aorta. *Ann Thorac Surg* 1998; 65(2): 461-464.
79. Holmes IV, Bloch RD, Hall RA, Carter YM, Karmy-Jones RC. Natural history of traumatic rupture of the thoracic aorta managed nonoperatively: a longitudinal analysis. *Ann Thorac Surg* 2002; 73(4): 1149-1154.
80. Langanay T, Verhoye JP, Corbineau H, Agnino A, Derieux T, Menestret P, *et al.* Surgical treatment of acute traumatic rupture of the thoracic aorta a timing reappraisal? *Eur J Cardiothorac Surg* 2002; 21(2):282-7.
81. Kwon CC, Gill IS, Fallon WF, Yowler C, Akhrass R, Temes RT, *et al.* Delayed operative intervention in the management of traumatic descending thoracic aortic rupture. *Ann Thorac Surg* 2002; 74(5): S1888-S1891.
82. Pierangeli A, Turinetto B, Galli R, Caldarera I, Fattori R, Gavelli G. Delayed treatment of isthmic aortic rupture. *Cardiovascular Surgery* 2000; 8(4): 280-283.
83. Laks H, Myers J, Odim J, Plunkett M, MD. Adult Congenital Heart Disease. In: *Cardiac Surgery in the Adult.* Cohn LH, Edmunds LH Jr, Eds. McGraw-Hill, New York, 2003: 1329-1358.
84. Knyshov GV, Sitar LL, Glagola MD, Atamanyuk MY. Aortic aneurysms at the site of the repair of coarctation of the aorta: a review of 48 Patients. *Ann Thorac Surg* 1996; 61(3): 935-939.
85. von Kodolitsch Y, Aydin MA, Koschyk DH, Loose R, Schalwat I, Karck M, *et al.* Predictors of aneurysmal formation after surgical correction of aortic coarctation. *J Am Coll Cardiol* 2002; 39(4): 617-624.
86. Fawzy ME, Awad M, Hassan W, Al Kadhi Y, Shoukri M, Fadley F. Long-term outcome (up to 15 years) of balloon angioplasty of discrete native coarctation of the aorta in adolescents and adults. *J Am Coll Cardiol* 2004; 43(6): 1062-1067.
87. Mehta RH, Suzuki T, Hagan PG, Bossone E, Gilon D, Llovet A, *et al.* Predicting death in patients with acute type A aortic dissection. *Circulation* 2002; 105(2): 200-206.
88. Ehrlich M, Grabenwoeger M, Cartes-Zumelzu F, Grimm M, Petzl D, Lammer J, *et al.* Endovascular stent graft repair for aneurysms on the descending thoracic aorta. *Ann Thorac Surg* 1998; 66(1): 19-24.
89. Shimono T, Kato N, Yasuda F, Suzuki T, Yuasa U, Onoda K, *et al.* Transluminal Stent-Graft Placements for the Treatments of Acute Onset and Chronic Aortic Dissections. *Circulation* 2002; 106(90121): 241l-247.

Chapter 24

Diagnosis and treatment of infective endocarditis

Brian M Fabri MD FRCS (Ed)
Consultant Cardiac Surgeon
David R Ramsdale MD FRCP
Consultant Cardiologist

THE CARDIOTHORACIC CENTRE, LIVERPOOL, UK

Introduction

Infective endocarditis (IE) is an uncommon condition. The yearly incidence in developed countries is reported to be between 1.8 and 6.2 per 100,000 of the population [1-5]. The incidence increases after 30 years of age and exceeds 10 per 100,000 for people aged over 50 years [6-10]. Despite improved diagnostic techniques, modern antibiotics and surgical therapy, it remains a life-threatening disease with a substantial morbidity and mortality (~20%) [11]. Prosthetic valve endocarditis (PVE) (incidence 0.1-2.3 per patient year), carries an even higher mortality rate [12-14]. Prevention of endocarditis is therefore of paramount importance [15].

Methodology

An electronic search of MEDLINE revealed 8,844 publications written in English between 1964 and 2002. Where possible, the strength of evidence and the recommendations drawn from it are classified according to the definitions used by the Scottish Intercollegiate Guidelines Network [16], derived from the US Agency for Health Care Policy and Research.

Pathology

Infective endocarditis predominantly affects individuals with underlying structural cardiac defects [17]. The incidence and risk of IE associated with various cardiac structural abnormalities or following cardiac surgical and interventional procedures has been well documented in the literature [18,19]. Experimental studies suggest that endothelial damage leads to platelet and fibrin deposition resulting in a non-bacterial thrombotic endocardial lesion [20-23]. Surgical / dental procedures or instrumentation involving mucosal surfaces contaminated by organisms can cause a bacteraemia. Bacteria settle on damaged or abnormal heart valves or on the damaged endocardium close to anatomic defects, resulting in endocarditis or endarteritis and the pathologic hallmark of IE - vegetations [24]. Vegetations are made up of masses of organisms enmeshed with fibrin, platelets, and a variable inflammatory cell infiltrate.

Patients at risk

Currently, patients with prosthetic cardiac valves, intravenous drug abusers and patients with mitral valve prolapse or other non-rheumatic heart disease (congenital heart defects, bicuspid aortic valves), account for most cases of IE [17,25-29], although rheumatic heart disease is still responsible for approximately 40-50% of cases. Such patients are at increased risk when undergoing invasive procedures. Elderly patients, chronic alcoholics, patients with chronic inflammatory bowel disease, poor dental hygiene, chronic haemodialysis, those with diabetes mellitus and those on immunosuppressive treatment are also at increased risk of IE [5,30-41]. Left-sided cardiac structures are most commonly affected (85% of cases): isolated aortic lesions in 55-60%, isolated mitral lesions in 25-30% and mitral and aortic lesions in 15% of cases. Right-sided IE accounts for only 10-15% of cases.

Symptoms and clinical findings

The clinical manifestations of IE depend on the nature of any predisposing condition, the type and virulence of the responsible organism and the portal of entry [42]. Typically, patients with acute IE present with an accelerated illness with high remitting pyrexia, rigors and prostration [43,44]. It is usually caused by virulent pathogens such as *Staph. aureus* and pre-existing valve disease can be minimal. In contrast, patients with subacute IE have a more insidious presentation with anorexia, weight loss, fever, chills, myalgia, arthralgia and fatigue [44,45]. It usually affects patients with major pre-existing heart valve defects and is caused by less virulent pathogens such as the viridans streptococci.

Cardiac manifestations

The clinical picture is usually dominated by cardiac manifestations with the presence of new or worsening cardiac murmurs or the development of heart failure resulting from advanced valvular infection and destruction [43,47,48]. Eighty per cent of patients present with a murmur whilst 15-20% develop one in hospital [49,50]. Pre-existing cardiac disease is found in 60-75% of cases of left-sided endocarditis, but is rarer in right-sided disease. The degree of valvular destruction depends on the organism responsible, the duration of infection and its anatomic site. It may consist of ulceration, tear and rupture of chordae tendineae and perforation of the cusps themselves, resulting in moderate or severe regurgitation [51]. Typically, vegetations occur on the atrial surface of the mitral valve, on the ventricular surface of the aortic valve, distal to a coarctation of the aorta, in the pulmonary artery in association with a patent ductus and on the right side of a ventricular septal defect. Occasionally, all four valves are affected and mural endocarditis occurs [52]. Abscesses of the heart are observed in 20-40% of cases, mainly in the aortic valve ring [53-57]. They can spread to surrounding structures such as the aorta, the anterior mitral valve leaflet and the interventricular septum, and can result in fistulae between the two ventricles, between the aorta and left atrium, between the left ventricle and the right atrium and even into the pericardial cavity causing tamponade [58-61]. These complications are associated with a high mortality [62]. Septal abscesses can cause progressive conduction defects evidenced by prolongation of the PR interval and complete heart block [63]. Conduction defects are more often associated with prosthetic (PVE) than native valve endocarditis (NVE) and more with native aortic than mitral valve endocarditis. Aortic root abscesses may produce a sinus of Valsalva aneurysm or involve the coronary ostia. Occasionally, chest pain due to pleurisy, pericarditis or myocardial infarction resulting from coronary arterial embolism can be a presenting symptom [64-67]. An inflammatory or septic pericardial effusion is more usually found in patients with aortic valve endocarditis, but pericardial abscess may occur as a result of infection on the mitral valve [55]. Primary involvement of the myocardium can occur with reduction in contractility, ST-T wave abnormalities and ventricular arrhythmias. Sudden death can occur when free wall myocardial abscesses rupture [68,69].

Extracardiac manifestations

Extracardiac clinical manifestations consist of embolic (13-40%) as well as vasculitic phenomena due to immune-complex deposition [66,70,71]. Embolic infarcts in the kidneys or spleen, present with focal pain in the flanks or left upper quadrant. Retinal and peripheral limb emboli also occur. Splenomegaly is found in 30-50% of patients [53,70,72]. Splenic abscesses can be fatal when they rupture [73,74]. Abdominal CT or MRI scans appear to be the best diagnostic tests for a splenic abscess, which if diagnosed, requires an urgent splenectomy.

Neurological manifestations

Neurological manifestations may be the presenting feature [5,75]. These include any symptoms and signs associated with focal cerebral infarcts, cerebritis or abscess, haemorrhage or mycotic aneurysm, including simple headache, confusion, stroke, or seizures [76-79]. Meningism/meningitis may occur and CSF cultures may be positive [80]. These are particularly serious and life-threatening features with a mortality rate of 40%.

Vascular, embolic or immune-mediated phenomena

Other vascular or immune-mediated phenomena may occur including petechiae, splinter haemorrhages (5-15%), retinal haemorrhages, Roth spots (5-10%), painful Osler's nodes (5-10%), painless red Janeway lesions on the palms and soles and finger clubbing – which occurs late in 10-20% of patients. Mycotic aneurysms, which occur in up to 15% of patients who have IE, involve mainly the sinuses of Valsalva, the cerebral and carotid arteries, the branches of the abdominal aorta (the mesenteric arteries, renal artery) and more rarely, limb and coronary arteries [3,65,81-91]. They occasionally rupture, causing subarachnoid or intraventricular haemorrhage or other vascular catastrophies [92-95]. Intracranial mycotic aneurysms (1.2-5% of cases) have an overall mortality of 60%, but 80% if rupture should occur [65,93,96-98]. Contrast-enhanced CT scanning and 3-D magnetic resonance imaging may provide adequate information, but angiography remains the diagnostic imaging test of choice [96,99].

Deposits of immune complexes with complement along the renal glomerular basement membrane may cause a focal or diffuse glomerulonephritis. This can be diagnosed by renal biopsy with appropriate glomerular staining [100-102]. Arthritis and Osler's nodes have also been attributed to the local deposit of immune complexes [103-107]. Besides immune complex glomerulonephritis and septic renal infarcts, haemodynamic instability as well as antibiotic, drug and contrast medium toxicity can also be responsible for acute renal failure and indicates a poor prognosis.

Emboli are more likely to occur with enterococci, staphylococci, Gram-negative aerobic bacilli and fungi, with large mobile vegetations and especially when the mitral valve is affected. They tend to occur early, usually before hospital admission or within the first two weeks of therapy. Fifty percent of all emboli occur within 20 days and 80% within the first month of the initial symptoms of IE. Embolic complications tend to be recurrent, especially if vegetations persist on echocardiography. In >50% of cases, recurrence of a thromboembolic event occurs within 30 days. Up to 65% of embolic events involve the central nervous system, the majority involving the middle cerebral artery territory, and are associated with a high mortality [108].

Right-sided endocarditis

The tricuspid is more frequently involved (80%) than the pulmonary valve (20%) in patients with right-sided endocarditis. Pulmonary infarcts are often followed by lung abscesses and pleural effusions may occur [109-112]. Haemoptysis can be fatal [95]. Peripheral emboli and immunologic vascular phenomena are unusual with right-sided disease. The main cause is intravenous drug abuse, but others include pacemaker infection, infected central lines, skin and gynaecological infections and bacteraemia in patients with congenital cardiac defects [113,114]. In patients with intravenous drug abuse, the prognosis of right-sided IE is favourable (4-5% mortality), but recurrence is frequent (30%) [115,116]. When IE is associated with infection of pacemakers, central lines or other foreign bodies such as septal occluder devices or tube grafts, the device needs to be removed in order to maximize the chance of successful treatment with antimicrobial therapy which is required for four to six weeks [117].

Prosthetic valve endocarditis

When mechanical valves are affected (5-15% of all cases in developed countries), abscesses are particularly frequent, extending beyond the prosthetic ring into the annulus and peri-annular tissue. Conduction system disturbance and even purulent pericarditis are serious complications. The diagnosis requires a high index of suspicion [118]. Ring or septal abscess, fistulous tracts and dehiscence of the prosthesis are frequent autopsy findings. Vegetations can interfere with disc function causing obstruction and/or regurgitation. In bioprosthetic valve IE, the anatomic lesions vary between limited leaflet infection and disseminated infection [119].

The microbiology of early PVE (<60 days) (0.4-1.2% of cases) and of those occurring within the first year of surgery is characteristic [120,121]. *Staph. aureus* and *Staph. epidermidis* predominate (45-50%), followed by Gram-negative aerobic bacilli and fungi. Streptococci and enterococci are less common, accounting for <10% of cases. Contamination can occur intra-operatively (via the wound or the extracorpoeal circulation) or postoperatively (intravenous catheters, arterial lines, urethral catheters, endotracheal tubes). Coagulase-negative staphylococci predominate, particularly *Staph. epidermidis* - an increasing number of which are methicillin-resistant. *Staph. aureus* PVE carries a high mortality and surgery should be considered early [122]. In late PVE (>60 days), the bacteriology more closely resembles that of community-acquired NVE [5,123], although staphylococci are still important causative organisms. The incidence may be higher in tissue than mechanical valves [124].

Fungal endocarditis

Fungal endocarditis is frequently characterized by negative blood cultures and a lack of physical signs [125-129]. Candida or aspergillus infection are the commonest causes. Fever, changing murmurs and the presence of peripheral embolism are the most common signs. Although blood cultures are generally negative, 83-95% are positive in those with candida infection. Culture of a peripheral arterial embolus may provide the diagnosis and the specimen should be examined microscopically for hyphae. Routine serology has been useful in deep-seated cryptococcosis and histoplasmosis. Although candida precipitins and aspergillus antigens and antibodies might provide supportive diagnostic evidence of fungal infection, their sensitivity and specificity are disappointing [130-133]. Fungal vegetations are frequently large (10-30mm diameter), bulky, friable and valvular or endocardial in position [134]. Echocardiography and transoesophageal echocardiography (TOE) in particular, are most important in establishing an aetiological diagnosis, for defining the anatomical extent of the valvular disease and for guiding the surgical strategy [135]. Emboli are frequently large and multiple, cause considerable functional and neurological damage and are associated with a high mortality [129]. Metastatic abscesses are another frequent complication - the heart and kidneys being involved most commonly [136,137]. Medical treatment combined with early surgery is the mainstay of treatment. Surgery should be performed as soon as the bulky vegetations are identified in order to prevent the high rate (68%) of embolisation. Fungal endocarditis may complicate prolonged antibiotic treatment of PVE and prophylactic oral nystatin may be valuable [138].

Blood culture-negative endocarditis

Blood culture-negative endocarditis (CNE)(5-10%) is usually due to patients having been treated with antibiotics prior to the blood cultures being taken. Other causes include fungal infections, fastidious slow-growing organisms eg. *Brucella* spp, *Neisseria* spp, *Legionella* spp, *Nocardia* spp, *Mycoplasma* spp, cell-dependent organisms eg. *Bartonella* spp, *Chlamydia* spp, *Histoplasma* spp and *Coxiella burnetii* and "non-infective" endocarditis as seen in systemic lupus erythematosus and in terminal malignant disease ("marantic endocarditis") [139-150]. However, systemic lupus erythematosus and IE can co-exist [151].

Some of the more unusual infections have clinical features that are suggestive. For example, Q-fever endocarditis often occurs in patients in contact with farm animals, frequently involving the aortic valve, but also the mitral and prosthetic valves. Liver involvement, thrombocytopaenia and purpura are common [152,153]. Vegetations are usually small. Brucella endocarditis is also found in patients in contact with cattle and goats, usually farmers and veterinary surgeons [154]. Again the aortic valve is more frequently affected and aneurysms of the sinus of Valsalva with intramyocardial spread is common. Serological tests (antibodies, precipitins) may be helpful in these situations, particularly for rickettsia such as *Coxiella* or *Chlamydia* [155]. Although *Coxiella* (a strict intracellular Gram-negative micro-organism) may be found by Giemsa staining of the excised valve, endocarditis is best diagnosed by IgG (>1/800) and

IgA (>1/100) titres to phase I antigen using the microimmunofluorescence (MIF) test [155-157]. For *Brucella* spp (a facultative intracellular Gram-negative bacillus), high titres of specific IgG and IgM antibodies by tube agglutination are diagnostic. Bacterial polymerase chain reaction (PCR) analysis can be crucial in confirming the diagnosis in CNE eg. *Tropherema whipelli* or *Bartonella* spp and such molecular analysis has been recently implemented into the newest revision of the Duke criteria [158,159]. These additional tests may not only improve the sensitivity of the diagnosis, but may also improve the outcome by increasing the specificity of the antibiotic treatment.

Investigations

Mild to moderate anaemia with a normochromic, normocytic picture is commonly present. Neutrophil leucocytosis is common and the ESR and CRP are elevated in 90% of patients [160-163]. Intraleucocyte bacteria can be seen in buffy coat preparations of blood in up to 50% of cases [164].

Microscopic haematuria and/or proteinuria occur in 50% of cases. In those developing immune complex glomerulonephritis, red blood cell casts and heavy proteinuria may be present. Frequent renal function monitoring is essential to detect dysfunction early. A polyclonal increase in gammaglobulins is characteristic of active endocarditis and an elevated rheumatoid factor may be of diagnostic help [165,166].

An ECG and chest x-ray are useful for assessing the extent and severity of the infection, its effects on cardiac size and function and for determining whether surgery may need to be considered early or whether prophylactic temporary pacemaker implantation is indicated. Significant conduction abnormalities, classically seen in the presence of aortic root abscesses, especially if new or progressive, warrant urgent temporary pacing.

A chest x-ray may show evidence of cardiomegaly and heart failure. In tricuspid valve endocarditis from intravenous drug abuse or in patients with serious permanent pacemaker infection, the chest radiograph may show infective pulmonary emboli and pulmonary abscesses.

Infection-related antiphospholipid antibodies may help in predicting risk of embolic events and the application of PCR technology to blood and tissue samples may be useful for identifying more unusual pathogens causing IE [167-171].

When valve replacement is undertaken, valvular tissue should be examined histologically and cultured for the presence of organisms that may allow postoperative antibiotics to be tailored accordingly. Bacterial DNA probe analysis of explanted tissue and amplification by PCR may be an alternative to histology and culture.

The key tests, however, are blood cultures and echocardiography.

Blood cultures

Between three and six sets of blood cultures should be obtained at intervals of over one hour within the first 24 hours from all patients suspected of having IE before commencing antibiotic treatment. Three sets of blood cultures should be taken if the patient is extremely unwell and the clinical features suggest that IE is very likely, and six sets if the patient is not acutely sick or when the diagnosis is not obvious clinically. Optimal aseptic technique is necessary to avoid false positive cases due to contaminating organisms from the skin [172,173]. Each set of blood cultures should be taken via a separate venepuncture.

The bacteraemia associated with IE is typically continuous, with 10-200 colony-forming units per ml of blood [174]. The number of positive culture results is directly related to the number of blood samples drawn and the volume of blood in each individual sample. Single samples should never be relied upon because the most common contaminants, coagulase-negative staphylococci can be responsible for IE and a positive culture will be difficult to interpret [175]. Ideally, cultures should be spaced at least 60 minutes apart to prove that bacteraemia is continuous. Blood cultures should be stored in an incubator at 37°C and not in a refrigerator. The possibility of IE should be made clear on the request form.

In general, about two-thirds of blood cultures are positive in patients with IE. Those patients with untreated IE and continuous bacteraemia will generally have positive culture results in all samples [176]. Ninety percent will be diagnosed by the first sample and 95% after three cultures [175-177]. Other patients will have a much lower incidence of positive cultures. These include patients who have already received antibiotic treatment, those with fungal endocarditis or with "difficult-to-culture" micro-organisms and those with CNE [178]. Blood cultures may be negative in as many as 25% of patients who received recent outpatient antibiotic therapy and it may be prudent to delay treatment (dependent on the patient's clinical status) in order to maximize the chance of obtaining positive blood cultures [179-182]. Culturing arterial rather than venous blood and drawing blood during spikes of temperature does not appear to be of any additional value [183]. When blood cultures are negative because of previous antibiotic therapy, the period of time required for the blood cultures to become positive again, varies from 24 hours to two weeks depending on the activity of the antibiotic against the organism and the duration of prior treatment. If treatment has been received for only 2-3 days, cultures will probably revert to positive quickly. It is important to indicate on the request form whether antibiotics have been received by the patient so that special culture methods for unusual micro-organisms, lysis centrifugation techniques or serology may be considered.

The yield of positive cultures of "slow-growing" organisms such as nutritionally variant streptococci (approximately 5% of streptococci in IE) and the fastidious Gram-negative aerobic bacilli such as *Haemophilus* spp. or *Bartonella* spp., may be improved by prolonged incubation (7-21 days) or by using optimized blood culture media [184-188]. The microbiology laboratory should be informed when such organisms are suspected.

Echocardiography

Echocardiography is the most useful tool for confirming the anatomical diagnosis and for demonstrating vegetations on valves or other structures [189-196]. It should be performed by appropriately trained echocardiographers.

Transthoracic M-mode echocardiography (TTE) has a specificity of 98%, a sensitivity of 60-75% and should be performed early in all patients clinically suspected of having IE, including those with negative blood cultures [197-201].

Transoesophageal echocardiography has proved most valuable in assessing patients with suspected IE - being more sensitive (95%) than TTE for detecting and sizing vegetations, abscesses, pseudoaneurysms and valvular perforations [191-206]. The absolute sensitivity depends upon the site and the size of the abnormalities [194,207-209].

TOE using biplanar and multiplanar probes with colour flow, continuous and pulse-wave Doppler is more sensitive than TTE for detecting abscesses in patients with both NVE and PVE (87% versus 28%) [210-212]. TOE is the technique of choice in evaluating a patient with suspected PVE (since it is more likely to demonstrate a perivalvular abscess, dehiscence and fistulas), for those with NVE who have a prolonged course of infection, for those with endocarditis at unusual sites eg. pacemaker leads, and for those who do not respond to adequate medical therapy [191,205,210-218]. It is perhaps more useful in biological PVE rather than mechanical PVE, as it is often difficult to interpret images because of intense interfering echoes from mechanical prostheses [219].

Echocardiography also provides information on left ventricular function and an estimate of the severity of regurgitant flow [220-222]. Moreover, repeat echocardiography is often useful for early detection of cardiac complications requiring surgical intervention.

For suspected NVE, a TTE should be performed initially. If the TTE is technically inadequate, then a TOE should be undertaken. If the TTE is clearly positive or clearly negative, no further echo is necessary. However, a TOE should be performed if the TTE is abnormal but non-diagnostic.

Cardiac catheterisation

The use of invasive catheter techniques is usually limited to coronary arteriography in those with a history of angina or risk factors for coronary artery disease and for the identification of fistulous communications between chambers if echocardiography is inconclusive. However, there is a risk of systemic embolisation if contact is made with loose or friable vegetations and crossing potentially infected aortic valves should be avoided [223].

Criteria for diagnosis of infective endocarditis

Criteria for the diagnosis of IE were proposed by Von Reyn and colleagues [224] depending upon the results of symptoms, clinical signs and blood cultures, and subsequently refined by Durack *et al* [225]. They take into account information obtained by echocardiography and introduce the concept of major and minor diagnostic features and are known as the Duke Criteria (Table 1).

The individual value of each of the Duke criteria for the diagnosis of IE has been studied and modified but echo data, serology and culture of excised tissue appear to improve the specificity and sensitivity of the diagnostic criteria [188,206,220-222,224-236]. Comparison has been made between the Duke and other criteria (Beth Israel) for the diagnosis of IE and although the modified Duke criteria appear to be superior, confirmatory studies are few and small [237,238].

More recently, it has been proposed that PCR amplification of specific gene targets and universal loci for bacteria and fungi and subsequent sequencing to identify the possible causative organisms in blood culture and excised tissue, should be considered as a major Duke criterion [239]. Such molecular methods have been validated in the diagnosis of CNE and recently included into the newest revision of the Duke criteria [159,240].

The diagnosis of "definite" IE requires the presence of two major or one major plus three minor criteria, or five minor criteria and has a specificity of around 99% and sensitivity of >80% [225,241].

Treatment

IE continues to cause significant mortality (20%) so prevention is a high priority. However, the early diagnosis and adequate treatment based on appropriate antibiotic therapy and in many cases cardiac surgery, is also of paramount importance.

Prophylaxis

Antimicrobial prophylaxis before selected procedures in patients at risk has become routine in most countries, despite the fact that there is no prospective study that proves that such therapy is definitely beneficial [242-244]. Animal experiments and some human studies have however suggested benefit from prophylactic antibiotics [245]. Current "best practice" continues to favour the use of antibiotic prophylaxis of selected patients at risk of IE who are undergoing procedures that can cause bacteraemia [246,247]. Guidelines have been published by expert groups both in Europe [15,248] and USA [249] and the differences in recommendations are minor.

Antimicrobial therapy for infective endocarditis

General management

IE requires prompt treatment with appropriate antibiotics, administered parenterally in doses sufficient to eradicate the organism from the blood, from vegetations and from local or metastatic foci of infection. Parenteral administration is essential to ensure complete bioavailability, high serum concentrations and good penetration into the vegetations.

The type and duration of antibiotic treatment is based on the organism responsible, its sensitivity, a history of penicillin allergy and whether the valve involved is a native or a prosthetic valve [250,251]. Microbiological consultation is advisable. Very high densities of organisms protected from host defences exist inside vegetations (10^9-10^{10} per gram), and cure requires sterilization of vegetations with bactericidal agents in high concentrations for long enough duration [252,253]. Usually, this requires a combination of antimicrobials with synergistic activity, such as a cell-wall-active agent (B-lactams and glycopeptides) and an aminoglycoside.

Table 1. Duke criteria and terminology used in the modified diagnostic criteria.

1. **Definite infective endocarditis**

Pathological criteria

- Micro-organisms: demonstrated by culture or histology in a vegetation that has embolised, or in a intracardiac abscess, or
- Pathologic lesions: vegetation or intracardiac abscess present, confirmed by histology showing active endocarditis.

Clinical criteria (see below)

- 2 major criteria, or
- 1 major and 3 minor criteria, or
- 5 minor criteria

2. **Possible infective endocarditis**

- Findings consistent with IE that fall short of "definite", but not "rejected"

3. **Rejected**

- Firm alternate diagnosis for manifestations of endocarditis, or
- Resolution of manifestations of endocarditis, with antibiotic therapy for 4 days or less, or
- No pathological evidence of IE at surgery or autopsy, after antibiotic therapy for 4 days or less

DEFINITIONS

Major criteria

1. Positive blood culture for IE

- Isolation of micro-organism known to cause IE from two separate blood cultures eg. viridans streptococci, *Strep. bovis*, *Staph. aureus*, *Staph. epidermidis*, enterococci, *Haemophilus* spp, *Actinobacillus* spp. etc
- Persistently positive blood culture - defined as recovery of a micro-organism consistent with endocarditis from:-
  - (i) at least two blood cultures drawn more than 12 hrs apart, or
  - (ii) all of three or a majority of four or more separate blood cultures, with first and last drawn at least one hr apart

2. Evidence of endocardial involvement

- Positive echo for IE:-
  - (i) mobile intracardiac mass on valve or supporting structures or in path of regurgitant jet, or on implanted material without any alternative anatomical explanation, or
  - (ii) abscess, or
  - (iii) new partial dehiscence of prosthetic valve, or new valve regurgitation

3. Clinical evidence of new valvular regurgitation
4. Positive serology for Q-fever and other causes of culture-negative endocarditis eg. *Bartonella* spp, *Chlamydia psittaci*.
5. Positive identification of a micro-organism from blood culture or excised tissue using molecular biology methods

Minor criteria

1. Predisposition: predisposing heart condition or IV drug abuse
2. Fever: >38.0°C
3. Vascular phenomena: major arterial emboli, septic pulmonary infarcts, mycotic aneurysm, intracranial haemorrhage, conjunctival haemorrhages, Janeway lesions, *newly diagnosed clubbing, splinter haemorrhages, splenomegaly* *
4. Immunologic phenomena: glomerulonephritis, Osler's nodes, Roth spots, +ve rheumatoid factor, *high ESR (>1.5 times upper limit of normal), high C-reactive protein level(>100mg/l)* *
5. Microbiologic evidence: positive blood culture, but not meeting major criteria as defined above

* additional modifications to the Duke criteria appear to improve diagnostic sensitivity whilst retaining specificity.

Dosing regimens

For B-lactams and glycopeptides with time-dependent activity and no post-antibiotic effect, serum levels must be maintained throughout the dosing interval to prevent re-growth of bacteria between doses. This interval is determined by the rate of drug elimination and the serum half-life. Benzylpenicillin and anti-staphylococcal penicillins should be administered every 3-4 hours. Ceftriaxone, which has a long serum half-life (eight hours), can be administered once a day in the case of highly susceptible organisms such as viridans streptococci. Vancomycin and teicoplanin are administered every 12 or 24 hours respectively, after a loading dose for teicoplanin because of its long half-life. Aminoglycosides can be administered twice a day for Gram-negative bacilli endocarditis, but are needed three times daily for Gram-positive and enterococcal endocarditis.

Maximising effectiveness of anti-microbial treatment

In evaluating the potential efficacy of an antibiotic, the MIC, or the minimum concentration that inhibits bacterial growth *in vitro*, must be considered [254]. With most streptococci or staphylococci, the MIC and minimal bactericidal concentration (MBC) of cell-wall active antibiotics (penicillins, cephalosporins and vancomycin) do not differ significantly [255]. However, the MBCs of these antibiotics are much higher than the MICs for a minority of strains of streptococci and staphylococci, and for many strains of enterococci. When the difference is 10-fold or more, or when the MBC/MIC ratio is >32, the strains are said to be tolerant which indicates a slower rate of kill [256]. Tolerance can be overcome by addition of an aminoglycoside, resulting in a more rapid bactericidal activity [257-259]. In the treatment of enterococcal endocarditis an aminoglycoside must be added to amoxicillin or ampicillin to obtain adequate bactericidal effect and cure, although this is probably not essential in tolerant streptococcal or staphylococcal infection [260-263]. Serum drug level monitoring during aminoglycoside therapy is recommended. Gentamicin peak serum concentration (one hour post-intravenous dose) should be 6-10mg/L, but the trough level should be <2.0mg/L to avoid renal or ototoxic effects. Optimum vancomycin effects are achieved if serum concentrations are kept at least two to four times above the MIC of the causative organism. Trough levels should be 10-15mg/L.

The frequency of dosing varies, depending on the organism and the antibiotic(s) being used and whether or not a post-antibiotic effect exists. Intravenous antibiotics should be commenced as soon as the diagnosis is made and after appropriate blood culture samples have been collected and sent to the microbiology laboratory. Initially, intravenous benzylpenicillin and gentamicin in the same dosage as for treatment of IE caused by penicillin-sensitive viridans streptococci should be used. If there is a strong possibility of staphylococcal infection (intravenous drug abuse, infected haemodialysis lines or pacemaker infection), then intravenous flucloxacillin and/or vancomycin should be considered instead of benzylpenicillin. Once the blood culture results are available, treatment can be modified and a decision made about its duration. In patients recently receiving antibiotics, treatment may be delayed for a few days so as to increase the chance of isolating the responsible organism on subsequent blood cultures. Such delay is only reasonable in closely monitored patients with subacute illness who have no evidence of severe or progressive valve dysfunction, heart failure or embolic complications.

Isolating the infecting organism is extremely important, so that an appropriate antimicrobial agent can be chosen and the antimicrobial susceptibility of the organism can be established. Both MIC and MBC may be useful, although there is no data to suggest that MBC is any better than the more simple and reproducible MIC test. The routine determination of MBC is therefore not recommended [264].

A peak serum bactericidal titre of 1:8 or greater usually indicates an adequate therapeutic effect. A peak bactericidal titre of 1/64 and a trough of 1/32 represents optimal therapy [265]. Determination of the titre is only useful when the response to treatment with recommended regimens is suboptimal, when IE is due to an unusual micro-organism or when an unconventional treatment regimen is used [261].

Specific treatment regimens

Specific treatment regimens for the less common micro-organisms and fungi are beyond the scope of this chapter but are available in the literature.

Prosthetic valve endocarditis

In early PVE, *Staph. epidermidis* and *Staph. aureus* are the most frequent organisms responsible. Vegetations are generally larger than those found in NVE and prosthetic material protects organisms against antimicrobial treatment, both making sterilization with antibiotics extremely difficult [266,267]. Consequently, antibiotics have to be used in dosages which result in maximum but non-toxic serum concentrations, in order to penetrate the vegetations, and the duration of treatment must also be longer. Antibiotic sterilization of large vegetations is unlikely with organisms that have a high MIC. A minimum of two months intravenous therapy may cure some cases but most will require further valve surgery and a further month's intravenous treatment. Beyond six months, the organisms causing "late" PVE are not dissimilar to those responsible for NVE [268]. When PVE is clinically apparent and blood cultures are not yet positive, empiric treatment should be initiated with intravenous vancomycin and gentamicin.

PVE has a poor prognosis and demands prompt and careful assessment of the need for early surgical intervention [268-275]. TOE is essential in order to recognise the presence of vegetations on the prosthesis and for diagnosing periprosthetic abscess formation, fistulas and prosthetic valve dysfunction not seen on a transthoracic study.

Surgery should be considered urgently in patients with PVE due to aggressive organisms such as *Staph. aureus*, those who fail to respond immediately to antibiotics, those with large periprosthetic leaks or abscesses, fistula formation and false aneurysms, vegetations on the prosthesis, new-onset conduction disturbance, heart failure due to prosthetic valve dysfunction and fungal infection [276-281].

It is generally a forlorn hope that these situations will be cured by medical treatment alone, but occasionally, medical treatment alone may be appropriate [270,282-288]. Conservative management can be considered in patients in whom the diagnosis is made early, those with streptococcal infection, a prompt antibiotic response, favourable TOE findings such as small or absent vegetations and in those with no periprosthetic abscesses or prosthetic dysfunction. However, these patients require careful clinical monitoring and should be reconsidered for surgery if complications arise – as happens not infrequently [270,286]. Patients in whom surgery is contraindicated or who refuse to consent for surgery may also be managed medically, but mortality is significant (26-70%) [289,290].

Other aspects of treatment

Penicillin allergy

Patients with a convincing history of immediate-type (IgE-mediated) hypersensitivity reaction to penicillin, including urticarial rash or angioneurotic oedema, should not receive penicillin, cephalosporin or other B-lactam antibiotics. Vancomycin or teicoplanin should be substituted and given with gentamicin, although the risk of nephrotoxicity increases and requires careful monitoring.

Monitoring of plasma drug levels

Most treatment regimens require regular monitoring of plasma antimicrobial concentrations. Peak and trough levels should be checked twice weekly, but more frequently in the elderly and in those with renal or hepatic impairment, in order to minimize the risk of toxicity and to ensure that bactericidal concentrations are maintained [291]. Monitoring of drug levels will generally require close liaison with the microbiologist.

Response to treatment

Patients should be monitored frequently to assess the response to treatment, to detect complications promptly and to reappraise the need for surgical intervention. Assessment should include clinical examination, ECG, blood count, ESR and CRP, renal and liver function tests and repeat echocardiograms.

Most patients improve during the first week of effective antimicrobial therapy. CRP values usually decrease rapidly during the first or second week but may remain slightly elevated for four to six weeks. A persistently elevated CRP suggests inadequately controlled infection with cardiac or septic complications. ESR is less useful for reflecting the therapeutic response, since high values may persist over several weeks despite clinical improvement. Persistence or recurrence of fever may not only be due to inadequate therapy, but also to myocardial or metastatic abscesses, recurrent emboli, venous thrombosis extending from the site of venous cannulation, superinfection or febrile reaction to the antibiotics (a common recurrence of fever) [292]. Persisting bacteraemia indicates persisting infection.

If a rash develops, the antibiotics should be changed unless the antimicrobial therapy options are very limited.

Weight gain, improvement of appetite and a rise in haemoglobin may not occur for weeks after treatment and splenomegaly takes months to resolve. New or changing heart murmurs due to valvular destruction may occur during or after therapy and must be sought by regular physical examination during the period of treatment. Heart failure may develop and is the principal cause of death, especially in aortic valve endocarditis. The natural history of vegetations during successful medical treatment of IE has been described by Vuille *et al* [293]. Echocardiography should be performed at any time during the course of treatment if the symptoms or physical signs change and at the end of treatment to document the site and extent of valvular damage and as a baseline for long-term follow-up.

Mycotic aneurysms may regress on antimicrobial therapy or rupture weeks or years later. Central nervous system symptoms/physical signs suggest cerebral aneurysm formation with leakage or enlargement and demand urgent investigation and treatment. Renal insufficiency from glomerulonephritis usually improves with treatment but not always, and a specialist opinion should be sought early.

Relapse/new episodes

If a primary focus responsible for IE is identified, it should be eliminated prior to an elective cardiac surgical procedure in an attempt to prevent relapse. Following medical or surgical treatment of IE, all patients require careful follow-up for signs of clinical relapse or haemodynamic deterioration. Most relapses occur within two months of stopping treatment and especially within four weeks. The reported relapse rate is <2% for streptococcal IE in native valves, but is considerably higher for virulent organisms such as staphylococci and enterococci (8-20%) and for PVE (10-15%). Difficult-to-treat organisms such as *Brucella, Chlamydia* and *Bartonella* and polymicrobial IE seen in drug abusers are associated with an increased relapse rate. Blood cultures two to four weeks after completion of treatment detect most relapses. Delayed relapses may occur with fungal and Q-fever endocarditis. When relapse occurs in patients with PVE after a course of medical therapy, a perivalvular infection is usually present and further surgery is usually required [294].

Surgery in patients with active infective endocarditis: indications, timing and results

Indications of surgery

Medical treatment alone can cure many patients with IE [295]. However, in 25-30% of patients, medical treatment alone is insufficient and must be combined with surgery. Surgery is indicated in patients with life-threatening congestive heart failure [296] or cardiogenic shock due to surgically treatable valvular heart disease. This applies even in cases of unproven IE if the patient has reasonable prospects of recovery and a satisfactory quality of life after surgery. Cardiac failure in patients with IE, managed with only medical treatment, carries a mortality of over 50% [295]. Many studies show that surgical intervention improves the prognosis of IE over medical treatment alone and a high early surgery rate is associated with good long-term results and no increase in-hospital mortality [17,297-302]. However, there are no randomised trials of medical versus surgical treatment and the conclusions that have emerged, although often well supported by case studies, can only be rated as evidence grade B. Surgery should be postponed or avoided if serious complications make the prospect of recovery unlikely.

In patients with stable haemodynamics, the indications for surgery for IE are less clear and depend also on whether native or prosthetic valves are involved. Early consultation with a cardiac surgeon is advisable in case the need for surgery becomes emergent. Surgery is indicated in patients with annular or aortic abscesses, those with fungal endocarditis and those with infections resistant to antibiotics. Indeed, persisting fever often represents an abscess of the valve ring and surrounding structures or widespread tissue destruction, and generally necessitates surgical intervention [303-305]. Peri-annular extension occurs in 10-40% of all NVE and complicates aortic IE more commonly than mitral or tricuspid IE [306-308]. It occurs in 56-100% of patients with PVE [309]. However, penicillin hypersensitivity is also a common cause of recurrent fever, with rash and eosinophilia suggesting such a reaction. Neutropenia and impaired renal function may suggest toxic overdosing. In such instances the fever usually disappears promptly after drug withdrawal. The emergence of antibiotic resistance in the infecting organism is seldom a cause and if the bacteria have been cultured and the patient given appropriate bactericidal antibiotics, then the temptation to change the treatment should be resisted. Patients with a vegetation >10mm in diameter have a significantly higher incidence of embolisation than those with smaller vegetations [310]. The risk is higher in mitral (25%) compared to aortic (10%) disease, especially if the anterior mitral leaflet is involved. However, surgery on the basis of vegetation size alone is controversial. Valvular vegetations can be identified and sized by echocardiography, especially TOE. Early surgery should be considered for aortic/mitral kissing vegetations.

Surgery is usually indicated if there is a history of prior systemic embolisation, recurrent emboli, persistent vegetation after a major systemic embolus or an associated perivalvular abscess. This is especially the case in patients who have endocarditis caused by *Staph. aureus*, fungi or *Haemophilus* spp.

Many of the important issues concerning the surgical management of PVE have been the subject of discussions and review articles [311-319]. Acute valvular regurgitation with pulmonary oedema, dehiscence of a prosthetic valve and abscess formation are absolute indications for surgery. Patients with PVE should have their warfarin replaced by heparin in case urgent surgery is required. Anticoagulant therapy is potentially hazardous in patients with IE [320].

Abdominal and splenic abscesses should be dealt with before cardiac surgery is undertaken.

In intravenous drug addicts with tricuspid valve endocarditis and tricuspid regurgitation, large vegetations can be treated by tricuspid valve repair, tricuspid valvectomy or vegetectomy [321-324].

Infection with certain organisms (fungi, *Coxiella burnetii* and enterococci for which there is no synergistic bactericidal combination) rarely respond to medical treatment alone and usually require surgery.

Timing of surgery

If early surgery is indicated in the course of active IE such as severe aortic regurgitation and progressive pulmonary oedema, there is little evidence that there is anything to be gained by delaying intervention for prolonged periods of antibiotics [325-327]. The frequency of early relapse and/or prosthetic infection after surgery is low [328,329]. However, the optimal timing of surgery remains controversial if heart failure improves, although two weeks of antibiotic therapy is generally considered ideal [330].

Early surgery for PVE reduces mortality even when the period of pre-operative antibiotic treatment has been brief [331,332]. Although ten days of antibiotic therapy prior to surgery is desirable, surgery should not be delayed as postoperative endocarditis is surprisingly uncommon [333,334].

The optimal timing of surgery after a cerebral embolism is often unclear because heparinization during bypass may exacerbate the clinical course of a recent cerebral infarction [335,336]. Ideally, ten days should be allowed to elapse in patients who have sustained a cerebral infarct although surgical results are good within the first 72 hours [337-340]. At least three weeks should be allowed to elapse in those who have

Table 2. Indications for surgery for native and prosthetic valve endocarditis.

Native

- Acute AR or MR with heart failure
- Acute AR with tachycardia and early closure of the mitral valve
- Fungal endocarditis.
- Annular or aortic abscess, true aneurysm of the sinus of valsalva, true or false aneurysm of the aorta
- Evidence of valvular dysfunction and persistent infection after a prolonged period (7-10 days) of appropriate antibiotics, as indicated by presence of **fever**, **leukocytosis**, **bacteraemia** – assuming that there are no non-cardiac causes for infection
- Recurrent emboli after appropriate antibiotic therapy
- Mobile vegetations >10mm diameter
- Early infection of the mitral valve - that can be repaired
- Persistent pyrexia and leukocytosis with negative blood cultures
- Relapse after an adequate course of antibiotics

Prosthetic

- Early prosthetic valve endocarditis (<2 months)
- Heart failure with prosthetic valve dysfunction
- Fungal endocarditis
- Staphylococcal endocarditis unresponsive to antibiotics
- Paravalvar leak, annular or aortic root abscess
- Sinus or aortic true/false aneurysm, fistula formation
- Infection with Gram -ve organisms or organisms with a poor response to antibiotics
- Persistent bacteraemia after 7-10 days of antibiotics
- Recurrent peripheral embolus
- Vegetation on prosthesis
- New-onset conduction disturbance
- Relapse after an adequate course of antibiotics

had an intracranial haemorrhage. CAT and MRI scanning should be performed prior to any possible surgery in order to exclude cerebral haemorrhage in patients with neurological signs or symptoms [341,342]. Contemporary approaches to the management of neurosurgical complications of IE have been presented in the literature [343-345].

The indications for surgery for NVE and PVE are shown in Table 2 [346-350]. Whether antibiotic-impregnation of heart valve sewing rings prevents IE or is useful in the surgical treatment of IE, remains unclear at present [351].

Results of surgery

Operative mortality varies from 4%-30%. The highest risk and poorest outcome appears to be in patients with *Staph. aureus* infection, heart failure, a perivalvular abscess or aortic root abscess as well as those with endocarditis due to certain Gram-negative aerobic bacilli (*E. coli*, *Serratia* spp., *P. aeruginosa*), fungi, *Staph. aureus* and *Staph. epidermidis* which are resistant to penicillin and sometimes methicillin [352,353]. Early surgical intervention is required in many of these cases, but the mortality may still be >20% [354]. Among patients who have NVE, survival ranges from 70%-80% at five years although it is less optimistic in those with PVE, where surgical treatment is generally better than medical therapy alone [355]. A relapse rate of IE of 5%-10% occurs when surgery is performed in the acute phase of the disease and paravalvular regurgitation occurs in 5-15% of cases. Long-term results of surgical treatment of active infective aortic valve endocarditis with associated peri-annular abscess have been recently presented [356,357].

The relative benefit of homografts or mechanical prostheses both in the short or long-term remains debatable. Randomised trials, although difficult in such circumstances, would be necessary to settle this issue [286,358-375]. Allograft aortic root replacement is a valuable technique in the complex setting of PVE with peri-annular involvement [364,373]. Antibiotics should be continued after surgery. The duration depends on the length of treatment pre-operatively, the susceptibility of the micro-organism to antibiotics, the presence of paravalvular lesions and the culture status of vegetations or valve removed.

Prognosis

The determinants of early and late survival in patients with IE have been well documented [376]. Several factors worsen the prognosis of IE and early surgical intervention may be necessary [377].

Clinical factors include old age, the presence of heart failure, renal failure, neurological symptoms, systemic emboli and delay in diagnosis. Persistent fever beyond the first week of treatment often indicates the development of complications such as progressive valve destruction, annular extension, development of perivalvular abscess or the presence of septic emboli.

Bacteriological factors include the causative organism with a worse prognosis if *Staph aureus*, certain Gram-negative aerobic bacilli or fungi are involved. These often present as acute IE and produce severe intracardiac destruction and major embolic complications. Early surgical intervention is frequently required and the mortality rate is >20% [43].

Echocardiographic factors include aortic valve endocarditis, PVE and ring abscesses when persisting infection is more likely and surgery often inevitable [216]. The presence of recent, large (>10mm), very mobile, pedunculated vegetations increase the risk of systemic embolisation which may significantly affect prognosis.

The cure rate for NVE is >90% for streptococci, 75-90% for enterococci and 60-75% for *Staph. aureus* [261,263,378]. The usual causes of death are heart failure, emboli, rupture of mycotic aneurysms, postoperative complications, renal failure and overwhelming infection. The prognosis is worse in PVE, and on rare occasions, only heart transplantation can resolve intractable infection on prosthetic valves [271]. Late PVE has a better prognosis than early PVE with mortality rates of 19-50% and 41-80% respectively [268,272-275,379]. Valvular dysfunction, dehiscence and intracardiac abscesses are commoner in early infection and the antibiotic-resistant micro-organisms associated with early disease contribute to the higher mortality.

In 1995, Delahaye *et al* reported on the long-term prognosis of IE [380]. In their series (1970-1986), global survival was 75% at six months and 57% at five years with an annual instantaneous risk of death being 0.55 at six months, 0.18 at one year and 0.03 thereafter. After one year, the only factor that influenced prognosis was age. The risk of recurrence appears to be 0.3-2.5/100 patient/years [380,381]. Castillo *et al* (1987-1997) reported a 5-year survival of 71% [301]. In NVE, 5-year survival has been reported to be 88-96% in contrast to PVE where 5-year survival rate is between 60-82% [301,382,383]. Late PVE may have 5-year survival rates of between 80-82% [301,384].

The long-term results of multivalvular surgery for IE have been recently reported [385].

Conclusions

IE is a life-threatening disease with substantial morbidity and mortality (=20%) despite improved techniques to aid diagnosis, modern antibiotics and surgical therapy (see recommendations).

Acknowledgements

We acknowledge the expertise of Prof. Tom SJ Elliott, Dr. Paul Wright, Prof. Graham J Roberts, Dr. Peter Wallace, Dr. Nicholas Palmer and Dr. Petros Nihoyannopoulos, whose opinions and advice are reflected herein.

Recommendations	Evidence level
◆ The diagnosis of IE should always be suspected in sick patients with known cardiac disease or new cardiac murmurs. The patient should be admitted to hospital for full investigation, including blood cultures, temperature monitoring, haematological and biochemical investigation, ECG, chest x-ray and echocardiography. If the diagnosis is confirmed by blood culture, the patient should be referred to an experienced cardiologist and the microbiologist should be involved from the outset.	III/C
◆ If transthoracic echocardiography is suboptimal, transoesophageal echocardiography (TOE) should be considered to obtain further information on the size, site or mobility of vegetations, abscess or fistula formation or valve perforation. TOE should be performed in all patients with PVE.	III/C
◆ The majority of NVE and of late PVE are caused by viridans streptococci (50-70%), *Staphylococcus aureus* (25%) and enterococci (10%). In early PVE, *Staphylococcus epidermidis* and *Staphylococcus aureus* are the commonest organisms.	III/C
◆ Once the diagnosis is established, treatment should be commenced according to published guidelines or with alternative antibiotics if microbiological tests suggest more appropriate agents are suitable. In a sick patient, antibiotic treatment should be commenced immediately after blood cultures have been collected and the regimen adjusted once the microbiological data is available. Generally, prolonged intravenous antibiotic therapy is necessary, administered via a large central vein. Only the most penicillin-sensitive streptococci should be considered for treatment with shorter courses of penicillin.	III/C
◆ CNE requires close scrutiny for unusual and slow-growing organisms and fungi. Serological tests for *Coxiella burnetii, Bartonella* spp and *Chlamydia* spp should be performed if the diagnosis is still suspected and there is still no growth after seven days. Microscopy and culture of any excised tissue is essential. Molecular assay for specific gene targets and universal loci for bacteria and fungi and subsequent sequencing may be applied to blood culture or excised material to help identify the causative organism. Treatment should involve antibiotics that are appropriate for the most likely organism for the particular clinical scenario, but should generally cover Gram-positive and Gram-negative organisms. Patients with a history of penicillin-allergy or who develop penicillin-allergy should be treated with (or changed to) vancomycin, teicoplanin and gentamicin or other appropriate antibiotics.	III/C
◆ Susceptible patients should be informed of the risk of IE and the need for antibiotic prophylaxis. They should inform any doctor or dentist who is responsible for providing care and they should carry a card reminding them of the importance of the risk and how to avoid IE. Patients at moderate or high risk of IE should be given antibiotic prophylaxis with appropriate antibiotics based upon the type of dental or surgical procedure being performed.	III/C

Recommendations continued.	**Evidence level**
◆ In haemodynamically-stable patients, early consultation with a cardiac surgeon is recommended in case surgery is required urgently. Patients with life-threatening congestive heart failure, left heart failure or cardiogenic shock due to treatable valvular disease should undergo emergency cardiac surgery, if the patient has reasonable prospects of recovery and a satisfactory quality of life. Surgery is indicated in patients with annular or aortic abscess, in those with infections resistant to antibiotics and in those with fungal endocarditis. Large mobile vegetations and recurrent emboli after appropriate antibiotic therapy are also indications for surgery and patients with PVE will generally require repeat operative intervention.	III/C

References

1. van der Meer JT, Thompson J, Valkenburg HA, Michel MF. Epidemiology of bacterial endocarditis in the Netherlands. 1. Patient Characteristics. *Arch Intern Med* 1992; 152: 1863-8.
2. Delahaye F, Goulet V, Lacassin F, *et al.* Epidemiology of infective endocarditis in France in 1991. *Arch Mal Coeur* 1993; 86(Suppl 12): 180-6.
3. Horstkotte D, Piper C. Endocarditis. In: *Textbook of acquired heart valve disease*, vol II. Acar J, Bodnar E, Eds. ICR Publishers, London, 1995: 596-677.
4. Karchmer AW. Infective endocarditis. *Braunwald's Heart Disease*, 5th ed, vol 2. WB Saunders, Philadelphia, 1997; 1077-104.
5. Mylonakis E, Calderwood SB. Infective endocarditis in adults. *N Engl J Med* 2001; 345: 1318-30.
6. O'Callaghan C, McDougall P. Infective endocarditis in neonates. *Arch Dis Child* 1988; 63: 53-7.
7. Lorber A, Luder AS, Dembo L. Acute bacterial endocarditis in early infancy. *Int J Cardiol* 1987; 17: 343-5.
8. Fukushige J, Igarashi H, Ueda K. Spectrum of infective endocarditis during infancy and childhood: 20 year review. *Pediatr Cardiol* 1994; 15: 127-31.
9. Dommisse J. Infective endocarditis in pregnancy. A report of 3 cases. *S Afr Med J* 1988; 73: 186-7.
10. Selton-Suty C, Hoen B, Grentzinger A, *et al.* Clinical and bacteriological characteristics of infective endocarditis in the elderly. *Heart* 1997; 77: 260-3.
11. Bouza E, Menasalvas A, Munoz P, *et al.* Infective endocarditis - a prospective study at the end of the twentieth century: new predisposing conditions, new etiologic agents and still a high mortality. *Medicine* 2001; 80: 298-307.
12. Schulz R, Werner J, Fuchs B, *et al.* Clinical outcome and echocardiographic findings of native and prosthetic valve endocarditis in the 1990s. *Eur Heart J* 1996; 17: 281-8.
13. Netzer ROM, Zollinger E, Seiler C, *et al.* Infective endocarditis: clinical spectrum, presentation and outcome. An analysis of 212 cases 1980-1995. *Heart* 2000; 84: 25-30.
14. Piper C, Korfer R, Horstkotte D. Prosthetic valve endocarditis. *Heart* 2001; 85: 590-3.
15. Leport C, Horstkotte D, Burckhardt D and the Group of Experts of the International Society for Chemotherapy. Antibiotic prophylaxis for infective endocarditis from an international group of experts towards a European consensus. *Eur Heart J* 1995; 16(Suppl B): 126-31.
16. Scottish Intercollegiate Guidelines Network (SIGN). http://www.sign.ac.uk
17. McKinsey DS, Ratts TE, Bisno AL. Underlying cardiac lesions in adults with infective endocarditis: The changing spectrum. *Am J Med* 1987; 82: 681-8.
18. Michel PL, Acar J. Native cardiac disease predisposing to infective endocarditis. *Eur Heart J* 1995; 16(Suppl B): 2-6.
19. de Gevigney G, Pop C, Delahaye JP. The risk of infective endocarditis after cardiac surgical and interventional procedures. *Eur Heart J* 1995; 16: (Suppl B) 7-14.
20. Ferguson DJ, McColm AA, Savage TJ, *et al.* A morphological study of experimental rabbit staphylococcal endocarditis and aortitis. I. Formation and effect of infected and uninfected vegetations on the aorta. *Br J Exp Pathol* 1986; 67: 667-78.
21. Ferguson DJP, McColm AA, Ryan DM, Acred P. A morphological study of experimental staphylococcal endocarditis and aortitis. II. Inter-relationship of bacteria, vegetation and cardiovasculature in established infections. *Br J Exp Pathol* 1986; 67: 679-86.
22. Lopez JA, Ross RS, Fishbein MC, Siegel RJ. Non bacterial thrombotic endocarditis. A review. *Am Heart J* 1987; 113: 773-84.
23. Rodbard S. Blood velocity and endocarditis. *Circulation* 1963; 27: 18-25.
24. Livornese IL Jr., Korzeniowski O. Pathogenesis of infective endocarditis. In: *Infective endocarditis*. Second edition. Kaye D, Ed. Raven Press, New York, 1992: 19-35.

25. Reisberg BE. Infective endocarditis in the narcotic addict. *Prog Cardiovasc Dis* 1979; 22: 193-204.
26. Korzeniowski OM, Kaye D. Infective endocarditis. In: *Heart Disease - A Textbook of Cardiovascular Medicine*, 4th Edition. Braunwald E, Ed. W.B. Saunders Co., PA, USA, 1992: 1078-1105.
27. Bayliss R, Clarke C, Oakley CM, Somerville W, Whitfield AG, Young SE. The microbiology and pathogenesis of infective endocarditis. *Br Heart J* 1983; 50: 513-9.
28. Piper C, Horstkotte D, Schulte HD, Schultheib HP. Mitral valve prolapse and infection: a prospective study for risk calculation. *Eur Heart J* 1996; 17: 210.
29. Bansal RC, *et al.* Infective endocarditis. *Med Clin North Am* 1995; 79: 1205-40.
30. Kaye D. Changing pattern of infective endocarditis. *Am J Med* 1985; 78(Suppl 6B): 157-62.
31. Buchbinder NA, Roberts WC. Alcoholism: an important but unemphasised factor predisposing to infective endocarditis. *Arch Intern Med* 1973; 132: 689-92.
32. Beales IL, Ledson M. Endocarditis in chronic liver disease. *Am J Gastroenterol* 1994; 89: 2279.
33. Kreuzpaintner G, Horstkotte D, Heyll A, *et al.* Increased risk of bacterial endocarditis in inflammatory bowel disease. *Am J Med* 1992; 92: 391-5.
34. Cross AS, Steigbigel RJ. Infective endocarditis and access site infections in patients on hemodialysis. *Medicine* 1976; 55: 453-66.
35. Dobkin JF, Miller MH, Steigbigel NH. Septicaemia in patients on chronic haemodialysis. *Ann Intern Med* 1978; 88: 28-33.
36. Rayfield EJ, Ault MJ, Keusch GT, *et al.* Infection and diabetes: The case for glucose control. *Am J Med* 1982; 72: 439-50.
37. Gallagher PG, Watanakunakorn C. Group B streptococcal endocarditis: Report of seven cases and review of the literature, 1962-1985. *Rev Infect Dis* 1986; 8: 175-88.
38. Wilkinson NM. Fatal bacterial endocarditis following aortic valve replacement in a patient being treated with methotrexate. *J Heart Valve Dis* 1999; 8: 591-2.
39. Hearn CJ, Smedira NG. Pulmonic valve endocarditis after orthotopic liver transplantation. *Liver Transpl Surg* 1999; 5: 456-7.
40. Strom BL, Abrutyn E, Berlin JA, *et al.* Risk factors for infective endocarditis: oral hygiene and non-dental exposure. *Circulation* 2000; 102: 2842-8.
41. Steckelberg JM and Wilson WR. Risk factors for infective endocarditis. *Infect Dis Clin North Am* 1993; 7: 9-19.
42. Bayer AS, Bolger AF, Taubert KA, *et al.* Diagnosis and management of infective endocarditis and its complications. *Circulation* 1998; 98: 2936-48.
43. Chambers HF, Korzeniowski OM, Sande MA. *Staphylococcus aureus* endocarditis: clinical manifestations in addicts and non-addicts. *Medicine* 1983; 62: 170-7.
44. Espersen F, Frimodt-Moller N. *Staphylococcus aureus* endocarditis. A review of 119 cases. *Arch Intern Med* 1986; 146: 1118-21.
45. Terpenning MS, Buggy BP, Kauffman CA. Infective endocarditis: clinical features in young and elderly patients. *Am J Med* 1987; 83: 626-34.
46. Durack DT. Infective and non-infective endocarditis. In: *The heart, arteries and veins.* 7th edn. Hurst JW, Ed. McGraw-Hill, New York, 1990: 1230-55.
47. Varma MP, McCluskey DR, Khan MM, *et al.* Heart failure associated with infective endocarditis. A review of 40 cases. *Br Heart J* 1986; 55: 191-7.
48. Mills J, Utley J, Abbott J. Heart failure in infective endocarditis: predisposing factors, course and treatment. *Chest* 1974; 66: 151-7.
49. Smith RH, Radford DJ, Clark RA, Julian DG. Infectious endocarditis: a survey of cases in the South East region of Scotland between 1969 and 1972. *Thorax* 1976; 31: 373-9.
50. Lerner PI, Weinstein L. Infective endocarditis in the antibiotic era. *N Engl J Med* 1966; 274: 199-206; 259-66; 388-93.
51. Weinstein L. Life-threatening complications of infective endocarditis and their management. *Arch Intern Med* 1986; 146: 953-7.
52. Lam D, Emilson B, Rapaport E. Four-valve endocarditis with associated right ventricular mural vegetations. *Am Heart J* 1988; 115: 189-92.
53. Thomas D, Desruennes M, Jault F, Isnard R, Gandjbakhch I. Cardiac and extracardiac abscesses in infective endocarditis. *Arch Mal Coeur* 1993; 86 (Suppl 12): 1825-37.
54. Arnett EN, Roberts WC. Valve ring abscess in active endocarditis. Frequency, location and clues to clinical diagnosis from the study of 95 necropsy patients. *Circulation* 1976; 54: 140-5.
55. Sandler MA, Kotler MN, Bloom RD, Jacobson L. Pericardial abscess extending from mitral vegetation: an unusual complication of infective endocarditis. *Am Heart J* 1989; 118: 857-9.
56. Oakley CM. Perivalvular abscesses in infective endocarditis. *Eur Heart J* 1999; 20: 170-1.
57. Hwang SW, Yucel EK, Bernard S. Aortic root abscess with fistula formation. *Chest* 1997; 111: 1436-8.
58. Piper C, Hetzer R, Korfer F, *et al.* The importance of secondary mitral valve involvement in primary aortic valve endocarditis: the mitral kissing vegetation. *Eur Heart J* 2002; 23: 79-86.
59. Vaghjimal A, Lutwick LI, Chapnick EK, Greengart A. Interventricular septal endocarditis. *South Med J* 1998; 91: 43-4.
60. Behnam R. Aortico-left atrial fistula in aortic valve endocarditis. *Chest* 1992; 102: 1271-3.
61. Anguera I, Quaglio G, Miro JM, *et al.* Aortocardiac fistulas complicating infective endocarditis. *Am J Cardiol* 2001; 87: 652-4.
62. Bussani R, Sinagra G, Poletti A, *et al.* Cardiac tamponade: an unusual, fatal complication of infective endocarditis. *G Ital Cardiol* 1999; 29: 1512-6.
63. DiNubile MJ, Calderwood SB, Steinhaus DM, Karchmer AW. Cardiac conduction abnormalities complicating native valve active infective endocarditis. *Am J Cardiol* 1986; 58: 1213-7.
64. McDonald CL, Crafton EM, Covin FA, *et al.* Pericarditis: a probable complication of endocarditis due to *Haemophilus influenzae. Clin Infect Dis* 1994; 18: 648-9.

65. Wilson WR, Giuliani ER, Danielson GK, Geraci JE. Management of complications of infective endocarditis. *Mayo Clinic Proc* 1982; 57: 162-70.
66. Perera R, Noack S, Dong W. Acute myocardial infarction due to septic coronary embolism. *N Engl J Med* 2000; 342: 977-8.
67. Jeremias A, Casserly I, Estess JM, *et al.* Acute myocardial infarction after aortic valve endocarditis. *Am J Med* 2001; 110: 417-8.
68. Anguera I, Quaglio G, Ferrer B, *et al.* Sudden death in Staphylococcus aureus-associated infective endocarditis due to perforation of a free-wall myocardial abscess. *Scand J Infect Dis* 2001; 33: 622-5.
69. Shackcloth MJ, Dihmis WC. Contained rupture of a myocardial abscess in the free wall of the left ventricle. *Ann Thorac Surg* 2001; 72: 617-9.
70. Ting W, Silverman NA, Arzouman DA, Levitsky S. Splenic septic emboli in endocarditis. *Circulation* 1990; 82(Suppl IV): 105-9.
71. Millaire A, Leroy O, Gaday V, *et al.* Incidence and prognosis of embolic events and metastatic infections in infective endocarditis. *Eur Heart J* 1997; 18: 677-84.
72. Weinstein L, Rubin RH. Infective endocarditis. *Prog Cardiovasc Dis* 1973; 16: 239-74.
73. Lutwick LI, Gradon JD, Chapnick EK, *et al. Haemophilus parainfluenzae* endocarditis treated with vegetectomy and complicated by late, fatal splenic rupture. *Pediatr Infect Dis J* 1991; 10: 778-81.
74. Pringle SD, McCartney AC, Cobbe SM. Spontaneous splenic rupture as complication of infective endocarditis. *Int J Cardiol* 1988; 19: 384-6.
75. Heiro M, Nikoskelainen J, Engblom E, *et al.* Neurological manifestations of infective endocarditis: a 17-year experience in a teaching hospital in Finland. *Arch Intern Med* 2000; 160: 2781-7.
76. Salgado AV, Furlan AJ, Keys TF, *et al.* Neurologic complications of endocarditis: a 12-year experience. *Neurology* 1989; 39: 173-8.
77. Delahaye JP, Poncet P, Malquarti V, *et al.* Cerebrovascular accidents in infective endocarditis: role of anticoagulation. *Eur Heart J* 1990; 11: 1074-8.
78. Weeks SG, Silva C, Auer RN, *et al.* Encephalopathy with staphylococcal endocarditis: multiple neuropathological findings. *Can J Neurol Sci* 2001; 28: 260-4.
79. Cabell CH, Pond KK, Peterson GE, *et al.* The risk of stroke and death in patients with aortic and mitral valve endocarditis. *Am Heart J* 20901; 142: 75-80.
80. Kelly J, Barnass S. *Staphylococcus aureus* endocarditis presenting as meningitis and mimicking meningococcal sepsis. *Int J Clin Pract* 1999; 53: 306-7.
81. Hubautt JJ, Albat B, Frapier JM, Chaptal PA. Mycotic aneurysm of the extracranial carotid artery: an uncommon complication of bacterial endocarditis. *Ann Vasc Surg* 1997; 11: 634-6.
82. Silver SG. Ruptured mycotic aneurysm of the superior mesenteric artery that was due to Cardiobacterium endocarditis. *Clin Infect Dis* 1999; 29: 1573-4.
83. Ohebshalom MM, Tash JA, Coll D, *et al.* Massive hematuria due to right renal artery mycotic pseudoaneurysm in a patient with subacute bacterial endocarditis. *Urology* 2001; 58: 607.
84. Cakalagaoglu C, Keser N, Alhan C. Brucella-mediated prosthetic valve endocarditis with brachial artery mycotic aneurysm. *J Heart Valve Dis* 1999; 8: 586-90.
85. McKee MA, Ballard JC. Mycotic aneurysm of the tibio-peroneal arteries. *Ann Vasc Surg* 1999; 13: 188-90.
86. Mann CF, Barker SG. Occluded mycotic popliteal aneurysm secondary to infective endocarditis. *Eur J Vasc Endovasc Surg* 1999; 18: 169-70.
87. Safar HA, Cina CS. Ruptured mycotic aneurysm of the popliteal artery. A case report and review of the literature. *J Cardiovasc Surg* 2001; 42: 237-40.
88. Jhirad R, Kalman PG. Mycotic axillary artery aneurysm. *J Vasc Surg* 1998; 28: 708-9.
89. WilsonWR, Lie JT, Houser OW, *et al.* The management of patients with mycotic aneurysms. *Curr Clin Top Infect Dis* 1981; 2: 151.
90. Mansur AJ, Grinberg M, Leao PP, *et al.* Extracranial mycotic aneurysms in infective endocarditis. *Clin Cardiol* 1986; 9: 65-72.
91. Reece IJ, al Tareif H, Tolia J, Saeed FA. Mycotic aneurysm of the left anterior descending coronary artery after aortic endocarditis. A case report and brief review of the literature. *Tex Heart Inst J* 1994; 21: 231-5.
92. Krapf H, Skalej M, Voight K. Subarachnoid hemorrhage due to septic embolic infarction in infective endocarditis. *Cerebrovasc Dis* 1999; 9: 182-4.
93. Bohmfalk GL, Story JL, Wissinger JP, Brown WE Jr. Bacterial intracranial aneurysm. *J Neurosurg* 1978; 48: 369-82.
94. Roach MR, Drake CG. Ruptured cerebral aneurysms caused by microorganisms. *N Engl J Med* 1965; 273: 240-4.
95. Cosmo LY, Risi G, Nelson S, *et al.* Fatal hemoptysis in acute bacterial endocarditis. *Am Rev Respir Dis* 1988; 137: 1223-6.
96. Camarata PJ, Latchaw RE, Rufenacht DA, Heros RC. Intracranial aneurysms. *Invest Radiol* 1993; 28: 373-82.
97. Lerner P. Neurologic complications of infective endocarditis. *Med Clin North Am* 1985; 69: 385-98.
98. Clare CE, Barrow DL. Infectious intracranial aneurysms. *Neurosurg Clin N Am* 1992; 3: 551-566.
99. Huston J III, Nichols DA, Luetmer PH, *et al.* Blinded prospective evaluation of sensitivity of MR angiography to known intracranial aneurysms: importance of aneurysm size. *Am J Neuroradiol* 1994; 15: 1607-14.
100. McKinsey DS, McMurray TI, Flynn JM. Immune complex glomerulonephritis associated with *Staphylococcus aureus* bacteremia: response to corticosteroid therapy. *Rev Infect Dis* 1990; 12: 125-7.
101. Eknoyan G, Lister BJ, Kim HS, Greenberg SD. Renal complications of bacterial endocarditis. *Am J Nephrol* 1985; 5: 457-69.
102. Weinstein L, Schlesinger JJ. Pathoanatomic, pathophysiologic and clinical correlations in endocarditis. *N Engl J Med* 1974; 291: 832-7.
103. Roberts-Thomson PJ, Rischmueller M, Kwiatek RA, *et al.* Rheumatic manifestations of infective endocarditis. *Rheumatol Int* 1992; 12: 61-3.

104. Churchill MA Jr., Geraci JE, Hunder GG. Musculoskeletal manifestations of bacterial endocarditis. *Ann Intern Med* 1977; 87: 754-9.
105. Yee J, McAllister CK. The utility of Osler's nodes in the diagnosis of infective endocarditis. *Chest* 1987; 92: 751-2.
106. Watanakunakorn C. Osler's nodes on the dorsum of the foot. *Chest* 1988; 94: 1088-90.
107. Alpert JS, Krous HF, Dalen JE, *et al.* Pathogenesis of Osler's nodes. *Ann Intern Med* 1976; 85: 471-3.
108. Pruitt AA, Rubin RH, Karchmer AW, Duncan GW. Neurologic complications of bacterial endocarditis. *Medicine* 1978; 57: 329-43.
109. Robbins MJ, Soeiro R, Frishman WH, Strom JA. Right-sided valvular endocarditis: etiology, diagnosis and an approach to therapy. *Am Heart J* 1986; 111: 128-35.
110. Cassling RS, Rogler WC, McManus BM. Isolated pulmonic valve infective endocarditis: a diagnostically elusive entity. *Am Heart J* 1985; 109: 558-67.
111. Dressler FA, Roberts WC. Infective endocarditis in opiate addicts: analysis of 80 cases studied at necropsy. *Am J Cardiol* 1989; 63: 1240-57.
112. Sexauer WP, Quezado Z, Lippmann ML, Goldberg SK. Pleural effusions in right-sided endocarditis: characteristics and pathophysiology. *South Med J* 1992; 85: 1176-80.
113. Federmann M, Dirsch OR, Jenni R. Pacemaker endocarditis. *Heart* 1996; 75: 446.
114. Tang DC, Huang TP. Internal jugular vein haemodialysis catheter-induced right atrial endocarditis - case report and review of literature. *Scand J Urol Nephrol* 1998; 32: 411-4.
115. Hecht SR, Berger M. Right-sided endocarditis in intravenous drug users. *Ann Intern Med* 1992; 117: 560-6.
116. Chambers HF, Morris DL, Tauber MG, Modin G. Cocaine use and the risk for endocarditis in intravenous drug users. *Ann Intern Med* 1987; 106: 833-6.
117. Cacoub P, Leprince P, Nataf P, *et al.* Pacemaker infective endocarditis. *Am J Cardiol* 1998; 82: 480-4.
118. Arvay A, Lengyel M. Incidence and risk factors of prosthetic valve endocarditis. *Eur J Cardiothoracic Surg* 1988; 2: 340-6.
119. Bortolotti U, Thiene G, Milano A, *et al.* Pathological study of infective endocarditis on Hancock porcine bioprostheses. *J Thorac Cardiovasc Surg* 1981; 81: 934-42.
120. Horstkotte D, Korfer R, Loogen F, *et al.* Prosthetic valve endocarditis: clinical findings and management. *Eur Heart J* 1984; 5(Suppl C): 117-22.
121. Chastre J, Trouillet JL. Early infective endocarditis in prosthetic valves. *Eur Heart J* 1995; 16(Suppl B): 32-8.
122. John MD, Hibberd PL, Marchmer AS, *et al.* *Staphylococcus aureus* prosthetic valve endocarditis: optimal management and risk factors for death. *Clin Infect Dis* 1998; 26: 1302-9.
123. Braunwald E. Infective endocarditis, Chapter 35. In: *Heart Disease. A textbook of cardiovascular medicine*, 4th edition. WB Saunders Co, 1992: 1082.
124. Horstkotte D, Piper C, Niehues R, *et al.* Late prosthetic valve endocarditis. *Eur Heart J* 1995; 16(Suppl B): 39-47.
125. Rubinstein E, Lang R. Fungal endocarditis. *Eur Heart J* 1995; 16(Suppl B): 84-9.
126. Moyer DV, Edwards Jr. JE. Fungal endocarditis. In: *Infective endocarditis*, 2nd edn. Kaye D, Ed. Raven Press, New York, 1992: 299-312.
127. Kammer RB, Utz JP. Aspergillus species endocarditis: the face of a not so rare disease. *Am J Med* 1974; 56: 506-21.
128. Seelig MS, Speth CP, Kozinn PJ, *et al.* Patterns of Candida endocarditis following cardiac surgery: importance of early diagnosis and therapy (an analysis of 91 cases). *Prog Cardiovasc Dis* 1974; 17: 125-60.
129. Rubinstein E, Noriega ER, Simberkoff MS, Holzman R, Rahal Jr. JJ. Fungal endocarditis: analysis of 24 cases and review of the literature. *Medicine* 1975; 54: 331-44.
130. Microbiology Resource Committee, College of American Pathologists. Memorandum to CAP Mycology Survey participants re 1987 Survey set F-B. Traverse City, Michigan 1987.
131. Paya CV, Roberts GD, Cockerill RF. Laboratory methods for the diagnosis of disseminated histoplasmosis. *Mayo Clinic Proc* 1987; 62: 480-5.
132. Bisbe J, Miro JM, Torres JM, *et al.* Diagnostic value of serum antibody and antigen detection in heroin addicts with systemic candidiasis. *Rev Inf Dis* 1989; 11: 310-5.
133. Weiner MH. Antigenaemia detected by radioimmunoassay in systemic aspergillosis. *Ann Int Med* 1980; 92: 793-6.
134. Donal E, Abgueguen P, Coisne D, *et al.* Echocardiographic features of Candida species endocarditis: 12 cases and a review of published reports. *Heart* 2001; 86: 179-82.
135. Lengyel M. The impact of transesophageal echocardiography on the management of prosthetic valve edocarditis: experience of 31 cases and review of the literature. *J Heart Valve Dis* 1997; 6: 204-11.
136. Walsh TJ, Hutchins GM, Bulkley BH, *et al.* Fungal infections of the heart: analysis of 51 autopsy cases. *Am J Cardiol* 1980; 45: 357-66.
137. Andriole VT, Kravetz HM, Roberts WC, *et al.* Candida endocarditis. *Am J Med* 1962; 32: 251-85.
138. Gregg CR, McGee ZA, Bodner SJ, *et al.* Fungal endocarditis complicating treatment of prosthetic valve bacterial endocarditis: value of prophylactic oral nystatin. *South Med J* 1987; 80: 1407-9.
139. Oakley CM. The medical treatment of culture-negative infective endocarditis. *Eur Heart J* 1995; 16(Suppl B): 90-3.
140. Brouqui P, Raoult D. Endocarditis due to rare and fastidious bacteria. *Clin Microbiol Rev* 2001; 14: 177-207.
141. Rolain JM, Maurin M and Raoult D. Bactericidal effect of antibiotics on Bartonella and Brucella spp.: clinical complications. *J Antimicrob Chemother* 2000; 46: 811-4.
142. Popat K, Barnardo D, Webb-Peploe M. Mycoplasma pneumoniae endocarditis. *Br Heart J* 1980; 44: 111-2.
143. Al-Kasab S, al-Fagih MR, al-Yousef S, *et al.* Brucella infective endocarditis. Successful combined medical and surgical therapy. *J Thorac Cardiovasc Surg* 1988; 95: 862-7.
144. Shafer RW, Braverman ER. Q-fever endocarditis: delay in diagnosis due to an apparent clinical response to corticosteroids. *Am J Med* 1989; 86: 729.
145. Jones RB, Priest JB, Kuo C. Subacute chlamydial endocarditis. *JAMA* 1982; 247: 655-8.

146. Fernandez-Guerrero ML, Muelas JM, Aguado JM, *et al.* Q-fever endocarditis on porcine bioprosthetic valves. Clinicopathologic features and microbiologic findings in three patients with doxycycline, cotrimoxazole and valve replacement. *Ann Intern Med* 1988; 108; 209-13.
147. Brearley BF, Hutchinson DN. Endocarditis associated with *Chlamydia trachomatis* infection. *Br Heart J* 1981; 46: 220-1.
148. Noseda A, Liesnard C, Goffin Y, Thys JP. Q-fever endocarditis: relapse 5 years after successful valve replacement for a first unrecognized episode. *J Cardiovasc Surg* 1988; 29: 360-3.
149. Stein A, Raoult D. Q fever endocarditis. *Eur Heart J* 1985; 16(Suppl B): 19-23.
150. Cohen JI, Sloss LJ, Kundsin R, Golightly L. Prosthetic valve endocarditis caused by *Mycoplasma hominis. Am J Med* 1989; 86: 819-21.
151. Demiricin M, Dogan R, Peker O, *et al.* Aortic insufficiency and enterococcal endocarditis complicating systemic lupus erythematosus. *Thorac Cardiovasc Surg* 1995; 43: 302-4.
152. Houpikian P, Habib G, Mesana T, Raoult D. Changing clinical presentation of Q fever endocarditis. *Clin Infect Dis* 2000; 34: E 28-31.
153. Musso D, Raoult D. *Coxiella burnetii* blood cultures from acute and chronic Q-fever patients. *J Clin Microbiol* 1995; 33: 3129-32.
154. Akinci E, Gol MK, Balbay Y. A case of prosthetic mitral valve endocarditis caused by *Brucella abortus. Scand Infect Dis* 2001; 33: 71-2.
155. Raoult D, Urvolgyi J, Etienne J, *et al.* Diagnosis of endocarditis in acute Q-fever by immunofluorescence serology. *Acta Virol* 1988; 32: 70-4.
156. Muhlemann K, Matter L, Meyer B, *et al.* Isolation of *Coxiella burnetti* from heart valves of patients treated for Q-fever endocarditis. *J Clin Microbiol* 1995; 33: 428-31.
157. Siegman-Igra Y, Kaufman O, Kaysary A, *et al.* Q-fever endocarditis in Israel and a worldwide review. *Scand J Infect Dis* 1997; 29: 41-9.
158. Nikkari S, Gotoff R, Bourbeau PP, *et al.* Identification of *Cardiobacterium hominis* by broad-range bacterial polymerase chain reaction analysis in a case of culture-negative endocarditis. *Arch Intern Med* 2002; 162: 477-9.
159. Lisby G, Gutschik E, Durack DT. Molecular methods for diagnosis of infective endocarditis. *Infect Dis Clin North Am* 2002; 16: 393-412.
160. McCartney AC, Orange GV, Pringle SD, *et al.* Serum C reactive protein in infective endocarditis. *J Clin Pathol* 1988; 41: 44-8.
161. Hogevik H, Olaison L, Andersson R, Alestig K. C-reactive protein is more sensitive than erythrocyte sedimentation rate for diagnosis of infective endocarditis. *Infection* 1997; 25: 82-5.
162. Olaison L, Hogevik H, Alestig K. Fever, C-reactive protein, and other acute-phase reactants during treatment of infective endocarditis. *Arch Intern Med* 1997; 157: 885-92.
163. Lamas CC, Eykyn SJ. Suggested modifications to the Duke criteria for the clinical diagnosis of native valve and prosthetic valve endocarditis: analysis of 118 pathologically proven cases. *Clin Inf Dis* 1997; 25: 713-9.
164. Powers DL, Mandell GL. Intraleukocytic bacteria in endocarditis patients. *JAMA* 1974; 227: 312-3.
165. Williams RC. Rheumatoid factors in subacute bacterial endocarditis and other infectious diseases. *Scand J Rheumatol Suppl* 1988; 75: 300-8.
166. Asherson RA, Tikly M, Staub H, *et al.* Infective endocarditis, rheumatoid factor and cardiolipin antibodies. *Ann Rheum Dis* 1990; 49: 107-8.
167. Roggenkamp A, Leitritz L, Baus K, Falsen E, Heesemann J. PCR for detection and identification of *Abiotrophia spp. J Clin Microbiol* 1998; 36: 2844-6.
168. Goldenberger D, Kunzli A, Vogt P, Zbinden R, Altwegg M. Molecular diagnosis of bacterial endocarditis by broad-range PCR amplification and direct sequencing. *J Clin Microbiol* 1997; 35: 2733-9.
169. Qin X and Urdahl KB. PCR and sequencing of independent genetic targets for the diagnosis of culture negative bacterial endocarditis. *Diagn Miucrobiol Infect Dis* 2001; 40: 145-9.
170. Wilck MB, Wu Y, Howe JG, *et al.* Endocarditis caused by culture-negative organisms visible by Brown and Brenn staining: utility of PCR and DNA sequencing for diagnosis. *J Clin Microbiol* 2001; 39: 2025-7.
171. Watkin RW, Lang S, Lambert PA, Littler WA, Elliott TSJ. The microbial diagnosis of infective endocarditis. *J Infect* 2003; (in press)
172. Washington JA II. The role of the microbiology laboratory in the diagnosis and antimicrobial treatment of infective endocarditis. *Mayo Clin Proc* 1982; 57: 22-32.
173. Washington JA II. The microbiological diagnosis of infective endocarditis. *J Antimicrob Chemother* 1987; 20: 29-39.
174. Werner AS, Cobbs CG, Kaye D, Hook EW. Studies on the bacteremia of bacterial endocarditis. *JAMA* 1967; 202: 199-203.
175. Weinstein M, Reller L, Murphy J, Lichenstein K. Clinical significance of positive blood cultures: a comprehensive analysis of 500 episodes of bacteraemia and fungemia in adults. I. Laboratory and epidemiologic observations. *Rev Infect Dis* 1983; 5: 35-53.
176. Belli J, Waisbren BA. The number of blood cultures necessary to diagnose most cases of bacterial endocarditis. *Am J Med Sci* 1956; 232: 284-8.
177. Weinstein M, Reller L, Murphy J, Lichenstein K. Clinical significance of positive blood cultures: a comprehensive analysis of 500 episodes of bacteraemia and fungemia in adults. I. Clinical observations, with special reference to factors influencing prognosis. *Rev Infect Dis* 1983; 5: 54-70.
178. Barnes PD, Crook DWM. Culture negative endocarditis. *J Infect* 1997; 35: 209-13.
179. Pesanti EL, Smith IM. Infective endocarditis with negative blood cultures. An analysis of 52 cases. *Am J Med* 1979; 66: 43-50.
180. Van Scoy RE. Culture-negative endocarditis. *Mayo Clin Proc* 1982; 57: 149-54.
181. Pazin GJ, Saul S, Thompson ME. Blood culture positivity: Suppression by outpatient antibiotic therapy in patients with bacterial endocarditis. *Arch Intern Med* 1982; 142; 263-8.
182. Hoen B, Selton-Suty C, Lacassin F, *et al.* Infective endocarditis in patients with negative blood cultures: analysis

of 88 cases from a one-year nationwide survey in France. *Clin Infect Dis* 1995; 20: 501-6.
183. Mallen MS, Hube EL Brenes M. Comparative study of blood cultures made from artery, vein and bone marrow in patients with subacute bacterial endocarditis. *Am Heart J* 1946; 692-5.
184. Geraci JE, Wilson WR. Endocarditis due to gram-negative bacteria: report of 56 cases. *Mayo Clin Proc* 1982; 57: 145-8.
185. Chen YC, Chang SC, Luh KT, Hsieh WC. Actinobacillus actinomycetemcomitans endocarditis: a report of four cases and review of literature. *Q J Med* 1992; 81: 871-8.
186. Drancourt M, Birtles R, Chaumentin G, *et al.* New serotype of *Bartonella henselae* in endocarditis and cat-scratch disease. *Lancet* 1996; 347: 441-3.
187. Doern GV, Davaro R, George M, Campognone G, *et al.* Lack of requirement for prolonged incubation of Septi-Chek blood culture bottles in patients with bacteremia due to fastidious bacteria. *Diagn Microbiol Infect Dis* 1996; 24: 141-3.
188. Raoult D, Fournier PE, Drancourt M, *et al.* Diagnosis of 22 new cases of Bartonella endocarditis. *Ann Intern Med* 1996; 125: 646-52.
189. Editorial. Vegetations, valves and echocardiography. *Lancet* 1988; 2: 1118-9.
190. Buda AJ, Zotz RJ, Le Mire MS, Bach DS. Prognostic significance of vegetations detected by two-dimensional echocardiography in infective endocarditis. *Am Heart J* 1986; 112; 1291-6.
191. Erbel R, Rohmann S, Drexler M, *et al.* Improved diagnostic value of echocardiography in patients with infective endocarditis by transoesophageal approach. A prospective study. *Eur Heart J* 1988; 9: 43-53.
192. Mugge A, Daniel WG, Franck G, Lichtlen PR. Echocardiography in infective endocarditis: Reassessment of prognostic implications of vegetation size determined by the transthoracic and the transesophageal approach. *J Am Coll Cardiol* 1989; 14: 631-8.
193. Schwinger ME, Tunick PA, Freedberg RS, Kronzon I. Vegetations on endocardial surfaces struck by regurgitant jets: diagnosis by transesophageal echocardiography. *Am Heart J* 1990; 119: 1212-5.
194. Taams MA, Gussenhoven EJ, Bos E, *et al.* Enhanced morphological diagnosis in infective endocarditis by transoesophageal echocardiography. *Br Heart J* 1990; 63: 109-13.
195. Steckelberg JM, Murphy JG, Ballard D, *et al.* Emboli in infective endocarditis: The prognostic value of echocardiography. *Ann Intern Med* 1991; 114: 635-40.
196. Birmingham GD, Rahko PS and Ballantyne F 3rd, *et al.* Improved detection of infective endocarditis with transesophageal echocardiography. *Am Heart J* 1992; 123: 774-81.
197. Gilbert BW, Haney RS, Crawford F, *et al.* Two-dimensional echocardiographic assessment of vegetative endocarditis. *Circulation* 1977; 55: 346-53.
198. Plehn JF. The evolving role of echocardiography in management of bacterial endocarditis. *Chest* 1988; 94: 904-6.
199. Stewart JA, Silimperi D, Harris P, *et al.* Echocardiographic documentation of vegetative lesions in infective endocarditis: clinical implications. *Circulation* 1980; 61: 374-80.
200. Irani WN, Grayburn PA, Alfredi I. A negative transthoracic echocardiogram obviates the need for transesophageal echocardiography in patients with suspected native valve active infective endocarditis. *Am J Cardiol* 1996; 78: 101-3.
201. Nihoyannopoulos P, Oakley CM, Exadactylos N, Ribeiro P, Westaby Foale RA. Duration of symptoms and the effects of a more aggressive surgical policy: two factors affecting prognosis of infective endocarditis. *Eur Heart J* 1985; 6: 380-90.
202. Kupferwasser LI, Darius H, Muller AM, *et al.* Diagnosis of culture-negative endocarditis: the role of the Duke criteria and the impact of transesophageal echocardiography. *Am Heart J* 2001; 142: 146-52.
203. Tingleff J, Egeblad H, Gotzsche CO, *et al.* Perivalvular cavities in endocarditis: abscesses versus pseudoaneurysms? A transesophageal Doppler echocardiographic study in 118 patients with endocarditis. *Am Heart J* 1995; 130: 93-100.
204. Tunick PA, Freedberg RS, Schrem SS, Kronzon I. Unusual mitral annular vegetation diagnosed by transesophageal echocardiography. *Am Heart J* 1990; 120: 444-6.
205. Jaffe WM, Morgan DE, Pearlman AS, Otto CM. Infective endocarditis. 1983-1988: echocardiographic findings and factors influencing morbidity and mortality. *J Am Coll Cardiol* 1990; 15: 1227-33.
206. Martin RP. The diagnostic and prognostic role of cardiovascular ultrasound in endocarditis: bigger is not better. *J Am Coll Cardiol* 1990; 15: 1234-7.
207. Rohmann S, Erbel R, Gorge G, *et al.* Clinical relevance of vegetation localization by transoesophageal echocardiography in infective endocarditis. *Eur Heart J* 1992; 12: 446-52.
208. Shapiro SM, Bayer AS. Transesophageal and Doppler echocardiography in the diagnosis and management of infective endocarditis. *Chest* 1991; 100: 1125-30.
209. Pedersen WR, Walker M, Olson JD, *et al.* Value of transesophageal echocardiography as an adjunct to transthoracic echocardiography in evaluation of native and prosthetic valve endocarditis. *Chest* 1991; 100: 351-6.
210. Daniel W, Mugge A, Martin R, *et al.* Improvement in the diagnosis of abscesses associated with endocarditis by transesophageal echocardiography. *N Engl J Med* 1991; 324: 795-800.
211. Job FP, Gronke S, Lethen H, *et al.* Incremental value of biplane and multiplane transesophageal echocardiography for the assessment of active infective endocarditis. *Am J Cardiol* 1995; 75: 1033-37.
212. Lowry RW, Zoghbi WA, Baker WB, *et al.* Clinical impact of transesophageal echocardiography in the diagnosis and management of infective endocarditis. *Am J Cardiol* 1994; 73: 1089-91.
213. Culver DL, Cacchione J, Stern D, *et al.* Diagnosis of infective endocarditis on a Starr-Edwards prosthesis by transesophageal echocardiography. *Am Heart J* 1990; 119: 972-3.
214. Shapiro S, Young E, De Guzman S, *et al.* Transesophageal echocardiography in diagnosis of infective endocarditis. *Chest* 1994; 105: 377-82.

215. Leung D, Cranney G, Hopkins A, Walsh W. Role of transesophageal echocardiography in the diagnosis and management of aortic root abscess. *Br Heart J* 1994; 72: 175-81.
216. Rohmann S, Erbel R, Mohr-Kahaly S, Meyer J. Use of transoesophageal echocardiography in the diagnosis of abscess in infective endocarditis. *Eur Heart J* 1995; 16(Suppl B): 54-62.
217. Vered Z, Mossinson D, Peleg E, *et al.* Echocardiographic assessment of prosthetic valve endocarditis. *Eur Heart J* 1995; 16(Suppl B): 63-7.
218. Mukhtari O, Horton CJ Jr., Nanda NC, *et al.* Transesophageal color Doppler three-dimensional echocardiographic detection of prosthetic aortic valve dehiscence: correlation with surgical findings. *Echocardiography* 2001; 18: 393-7.
219. Martin RP, French JW, Popp RL. Clinical utility of two-dimensional echocardiography in patients with bioprosthetic valves. *Adv Cardiol* 1980; 27: 294-304.
220. Shapiro S, Kupferwasser LI. Echocardiography predicts embolic events in infective endocarditis. *J Am Coll Cardiol* 2001; 37: 1077-9.
221. Di Salvo G, Habib G, Pergola V, *et al.* Echocardiography predicts embolic events in infective endocarditis. *J Am Coll Cardiol* 2001; 37: 1069-76.
222. Heinle S, Wilderman N, Harrison JK, *et al.* Value of transthoracic echocardiography in predicting embolic events in active endocarditis. Duke Endocarditis Service. *Am J Cardiol* 1994; 74: 799-801.
223. Ward C. Cardiac Catheterisation in patients with infective endocarditis. *J R Coll Physicians Lond* 1997; 31: 341-2.
224. von Reyn C, Levy B, Arbeit R, Friedland G, Crumpacker C. Infective endocarditis: an analysis based on strict case definitions. *Ann Intern Med* 1981; 94: 505-18.
225. Durack D, Lukes A, Bright D. The Duke Endocarditis Service. New criteria for diagnosis of infective endocarditis: utilization of specific echocardiographic findings. *Am J Med* 1994; 96: 200-9.
226. Heiro M, Nikoskelainen J, Hartiala JJ, *et al.* Diagnosis of infective endocarditis. Sensitivity of the Duke vs von Reyn criteria. *Arch Intern Med* 1998; 158: 18-24.
227. Habib G, Derumeaux G, Avierinos JF, *et al.* Value and limitations of the Duke criteria for the diagnosis of infective endocarditis. *J Am Coll Cardiol* 1999; 33: 2023-9.
228. Muhlestein JB. Infective endocarditis: how well are we managing our patients? *J Am Coll Cardiol* 1999; 33: 794-5.
229. Delahaye F, Rial MO, de Gevigney G, *et al.* A critical appraisal of the quality of the management of infective endocarditis. *J Am Coll Cardiol* 1999; 33: 788-93.
230. Hoen B, Beguinot I, Raboud C, *et al.* The Duke criteria for diagnosing infective endocarditis are specific: analysis of 100 patients with acute fever or fever of unknown origin. *Clin Infect Dis* 1996; 23: 298-302.
231. Cecchi E, Parrini I, Chinaglia A, *et al.* New diagnostic criteria for infective endocarditis. A study of sensitivity and specificity. *Eur Heart J* 1997; 18: 1149-56.
232. Olaison L, Hogevik H. Comparison of the von Reyn and Duke criteria for the diagnosis of infective endocarditis: a critical analysis of 161 episodes. *Scand J Infect Dis* 1996; 28: 399-406.
233. Dodds GA, Sexton DJ, Durack DT, *et al.* Negative predictive value of the Duke criteria for infective endocarditis. *Am J Cardiol* 1996; 77: 403-7.
234. Rognon R, Kehtari R. Individual value of each of the Duke criteria for the diagnosis of infective endocarditis. *Clin Microbiol Infect* 1999; 5: 396-403.
235. Fournier PE, Casalta JP, Habib G, *et al.* Modification of the diagnostic criteria proposed by the Duke Endocarditis Service to permit improved diagnosis of Q fever endocarditis. *Am J Med* 1996; 100: 629-33.
236. Lamas CC, Eykyn SJ. Blood culture negative endocarditis: analysis of 63 cases presenting over 25 years. *Heart* 2003; 89: 258-62.
237. Hoen B, Selton-Suty C, Danchin N, *et al.* Evaluation of the Duke criteria versus the Beth Israel criteria for the diagnosis of infective endocarditis. *Clin Infect Dis* 1995; 21: 905-9.
238. Naber CK, Bartel T, Eggebrecht H, *et al.* Diagnosis of endocarditis today: Duke criteria or clinical judgement? *Herz* 2001; 26: 379-90.
239. Millar BC, Moore JE, Mallon P, *et al.* Molecular diagnosis of infective endocarditis - a new Duke's criterion. *Scand J Infect Dis* 2001; 33: 673-80.
240. Grijalva M, Horvath R, Dendis M, *et al.* Molecular diagnosis of culture-negative infective endocarditis: clinical validation in a group of surgically treated patients. *Heart* 2003; 89: 263-8.
241. Li JS, Sexton DJ, Mick N, *et al.* Proposed modifications to the Duke's criteria for the diagnosis of infective endocarditis. *Clin Infect Dis* 2000; 30: 633-8.
242. Horstkotte D, Rosin H, Friedrichs W, Loogen F. Contribution for choosing the optimal prophylaxis of bacterial endocarditis. *Eur Heart J* 1987; 8(Suppl J): 379-81.
243. Imperpale T, Horwitz T. Does prophylaxis prevent post-dental infective endocarditis? A controlled evaluation of predictive efficacy. *Am J Med* 1990; 88: 131-6.
244. van de Meer J, van Wijk W, Thompson J, *et al.* Efficacy of antibiotic prophylaxis for prevention of native valve endocarditis. *Lancet* 1992; 339: 135-9.
245. Durack D. Prevention of infective endocarditis. *N Engl J Med* 1995; 332: 38-44.
246. Simmons NA, Ball AP, Cawson RA, *et al.* Antibiotic prophylaxis and infective endocarditis. *Lancet* 1992; 339: 1292-3.
247. Simmons NA. Recommendations for endocarditis prophylaxis. The Endocarditis Working Party for Antimicrobial Chemotherapy. *J Antimicrob Chemother* 1993; 31: 437-8.
248. Working Party of the British Society for Antimicrobial Chemotherapy. Antibiotic treatment of Streptococcal, Enterococcal and Staphylococcal endocarditis. Guidelines. *Heart* 1998; 79: 207-210.
249. Dajani A, Taubert K, Wilson W, *et al.* Prevention of bacterial endocarditis. Recommendations by the American Heart Association. *Circulation* 1997; 96: 358-66.
250. Wilson W, Karchmer A, Dajani A, *et al.* Antibiotic treatment of adults with infective endocarditis due to streptococci, enterococci, staphylococci and HACEK microorganisms. *JAMA* 1995; 274: 1706-13.

251. Besnier JM, Choutet P. Medical treatment of infective endocarditis: general principles. *Eur Heart J* 1995; 16(Suppl B): 72-4.
252. Scheld WM. Pathogenesis and pathophysiology of infective endocarditis. In: *Endocarditis*. Sande MA, Kaye D, Root RK Eds. Churchill Livingstone, New York, 1984: 1-32.
253. Durack DT, Beeson PB. Experimental bacterial endocarditis. II. Survival of bacteria in endocardial vegetations. *Br J Exp Pathol* 1972; 53: 50-3.
254. Washington JA. *In vitro* testing of antimicrobial agents. *Infect Dis Clin North Am* 1989; 3: 375-87.
255. Mulligan MJ, Cobbs CG. Bacteriostatic versus bactericidal activity. *Infect Dis Clin North Am* 1989; 3: 389-98.
256. Holloway Y, Dankert J, Hess J. Penicillin tolerance and bacterial endocarditis. *Lancet* 1980; 1: 589.
257. Eliopoulos GM. Synergism and antagonism. *Infect Dis Clin North Am* 1989; 3: 399-406.
258. Watanakunakorn C, Glotzbecker C. Synergism with aminoglycosides of penicillin, ampicillin and vancomycin against non-enterococcal group-D streptococci and Viridans streptococci. *J Med Microbiol* 1976; 10: 133-8.
259. Sande MA and Irvin RG. Penicillin-aminoglycoside synergy in experimental *Streptococcus viridans* endocarditis. *J Infect Dis* 1974; 129: 572-6.
260. Mandell GL, Kaye D, Levison ME, Hook EW. Enterococcal endocarditis: an analysis of 38 patients observed at the New York Hospital-Cornell Medical Center. *Arch Intern Med* 1970; 125: 258-64.
261. Bisno AL, Dismukes WE, Durack DT, *et al.* Antimicrobial treatment of infective endocarditis due to viridans streptococci, enterococci and staphylococci. *JAMA* 1989; 261: 1471-7.
262. Moellering RC. Treatment of enterococcal endocarditis. In: *Endocarditis.* Sande MA, Kaye D, Root RK, Eds. Churchill Livingstone, New York, 1984: 113-133.
263. Wilson WR, Geraci JE. Treatment of streptococcal infective endocarditis. *Am J Med* 1985; 78(Suppl 6B): 128-37.
264. Gutschik E and the Endocarditis Working Group of the International Society of Chemotherapy. Microbiological recommendations for the diagnosis and follow-up of infective endocarditis. *Clin Microbiol Infect* 1998; 4(Suppl 3): S10-16.
265. Weinstein MP, Stratton CW, Ackley A, *et al.* Multicenter collaborative evaluation of a standardized serum bactericidal test as a prognostic indicator in infective endocarditis. *Am J Med* 1985; 78: 262-9.
266. Horstkotte D, Weist K, Rueden H. Better understanding of the pathogenesis of prosthetic valve endocarditis - recent perspectives for prevention strategies. *J Heart Valve Dis* 1998; 7: 313-15.
267. Hyde JAJ, Darouiche RO, Costeron JW. Strategies for prophylaxis against prosthetic valve endocarditis. A review article. *J Heart Valve Dis* 1998; 7: 316-26.
268. Cowgill LD, Addonizio VP, Hopeman AR, Harken AH. Prosthetic valve endocarditis. *Curr Probl Cardiol* 1986; 11: 617-64.
269. Tornos P. Management of prosthetic valve endocarditis: a clinical challenge. *Heart* 2003; 89: 245-6.
270. Akowuah EF, Davies W, Oliver S, *et al.* Prosthetic valve endocarditis: early and late outcome following medical or surgical treatment. *Heart* 2003; 89: 269-72.
271. DiSesa VJ, Sloss LJ, Cohn LH. Heart transplantation for intractable prosthetic valve endocarditis. *J Heart Transplant* 1990; 9: 142-3.
272. Brottier E, Gin H, Brottier L, *et al.* Prosthetic valve endocarditis: diagnosis and prognosis. *Eur Heart J* 1984; 5(Suppl C)123-7.
273. Cowgill LD, Addonizio VP, Hopeman AR, Harken AH. A practical approach to prosthetic valve endocarditis. *Ann Thorac Surg* 1987; 43: 450-7.
274. Leport C, Vilde JL, Bricaire F, *et al.* Fifty cases of late prosthetic valve endocarditis: improvement in prognosis over a 15 year period. *Br Heart J* 1987; 58: 66-71.
275. Dismukes WE. Prosthetic valve endocarditis. Factors influencing outcome and recommendations for therapy. In: *Treatment of infective endocarditis.* Bisno AL, Ed. Grune & Stratton, New York, 1981: 167-191.
276. Durack DT. Infective endocarditis. In: *The Heart,* 7th edition companion handbook. Schlant R, Hurst WJ, Eds. McGraw Hill, New York, 1990: 153-67.
277. Scheld WM, Sande MA. Endocarditis and intravascular infections. In: *Principles and practice of infectious diseases*, 4th edn. Mandell GL, Douglas RG Jr, Dolin R, Eds. Churchill Livingstone, New York, 1995: 740-83.
278. DiNubile MJ, Calderwood SB, Steinhaus DM, Karchmer AW. Cardiac conduction abnormalities complicating native valve active endocarditis. *Am J Cardiol* 1986; 58: 1213-17.
279. Tucker KJ, Johnson JA, Ong T, *et al.* Medical management of prosthetic aortic valve endocarditis and aortic root abscess. *Am Heart J* 1993; 125: 1195-7.
280. Guzman F, Cartmill I, Holden MP, Freeman R. Candida endocarditis: report of four cases. *Int J Cardiol* 1987; 16: 131-6.
281. Douglas JL, Cobbs CG. Prosthetic valve endocarditis. In: *Infective endocarditis*, 2nd edn. Kaye D, Ed. Raven Press, New York, 1992: 375-96.
282. Yu VL, Fang GD, Keys TF, *et al.* Prosthetic valve endocarditis: superiority of surgical valve replacement versus medical therapy only. *Ann Thorac Surg* 1994; 58: 1073-7.
283. Saffle JR, Gardner P, Schoenbaum SC, *et al.* Prosthetic valve endocarditis: the case for prompt valve replacement. *J Thorac Cardiovasc Surg* 1977; 3: 416-20.
284. Lytle BW, Taylor PC, Sapp SK, *et al.* Surgical treatment of prosthetic valve endocarditis. *J Thorac Cardiovasc Surg* 1996; 111: 198-210.
285. Farina G, Vitale N, Piaza L, *et al.* Long-term results of surgery for prosthetic valve endocarditis. *J Heart Valve Dis* 1994; 2: 165-71.
286. Moon MR, Miller DL, Moore KA, *et al.* Treatment of endocarditis with valve replacement: the question of tissue versus mechanical prosthesis. *Ann Thorac Surg* 2001; 71: 1164-71.
287. Trunninger K, Attenhofer CH, Seifert B, *et al.* Long-term follow-up of prosthetic valve endocarditis: what characteristics identify patients who were treated successfully with antibiotics alone. *Heart* 1999; 82: 714-20.
288. Karchmer AW, Dismuke WE, Buckley MJ, *et al.* Late prosthetic valve endocarditis: clinical features influencing therapy. *Am J Med* 1978; 64: 199-206.

289. Kuyvenhoven P, Rijk-Zwikkere GL, Hermans J, *et al.* Prosthetic valve endocarditis: analysis of risk factors for mortality. *Eur J Cardiothoracic Surg* 1994; 8: 420-4.
290. Ivert TS, Dismukes WE, Cobbs CG, *et al.* Prosthetic valve endocarditis. *Circulation* 1984; 69: 223-32.
291. Chow AW, Azar RM. Glycopeptides and nephrotoxicity. *Intensive Care Med* 1994; 20(Suppl 4): 23-9.
292. Blumberg EA, Robbins N, Adimora A, Lowy FD. Persistent fever in association with infective endocarditis. *Clin Infect Dis* 1992; 15: 983-90.
293. Vuille C, Nidorf M, Weyman AE, Picard MH. Natural history of vegetations during successful medical treatment of endocarditis. *Am Heart J* 1994; 128: 1200-9.
294. Mansur AJ, Dal Bo CM, Fukushuma JT, *et al.* Relapses, recurrence, valve replacement and mortality during the long-term follow-up after infective endocarditis. *Am Heart J* 2001; 141: 78-86.
295. Verheul HA, van den Brink RB, van Vreeland T, *et al.* Effects of changes in management of active infective endocarditis on outcome in a 25-year period. *Am J Cardiol* 1993; 72: 682-7.
296. Middlemost S, Wisenbaugh T, Meyerowitz C, *et al.* A case for early surgery in native left-sided endocarditis complicated by heart failure: results in 203 patients. *J Am Coll Cardiol* 1991; 18: 663-7.
297. Bogers AJJC, van Vreeswijk H, Verbaan CJ, *et al.* Early surgery for active infective endocarditis improves early and late results. *Thorac Cardiovasc Surg* 1991; 39: 284-7.
298. Jubair KA, Al Fagih MR, Ashmeg A, *et al.* Cardiac operations during active endocarditis. *J Thoracic Cardiovasc Surg* 1992; 104: 487-90.
299. Vlessis AA, Hovaguimian H, Jaggers J, *et al.* Infective endocarditis: ten-year review of medical and surgical therapy. *Ann Thorac Surg* 1996; 61: 1217-22.
300. Dehler S, Elert O. Early and late prognosis following valve replacement for bacterial endocarditis of the native valve. *Thorac Cardiovasc Surg* 1995; 43: 83-9.
301. Castillo JC, Anguita MP, Ramirez A, *et al.* Long-term outcome of infective endocarditis in patients who were not drug addicts: a 10 year study. *Heart* 2000; 83: 525-30.
302. Alexiou C, Langley SM, Stafford H, *et al.* Surgery for active culture-positive endocarditis: determinants of early and late outcomes. *Ann Thorac Surg* 2000; 69: 1448-54.
303. Douglas A, Moore-Gillon J, Eykyn SJ. Fever during treatment of infective endocarditis. *Lancet* 1986; I: 1341-3.
304. Graupner C, Vilacosta I, SanRoman J, *et al.* Periannular extension of infective endocarditis. *J Am Coll Cardiol* 2002; 39: 1204-11.
305. Choussat R, Thomas D, Isnard R, *et al.* Perivalvular abscess associated with endocarditis: clinical features and prognostic factors of overall success in a series of 233 cases. Perivalvular Abscess French Multicentre Study. *Eur Heart J* 1999; 20: 232-41.
306. Stinson EB. Surgical treatment of infective endocarditis. *Prog Cardiovasc Dis* 1979; 22: 145-68.
307. Becher H, Hanrath P, Bleifeld W, Bleese N. Correlation of echocardiographic and surgical findings in acute bacterial endocarditis. *Eur Heart J* 1984; 5(Suppl C): 67-70.
308. Arnett EN, Roberts WC. Prosthetic valve endocarditis: clinicopathologic analysis of 22 necropsy patients with comparison of observations in 74 necropsy patients with active endocarditis involving natural left-sided cardiac valves. *Am J Cardiol* 1976; 38: 281-92.
309. Blumberg EA, Karalis DA, Chandrasekaran K, *et al.* Endocarditis-associated paravalvular abscesses: do clinical parameters predict the presence of abscess? *Chest* 1995; 107: 898-903.
310. Scarvelis D, Malcolm I. Embolization of a huge tricuspid valve bacterial vegetation. *J Am Soc Echocardiogr* 2002; 15: 185-7.
311. Stewart WJ, Shan K. The diagnosis of prosthetic valve endocarditis by echocardiography. *Semin Thorac Cardiovasc Surg* 1995; 7: 7-12.
312. Ergin MA. Surgical techniques in prosthetic valve endocarditis. *Semin Thorac Cardiovasc Surg* 1995; 7: 54-60.
313. David TE. The surgical treatment of patients with prosthetic valve endocarditis. *Semin Thorac Cardiovasc Surg* 1995; 7: 47-53.
314. Joyce F, Tingleff J, Pettersson G. The Ross operation in the treatment of prosthetic aortic valve endocarditis. *Semin Thorac Cardiovasc Surg* 1995; 7: 38-46.
315. Camacho MT, Cosgrove DM 3rd. Homografts in the treatment of prosthetic valve endocarditis. *Semin Thorac Cardiovasc Surg* 1995; 7: 32-7.
316. McGiffin DC, Kirklin JK. The impact of aortic valve homografts on the treatment of aortic prosthetic valve endocarditis. *Semin Thorac Cardiovasc Surg* 1995; 7: 25-31.
317. Gordon SM, Keys TF. Bloodstream infections in patients with implanted prosthetic cardiac valves. *Semin Thorac Cardiovasc Surg* 1995; 7: 2-6.
318. Lytle BW. Surgical treatment of prosthetic valve endocarditis. *Semin Thorac Cardiovasc Surg* 1995; 7: 13-9.
319. Lytle BW. Prosthetic valve endocarditis. Introduction. *Semin Thorac Cardiovasc Surg* 1995; 7: 1.
320. Tornos P, Alnurante B, Mirabet S. Infective endocarditis due to *Staphylococcus aureus*: deleterious effect of anticoagulant therapy. *Arch Intern Med* 1999; 159: 473-5.
321. Nihoyannopoulos P. Tricuspid valvectomy following tricuspid valve endocarditis in an intravenous drug addict. *Heart* 2001; 86: 144.
322. Carozza A, Penzulli A, De Feo M, *et al.* Tricuspid repair for infective endocarditis: clinical and echocardiographic results. *Tex Heart Inst J* 2001; 28: 96-101.
323. Yee ES, Khonsari S. Right-sided infective endocarditis: valvuloplasty, valvectomy or replacement. *J Cardiovasc Surg* 1989; 30: 744-8.
324. Hughes CF, Noble N. Vegetectomy: an alternative surgical treatment for infective endocarditis of the atrioventricular valves in drug addicts. *J Thorac Cardiovasc Surg* 1988; 95: 857-61.
325. Reinhartz O, Herrmann M, Redling F, Zerkowski HR. Timing of surgery in patients with acute infective endocarditis. *J Cardiovasc Surg* 1996; 37: 397-400.
326. Wilson WR, Davidson GK, Giuliani ER, *et al.* Cardiac valve replacement in congestive heart failure due to infective endocarditis. *Mayo Clin Proc* 1979; 54: 223-6.

327. Moon MR, Stinson EB, Miller DC. Surgical treatment of endocarditis. *Prog Cardiovasc Dis* 1997; 40: 239-64.
328. Karchmer AW, Stinson EB. The role of surgery in infective endocarditis. In: *Current Clinical Topics in Infectious Diseases*. Remington JS, Schwartz MN, Eds. McGraw-Hill, New York, 1980: 124-157.
329. Jung JY, Saab SB, Almond CH. The case for early surgical treatment of left-sided primary infective endocarditis: a collective review. *J Thorac Cardiovasc Surg* 1975; 70: 509-18.
330. Acar J, Michel PL, Varenne O, Michaud P, Rafik T. Surgical treatment of infective endocarditis. *Eur Heart J* 1995; 16(Suppl B): 94-8.
331. Saffle JR, Gardner P, Schoenbaum SC, Wild W. Prosthetic valve endocarditis: the case for prompt valve replacement. *J Thorac Cardiovasc Surg* 1977; 73: 416-20.
332. Peri CM, Vuk F, Huski CR. Active infective endocarditis: low mortality associated with early surgical treatment. *Cardiovasc Surg* 2000; 8: 208-13.
333. Karchmer AW. Treatment of prosthetic valve endocarditis. In: *Endocarditis*. Sand MA, Kaye D and Root RT, Eds. Churchill Livingstone, New York, Edinburgh, London and Melbourne, 1984.
334. Richardson JV, Karp RB, Kirklin JW, Dismukes WE. Treatment of infective endocarditis: a 10-year comparative analysis. *Circulation* 1978; 58: 589-97.
335. Parrino PE, Kron IL, Ross SD, *et al*. Does a focal neurological deficit contraindicate operation in a patient with endocarditis? *Ann Thorac Surg* 1999; 67: 59-64.
336. Gillinov AM, Shah RV, Cxurtis WE, *et al*. Valve replacement in patients with endocarditis and acute neurologic deficit. *Ann Thorac Surg* 1996; 61: 1125-9.
337. Parrino PE, Kron IL, Ross SD, *et al*. Does a focal neurologic deficit contraindicate operation in a patient with endocarditis. *Ann Thorac Surg* 1999; 67: 59-64.
338. Eishi K, Kawazoe K, Kuriyama Y, *et al*. Surgical management of infective endocarditis associated with cerebral complications. Multi-center retrosective study in Japan. *J Thorac Cardiovasc Surg* 1995; 110: 1745-55.
339. Ting W, Silverman N, Levitsky S. Valve replacement in patients with endocarditis and cerebral septic embolism. *Ann Thorac Surg* 1991; 51: 18-21.
340. Piper C, Wiemer M, Schulte HG, Horstkotte D. Stroke is not a contraindication for urgent valve replacement in acute infective endocarditis. *J Heart Valve Dis* 2001; 10: 703-11.
341. Vilacosta I, Gomez J. Complementary role of MRI in infectious endocarditis. *Echocardiography* 1995; 12: 673-6.
342. Bertorini TE, Laster RE Jr., Thompson BF, Gelfand M. Magnetic resonance imaging of the brain in bacterial endocarditis. *Arch Intern Med* 1989; 149: 815-7.
343. Turtz AR, Yocom SS. Contemporary approaches to the management of neurosurgical complications of infective endocarditis. *Curr Infect Dis Rep* 2001; 3: 337-46.
344. Utoh J, Miyauchi Y, Goto H, *et al*. Endovascular approach for an intracranial mycotic aneurysm associated with infective endocarditis. *J Thorac Cardiovasc Surg* 1995; 110: 557-9.
345. Salgado AV, Furlan AJ, Keys TF. Mycotic aneurysm, subarachnoid hemorrhage, and indications for cerebral angiography in infective endocarditis. *Stroke* 1987; 18: 1057-60.
346. Dodge A, Hurni M, Ruchat P, *et al*. Surgery in native valve endocarditis: indications, results and risk factors. *Eur J Cardiothoracic Surg* 1995; 9: 330-4.
347. Aranki SF, Santini F, Adams DH, *et al*. Aortic valve endocarditis. Determinants of early survival and late morbidity. *Circulation* 1994; 90(Suppl II): 175-82.
348. Olaison L, Hogevik H, Myken P, *et al*. Early surgery in infective endocarditis. *QJM* 1996; 89: 267-78.
349. Reinhartz O, Herrmann M, Redling F, *et al*. Timing of surgery in patients with acute infective endocarditis. *J Cardiovasc Surg* 1996; 37: 397-400.
350. Lytle BW, Priest BP, Taylor PC, *et al*. Surgical treatment of prosthetic valve endocarditis. *J Thorac Cardiovasc Surg* 1996; 111: 198-207.
351. Cimbollek M, Nies B, Wenz R, Kreuter J. Antibiotic-impregnated heart valve sewing rings for treatment and prophylaxis of bacterial endocarditis. *Antimicrob Agents Chemother* 1996; 40: 1432-7.
352. Mullany C, Chau Y, Schaff H, *et al*. Early and late survival after surgical treatment of culture-positive active endocarditis. *Mayo Clin Proc* 1995; 70: 517-25.
353. Middlemost S, Wisenbaugh T, Meyerowitz C, *et al*. A case for early surgery in native left-sided endocarditis complicated by heart failure:results in 203 patients. *J Am Coll Cardiol* 1991; 18: 663-7.
354. Espersen F, Frimodt-Noller N. *Staphylococcus aureus* endocarditis. A review of 119 cases. *Arch Intern Med* 1986; 146: 1118-21.
355. Delany D, Pellerini M, Carrier M, *et al*. Immediate and long-term results of valve replacement for native and prosthetic valve endocarditis. *Ann Thorac Surg* 2000; 70: 1219-23.
356. Knosalla C, Weng Y, Yankah AC, *et al*. Surgical treatment of active infection aortic valve endocarditis with associated periannular abscess - 11 year results. *Eur Heart J* 2000; 21: 490-7.
357. d'Udekem Y, David TE, Feindel CM, *et al*. Long-term results of operation for paravalvular abscess. *Ann Thorac Surg* 1996; 62: 48-53.
358. Niwaya K, Knott-Craig CJ, Santangelo K, *et al*. Advantage of autograft and homograft valve replacement for complex aortic valve endocarditis. *Ann Thorac Surg* 1999; 67: 1603-8.
359. Grandmougin D, Prat A, Fayad G, *et al*. Acute aortic endocarditis with annular destruction: assessment of surgical treatment with cryopreserved valvular homografts. *J Heart Valve Dis* 1999; 8: 234-41.
360. Haydock D, Barratt-Boyes B, Macedo T, *et al*. Aortic valve replacement for active infectious endocarditis in 108 patients. A comparison of freehand allograft valves with mechanical prostheses and bioprostheses. *J Thorac Cardiovasc Surg* 1992; 103: 130-9.
361. Petrou M, Wong K, Albertucci M, *et al*. Evaluation of unstented aortic homografts for the treatment of prosthetic aortic valve endocarditis. *Circulation* 1994; 90(part 2): 198-204.
362. Zwischenberger JB, Shalaby TZ, Conti VR. Viable cryopreserved aortic homograft for aortic valve endocarditis and annular abscesses. *Ann Thorac Surg* 1989; 48: 365-70.

363. Pagano D, Allen SM, Bonser RS. Homograft aortic valve and root replacement for severe destructive native or prosthetic endocarditis. *Eur J Cardiothorac Surg* 1994; 8: 173-6.
364. Dossche KM, Defauw JJ, Ernst SM, *et al.* Allograft aortic root replacement in prosthetic aortic valve endocarditis: a review of 32 patients. *Ann Thorac Surg* 1997; 63: 1644-9.
365. O'Brien MF, Stafford EG, Gardner MA, *et al.* A comparison of aortic valve replacement with viable cryopreserved and fresh allograft valves, with a note on chromosomal studies. *J Thorac Cardiovasc Surg* 1987; 94: 812-23.
366. McGiffin DC, Galbraith AJ, McLachlan GL, *et al.* Aortic valve infection. Risk factors for death and recurrent endocarditis after aortic valve replacement. *J Thorac Cardiovasc Surg* 1992; 104: 511-20.
367. Dearani JA, Orszulak TA, Schaff HV, *et al.* Results of allograft aortic valve replacement for complex endocarditis. *J Thorac Cardiovasc Surg* 1997; 113: 285-91.
368. Edwards MB, Ratnatunga CP, Dore CJ, *et al.* Thirty-day mortality and long-term survival following surgery for prosthetic endocarditis: a study from the UK heart valve registry. *Eur J Cardiothorac Surg* 1998; 14: 156-64.
369. D'Udekem Y, David TE, Feindel CM, *et al.* Long-term results of surgery for active infective endocarditis. *Eur J Cardiothorac Surg* 1997; 11: 46-52.
370. Jault F, Gandjbakhch I, Rama A, *et al.* Active native valve endocarditis: determinants of operative death and late mortality. *Ann Thorac Surg* 1997; 63: 1737-41.
371. Ladowski JS, Deschner WP. Allograft replacement of the aortic valve for active endocarditis. *J Cardiovasc Surg* 1996; 37(Suppl 1): 61-2.
372. Wos S, Jasinski M, Bachowski R. Results of mechanical prosthetic valve replacement in active valvular endocarditis. *J Cardiovasc Surg* 1996; 37(Suppl 1): 29-32.
373. Robi C, Sek E. Are allografts the "choice" in infectious endocarditis with perivalvular abscess? *Eur Heart J* 2000; 21: 421.
374. Yankah AC, Klose H, Petzina R, *et al.* Surgical management of acute aortic root endocarditis with valve homograft: 13-year experience. *Eur J Cardiovasc Surg* 2002; 21: 260-7.
375. Guerra JM, Tornos MP, Permanye-Miralda G, *et al.* Long-term results of mechanical prostheses for treatment of active endocarditis. *Heart* 2001; 86: 63-8.
376. Aranki SF, Adams DH, Rizzo RJ, *et al.* Determinants of early mortality and late survival in mitral valve endocarditis. *Circulation* 1995; 92: 143-9.
377. Mansur AJ, Grinberg M, Cardoso RH, *et al.* Determinants of prognosis in 300 episodes of infective endocarditis. *Thorac Cardiovasc Surg* 1996; 44: 2-10.
378. Malquarti V, Saradarian W, Etienne J, *et al.* Prognosis of native valve infective endocarditis. A review of 253 cases. *Eur Heart J* 1984; 5(Suppl C): 11-20.
379. Bayliss R, Clark C, Oakley CM, *et al.* Incidence, mortality and prevention of infective endocarditis. *J R Coll Physicians* 1986; 20: 15.
380. Delahaye F, Echchard R, de Gevigney G, *et al.* The long-term prognosis of infective endocarditis. *Eur Heart J* 1995; 16(Suppl B): 48-53.
381. Renzulli A, Carozza A, Romano G, *et al.* Recurrent infective endocarditis: a multivariate analysis of 21 years of experience. *Ann Thorac Surg* 2001; 72: 39-43.
382. Tornos MP, Permanyer-Miralda G, Olona M, *et al.* Long term complications of native valve infective endocarditis in non addicts. *Ann Intern Med* 1992; 117: 567-72.
383. Calderwood SP, Swinsky LA, Karchmer AW, *et al.* Prosthetic valve endocarditis. Analysis of factors affecting outcome of therapy. *J Thorac Cardiovasc Surg* 1986; 92: 776-83.
384. Tornos P, Almirante B, Olona M, *et al.* Clinical outcome and long-term prognosis of late prosthetic valve endocarditis: a 20-year experience. *Clin Infect Dis* 1997; 24: 381-6.
385. Mihaljevic T, Byrne JG, Cohn LH, Aranki SF. Long-term results of multivalvar surgery for infective multivalve endocarditis. *Eur J Cardiothoracic Surg* 2001; 20: 842-6.

Chapter 25

Blood conservation techniques in cardiothoracic surgery

Artyom Sedrakyan MD ScC
Honorary Lecturer and Research Scholar

THE ROYAL COLLEGE OF SURGEONS OF ENGLAND AND
THE LONDON SCHOOL OF HYGIENE AND TROPICAL MEDICINE, LONDON, UK

Introduction

It is well documented that postoperative bleeding leading to re-operation occurs in up to 6% of cardiac surgical patients and increases mortality [1,2]. Blood loss often necessitates allogeneic blood product transfusions which are very common after major cardiothoracic surgery. Over 60% of more than 11 million blood units used in the United States are transfused in the surgical setting [3]. However, transfusions are associated with risks such as transfusion reaction, sepsis, febrile reactions, immunosuppression, viral and bacterial infections [4]. These problems can be more pronounced in developing countries where universal antibody screening is not always possible, due to equipment shortages and costs [3].

Given widespread shortage of safe allogeneic blood products and concern over adverse consequences of blood transfusion, blood conservation techniques are becoming increasingly important in the peri-operative management of cardiothoracic patients.

In this chapter we will cover:-

1. Anti-fibrinolytic medications:-
   a. Aprotinin.
   b. Epsilon aminocaproic acid.
   c. Tranexamic acid.
2. Desmopressin.
3. Other blood conservation techniques.

Methodology

We searched for systematic reviews and randomised clinical trials by using MEDLINE, EMBASE and the Cochrane Controlled Trials Register. We abstracted the estimates of risk from the original reports and meta-analytic estimates from systematic reviews. For trials addressing aprotinin use in coronary artery bypass grafting (CABG), specific meta-analyses were performed. We combined the relative risk estimates acquired from the trials using a fixed effect model. RevMan 4.1 was used for all statistical analyses.

Anti-fibrinolytic medications

Aprotinin

Aprotinin (trasylol) is the only US Food and Drug Administration (FDA) approved pharmacological treatment to reduce blood transfusion in coronary artery bypass grafting (CABG). The use of aprotinin in coronary artery bypass surgery has been associated with more than a 45% reduction in the odds of blood transfusion as compared to placebo in many large multicentre trials [5-7]. Although there were some side effects (myocardial infarction [MI] and renal failure) reported in the literature [8,9], the evidence supporting these associations is very limited and primarily based on case series. Systematic reviews of the randomised clinical trials (RCT) conducted by Levi *et al* [10], Munoz *et al* [11], and the Cochrane Collaboration [12] attempted to address safety and efficacy of aprotinin use in cardiac surgery. These reviews combined a mixture of cardiac surgical procedures, the incidence of stroke was incompletely evaluated and the incidence of atrial fibrillation was not addressed. To complement these findings we performed our own rigorous review with particular emphasis on CABG patients.

Blood transfusion benefits

The earliest meta-analysis by Levi *et al* [10] reported a 63% reduction in the proportion of patients requiring blood transfusion based on 40 trials of aprotinin. However, the odds ratio (OR) and not the relative risk (RR) was used by these authors, which could overestimate the effect of aprotinin for prevalent outcomes such as blood transfusion [13]. Later meta-analysis [12], which was based on a larger number of trials and calculated relative risk of requiring transfusion, has shown only a 31% reduction in the proportion of patients requiring blood transfusion (95% CI 24%-36%). In our meta-analysis based on CABG population, the total number of people requiring any blood transfusion was 40.33% in the aprotinin group and 63.34% in the placebo group. There was a 39% risk reduction of blood transfusion associated with the use of aprotinin (RR 0.61; 95% CI 0.58-0.66). This meant that over 250 people will be prevented from receiving any blood transfusion per 1000 CABG procedures. On average, there was one unit of blood saved per cardiac surgical procedure [10].

Levi *et al* also reported that full-dose aprotinin was associated with a 25% reduction in the odds of blood transfusion compared to low-dose. Additionally, Munoz *et al* [11] reported that patients treated with aprotinin were less likely to undergo re-exploration for bleeding than controls (1.1% vs 4.2%, p<0.001).

Safety and other effects

Mortality

Levi *et al* [10] reported a 45% reduction in the odds of mortality (95% CI 10%-66%), when information from 26 trials of aprotinin was combined. However, there were some numerical discrepancies in this study [14] and further reviews did not support this finding. One of the reviews has reported 2.7% vs 3.1% mortality in high-dose and placebo groups and 3.3% vs 2.2% in low-dose and placebo groups [11]. The Cochrane review[12] found a statistically insignificant 13% reduction in mortality and our review of coronary bypass RCTs has shown no significant increased or decreased risk of mortality associated with the use of aprotinin (RR 0.96; 95% CI 0.65-1.40).

Myocardial infarction

Levi *et al* reported a RR of 1.13 in 18 trials of aprotinin (95% CI 0.76-1.67) and also found a statistically significant difference between high and low doses of aprotinin favouring low-dose (RR 0.46; 95% CI 0.24-0.89). Munoz *et al* [11] did not compare high and low doses of aprotinin and similarly reported no statistically significant higher risk of MI. Our systematic review of only CABG trials, which nevertheless was based on a considerably larger number of studies (28 trials), has shown a tendency toward reduction of the risk of MI in the aprotinin group as compared to placebo (RR 0.85; 95% CI 0.63-1.14).

Renal failure

Renal failure was addressed by Henry *et al* [12] who reported no increased or decreased risk in 13 trials (RR 1.19; 95% CI 0.79-1.79). We were able to acquire data from 17 trials of CABG that enrolled 3003 patients. Meta-analytic estimates for renal failure again did not show increased risk associated with aprotinin therapy (RR 1.01; 95% CI 0.55-1.83).

Stroke

Munoz *et al* [11] reported a tendency towards a stroke incidence reduction, that did not reach statistical significance (p=0.07). A similar tendency was reported by Henry *et al* [12] (RR 0.43; 95% CI 0.16-1.19) who combined eight trials. Our review of CABG trials was based on 13 reports [5-9,15-22] and stroke incidence was evaluated in 2976 patients. Aprotinin use was associated with a 47% relative risk reduction (RR 0.53; 95% CI 0.31-0.90) as compared to placebo (see Figure 1).

Atrial fibrillation

Our review of 11 studies involving 2460 patients has shown a tendency towards risk reduction associated with aprotinin use (RR 0.90; 95% CI 0.78- 1.04).

Other safety information

No increased or decreased risk of deep venous thrombosis, pulmonary embolism or any other thrombosis was found to be associated with aprotinin in the Cochrane review [12].

Epsilon aminocaproic acid

Epsilon aminocaproic acid (EACA) acts as an effective inhibitor of fibrinolysis. The beneficial effects of this medication are linked to inhibition of plasminogen activator substances and possibly, to antiplasmin. EACA appears to penetrate red blood cells as well as other tissue cells [23]. It should be noted that EACA is much cheaper than aprotinin [11].

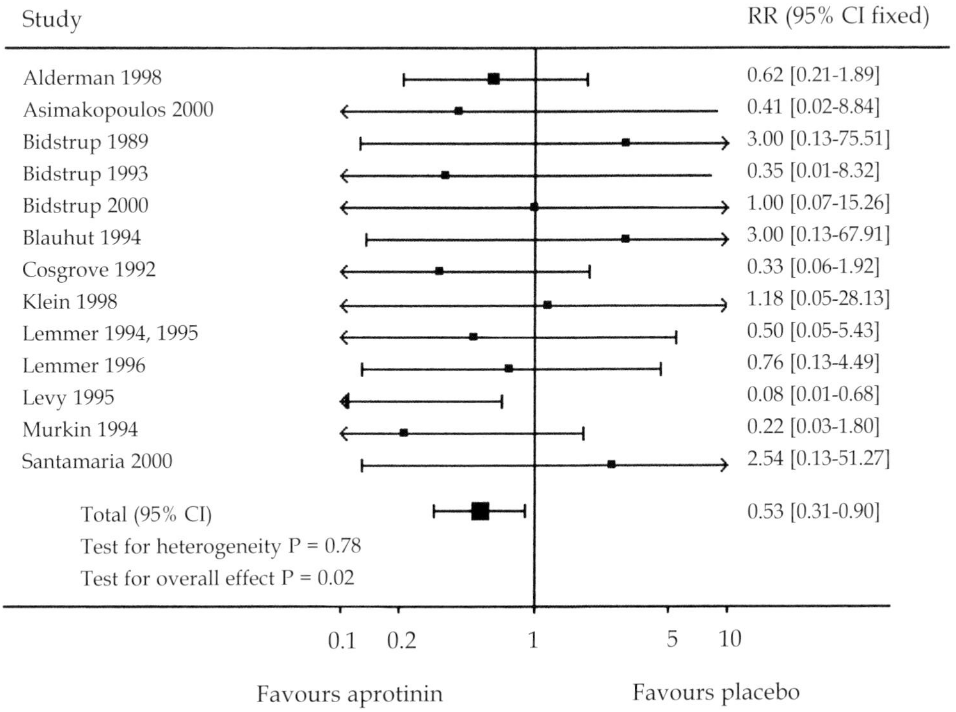

Figure 1. **Stroke benefit observed in the trials of aprotinin use in CABG.**

Blood transfusion benefits

Levi *et al* [10] did not separate EACA and tranexamic acid and reported a 51% reduction in the odds of blood transfusion associated with these lysine analogues. There was an average of approximately one unit of blood saved, compared to placebo. As confirmation, both Henry *et al* [12] and Munoz *et al* [11], reported an approximate 50% reduction in the need for blood transfusion associated with EACA. However, the reduction of the re-exploration rate for bleeding was not statistically significant for EACA [11]. Moreover, lysine analogues were found to be inferior to aprotinin in seven trials comparing these medications (OR 1.45; 95% CI 1.02-2.08) as reported by Levi *et al.*

Safety and other effects

Mortality

Munoz *et al* [11] reported no statistically significant difference in mortality between EACA and placebo after combining four trials (1.8% vs 1.4%, p=0.7). Similar results were found in the Cochrane Review by Henry *et al* [12] who reported a statistically insignificant tendency towards a 66% higher risk of mortality (RR 1.66; 95% CI 0.46-6.01) in the same four trials.

Myocardial infarction

Munoz *et al* specifically addressed this outcome and did not report increased or decreased risk of MI when EACA was compared to placebo in four trials (3.9% vs 3.8%, p=0.9). Henry *et al* [12] also reported no increased risk of MI (RR 0.9; 95% CI 0.30-2.76) in three trials.

Renal failure

There were no trials or systematic reviews reporting data on this outcome.

Stroke

There were too few number of events to reach valid conclusions regarding this outcome.

Atrial fibrillation

No data is reported regarding this outcome.

Other safety information

Only information on thrombosis was available, based on 194 patients as reported by Henry *et al* [12]. No valid conclusions can be made.

Tranexamic acid

Tranexamic acid (TA) is a competitive inhibitor of substances responsible for plaminogen activation. At higher doses it is a non-competitive inhibitor of plasmin, acting as an inhibitor to fibrinolysis. It has been shown to be at least ten times more potent than EACA [23] and is cheaper than both aprotinin and EACA [24].

Blood transfusion benefits

Henry *et al* [12] calculated a 34% relative reduction of the risk of blood transfusion and approximately one unit of blood saved associated with TA. This is more likely to be accurate than combined estimates for lysine analogues reported by Levi *et al* [10] (see EACA section).

However, similarly to EACA, TA was not shown to be associated with a statistically significant reduction of re-exploration for bleeding [12]. The same author reported a tendency towards a 21% higher risk of blood transfusion associated with TA when it was compared to aprotinin in seven small trials.

Safety and other effects

Mortality

Mortality data was combined in seven trials by Henry *et al* [12] who reported a statistically insignificant 22% higher risk of mortality associated with TA (RR 1.21; 95% CI 0.83-1.76). Other reviewers did not address this issue or did not report separate results.

Myocardial infarction

Only Henry *et al* [12] reported a RR of 0.69 (95% CI 0.21-2.29) in eight trials of this medication.

Renal failure

Henry *et al* [12] reported a RR of 0.87 (95% CI 0.08-9.78 in two trials of this medication.

Stroke

Henry *et al* [12], reported a tendency towards a higher risk of stroke in six trials (RR 2.27; 95% CI 0.65-7.99). However, there were too few events to reach valid conclusions.

Atrial fibrillation

No data is reported regarding this outcome.

Other safety information

No increased or decreased risk of deep venous thrombosis, pulmonary embolism or any other thrombosis was found to be associated with TA in the Cochrane review [12].

Desmopressin

Desmopressin is a vasopressin analogue that is associated with a reduced release of the contents of Weibel-Palade bodies, including von Willebrand factor, thus its action is mostly associated with increased levels of von Willebrand factor and factor VIII [11]. Desmopressin is a valuable treatment for mild haemophilia and it was proposed that it might be beneficial in reducing bleeding after cardiopulmonary bypass (CPB), given the changes in platelet function occurring during and after CPB [25].

Blood transfusion benefits

The review by Henry *et al* [25] specifically addressing the effectiveness of desmopressin found no reduction in the proportion of people requiring a blood transfusion (RR 0.98; 95% CI 0.88-1.10). Similarly, a reduction in the volume of transfused blood was minimal and not statistically significant (on average, 0.05 units). Although there was a tendency towards a reduction of re-exploration for bleeding, the effect was not statistically significant.

Safety and other effects

Mortality

Desmopressin has not been shown to be associated with a reduced or increased mortality in one systematic review (RR 1.02, 95% CI 0.29-3.56) [10]. However, another review found a tendency towards a higher mortality associated with desmopressin after combining nine trials (RR 1.58; 95% CI 0.58-4.05) [25].

Myocardial infarction

Levi *et al* reported a 2.4 fold increase of MI (95% CI 1.2-5.6) associated with desmopressin in five trials, while Henry *et al* reported only a tendency towards a 1.5 times increase in the risk of MI (95% CI 0.67-3.49) in seven trials.

Renal failure

There were no trials or systematic reviews reporting information on this outcome.

Stroke

No information is available about the incidence of stroke in the trials of desmopressin.

Atrial fibrillation

No information is available about this outcome in the trials of desmopressin.

Other blood conservation techniques

Cell salvage use

A systematic review by Carless *et al* [26] reported that cell salvage is associated with an 18% reduction (95% CI 5%-30%) in the number of patients requiring blood transfusion. This meta-analysis was based on 12 trials comparing cell salvage with controls that did not receive any other active treatment to reduce exposure to blood transfusion. When cell salvage was combined with another blood conservation technique (eg. anti-fibrinolytic use), it was still associated with over a 30% reduction (95% CI 13%-44%) in the risk of blood transfusion compared to blood conservation (eg. anti-fibrinolytic use) without cell salvage.

The review reported that washed cell salvage is superior to unwashed and there was no difference between intra-operative versus postoperative use. However, these data as well as data on safety in cardiac surgery was not separately analysed and is inadequate to reach valid conclusions.

Platelet rich plasmapheresis

This technique produces a concentrated autologous platelet product and is recently being considered as an alternative approach to blood conservation in the surgical setting. The most recent systematic review with a meta-analysis [27] combined results from 19 clinical trials and has shown a 29% reduction (95% CI 10%-44%) in the risk of blood transfusion associated with this technique. However, when it was investigated in combination with cell salvage, it was not associated with a statistically significant reduction in blood transfusion compared to cell salvage alone (RR 0.80; 95% CI 0.60-1.08). There were too few trials reporting safety data for this intervention.

Recommendations	Evidence level
◆ Aprotinin is one of the most extensively investigated treatments to reduce blood transfusion requirements in cardiac surgery. It seems to be safe and is associated with a reduced risk of stroke.	I/A
◆ Superiority of aprotinin compared to lysine analogues (EACA and TA) is not yet well established. However, safety data for lysine analogues is still inadequate, and although these medications are much cheaper, until further studies establish their non-inferiority, safety and cost-effectiveness, aprotinin should be considered a first choice as an anti-fibrinolytic. Further studies should also address optimal and cost-effective dosage of aprotinin use.	I/A
◆ Desmopressin is of no use as a pharmacologic therapy to reduce blood conservation in cardiac surgery.	I/A
◆ Combining anti-fibrinolytic medications with either cell salvage techniques or platelet rich plasmapheresis seems to be a pragmatic choice. However, costs-effectiveness analyses are crucial when using these combined techniques. Combining anti-fibrinolytic medications with both cell salvage and platelet rich plasmapheresis is unlikely to be cost-effective.	I/A

References

1. Unsworht-White MJ, Herriot A, Valencia O, *et al.* Resternotomy for bleeding after cardiac operation: a marker for increased morbidity and mortality. *Ann Thorac Surg* 1995; 59: 664-667.
2. Dacey LJ, Munoz JJ, Baribeau YR, *et al.* Re-exploration for hemorrhage following coronary artery bypass grafting: incidence and risk factors. Northern New England Cardiovascular Disease Study Group. *Arch Surgery* 1998; 133(4): 442-7.
3. Hill SR, Carless PA, Henry DA, *et al.* Transfusion thresholds and other strategies guiding allogenic red blood cell transfusion (Cochrane review). In: *The Cochrane Library*, issue 4, 2003. John Wiley & Sons, Ltd., Chichester, UK.
4. Spiess BD. Cardiac anesthesia risk management. Hemorrhage, coagulation, and transfusion: a risk-benefit analysis. *J Cardiothorac Vasc Anesth* 1994; 8(1 suppl 1): 19-22.
5. Alderman EL, Levy JH, Rich JB, *et al.* Analyses of coronary graft patency after aprotinin use: results from the International Multicenter Aprotinin Graft Patency Experience (IMAGE) trial. *J Thorac Cardiovasc Surg* 1998; 116(5): 716-30.
6. Levy JH, Pifarre R, Schaff HV, *et al.* A multicenter, double-blind, placebo-controlled trial of aprotinin for reducing blood loss and the requirement for donor-blood transfusion in patients undergoing repeat coronary artery bypass grafting. *Circulation* 1995; 92(8): 2236-44.
7. Lemmer JHJ, Dilling EW, Morton JR, *et al.* Aprotinin for primary coronary artery bypass grafting: a multicenter trial of three dose regimens. *Ann Thorac Surg* 1996; 62(6): 1659-68.
8. Cosgrove DM, Heric B, Lytle BW, *et al.* Aprotinin therapy for re-operative myocardial revascularization: a placebo-controlled study. *Ann Thorac Surg* 1992; 54(6): 1031-6.
9. Lemmer JHJ, Stanford W, Bonney SL, *et al.* Aprotinin for coronary bypass operations: efficacy, safety, and influence on early saphenous vein graft patency. A multicenter, randomized, double-blind, placebo-controlled study. *J Thorac Cardiovasc Surg* 1994; 107(2): 543-51.
10. Levi M, Cromheecke ME, de Jonge E, *et al.* Pharmacological strategies to decrease excessive blood loss in cardiac surgery: a meta-analysis of clinically relevant endpoints. *Lancet* 1999; 354(9194): 1940-7.
11. Munoz JJ, Birkmeyer NJO, Birkmeyer JD, O'Connor GT, Dacey LJ. Is aminocaproic acid as effective as aprotinin in reducing bleeding with cardiac surgery? A meta-analysis. *Circulation* 1999; 99: 81-89.
12. Henry DA, Moxey AJ, Carless PA, *et al.* Anti-fibrinolytic use for minimizing peri-operative allogenic blood transfusion (Cochrane Review). In: *The Cochrane Library*, Issue 4, 2003. John Wiley & Sons, Ltd., Chichester, UK.
13. Petitti D. *Decision Analysis and Cost-effectiveness Analysis: Methods for Quantitative Synthesis in Medicine.* Oxford University Press Inc, New York, 1994.
14. Weightman WM, Gobbs NM. Pharmacological strategies for blood loss (letter). *Lancet* 2001; 357: 1131.
15. Asimakopoulos G, Kohn A, Stefanou DC, Haskard DO, Landis RC, Taylor KM. Leukocyte integrin expression in patients undergoing cardiopulmonary bypass. *Ann Thorac Surg* 2000; 69(4): 1192-7.
16. Bidstrup BP, Royston D, Sapsford RN, Taylor KM. Reduction in blood loss and blood use after cardiopulmonary bypass with high-dose aprotinin (Trasylol). *J Thorac Cardiovasc Surg* 1989; 97(3): 364-72.
17. Bidstrup BP, Underwood SR, Sapsford RN, Streets EM. Effect of aprotinin (Trasylol) on aorto-coronary bypass graft patency. *J Thorac Cardiovasc Surg* 1993; 105(1): 147-52; discussion 153.
18. Bidstrup BP, Hunt BJ, Sheikh S, Parratt RN, Bidstrup JM, Sapsford RN. Amelioration of the bleeding tendency of pre-operative aspirin after aortocoronary bypass grafting. *Ann Thorac Surg* 2000; 69(2): 541-7.
19. Blauhut B, Harringer W, Bettelheim P, Doran JE, Spath P, Lundsgaard-Hansen P. Comparison of the effects of aprotinin and tranexamic acid on blood loss and related variables after cardiopulmonary bypass. *J Thorac Cardiovasc Surg* 1994; 108(6): 1083-91.
20. Klein M, Keith PR, Dauben HP, *et al.* Aprotinin counterbalances an increased risk of peri-operative hemorrhage in CABG patients pre-treated with aspirin. *Eur J Cardiothorac Surg* 1998; 14(4): 360-366.
21. Murkin JM, Lux J, Shannon NA, *et al.* Aprotinin significantly decreases bleeding and transfusion requirements in patients receiving aspirin and undergoing cardiac operations. *J Thorac Cardiovasc Surg* 1994; 107(2): 554-61.
22. Santamaria A, Mateo J, Oliver A, *et al.* The effect of two different doses of aprotinin on hemostasis in cardiopulmonary bypass surgery: similar transfusion requirements and blood loss. *Haematologica* 2000; 85: 1277-1284.
23. Faught C, Wells P, Ferguson D, Laupacis A. Adverse effects of methods for minimizing peri-operative allogeneic transfusion: a critical review of the literature. *Transfus Med Rev* 1998; 12(3): 206-25.
24. Casati V, Guzzon D, Oppizzi M, *et al.* Hemostatic effects of aprotinin, tranexamic acid, and epsilon-aminocaproic acid in primary cardiac surgery. *Ann Thorac Surg* 1999; 68(6): 2252-6.
25. Henry DA, Moxey AJ, Carless PA, *et al.* Desmopressin for minimizing peri-operative allogeneic blood transfusion (Cochrane Review). In: *The Cochrane Library*, Issue 4, 2003. John Wiley & Sons, Ltd., Chichester, UK.
26. Carless PA, Henry DA, Moxey AJ, O'Connell D, Ferguson D. Cell salvage for minimizing peri-operative allogeneic blood transfusion (Cochrane Review). In: *The Cochrane Library*, Issue 4, 2003. John Wiley & Sons, Ltd., Chichester, UK.
27. Carless PA, Rubens FD, Antony DM, O'Connell D, Henry DA. Platelet-rich-plasmapheresis for minimizing peri-operative allogeneic blood transfusion (Cochrane Review). In: *The Cochrane Library*, Issue 4, 2003. John Wiley & Sons, Ltd., Chichester, UK.

Chapter 26

Interventions during cardiac surgery to reduce cognitive decline

Donald C Whitaker FRCS (Ed)
Specialist Registrar, Cardiothoracic Surgery

Guy's and St Thomas' Hospitals, London, UK

Introduction

Cardiac surgery with or without cardiopulmonary bypass (CPB) may cause in some patients a global cerebral injury manifest as impaired postoperative cognitive functioning [1,2]. This is a separate issue from discrete stroke. A deterioration in cognitive function can be detected by neuropsychological (NP) testing of concentration, memory, learning or the speed of mental and visuo-motor responses. Although reports on the effect of such deterioration on everyday functioning of patients are often anecdotal, there is objective evidence that tasks such as driving may be adversely affected [3].

The incidence of deficits varies widely depending on the methods and timing of NP assessment and on the subjects studied. Incidences of up to 80% have been reported [1]. However, recent studies in low-risk populations, in which neuroprotective techniques are used, report incidences of about 7% [4,5]. A recent systematic review suggests that an approximate 20% incidence of decline is to be expected two months after surgery [2]. These deficits have been shown to persist in studies up to five years post-surgery [6-8]. Although any resulting disability must be seen in the context of the overall benefits of cardiac surgery, there is good evidence that the use of arterial line filters and alpha stat acid base control during CPB reduce the cognitive decline and are therefore recommended. The evidence for other techniques such as off-pump surgery is less convincing, but will also be reviewed in this chapter. The evidence for various theoretical mechanisms (micro-emboli, altered cerebral blood flow and the inflammatory response) to explain the NP decline which can occur, although fascinating, is beyond the scope of this chapter which concentrates solely on the interventions which a surgeon, with the help of anaesthetic and perfusion staff, can implement to protect patients from cognitive decline. Patient factors which will inevitably contribute to NP outcome are also not discussed here.

Filters

Arterial line filters have gained in popularity because they have been shown to remove both micro-emboli and, in the event of a perfusion accident, large air emboli [9]. Five studies (Table 1) have examined the effect of filtration on neuropsychological outcome. Garvey *et al* [10] compared 46 unselected open heart

Table 1. Filter studies.

	Garvey	Aris	Sellman	Pugsley	Whitaker
Year	1983	1986	1993	1994	2004
n	46	100	54	100	198
Type of study	Retrospective Uncontrolled	RCT	RCT	RCT	RCT
Test group	Pall 40 micron or Bentley 25 micron	Shiley 20 micron	Swank 10 micron and bubble oxygenator (1)	Pall 40 micron	40 micron plus leucocyte depletion
Control group(s)	No filter	No filter	No filter, bubble oxygenator (2), no filter, membrane oxygenator (3)	No filter	40 micron
Outcome measure	CLAT	NP battery	NP battery	NP battery	NP battery
Definition of NP decline	Decline in CLAT score 1 SD below pre-op score	Decline below 1 SD in at least 1 of 3 domains	Decline by 1 SD in 2 or more tests	Decline by 1 SD in 2 or more tests	Decline by 1 SD in 2 or more tests
Timing of tests	Pre-operatively, one week post surgery	Pre-operatively, 10 days post surgery	Pre-operatively, 1 and 6 months post surgery	Pre-operatively, 8 weeks post surgery	Pre-operatively, 6 weeks post surgery
Result (% NP decline)	40 micron - 0% 25 micron - 24% no filter - 14%	20 micron - 64% No filter - 56%	(1) - 12% and 6% (2) - 24% and 12% (3) - 15% and 5%	40 micron - 8% No filter - 27%	40 micron / LD - 6% 40 micron - 8%

RCT = Randomised controlled trial; CLAT = Willner's conceptual level analogy test; NP= Neuropsychological; SD = Standard deviation

surgery patients who received either a Pall 40µm or Bentley AF-10 (25µm) filter with a historical group from nine years previously which had received no filtration. Neither anaesthesia, surgical or perfusion protocols are mentioned in this paper and the fact that the controls are historical makes comparison unreliable. Additionally, intellectual brain function was assessed using the CLAT (conceptual level analogy test), which is a single global measure of cognitive function. This type of assessment is unlikely to have the sensitivity required to detect changes following cardiac surgery. The decreased impairment found with the filter group could be due to many changes which could have occurred in the nine years between sampling the different groups.

In his RCT of 100 cases, Aris *et al* [11] used a more comprehensive battery of neuropsychological tests giving this study more credibility. Aris *et al* compared patients who had a Shiley 20µm nylon screen filter with a non-filter control group, but was unable to show any difference in outcome between the two. A negative result in a study of this size is unlikely to be the result of a type II error, but could be due to a number of other factors. The filter could have no effect or the filter could have a detrimental effect due to its small pore size or unusual form (nylon). More relevant is the possibility that the neuropsychological tests were performed at too early a stage postoperatively. Aris *et al* performed these tests at ten days postoperatively when many peri-operative factors such as anaesthesia, analgesia, pain or anxiety may continue to cloud the patients' neuropsychological function. The 1995 consensus[12] suggests that the ideal time to perform postoperative testing is three months post-surgery. Many studies use four to 12 weeks for convenience.

A better NP assessment technique was used by Sellman *et al*[13] who tested three groups with a battery of NP tests before surgery and at one and six months post-surgery. The postoperative testing was therefore likely to be far more specific than Aris *et al.* Sellman *et al* did not find a significant difference between the bubble oxygenator group with 10µm in-depth adsorption filter and the bubble oxygenator group without a filter. However, the membrane oxygenator group (without filter) was found to perform better than the bubble oxygenator group without filter at one month post-surgery on certain NP tests. Unfortunately, the value of this study is limited by the small numbers (17 to 20 in each group).

It was not until the study of Pugsley *et al*[14] a year later which used a greater number of subjects and a neuropsychological battery at appropriate times, that more convincing evidence of a neuroprotective effect of filtration was produced. One hundred patients having bubble oxygenated CPB were randomised to receive either the Pall 40µm (polyester screen) arterial line filter or no filter. Perfusion, anaesthesia and surgical technique were all well controlled. NP function was assessed pre-operatively, at eight days and eight weeks postoperatively. Transcranial doppler (TCD) was used to assess the number of micro-emboli in the middle cerebral artery intra-operatively. Pugsley showed that the 40µm filter significantly reduced the number of micro-emboli. Most importantly, Pugsley demonstrated a correlation between the number of micro-emboli detected and the incidence of a NP deficit postoperatively. Of those with a micro-emboli count <200, 8.6% (5/58 95% CI 3%-19%) had a deficit whereas of those with counts >1000, 43% (3/7 95% CI 10%-82%) had deficits. Filtered patients showed less deterioration on eight out of ten NP tests at eight weeks post-surgery compared to the non-filtered group. A deficit in performance (defined in Pugsley's study as a reduction in one SD of test score in two or more tests) occurred in four of 49 filtered patients and 12 of 45 non-filtered patients ($p<0.03$). Although Pugsley used bubble oxygenators and pH stat acid base control, both of which are little used today, the study provides good support for the value of arterial line filtration.

Most recently, a study compared NP outcome in 198 patients randomised to receive either a leucocyte depleting (LD) arterial line filter or one of two control standard filters [5]. Although there was a reduction in micro-emboli with the LD filter and a trend across a battery of NP tests towards improved NP outcome, there was not a statistically significant improvement in overall NP outcome. There is therefore, no clear advantage to using a LD filter rather than a conventional screen filter.

Oxygenators

Because membrane oxygenators produce less micro-emboli (as detected by transcranial doppler, TCD) than bubble oxygenators[15], their almost universal use these days is likely to have a beneficial effect on neuropsychological outcome. There is one study which suggests that there are reduced neuropsychological deficits when membrane oxygenators are used [16].

Pharmacological

There is an ongoing search for an effective neuroprotective drug for use in cardiac surgery. Surgery may be the ideal time to test such a drug because the injury is anticipated and treatment can be prophylactic. Two commonly used anaesthetic drugs, propofol and thiopentone, have been studied the most.

Nussmeir *et al*[17] first reported neuroprotective effects of thiopentone. They studied 182 patients having true open-heart surgery and randomised patients to receive either a thiopentone infusion during bypass or fentanyl. The dose of thiopentone was sufficient to maintain electroencephalographic silence throughout bypass. It was found that the thiopentone group had less "neuropsychiatric" (actual tests were neurological, psychiatric and the trailmaking tests) abnormalities at day one and day ten post-surgery. Unfortunately, longer-term effects were not studied. A later randomised trial [18] of 300 coronary artery bypass surgery patients found no neuroprotective effect but delayed awakening and greater inotrope dependence in the thiopentone group. A recent retrospective review by Pascoe *et al* [19] also found no benefit of thiopentone in open-chamber cardiac surgery. The evidence is therefore on the whole not supportive of thiopentone having a useful neuroprotective effect.

The evidence that propofol has a neuroprotective effect is equally unconvincing. Although propofol has physiological effects on the brain similar to thiopentone, reducing cerebral metabolic rate for oxygen ($CMRO_2$) and cerebral blood flow and inducing electroencephalographic (EEG) burst suppression [20], this does not seem to lead to clinically improved neurological or neuropsychological outcomes. In a trial of 225 patients having valve surgery, randomised to receive propofol or no propofol, NP outcome was the same at five to seven days and three months post-operation in both test and control groups [21]. In a recent RCT, Kadoi *et al* [4] found that there was no difference in NP outcome in 90 patients randomised to receive propofol compared to 90 patients receiving fentanyl.

Calcium channel antagonists such as nimodipine have been shown to reduce ischaemic cerebral injury in animals by limiting the amount of ischaemia-induced calcium entry which precedes cell death. A small randomised study of 35 patients having CABG or valve surgery from 1990 suggested an improvement in certain neuropsychological tests at six months post-surgery in the group given peri-operative nimodipine [22]. A later, larger randomised study [23] was halted prematurely when an increased mortality and bleeding rate was found in the nimodipine group. In the 150 patients randomised, no difference in neuro-psychological outcome was found.

Remacemide is an NMDA receptor antagonist which has been shown to reduce cerebral injury in animal models of focal ischaemia. Arrowsmith *et al* [24] using a battery of nine neuropsychological tests before and then eight weeks after surgery, assessed its clinical effects in a RCT of 171 patients having CABG surgery. The group of patients who received remacemide had a significantly better global change (Z) score of neuropsychological function compared to the control group. This probably reflects an increased capacity for learning in the remacemide group who have suffered less cerebral injury and therefore, provides evidence that remacemide is protective during cardiac surgery. Although, in contrast to previous studies of nimodipine or thiopentone, there were no serious adverse effects associated with remacemide, it should be noted that its use was associated with an increased frequency of dizziness, nausea and ataxia in the short-term.

It has been known for about 20 years that cardiac surgery with CPB is associated with an abnormal systemic inflammatory response. It is also likely that local inflammatory processes contribute to brain injury, but it is extremely difficult to study this, at least in humans. Aprotinin is a non-specific serine protease inhibitor, used mainly to reduce peri-operative bleeding due to its anti-fibrinolytic effects. However, aprotinin's lack of specificity at inhibiting enzymes has also resulted in a number of other anti-inflammatory properties being discovered. As yet, there are no randomised trials assessing the effect of aprotinin on neuropsychological outcome. Retrospective analysis of data from trials investigating aprotinin's effects on other outcomes suggests that aprotinin may reduce stroke rate [25]. Therefore, while there is potential for aprotinin to be neuroprotective, this concept remains untested.

Clomethiazole is the most recently tested potentially neuroprotective drug. In a randomised controlled trial of 245 patients using a thorough pre-operative and postoperative battery of neuro-psychological tests, Kong *et al* [26] found no improvement in neuropsychological outcome using clomethiazole.

Acid base management

The solubility of a gas in blood increases as the temperature falls. Therefore, during hypothermic bypass, when blood gas samples, which are always brought to 37°C in the blood gas analyser are back corrected to the temperature of the patient at the time the sample was taken, the patient appears to have a low $PaCO_2$ and a high pH. It is possible to correct the pH to the normal range by increasing the $PaCO_2$ and this method is known as pH stat control. However it is normal in nature for the neutral point of water to change with temperature and this is matched by the intracellular imidazole groups Allowing this to occur without the addition of CO_2 to "correct" it, is known as alpha stat control. There is evidence that alpha stat management leads to a better neurological and neuropsychological outcome. Bashein *et al*[27] in 1990, found no difference in neuropsychological outcome when either pH stat or alpha stat was used, but Stephan *et al*[28] found in 65 patients that hypothermia with pH stat management was associated with marked cerebral hyperaemia and an increase in neurological events by day seven post-surgery. This finding was supported by a later study of 316 patients by Murkin *et al*[29] in 1995 which found that there was improved neuropsychological outcome at two months post-surgery in a group randomised to receive alpha stat rather than pH stat. However, this significant difference was only found on *post hoc* analysis of a subgroup of patients whose CPB time was greater than 90 minutes.

Patel *et al*[30] (1996) randomised 70 patients to receive pH stat or alpha stat control with both groups cooled to 28°C. A significantly greater proportion of the pH stat patients showed deterioration in NP function at six weeks post-surgery. Interestingly, Patel also measured cerebral blood flow and found that it was greater in the pH stat group as was cerebral artery blood flow velocity. Although there was hyperaemia, as measured by cerebral extraction ratio for oxygen, in both groups it was more pronounced in the pH stat group. This study therefore suggested that the pH stat control disrupted the normal cerebral autoregulation and that the increased blood flow was harmful.

In summary, alpha stat acid-base balance reduces cognitive decline compared to pH stat (Table 2).

Table 2. Acid-base management studies.

	Bashein	Stephan	Murkin	Patel
Year	1990	1992	1995	1996
n	86	65	316	70
Type of study	RCT	RCT	RCT	RCT
Test group	Alpha stat	Alpha stat	Alpha stat	Alpha stat
Control group(s)	pH stat	pH stat	pH stat	pH stat
Outcome measure	NP battery	Neurological exam	NP battery	NP battery
Definition of NP decline	Decline by 1 SD in 2 or more tests	NA	Decline in change score in 1 or more of 4 test domains	Decline by 1 SD in 2 or more tests
Timing of tests	Pre-operatively, 8 days and 7 months post surgery	Pre-operatively, 7 days post surgery	Pre-operatively, 7 days and 2 months post surgery	Pre-operatively, 6 weeks post surgery
Result (% NP decline)	No difference between groups	Neurological dysfunction occurred more often in the pH-stat group (p=0.036)	Alpha stat - 78% and 30% pH stat - 80% and 36% (p=ns) Subgroup analysis (patients with CPB time greater than 90 mins: alpha stat - 83% and 27% pH stat - 86% and 44% (p=0.047)	Alpha stat - 20% pH stat - 49% (p=0.02)

RCT = Randomised controlled trial; NP = Neuropsychological; NA = Not applied

Table 3. **Hypothermia studies.**

	Mora	Regragui	Plourde	Heyer	Grimm	Nathan
Year	1996	1996	1997	1997	2000	2001
n	86	96	62	99	144	223
Type of study	RCT	RCT	RCT	RCT	RCT	RCT
Test groups#	28° C	28° C	28° C	28° C	32° C	34° C after XC release
	34° C	32° C 37° C	36° C	34° C	37° C	37° C after XC release
Outcome measure	NP battery (5)	NP battery (7)	NP battery (12)	NP battery (8)	P300 auditory evoked potentials and 1 NP test	NP battery (11)
Definition of NP decline	Each test analysed individually	ANOVA used	Decline by 1 SD in 1 or more tests	25% decrease in overall post-operative performance	NA	Decline by 0.5 SD in 1 or more of 3 domains
Timing of tests	Pre-operatively, 7-10 days and 4-6 weeks post surgery	Pre-operatively, 6 weeks post surgery	Pre-operatively, 7 days post surgery	Pre-operatively, 6 days and 6-9 weeks post surgery	Pre-operatively, 7 days and 4 months post surgery	Pre-operatively, 1 week and 3 months post surgery
Result (% NP decline)	No difference between groups However, none of the hypo-thermia group had strokes but 10% in the warm group did (p=0.006)	The 28° C and 32° C had less NP decline than the 37° C group (p=0.015)	28° C - 67% 36° C - 67%	No difference between groups using either event rate or group rate analysis	Trend towards improved P300 at 7 days in 37° C group (p=0.06) No difference by 4 months	34° C - 48% at 1 week 37° C - 62% at 1 week (p=0.048) No difference at 3 months

RCT = randomised controlled trial; NP = neuropsychological; # = temperature while on cardiopulmonary bypass unless stated otherwise; XC = cross-clamp; ANOVA = analysis of variance; SD = standard deviation; NA = not applied

Temperature

The two main issues regarding temperature management and subsequent cognitive outcome are the degree of hypothermia at which bypass is conducted and then the rate and extent to which subsequent rewarming occurs. There are a number of studies investigating the former issue (Table 3), with no clear overall outcome, but none, as far as the author is aware, investigating the latter.

Hypothermia has been used as both a cardio-protective and a neuroprotective strategy throughout the history of cardiac surgery. More recently, normothermia and normothermic cardioplegia have been investigated as a means of myocardial protection, leading to concern regarding possible compromise of cerebral protection using this technique. The following studies that have investigated the effect of normothermic compared to hypothermic bypass on neurological and neuropsychological outcome reveal conflicting results.

Singh *et al* [31] and also Mclean *et al* [32] found no difference in neurological outcome when normothermic or hypothermic bypass was used. In contrast Martin *et al* [33] found a marked increase in neurological events when normothermia was used. One criticism of all three of these studies is that the actual brain temperature was not measured. Depending on what bypass strategies are used, the actual brain temperature may be little different whether or not hypothermia is used. Also, it is possible that diffuse and focal cerebral injury (producing NP and neurological deficits respectively) may be differently affected by hypothermia. This is supported by a study of Mora *et al* [34] in which 138 patients were randomised to hypothermic or normothermic bypass and both neurological and neuropsychological outcomes were measured. Normothermic bypass increased the risk of stroke but not NP deficit. Regragui *et al* [35] randomised 96 adults to receive bypass at 37°C, 32°C and 28°C. There was a lower incidence of cognitive deficit in the 32°C group compared to the 37°C group, but cooling to 28°C conferred no additional benefit. Plourde *et al* [36] and Heyer *et al* [37] in two RCTs, did not find any difference between mild hypothermia and normothermia. More recently, a study by Grimm *et al* [38], suggested that normothermia may be less harmful than hypothermia. However, this study is seriously limited by a number of flaws. Grimm *et al* measured P300 auditory evoked potentials, the Mini Mental State exam and Trailmaking A tests to assess neuropsychological outcome in patients randomised to normothermia (37°C) and hypothermia (32°C). There was no difference in Mini Mental State exam and Trailmaking A tests, but there was a prolongation of P300 potentials in the hypothermia group four months after surgery. They failed to use a battery of tests as is recommended, and the relationship of P300 potentials to cognitive function in the setting of cardiac surgery is unknown. Also, the paper does not explain the important issue of exactly how temperature was managed and it is possible that the hypothermia group received damagingly rapid or excessive rewarming.

Nathan *et al* [39] studied the effects of two different rewarming strategies at the end of CPB. In a randomised controlled clinical trial, all patients were cooled to 32°C on CPB and then rewarmed to either 37°C or 34°C with no further rewarming. Although it was found that the 34°C group had less cognitive deficit at one week and three months postoperatively, the method of analysing cognitive change was unusual. A battery of 11 tests was used but these were then grouped into three domains and patients were classified as having a deficit if there was a deterioration in 0.5 of a standard deviation or greater in a domain. At three months a difference in only one of the 11 tests was seen. This suggests that the difference between groups at one week was a temporary effect which had worn off by three months.

In summary, although hypothermia itself may be neuroprotective, the evidence is not conclusive.

Surgical techniques and "off-pump" surgery

It is possible that surgical techniques may have a profound effect on both neurological and NP outcome following surgery. Although strong opinions tend to be expressed with regard to surgical technique, there has been relatively little scientific study of this issue. The common and logical view is that manipulating a calcific or atheromatous aorta is harmful. Such manipulation may dislodge macro- and micro-emboli with the subsequent adverse effects. There are three main manipulations to the aorta during CABG surgery which need to be considered. The first is the cannulation of the aorta necessary to initiate CPB. The second is the cross-clamping of the aorta which precedes either cross-clamp fibrillation or cardioplegic arrest. The third manipulation is the application of a side-biting clamp to perform proximal aorto-coronary anastamoses. Off-pump CABG avoids cannulation and cross-clamping, but unless a Y-graft technique is used, so that all grafts are fed from the

Table 4. Off-pump studies.

	Malheiros	BhaskerRao	Taggart	Diegeler	Lloyd	Van Dijk	Zamvar
Year	1995	1998	1999	2000	2000	2002	2002
n	81	322	75	40	60	281	60
on-pump	48	305	50	20	30	139	30
off-pump	33	17	25	20	30	142	30
Type of study	Prospective non-randomised	Prospective non-randomised	Prospective non-randomised matched groups	RCT	RCT	RCT	RCT
Outcome measure	NP battery (6) (non-standard)	ASEM test	NP battery (10) (standard)	NP battery (9) (non-standard) (Syndrom Kurz Test)	NP battery (7) (standard)	NP battery (10) (standard)	NP battery (9) (standard)
Definition of NP decline	Group mean analysis	NA	Group mean analysis	Group mean analysis	Group mean analysis	20% decline in 20% of test variables	1 SD decline in 2 or more tests
Timing of tests	Pre-operatively and up to 7 days post surgery	Pre-operatively and 1 day before discharge	Pre-operatively and at discharge and 3 months post surgery	Pre-operatively and 7 days post surgery	Pre-operatively and 12 weeks post surgery	Pre-operatively and 3 and 12 months post surgery	Pre-operatively and 1 and 10 weeks post surgery
Result (% NP decline)	No difference in NP outcome	Off-pump 94% On-pump 35% ($p<0.05$)	No difference in NP outcome	Significantly better NP outcome in off-pump group in terms of higher scores on Syndrom Kurz Test	No difference in NP outcome	At 3 months 21% in off-pump and 29% in on-pump groups ($p=0.15$). At 12 months 31% in off-pump and 34% in on-pump groups ($p=0.69$)	At 1 week 27% in off-pump and 63% in on-pump groups ($p=0.004$). At 10 weeks 10% in off-pump and 40% in on-pump groups ($p=0.0017$)

internal thoracic artery to avoid aorto-coronary anastamoses, side-biting clamps remain necessary.

Performing coronary artery bypass surgery without the use of cardiopulmonary bypass has a number of theoretical advantages and elimination of cerebral injury is potentially one of the most significant of these. There is some evidence for a reduction in both micro-emboli production and the inflammatory response, thought to have a major role in causing cerebral injury on bypass, in patients who have CABG without CPB. However, most of the studies carried out so far (Table 4) do not show any difference in neuropsychological outcome in on-bypass and off-bypass patients.

Malheiros *et al* [40] studied 81 patients who had CABG either with or without CPB according to surgical technical selection criteria. The CPB group had a mean of 2.9 grafts and a mean operative time of 325 minutes, whereas the non-CPB group had a mean of 1.7 grafts and a mean operative time of 251 minutes. The groups were not matched therefore, in terms of surgical trauma. No differences were found in early (five to seven days postoperatively) tests of neurological or neuropsychological outcome. Although the neuropsychological tests were not conventional they were reasonably comprehensive. However, at such an early postoperative stage many factors cloud neuropsychological performance, and tests at this stage without later testing, cannot be relied upon.

Bhasker-Rao *et al* [41] used ASEM (anti-saccadic eye movement) as a test of pre- and postoperative neurocognitive function in 322 CABG patients, 17 of whom had no CPB. Unfortunately, although ASEM is a good test of frontal lobe dysfunction in patients with dementia, it has not been validated in cardiac surgery patients. Therefore, the fact that the off-pump cases had fewer ASEM deficits after surgery is of extremely doubtful significance. A short report by Malheiros *et al* [42] in 1999, recorded no micro-embolic signals in a "series" of six patients. They did however, note fairly marked disturbances in middle cerebral artery blood velocity during manipulation of the heart. Off-pump surgery thus has the potential for a deleterious effect on cognitive function by compromising cerebral blood flow despite the relative lack of micro-emboli.

More recently, a number of studies have continued to give conflicting results regarding cognitive outcome after off-pump surgery. Diegeler *et al* [43] randomised 40 patients to off-pump or conventional CABG with CPB surgery. Unfortunately, the tests they used to assess cognitive outcome (a "standardised *psychiatric* assessment" and the Syndrom Kurz Test) are unvalidated in cardiac surgery and were performed only early after surgery (at seven days). Diegler *et al*'s finding that there was a marked increase in cognitive impairment in the conventional group and no impairment at all in the off-pump group must therefore be interpreted cautiously. In contrast, Taggart *et al* [44], in a study using a conventional neuropsychological test battery pre-surgery, at discharge and at three months post-surgery, were unable to find any difference in medium-term cognitive outcome between either on-pump or off-pump cases. Taggart's study however, was not randomised but studied 25 off-pump patients compared to 50 matched on-pump controls. The fact that Taggart used a validated battery of neuropsychological tests lends that study more overall weight. Lloyd *et al*'s RCT of 60 patients [45] found no difference in NP outcome 12 weeks after on-pump or off-pump surgery.

Van Dijk *et al* [46] randomised 281 patients and measured cognitive outcome using a recognised battery of ten tests at three and 12 months after surgery. They found no difference in the two groups at three months post-surgery using incidence analysis (21% in the off-pump group and 29% in the on-pump group), but there was a significant difference in the overall standardised change score at three months (0.19 vs 0.13, p=0.03). There was no difference at 12 months using either method of analysis. Van Dijk *et al*'s follow-up rate was good overall, but the follow-up rate was 90% in the on-pump group and 98% in the off-pump group at three months. It is therefore possible that a greater difference between the groups was missed because those patients with the greater cognitive impairment are more likely to drop out. The latest study to be published does suggest that surgery without cardiopulmonary bypass causes less cognitive impairment than with bypass. Zamvar *et al* [47] (2002) randomised 60 patients to on- or off-CPB and performed pre-operative and one and 10-week postoperative NP testing with a battery of nine standard tests. Although the number of patients studied was relatively low, an impressive 100% follow-up rate at ten weeks was achieved. In a relatively low-risk group (patients with previous TIAs and CVAs were excluded) incidence of decline (defined as deterioration by more than one SD in two or more tests) was 40% in the on-pump group and 10% in the off-pump group (a highly significant difference). Such a high incidence is difficult to explain and unfortunately, Zamvar *et al* give very little detail of operative procedures in either of their groups, thus limiting the applicability of their study.

Most of the studies investigating NP outcome after on-pump or off-pump surgery, have had small numbers so the lack of difference in Taggart *et al* [44] and Lloyd *et al*'s [45] studies may have been the result of type 2 errors. The positive results of Diegler *et al* [43] and Zamvar *et al* [47] also come from relatively small but, as discussed, flawed studies. The largest of the well conducted studies (Van Dijk *et al* [46]) showed no difference in NP outcome. Off-pump surgery cannot therefore be recommended as a technique to reduce cognitive decline.

Interventions during cardiac surgery to reduce cognitive decline

Recommendations	Evidence level
◆ Arterial line filters reduce cognitive decline.	Ib/A
◆ Alpha stat acid base balance reduces cognitive decline.	Ib/A
◆ The evidence for hypothermia and off-pump surgery is high, but conflicting. They are therefore, not recommended as a means to reduce cognitive decline.	Ib/A

References

1. Borowicz LM, Goldsborough MA, Selnes OA, McKhann GM. Neuropsychologic change after cardiac surgery: a critical review. *J Cardiothorac Vasc Anaes* 1996; 10: 105-112.
2. van Dijk D, Keizer AMA, Diephuis JC, Durand C, Vos LJ, Hijman R. Neurocognitive dysfunction after coronary artery bypass surgery: a systematic review. *J Thorac Cardiovasc Surg* 2000; 120: 632-639.
3. Ahlgren E, Lundqvist A, Nordlund A, Aren C, Rutberg H. Neurocognitive impairment and driving performance after coronary artery bypass surgery. *Eur J Cardiothorac Surg* 2003; 23: 334-40.
4. Kadoi Y, Saito S, Kunimoto F, Goto F, Fujita N. Comparative effects of propofol versus fentanyl on cerebral oxygenation state during normothermic cardiopulmonary bypass and postoperative cognitive dysfunction. *Ann Thorac Surg* 2003; 75: 840-6.
5. Whitaker DC, Newman SP, Stygall J, Hope-Wynne C, Harrison MJG, Walesby RK. The Effect of Leucocyte Depleting Arterial Line Filters on Cerebral Microemboli and Neuropsychological Outcome Following Coronary Artery Bypass Surgery. *Eur J Cardiothorac Surg* 2004; 25: 267-274.
6. Newman MF, Kirchner JL, Phillips-Bute B. Longitudinal assessment of neurocognitive function after coronary artery bypass surgery. *New Engl J Med* 2001; 344: 395-402.
7. Selnes OA, Royall RM, Grega MA, Borowicz LM Jr., Quaskey S, McKhann GM. Cognitive changes 5 years after coronary artery bypass grafting: is there evidence of late decline? *Arch Neurol* 2001; 58: 598-604.
8. Stygall J, Newman SP, Fitzgerald G, Steed L, Mulligan K, Arrowsmith JE, *et al.* Cognitive change 5 years after coronary artery bypass surgery. *Health Psychol* 2003; 22: 579-86.
9. Mejak BL, Stammers A, Rauch E, Vang S, Viessman T. A retrospective study on perfusion incidents and safety devices. *Perfusion* 2001; 15: 51-61.
10. Garvey JW, Willner A, Wolpowitz A, Caramonte L, Rabiner CJ, Weisz D, Wisoff BG. The effect of arterial filtration during open heart surgery on cerebral function. *Circulation* 1983*; 68* (Suppl 2):125-128.
11. Aris A, Solanes H, Camara ML, Junque C, Escartin A, Caralps JM. Arterial line filtration during cardiopulmonary bypass: neurologic, neuropsychologic, and haematologic studies. *J Thorac Cardiovasc Surg* 1986; 91: 526-533.
12. Murkin JM, Newman SP, Stump DA, Blumenthal JA. Statement of consensus on assessment of neurobehavioural outcomes after cardiac surgery. *Ann Thorac Surg* 1995; 59 : 1289-1295.
13. Sellman M, Holm L, Ivert T, Semb BKH. A randomised study of neuropsychological function in patients undergoing coronary bypass surgery. *Thoracic Cardiovascular Surgeon* 1993; 41: 349-354.
14. Pugsley WB, Klinger L, Paschalis C, Treasure T, Harrison M, Newman S. The impact of microemboli during cardiopulmonary bypass on neuropsychological functioning. *Stroke* 1994; 25: 1393-1399.
15. Padayachee TS, Parsons S, Theobald R, Linley JJ, Gosling RG, Deverall PB. The detection of microemboli in the middle cerebral artery during cardiopulmonary bypass; a transcranial Doppler ultrasound investigation using membrane and bubble oxygenators. *Ann Thorac Surg* 1987; 44: 298-302.
16. Smith PL, Blauth CI, Newman S. Cerebral microembolisation and neuropsycholgical outcome following coronary artery bypass surgery (CABS) with either a membrane or a bubble oxygenator. In: *Impact of cardiac surgery on the quality of life.* Willner A, Rodewald G, Eds. Plenum Press, New York, 1990: 337-342.
17. Nussmeier NA, Arlund C, Slogoff S. Neuropsychiatric complications after cardiopulmonary bypass: cerebral protection by a barbiturate. *Anesthesiology* 1986; 64: 165-70.
18. Zaidan JR, Klochany A, Martin WM, Zeigler JS, Harless DM, Andrews RB. Effect of thiopental on neurological outcome following coronary artery bypass grafting. *Anaesthesiology* 1991; 74: 406-411.
19. Pascoe EA, Hudson RJ, Anderson BA. High-dose thiopentone for open-chamber cardiac surgery: a retrospective review. *Can J Anaesth* 1996; 43: 575-579.
20. Newman MF, Murkin JM, Roach GW, Croughwell ND, White WD, Clements FM. Cerebral psychologic doses of propofol during nonpulsatile cardiopulmonary bypass. CNS Subgroup of McSPI. *Anaesth Analg* 1995; 81: 452-547.
21. Roach GW, Mewman MF, Murkin JM, Martzke JS, Ruskin A, Li J, Guo A, Wisniewski A, Mangano DT. Ineffectiveness of burst suppression therapy in mitigating perioperative cerebrovascular dysfunction. *Anaesthesiology* 1999; 90: 1255-1264.
22. Forsman M, Tubylewicz Olnes B, Semb G, Steen PA. Effects of nimodipine on cerebral blood flow and neuropsychological outcome after cardiac surgery. *Br J Anaes* 1990; 65: 514-520.

23. Legault C, Furberg CD, Wagenknecht LE, Rogers AT, Stump DA, Coker L, *et al.* Nimodipine neuroprotection in cardiac valve replacement: report of an early terminated trial. *Stroke* 1996; 27: 593-8.
24. Arrowsmith JE, Harrison MJG, Newman SP, Stygall J, Timberlake N, Pugsley WB. Neuroprotection of the brain during cardiopulmonary bypass: a randomised trial of Remacemide during coronary artery bypass in 171 patients. *Stroke* 1998; 29: 2357-2362.
25. Murkin JM. Attenuation of neurologic injury during cardiac surgery. *Ann Thorac Surg* 2001; 72: S1838-S1844.
26. Kong RS, Butterworth J, Aveling W, Stump DA, Harrison MJ, Hammon J, *et al.* Clinical trial of the neuroprotectant clomethiazole in coronary artery bypass graft surgery: a randomized controlled trial. *Anesthesiology* 2002; 97: 585-91.
27. Bashein G, Townes BD, Nessley M. A randomised trial of carbon dioxide management during hypothermic cardiopulmonary bypass. *Anaesthesiology* 1990; 72: 7-15.
28. Stephan H, Weyland A, Kazmaier S, Henze T, Menck S, Sonntag H. Acid-base management during hypothermic cardiopulmonary bypass does not affect cerebral metabolism but does affect blood flow and neurological outcome. *Br J Anaes* 1992; 69: 51-57.
29. Murkin JM, Martzke JS, Buchan AM, Bentley C, Wong CJ. A randomised study of the influence of perfusion technique and pH management strategy in 316 patients undergoing coronary artery bypass surgery: II. Neurologic and cognitive outcomes. *J Thorac Cardiovasc Surg* 1995; 110: 346-362.
30. Patel RL, Turtle MR, Chambers DJ, James DN, Newman S, Venn GE. Alpha-stat acid-base regulation during cardiopulmonary bypass improves neuropsychologic outcome in patients undergoing coronary artery bypass grafting. *J Thorac Cardiovasc Surg* 1996; 111: 1267-1279.
31. Singh AK, Feng WC, Bert AA, Rotenberg FA. Stroke during coronary artery bypass grafting using hypothermic versus normothermic perfusion. *Ann Thorac Surg* 1995; 59: 84-89.
32. McLean RF, Wong BI. Normothermic versus hypothermic cardiopulmonary bypass: central nervous system outcomes. *J Cardiothorac Vasc Anaes* 1996; 10: 45-53.
33. Martin TD, Craver JM, Gott JP, Weintraub WS, Ramsay J, Mora CT, Guyton RA. Prospective, randomised trial of retrograde warm blood cardioplegia: myocardial benefit and neurologic threat. *Ann Thorac Surg* 1994; (57): 298-302.
34. Mora CT, Henson MB, Weintraub WS, Murkin JM, Martin TD, Carver JM, Gott JP, Guyton, RA. The effect of temperature management during cardiopulmonary bypass on neurologic and neuropsychologic outcomes in patients undergoing coronary revascularisation. *J Thorac Cardiovasc Surg* 1996; 112: 514-522.
35. Regragui I, Birdi I, Bashar M, Izzat MB, Black AMS, Lopatatzidis A, Day CJE, Gardner F, Bryan AJ, Angelini GD. The effects of cardiopulmonary bypass temperature on neuropsychological outcome after coronary artery operations: a prospective randomised trial. *J Thorac Cardiovasc Surg* 1996; 112: 1036-1045.
36. Plourde G, Leduc AS, Morin JE, DeVarennes B, Latter D, Symes J, *et al.* Temperature during cardiopulmonary bypass for coronary artery operations does not influence postoperative cognitive function: a prospective, randomized trial. *J Thorac Cardiovasc Surg* 1997; 114: 123-8.
37. Heyer EJ, Adams DC, Delphin E, McMahon DJ, Steneck SD, Oz MC, *et al.* Cerebral dysfunction after coronary artery bypass grafting done with mild or moderate hypothermia. *J Thorac Cardiovasc Surg* 1997; 114: 270-7.
38. Grimm M, Czerny M, Baumer H, Kilo J, Madl C, Kramer L, *et al.* Normothermic cardiopulmonary bypass is beneficial for cognitive brain function after coronary artery bypass grafting – a prospective randomized trial. *Eur J Cardiothorac Surg* 2000; 18: 270-5.
39. Nathan HJ, Wells GA, Munson JL, Wozny D. Neuroprotective effect of mild hypothermia in patients undergoing coronary artery surgery with cardiopulmonary bypass: a randomized trial. *Circulation* 2001; 104: I85-91.
40. Malheiros SMF, Brucki SMD, Gabbi AA, Bertolucci PHF, Juliano Y, Carvalho AC, Buffolo E. Neurological outcomes in coronary artery surgery with and without cardiopulmonary bypass. *Acta Neurologica Scandinavica* 1995; 92: 256-260.
41. BhaskerRao B, VanHimbergen D, Edmonds HL Jr., Jaber S, Ali AT, Pagni S, *et al.* Evidence for improved cerebral function after minimally invasive bypass surgery. *J Card Surg* 1998; 13: 27-31.
42. Malheiros SMF, Massaro AR, Carvalho AC, Moises VA, Mussi A, Fredrico D, Teles CA, Buffolo E, Gabbai AA. Transesophageal echocardiography and transcranial Doppler monitoring in coronary surgery without cardiopulmonary bypass: preliminary results. *Cerebrovascular Diseases* 1999; 9: 358-360.
43. Diegeler A, Hirsch R, Schneider F, Schilling LO, Falk V, Rauch T, Mohr FW. Neuromonitoring and neurocognitive outcome in off-pump versus conventional coronary bypass operation. *Ann Thorac Surg* 2000; 69: 1162-1166.
44. Taggart DP, Browne SM, Halligan PW, Wade DT. Is cardiopulmonary bypass still the cause of cognitive dysfunction after cardiac operations? *J Thorac Cardiovasc Surg* 1999; 118: 414-420.
45. Lloyd CT, Ascione R, Underwood MJ, Gardner F, Black A, Angelini GD. Serum S100 protein release and neuropsychological outcome during coronary revascularisation on the beating heart: a prospective randomised study. *J Thorac Cardiovasc Surg* 2000; 119: 148-154.
46. Van Dijk D, Jansen EW, Hijman R, Nierich AP, Diephuis JC, Moons KG, *et al.* Cognitive outcome after off-pump and on-pump coronary artery bypass graft surgery: a randomized trial. *JAMA* 2002; 287: 1405-12.
47. Zamvar V, Williams D, Hall J, Payne N, Cann C, Young K, *et al.* Assessment of neurocognitive impairment after off-pump and on-pump techniques for coronary artery bypass graft surgery: prospective randomised controlled trial. *BMJ* 2002; 325: 1268.

Chapter 27

Indications for cardiac transplantation

Kiran CR Patel MA PhD MRCP
Specialist Registrar, Cardiology
Robert S Bonser FRCP FRCS FESC
Consultant Cardiothoracic Surgeon

Queen Elizabeth Hospital, University Hospital Birmingham NHS Trust, Birmingham, UK

Introduction

Cardiac transplantation activity worldwide is currently static, but in the UK, activity is declining [1] (Figure 1). In the developed world, where the extent of cardiac transplantation activity is limited by donor organ availability, there is a significant supply-demand imbalance [2]. Such an imbalance is unlikely to change in the near future, although the advent of device therapy for heart failure may have an impact on timing and perhaps need of transplantation in selected cases. As the supply of organs is unlikely to increase significantly, any expansion in the indications or threshold for cardiac transplantation would inevitably lead to two phenomena. Firstly, the number of patients dying on the waiting list for transplantation (currently in the region of 25%) will increase, and secondly, the percentage of patients on the waiting list receiving a transplant will decrease from the currently observed 60% within two years of listing, to a much lower level. In this chapter, we review the current evidence and indications for cardiac transplantation and also highlight non-conventional cases where successful outcome has been reported. We do not review the ethical dilemmas of attempting to expand the donor pool in order to accommodate and expand upon the currently accepted indications for transplantation, as this is outside the remit of this text.

Between 1967, when Barnard reported the first case of orthotopic cardiac transplantation in man, and 1995, there were over 3000 cardiac transplants and over 250 combined heart and lung transplants worldwide. In the USA alone, in 2001, there were 2202 heart transplants [3]. In the UK, the first three cardiac transplant procedures, performed between 1968 and 1970, were unsuccessful and a moratorium was imposed until 1979, when the cardiac community witnessed the development of, and meticulous evaluation of programmes at Papworth and Harefield. Improved success was attributed to improved surgical techniques, the use of endomyocardial biopsy in the diagnosis of rejection and the advent of cyclosporin use. Following early reported success, it was accepted that cardiac transplantation should be available, but deferred until all other treatment options had been exhausted, a principle which still applies today. In addition, today's clinician must evaluate whether the transplant recipient will likely return to normal or near-normal existence i.e. not be constrained by any other comorbid illnesses following transplantation, in order to make best use of scarce donor organs [4].

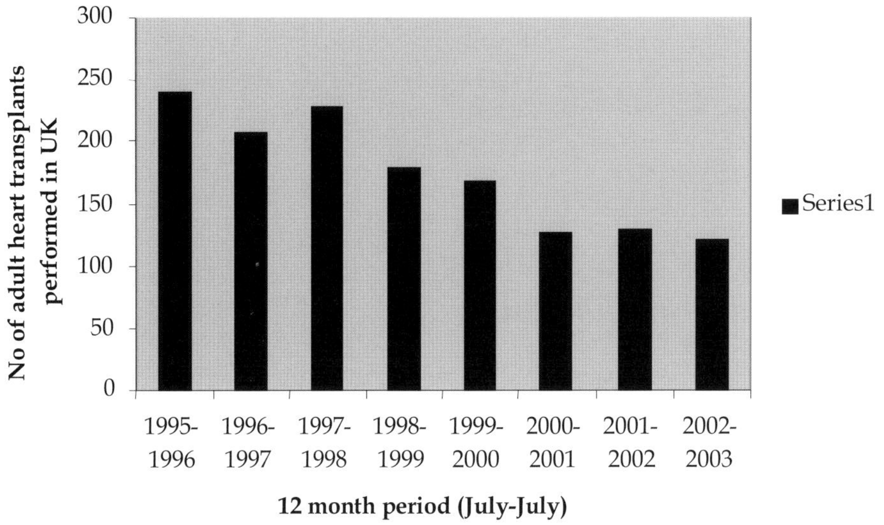

Figure 1. UK Cardiac transplant activity [1].

Methodology

A systematic review of the current literature on indications for cardiac transplantation was completed with a search of databases including PubMed between 1966 to 2004. In total, 66 publications were identified, of which three were recent systematic reviews and a further three were non-systematic reviews. There were no randomised controlled studies and the remaining papers were a mixture of observational and population-based publications, registry data, case reports and proceedings from annual congresses. Thus, the evidence base for cardiac transplantation is derived from comparisons of the natural history of heart failure and the outcome data for transplantation.

Death in heart failure

Most patients with heart failure die eventually of multi-organ failure as a consequence of low cardiac output or sudden death. Sudden death occurs in the context of malignant ventricular arrhythmias. This explains the benefit of added defibrillator activity to cardiac resynchronisation therapy in the recent COMPANION study [5]. Sudden cardiac death is more common in severe heart failure due to electrical remodelling, electrolyte changes and the use of anti-arrhythmic drugs which in themselves may prove to be pro-arrhythmic. The final demise of other heart failure patients may be accelerated by intercurrent infection, pulmonary embolism, myocardial infarction or stroke.

Treatment beyond medical therapy in heart failure

When conventional pharmacotherapy (fluid management, salt intake, weight management, exercise regimens and drug therapy [angiotensin converting enzyme inhibitors, β–blockers, aspirin, HMG COA reductase inhibitors]) is optimised in the individual patient, yet symptoms persist or quality of life is impaired, alternative therapies may be considered. One of these alternative therapies is cardiac transplantation, which should be entertained as a potential therapy when the likely prognosis following transplantation is predicted to be significantly superior to continuing conventional medical therapy. This requires specialist assessment of heart failure patients by clinicians with expertise in the knowledge of appropriate application of advanced therapies in heart failure, including transplantation. Alternatives to transplantation are exempt from the constraints of donor shortage, but may be viable alternatives in select patients.

Evidence for cardiac transplantation as a therapy

From a public health and political perspective it is rational to argue that transplantation is too expensive and serves too few individuals to be in the best public interests in terms of healthcare expenditure. However, such a belief must be balanced against the significant impact of heart failure on healthcare expenditure. Heart failure is a leading cause of hospitalisation and is one of the most expensive components of healthcare and this expense increases with increasing severity of heart failure. In terms of cost per year of life saved, cardiac transplantation compares favourably with other life-extending therapies such as haemodialysis [6]. There is therefore, evidence from a public health perspective that cardiac transplantation is a cost-effective treatment. Is there clinical evidence of benefit?

The COCPIT study [7] performed in a national cohort of adult patients listed for cardiac transplantation in Germany in 1997, found a beneficial effect only in a group of patients that was at high risk of dying from heart failure without transplantation. If these results can be reproduced in other countries, the discussion on the respective roles of pharmacological and organ-saving surgical therapies for advanced heart failure, medical urgency and waiting time as heart transplantation allocation criteria, and the feasibility of a randomised clinical trial testing the survival benefit of transplantation must be reopened. The listing of more critically ill patients and increasing use of marginal donor hearts, driven by the supply-demand imbalance of donor organs has been associated with a maintenance of outcomes after cardiac transplantation, but no significant improvement, even with better transplant management [8,9]. As a result, the survival benefit of transplantation in ambulant patients is now less clear than it seemed over a decade ago. The COCPIT study argues for cessation of or at least restricting the practice of listing low-risk ambulant patients with heart failure, for transplantation, until clear evidence of benefit is available by means of a clinical trial. However, most centres continue to provide ambulant patients access to transplantation and justify this practice on the basis of patient-specific prognosis eg. the heart failure survival score (the only validated survival index for predicting mortality in stable patients awaiting a heart transplant), versus predicted survival post-transplantation. Therefore, although originally considered only for patients with NYHA class IV symptoms, the 82% and 74% one- and 3-year cardiac transplantation survival rates respectively, compare favourably to the 15% to 20% annual mortality rates for patients with NYHA class III heart failure [10].

The survival benefit of cardiac transplantation as compared with current medical treatment in advanced heart failure has not been tested in a prospective randomised trial and such a trial, as well as being ethically unjustifiable, is unlikely to occur with the extremely poor prognosis of most patients referred for consideration of transplantation, despite the COCPIT study ramifications [11]. At best, one might hope to obtain registry data of patients referred for transplantation, some of whom might be offered alternative therapies either when transplantation has been deemed inappropriate or unavailable (i.e. patients offered alternative therapies whilst on a waiting list for transplantation). Overall, there is ample evidence of a mortality benefit of transplantation in non-ambulant patients, but clinical trial evidence in ambulant patients is lacking. The evidence for transplantation in this cohort is based upon predictive modelling of prognostic factors.

Higher risk non-transplant operative procedures as an alternative strategy

The critical issues determining whether patients should be offered high-risk conventional surgery as an alternative to transplantation are the underlying condition, the extent of irreversible disease and risk factors for poor outcome. In general, ischaemic cardiomyopathy, LV (left ventricular) aneurysm and valvular disease are the most common conditions where conventional surgery is considered as an alternative to transplantation.

Revascularisation

Survival of patients with ischaemic cardiomyopathy and heart failure is poor, with an annual mortality ranging from 30-50% [12]. Numerous studies [13,14] have shown that coronary artery bypass surgery (CABG) in patients with severe LV impairment may be performed with relatively low risk. However, surgery requires evidence of reversible ischaemia, good distal vessels to graft and the presence of occlusive coronary artery disease. An informal comparison [15] dictates that patients with severe heart failure perform comparably to, or better than patients offered transplantation, and although no randomised controlled trial exists, all patients with ischaemic cardiomyopathy should have the option of being considered for revascularisation prior to transplant assessment, in order to enable comparison of the risk of an available treatment against the risk of being placed on a waiting list for transplantation. The basis for surgical revasularisation is that not all ventricular dysfunction secondary to coronary artery disease is irreversible. Revascularisation in certain patients would appear to improve ventricular function [16,17]. These patients are said to demonstrate myocardial "hibernation" and ideally, evidence of reversible ischaemia selects those patients most likely to derive benefit from revascularisation [18-20]. Revascularisation in these patients may provide a further treatment option in the treatment of heart failure. The ongoing STICH [21] and HEART UK [22] trials aim to address the roles of ventricular restoration and revascularisation in ischaemic heart failure and will clarify the use of bypass surgery in chronic heart failure.

Valve surgery

The aims of valve surgery are to improve symptoms, prolong survival and prevent deterioration of cardiac function. It is beyond the scope of this chapter to discuss the situation when transplantation might be considered over high-risk valve surgery, but in general, patients with very severe LV dysfunction in combination with severe mitral regurgitation, aortic stenosis or aortic regurgitation require very careful evaluation before any surgical option, including transplantation, is considered.

Aneurysmectomy

In patients with heart failure, aneurysmectomy can improve systolic and diastolic function as well as provide symptomatic relief [23]. However, it is unclear whether surgery improves survival in the majority of patients. Those patients with extensive LV dysfunction and higher LV end diastolic pressure (LVEDP) appear to derive the greatest benefit. Dor *et al* showed that patients with an ejection fraction below 30%, LV dilatation and frequent ventricular arrhythmias derived most benefit from aneurysmectomy [24]. However, these are selected case series and further trial evidence is required to establish the role of surgery.

Transmyocardial laser revascularisation

Transmyocardial laser revascularisation is theoretically promising, but is unlikely to become a valid treatment in advanced ischaemic heart failure.

Ventricular assist devices

Ventricular assist devices represent an important advance in heart failure therapy. Their role in providing a bridge to transplantation appears established and there is now development of destination therapy programmes which have great promise [25,26]. Description of these devices is beyond the scope of this chapter, but ongoing studies will inevitably bring more attention to these devices in the near future.

Left ventricular restoration procedures

Partial LV resection (also known as LV reduction) was pioneered by Batista [27] to improve left ventricular function by improving haemodynamics according to Laplace's law, in patients with severe dilated cardiomyopathy in a region of the world where transplantation was not an available alternative. Despite early optimism, 12-month freedom from death or the need for relisting for transplantation was only 56% in a series of patients with idiopathic dilated cardiomyopathy [28]. The procedure is therefore an inferior alternative to transplantation. Endoventricular circular patch plasty is another form of surgical reduction, removing akinetic or dyskinetic scar tissue, but again, is associated with poor late survival when compared to transplantation, despite earlier claims that survival of patients with severe heart failure is similar to that of patients undergoing LV reduction surgery [29].

Cardiomyoplasty

Despite improvement in clinical symptoms, multiple studies failed to show any significant and sustained improvement in LV function with cardiomyoplasty [30]. High early mortality has been encountered, as the haemodynamic benefit of surgery takes up to 12 weeks to develop due to the obligatory period of muscle training. Cardiomyoplasty, if still used, should only be considered in patients with NYHA class III heart failure, without significant valvular disease, ischaemia or arrhythmias [31].

Cardiac resynchronisation therapy (± automated implantable cardioverter defibrillator therapy)

Although there are no long-term mortality studies in the use of device therapy, there is strong evidence that patient hospitalisation is decreased, quality of life is improved and early mortality is reduced [5,32-36]. These therapies may improve short-term survival, but have a limited effect on quality of life and exercise tolerance at present. In future, as cardiac resynchronisation therapy (CRT) and automated implantable cardiovertor defibrillator (AICD) therapy develop, the role of transplantation may need to be refined further. Also, these device therapies should not be considered alternatives to transplantation, but may serve as adjunctive therapy in some patients awaiting transplantation to improve short-term symptoms and prognosis whilst awaiting a suitable donor organ.

Survival following orthotopic cardiac transplantation

Early survival statistics following transplantation were poor, but the advent of endomyocardial biopsy to diagnose rejection and more significantly, cyclosporin and multi-drug immunosuppressant regimens dramatically improved survival rates (Tables 1 and 2) [37,38]. The most significant reduction in mortality over the past three decades has occurred in the early months following transplantation, which inevitably has an impact on improving long-term prognosis. At most institutions, survival at one month post-transplantation approaches 90% and declines to 50-60% at ten years. Mid- and long-term survival is dependent upon donor and recipient factors influencing rejection, infection, allograft vasculopathy and development of malignancy (Table 3). For the individual patient, it is possible to predict with some degree of accuracy the outcome from cardiac transplantation utilising the known risk factors for adverse events illustrated in

Table 1. Survival rates following cardiac transplantation (adapted from [39]).

Years post-transplantation	% Survival
1/12 (1 month)	93
1	85
3	78
5	72
7	66
10	55

Table 2. Causes of death following cardiac transplantation (adapted from [39]).

Cause of death	Interval to death and % of deaths in that period		
	<1yr	1-5 yrs	5-10 yrs
Early graft failure	23	0	0
Infection	24	9	9
Rejection	17	11	3
Allograft vasculopathy	5	25	27
Malignancy	3	20	33
Other	29	33	29

Table 3. Risk factors for death post-cardiac transplantation (adapted from [39]).

Risk factors for death post-cardiac transplantation	Cause of death				
	EGF	Infection	Rejection	Vasculopathy	Malignancy
RECIPIENT FACTORS					
Older age		X			X
Younger age			X	X	
White male					X
Non-white male			X	X	
Obesity		X	X		
Cachexia		X			
Ischaemic aetiology				X	
Insulin dependent DM				X	
Any DM		X			
Pulmonary disease		X			
PVD ($\uparrow$overall mortality)					
Herpes -ve			X		
Smoker				X	X
Gout					X
$\uparrow$CrCl	X	X			
$\uparrow$TPG	X		X		
$\uparrow$RAP	X	X			
PRA >10%	X				X
Previous sternotomy	X	X			
Ventilated	X	X			
IABP		X			
LVAD		X			
Early transplant			X	X	
DONOR FACTORS					
Older age	X	X	X	X	
Hep C +ve			X		
Abnormal echo	X				
DM	X				
CMV +ve				X	
$\uparrow$ischaemic time	X	X			
DONOR-RECIPIENT MISMATCH					
BMI	X				
CMV			X		
HLA			X		

EGF = Early graft failure; DM = diabetes mellitus; PVD = peripheral vascular disease; CrCl = creatinine clearance; TPG = transpulmonary gradient; RAP = right atrial pressure; PRA = panel reactive antibody; IABP = intra-aortic balloon pump; LVAD = LV assist device; CMV = cytomegalovirus; BMI = body mass index; HLA = human leukocyte antigen.

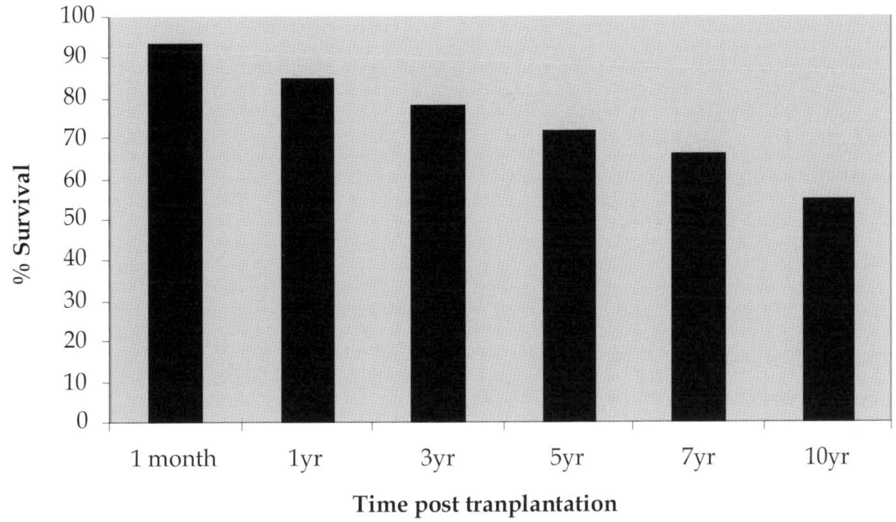

Figure 2. **Survival of patients post cardiac transplantation.**

Table 3, i.e. establishing patient-specific predictive models. Transplantation may thus be offered to those patients profiled to derive the highest long-term expected survival and lowest incidence of adverse events.

The major causes of death following cardiac transplantation are shown in Table 2 and are predominantly transplant-related, either from graft failure (early or late) or the side effects of long-term immunosuppression (infection, renal failure, malignancy). One should approach these listed causes with caution, since many will be inter-linked eg. early graft failure and infection, recurrent rejection and malignancy [39]. Different risk factors predispose to different causes of death and these are highlighted in Table 3.

For transplantation to be an effective long-term alternative in patients with advanced heart failure, estimated post-transplantation survival must be superior to prognosis without transplantation. One simplified approach is to compare prognosis in patients according to NYHA failure status to prognosis of patients post-transplantation. Using such survival statistics, it is clear that transplantation certainly offers improved prognosis in NYHA class IV heart failure, but in less severe, ambulant functional NYHA class II or III heart failure, its benefit is contentious. Transplantation incurs a significant hazard (~12%) of death within 30 days of the procedure. This early mortality together with a further risk of approximately 8% between 30 days and one year, and an attrition rate of 3-4% per annum thereafter, erodes the potential survival advantage. This hazard also delays the time-point at which additional life is achieved for the individual patient. Patients in NYHA class IV heart failure, on inotropic support, with an estimated survival measured in days or weeks, will derive survival advantage within the first months post-procedure. Alternatively, a stable ambulant patient with less severe heart failure might need several months or indeed years to begin to derive hypothetical additional life benefit. If the use of "marginal" donor organs is added to the balance, true survival benefit for these ambulant patients may be further delayed. Thus, in order to identify those patients most likely to benefit most from transplantation, a range of indices that predict heart failure prognosis and post-transplantation outcome are essential to identify those in most need and those most likely to benefit.

Table 4. Indications for cardiac transplantation as recommended by the International Society of Heart and Lung Transplantation (adapted from [40]).

Consider transplantation in advanced heart failure if:-
Functional limitation (NYHA class III or IV) despite maximal medical therapy
Refractory angina or life-threatening arrhythmia
Alternatives to transplantation are unavailable
Indications for transplantation in patients with optimal medical therapy:-
Definite indications
◆ VO_2 max <10 ml/Kg/min
◆ NYHA class IV
◆ Recurrent hospitalisations for heart failure
◆ Refractory ischaemia, LVEF <20% and coronary disease not amenable to revascularisation
◆ Recurrent symptomatic arrhythias
Probable indications
◆ VO_2 max <14 ml/Kg/min with other risk factors
◆ NYHA class III-IV
◆ Recent hospitalisations for heart failure
◆ Unstable angina not amenable to revascularisation and LVEF <25%

Patient selection and factors determining prognosis in heart failure and post-transplantation

Several clinical and laboratory indices are available that act as prognostic indicators in heart failure, while other factors are used to identify and triage patients who may derive the greatest benefit from transplantation. Decisions are based upon the balance between survival from cardiac disease (which is sometimes unknown with the advent of newer therapies eg. CRT, AICDs, ventricular assist devices, etc.) and non-cardiac disease, which might decrease patient and graft survival. There is a general agreement that cardiac transplantation be reserved for those in whom life expectancy AND quality of life are expected to improve. General recommendations regarding indications and contraindications to cardiac transplantation as recommended by the International Society of Heart and Lung Transplantation [40] are shown in Tables 4 and 5 and these largely agree with guidance from other publications [41-44].

Life expectancy

The best overall life expectancy post-transplantation is potentially achievable in those patients without comorbidity and with least need. On the contrary, those who are most in need, i.e. critically ill with end-stage cardiac disease and secondary organ dysfunction (eg. renal impairment), are likely to have a worse outcome post-transplantation, but may derive the greatest individual increase in survival. Hence, transplant recipient identification ideally identifies those patients with advanced cardiac disease but without comorbidity that would jeopardise post-transplant outcome. The "survival benefit margin" is the expected patient survival with transplantation minus the expected survival without transplantation [31]. If a patient with severe heart failure has a survival expectancy of 70% at one year with transplantation and 10% without, his survival benefit margin is 60%. If a patient with less severe heart failure is considered, with an expected survival of 80% at one year, his survival benefit margin is much less and in fact, worse with transplantation, at -10%. Clearly, the presence of other comorbid conditions intrudes upon the calculation, by virtue of affecting survival both in the transplanted and non-transplanted patient.

Table 5. Contraindications to cardiac transplantation as recommended by the International Society of Heart and Lung Transplantation (adapted from [40]).

General contraindications

- Any non-cardiac condition expected to reduce life expectancy or increase the risks of rejection or complications of immunosuppression

Specific contraindications

- Age over ~65 years
- Active infection
- Active peptic ulcer disease
- Diabetes mellitus with end organ damage
- Cerebrovascular or peripheral vascular disease
- Recent history of neoplasia
- Obesity
- Reduced creatinine clearance (<50 ml/min)
- Liver disease (not due to reversible hepatic congestion)
- Severe lung disease
- Pulmonary hypertension (>60mm Hg), raised transpulmonary gradient (>15mm Hg) and/or raised pulmonary vascular resistance (>5 Wood Units)
- Active pulmonary thromboembolic disease
- Smoking within last six months
- High risk of non-compliance
- Lack of independent family or poor social support

Relative contraindications

- Amyloidosis

Quality of Life

Actual quality of life (QOL) pre-transplantation and predicted QOL post-transplantation is of vital importance when undertaking the task of patient selection. Patients who by virtue of their illness are prevented from undertaking activities and interactions which improve their physical, psychological and social well-being, might be deemed to derive the greatest benefit in terms of improvement in quality of life post-transplantation [28].

Aetiology

Up to 6% of patients referred for cardiac transplantation may be amenable to the alternative treatment options discussed previously, such as valve surgery or CABG. Careful screening of these patients is therefore mandatory and necessitates revisiting and entertaining options which may originally have been deemed non-viable by the referring physician. Aetiology of the presenting illness must therefore be sought, clarified and confirmed (Table 6) in order to consider potential alternatives to transplantation. With the advent of newer therapies for cardiac failure such as CRT ± AICD and left ventricular assist devices, a significant number of patients might benefit from alternative therapies which might serve as a bridge to transplantation if not a destination therapy *per se*.

Ischaemic cardiomyopathy

Ischaemic cardiomyopathy has a worse prognosis than patients with non-ischaemic cardiomyopathy [46] and such patients have a higher waiting list mortality than patients with comparable prognostic indices.

Table 6. Aetiology of disease in patients referred for cardiac transplantation.

Cardiomyopathies	Other
Dilated cardiomyopathy (50%)	Severe valvular disease
Ischaemic cardiomyopathy (40%)	Severe angina not amenable to revascularisation
Hypertrophic cardiomyopathy	Arrhythmias refractory to medical therapy or devices
Restrictive cardiomyopathy	Congenital heart disease
Puerperal cardiomyopathy	

Thus there may be a need to list patients with ischaemic cardiomyopathy earlier in their illness than patients with dilated cardiomyopathy. Only a small fraction of patients with advanced heart failure secondary to ischaemic heart disease have coronary arteries amenable to percutaneous or surgical revascularisation techniques. However, this small fraction can derive improved symptomatic and survival benefit from CABG provided the graftable coronary arteries subtend a significant mass of "hibernating" myocardium [19-20]. However, in very severe left ventricular dysfunction with poor quality distal vessels and limited viability, surgical mortality increases and any survival advantage declines [47,48]. Thus, transplantation becomes the main option for many patients with end-stage ischaemic heart failure.

Non-ischaemic dilated cardiomyopathy

Clinical, functional and haemodynamic indices determine prognosis in this heterogeneous group of patients, grouped together due to the absence of significant coronary artery disease. An attempt to define aetiology is of paramount importance since some forms of dilated cardiomyopathy can show improved prognosis and even remission with appropriate medical therapy and meticulous surveillance over an indefinite time period eg. lymphocytic myocarditis, alcoholic cardiomyopathy, peri-partum cardiomyopathy and hypertensive cardiomyopathy.

Age

Increasing recipient age is associated with worse outcome following transplantation. Historically, there were arbitary age thresholds, above which transplantation was not considered (>55 years for ischaemic heart failure, >60 years for DCM). However, satisfactory long-term outcome can be achieved in the older patient and modern practice allows the careful assessment of a wide age range. Inevitably, a greater burden of comorbidity may preclude listing. Older patients are also at increased risk of complications post-transplantation eg. infection, rejection and steroid side effects (osteoporosis and fractures, diabetes, cataracts, myopathy, etc).

Despite these complications, some programs serve the older population by allocating older donor hearts (which are also associated with a worse long-term post-transplantation outcome) to older recipients who have no contraindication to suitability, other than an arbitrarily set age threshold. This increase in recipient and donor age limits may increase overall activity and may direct younger organs to recipients deemed to derive greatest benefit [49].

Duration of illness

Although mortality and decompensation are most likely in the immediate period after referral for transplantation, those individuals with a relatively acute history and short duration of symptomatic heart failure appear to have the greatest likelihood of remission with intensive observation and medical therapy [50,51]. In addition, those patients who remain stable for >6 months whilst awaiting transplantation have a superior prognosis.

Functional capacity

The New York Heart Association (NYHA) functional class in heart failure is widely accepted as a standard classification. Although the mortality prediction in an individual may be further refined by the other prognostic indices discussed below, in general, persistent NYHA class IV status, despite maximal medical therapy, is an unchallenged indication for considering cardiac transplantation [52]. The 1-year mortality rates in heart failure according to NYHA class are:-

- NYHA class II 3-25%
- NYHA class III 10-45%
- NYHA class IV 50-80%

Haemodynamic factors

Left ventricular ejection fraction (LVEF)

LVEF below 20% has been shown in multiple studies to be an independent risk factor for predicting morbidity and mortality in heart failure [53,54]. However, ejection fraction, as well as showing inter-observer variability, correlates poorly with clinical status and NYHA class. While some patients with a LVEF of 20% might be NYHA functional class II, others might be dependent upon inotropic support or mechanical support devices. This spectrum of symptomatology arises from the fact that LVEF is determined by multiple physiological factors such as preload, afterload, chronotropic status and inotropic state [55]. More relevant in assessment of the heart failure patient is the serial assessment of LVEF, which incorporates physiological changes and remodelling over time. A decrease in LVEF by 5% or more annually is associated with twice the mortality of patients in whom LVEF increases <5% per annum [56]. In patients with a relatively acute presentation, failure of LVEF to improve within six to eight months identifies a group at high risk of death within one year [57]. The variability of LVEF measurement and its poor discriminatory value necessitates the use of other measurements of haemodynamic function in addition to LVEF to refine prognosis.

Right ventricular ejection fraction (RVEF)

Impaired right ventricular function is detrimental to overall status in two ways. Firstly, it serves to increase the risk of visceral congestion, and secondly, impaired increase in RVEF upon exertion impairs LV filling and accentuates already compromised LVEF. In patients with NYHA class III or IV heart failure and severe LV dysfunction, RV function is an independent predictor of mortality. RVEF <35% is associated with a 70% 1-year mortality as opposed to a 23% 1-year mortality when RVEF was >35%. Resting and peak RVEF appears as sensitive a prognostic index as peak oxygen consumption [58].

Right heart catheterisation data

High measurements of right atrial pressure (RAP), pulmonary artery systolic (PAP_s) and diastolic (PAP_d) pressure and pulmonary capillary wedge pressures (PCWP) have all been associated with increased mortality. These measurements are a good measure of the physiological response to medical therapy and hence prognosis [31].

Cardiac index (CI)

A CI index below $2l/min/m^2$ is associated with a poor prognosis from heart failure [59].

Pulmonary hypertension and pulmonary vascular resistance (PVR)

The presence of significant and irreversible pulmonary hypertension increases heart failure and transplant mortality. A transpulmonary gradient (TPG) over 14mm Hg carries a 5-fold increase in post-transplant mortality at six months. Right ventricular dysfunction is a major component of overall early graft failure that is the main cause of early death post-transplantation. Any increase in pulmonary vascular resistance (PVR) will increase both early and long-term risks of transplantation. Thus, if a significant TPG is discovered (indicating an increased PVR), an attempt is made to manipulate this PVR using oxygen, nitric oxide donors, β adrenoceptor agonists or prostacyclin, to determine whether the TPG is fixed or reversible (with reversibility being seen before the onset of systemic hypotension). Often, in severe heart failure, elevated PVR is reactive to a high PCWP and falls to normal within one week following transplantation. If pulmonary artery pressure remains elevated despite medical therapy, this indicates the presence of a fixed component to the TPG which may contraindicate transplantation. Once listed, patients with increased but reversible PVR require TPG and PVR measurement prior to embarking upon a transplant operation.

Cardiopulmonary exercise testing (CPET)

Cardiopulmonary exercise testing measures the combined ability of the heart, lungs and blood to provide the body with oxygen to meet aerobic demand and identifies a threshold at which anaerobic metabolism begins to occur. Oxygen uptake abnormalities in heart failure patients were initially described by Weber in 1982 [60]. Since then, there have been many studies of the pathophysiology of oxygen uptake in heart failure patients and how this correlates to morbidity and mortality. In isolated heart failure, a reduction in peak oxygen consumption on exercise (VO_2 max) is attributable to an inability to increase cardiac output upon demand and hence is a reliable indicator of heart failure severity [61,62]. A peak VO_2 of less than 12ml/Kg/min is associated with a poor prognosis [59]. The study of Mancini *et al* [58] recommended that cardiac transplantation can be safely deferred in patients with a VO_2 max >14ml/Kg/min, as peak VO_2 max >14ml/Kg/min is associated with a 2-year survival in excess of 80%. Indexing the peak VO_2 max as a percentage of that expected at a certain age may be a more useful prognostic indicator. A value of <50% predicted for age is an important index, as clearly a VO_2 max of 14ml/Kg/min represents 60% of that predicted for a 60-year-old male, but only 30% of that predicted for a 30-year-old male. However, the association between VO_2 max and 1-year mortality is consistent across age ranges in most studies and is as follows:-

- <10ml/Kg/min associated with a 1-year survival of <30%.
- 10-18ml/Kg/min associated with a 1-year survival of 30-80%.
- >18ml/Kg/min associated with a 1-year survival of >80%.

Interpretation of a VO_2 max in the range of 12-14ml/Kg/min is less well defined. In these circumstances, repeated assessment and evaluation of a trend in measurements is likely to guide management.

In addition to peak oxygen consumption, the anaerobic threshold (the point at which oxygen delivery to peripheral tissues is insufficient to maintain oxidative metabolism) provides further prognostic information. It is identifiable as the point during exercise when venous lactate levels begin to rise rapidly and the more severe the heart failure, the earlier this occurs. In parallel with increased carbon dioxide production during anaerobic metabolism, minute ventilation also rises and this is of further discriminatory value. The presence of lung disease may also affect peak O_2 consumption and anaerobic threshold. Hence, lung function tests to assess lung volumes and diffusion capacity should be considered in parallel with CPET to ensure accurate data accrual regarding cardiac function uninfluenced by comorbid pulmonary disease (Table 7). Pulmonary function measurements such as FEV_1, FVC and DL_{CO} can all be reduced in heart failure, and, in the absence of known lung disease, do not influence outcome [63,64].

Table 7. Distinguishing between cardiac and pulmonary causes of dyspnoea using cardiopulmonary exercise testing (adapted from [65]).

Parameter	Cardiac causes	Pulmonary causes
VO_2 max	Reduced	Not achieved usually
Anaerobic threshold	Reduced	Rarely achieved
Maximal minute ventilation	50% of maximum minute ventilatory volume	>50% of maximum minute ventilatory volume
O_2 saturation of blood	Remains >90%	Falls

Metabolic factors

Serum sodium (Na)

Hyponatraemia is not only the result of neurohormonal activation (increased renin activity), but also reflects the intensity of diuretic therapy required to stabilise the patient. Independently, a Na level below 130mmol/L is associated with a 1-year survival rate of <20% [66].

Plasma noradrenaline (NorA)

Elevation of plasma NorA reflects an increasing use of adrenergic reserve and correlates with poor outcome in heart failure. Levels above 1200pg/ml have been shown to be associated with 2-year mortality levels over 80% [67].

B-type natriuretic peptide

This marker of cardiac dysfunction has been well validated in heart failure with levels of BNP being correlated with severity of heart failure as well as being of prognostic value [68], both in heart failure and post-transplantation [69]. The role of BNP testing as a guide to selection, listing, and monitoring of alternative therapies in the patient referred for transplant assessment requires further evaluation.

Comorbid illnesses

Chronic renal dysfunction

Chronic renal dysfunction with a creatinine clearance (CrCl) below 30ml/minute increases the risk of renal failure and death post-transplantation. Prognosis in transplant renal dysfunction appears primarily related to the early functional integrity of the donor heart and the long-term use of calcineurine inhibitors. Even in patients with relatively normal CrCl, renal dysfunction following cardiac transplantation is common. At three years, 44% of patients have a calculated glomerular filtration rate of <40ml/min and 64% have mild-to-moderate renal dysfunction [31]. Some 10% of transplant recipients progress to dialysis requirement. Thus, pre-operative renal dysfunction is an important relative contraindication to heart transplantation. A frequently encountered dilemma arises when it cannot be certain that a reduced CrCl is not due to poor cardiac output. In this situation, effective renal plasma flow (ERPF) using nuclear medicine techniques and urinary protein loss may be useful tools in identifying the presence of intrinsic renal disease.

Peripheral vascular disease (PVD)

PVD limits rehabilitation and impairs a return to "normal" activity and lifestyle post-transplantation. In addition, its progression may be accelerated post-transplantation.

Cerebrovascular disease

A history of cerebrovascular disease not only increases the peri-operative risk of events, but also increases the risk of future events which would attenuate the longevity of a transplant recipient. Long-term steroid therapy may accelerate atheromatous disease and unless the vascular disease is discrete and amenable to pre-operative treatment, it remains a relative contraindication to transplantation.

Liver disease

Hepatic dysfunction due to congestive cardiac failure generally improves within weeks of cardiac transplantation. The absence of cirrhosis and other progressive liver diseases is important to ascertain if at assessment there is any derangement of biochemical liver function tests or coagulation abnormalities.

Diabetes

In recipients free of pre-operative nephropathy, the presence of diabetes *per se* does not increase the risk of allograft vasculopathy, infections or rejection. Nevertheless, it remains a risk factor for death due to infection or vasculopathy.

Osteoporosis

If severe, this may pose increased risks during steroid therapy post-transplantation. Although not a contraindication *per se,* osteoporosis should be carefully evaluated prior to transplantation.

Body mass index (BMI)

Obesity carries a risk of increased morbidity and mortality both in the peri-operative and postoperative period. In the long-term, obesity, which may be accentuated by steroid therapy, increases the risk of infection, osteoporosis, diabetes and deconditioning. A body weight greater than 140% predicted is an independent risk factor for death and infection post-transplantation [70].

Smoking and alcohol abuse

Smoking and alcohol abuse are both associated with poor compliance to drug therapy. Smokers in addition, are at an increased risk of developing post-transplant lung cancer and accelerated atherosclerosis [71].

Psychological and social aspects

A positive attitude, unquestionable motivation and good social support appear to be pivotal to a good outcome after cardiac transplantation. These aspects are difficult to quantify, but are required to cope with:-

- Intensive follow-up.
- Frequent endomyocardial biopsies.
- An intensive regime of self-medication.
- Inevitable recurrent illnesses eg. infection.

Active infection

Active infection is an important contraindication to transplantation, as intense immunosuppression may lead to overwhelming sepsis. Recent pulmonary embolism is also a concern, as lung infarction may become the site of bacterial or fungal abscess formation. Transplantation has been performed in a Human Immunodeficiency virus positive recipient, but long-term outcome is not known [72]. Most transplant centres would assume the presence of HIV, Hepatitis B or systemic infection to preclude transplantation.

Active peptic ulcer disease

This remains a relative contraindication due to the risks of exacerbation of ulceration and bleeding complications on immunosuppression. Such patients ideally require intensive medical therapy including *Helicobacter pylori* eradication and endoscopic proof of ulcer healing prior to listing for transplantation. The presence of gallstones was also previously felt to be a relative contraindication to transplantation. In the current era, asymptomatic gallbladder disease can be dealt with electively a few months post-transplantation.

Prior malignancy

Immunosuppression increases the risk of tumour development and/or progression. All patients are screened by chest radiography and abdominal ultrasonography, and it could be argued that mammography and serum PSA (prostate specific antigen) levels should also be performed. Patients with a prior history of malignancy should ideally have a 5-year period free of disease before listing.

Specific diseases involving the heart

There are many less common disease processes involving the heart which may require transplantation, but have even less evidence to support this therapy than ischaemic and dilated cardiomyopathy.

Sarcoidosis

Cardiac sarcoidosis leading to restrictive cardiomyopathy is not a contraindication to transplantation since the recurrence of cardiac sarcoidosis post-transplantation is slow and may be partially ameliorated with steroid therapy. Clearly, the absence of significant multisystem disease from sarcoidosis is preferable in order to improve survival [31].

Amyloidosis

Even with limited experience of transplantation for this condition, there is clear evidence that most recipients will develop recurrent cardiac amyloidosis. In one survey, 4-year survival was less than 40% [73]. Despite this poor prognosis, there are isolated case reports of prolonged survival post-transplantation. As amyloid appears to be a pre-malignant process, management might include (peri-cardiac transplantation), bone marrow ablation and transplantation. However, once symptomatic, the deterioration in patients with cardiac amyloid is rapid and this may preclude the difficult logistics of such a strategy.

Peri-partum cardiomyopathy

Of all patients with peri-partum cardiomyopathy, 50% improve within six weeks of developing symptoms, while 50% develop progressive heart failure. Careful and repeated observation is needed to identify those failing to improve to allow early listing for transplantation.

Acute myocarditis

In this condition, most patients recover spontaneously, regardless of medical therapy [31]. A small proportion may progress to development of a dilated cardiomyopathy and subsequent refractory heart failure, which may necessitate assessment for transplantation. Survival following transplantation is inferior to patients transplanted for other aetiologies [74] and there is a growing body of opinion that in such cases, ventricular assist device deployment, as a bridge to recovery, may be a preferred treatment. Transplantation should be considered if cardiac biopsy reveals an absence of active inflammation in the face of continuing requirement for circulatory support [31].

Malignant cardiac tumours

Crespo *et al* [75] have reported two cases of transplantation in young males with cardiac angiosarcoma, both of whom died within 1-year post-transplantation of cerebral metastases. Cardiac malignancy, the authors recommend, should therefore, be a contraindication to transplantation.

Pericarditis

A single case report highlights successful transplantation for this condition [76].

Iron overload

Survival ranged from 14-74 months in a series of seven patients transplanted for iron overload cardiomyopathy reported by Koerner *et al* [77].

Isolated non-compaction

This is a condition where embryonic compaction of the myocardium fails to occur. There are only six reported cases of transplantation for this condition, which predisposes to thromboembolism and malignant arrhythmias [78].

Prognostic factors in heart failure and the Heart Failure Survival Score

Deciding upon the need for transplantation is a complex process in which the multiple indications and contraindications to transplantation must be addressed. Prediction of prognosis remains difficult (Table 8). Despite numerous clinical studies, no single variable is consistently able to predict survival or event rates in patients with heart failure and thus, convergence of a number of separate prognostic indicators is used to identify ambulant patients in greatest need. The importance of each prognostic index can be weighted and several variables combined to develop a composite risk score. The most commonly used score is the Heart Failure Survival Score (HFSS, Table 9). This score has been shown to be a good predictor of survival and event rates in heart failure and may be used as a guide to timing of listing. One-year event-free survival for ranges of HFSS revealed three distinct strata: low-risk (HFSS $\geq$8.10), medium-risk (HFSS 7.20 to 8.09), and high-risk (HFSS $\leq$7.19). The odds of an outcome

Table 8. Factors correlating with increased mortality rates in patients with heart failure.

Factor class	Variable
Patient demographics	Age
	Race
	Gender
Clinical	Aetiology
	NYHA status
	Illness duration
	Syncope
	Electrocardiography: signal averaged ECG, QT prolongation, arrhythmias
	Thyroid function
	Diabetes
	Renal failure
	Liver failure
Haemodynamic	Ejection fraction (LV and RV)
	LV end diastolic dimension
	Right atrial pressure
	Pulmonary capillary wedge pressure
	Cardiopulmonary - VO_2 max, 6-minute walk, anaerobic threshold
	Transpulmonary gradient
	Cardiac index
	Systemic hypertension
	Inotrope dependence
	Intra-aortic balloon pump dependence
Functional	NYHA class
	VO_2 max
	6-minute walk distance
Neurohormonal	Serum sodium
	Plasma renin activity
	Plasma aldosterone
	Natriuretic peptide levels (A and B type)
	Plasma noradrenaline
Haematological	Leukocytosis

event at one year for the low-risk stratum were five and 21 times less than for the medium- and high-risk strata respectively. Event-free survival rates at 1-year for the low-, medium-, and high-risk HFSS strata were 93±2%, 72±5%, and 43±7%, respectively. Event-free survival rates for the medium- and high-risk strata were much worse than would be expected after cardiac transplantation; the low-risk stratum had an event-free survival rate that was better than would be expected with transplantation, giving strong evidence for withholding transplantation in this low-risk group, but strongly considering transplantation in medium- and high-risk strata. To date, the HFSS has been shown to be the only validated tool in the evaluation of patients with heart failure referred for transplantation. Moreover, the score has been additionally validated in patients receiving β–blocker therapy [79,80].

Table 9. A model for predictors of mortality in heart failure (adapted from [81]).

Variable	Coefficient
Ischaemic cardiomyopathy (yes or no)	0.6931
Resting heart rate (bpm)	0.0216
LVEF (%)	- 0.0464
Mean arterial blood pressure (mm Hg)	- 0.0255
Interventricular conduction delay	0.6083
Peak VO_2 max (ml/Kg/min)	- 0.0546
Serum sodium (mM)	- 0.0470

HFSS - Heart failure survival score.

HFSS = (0.6931x (1 or 0) + (0.0216x HR) + (-0.0464xLVEF) + (-0.0255x MABP) + (0.6083x 1 or 0) + (-0.0546x VO_2 max) + (-0.0470x serum [Na])

Waiting list management

Ambulant and support dependent patients are placed on waiting lists for transplantation. The urgent group are more likely both to receive organs and to receive them sooner [31]. Ambulant outpatients require frequent review as the period of highest morbidity and mortality risk occurs in the first few months following listing for cardiac transplantation [82]. This accounts for much of the 10-30% waiting list mortality risk stated by most transplant programs. The majority, up to two thirds, of deaths on the waiting list, are sudden cardiac death. Such a statistic argues for the use of proven AICD therapy in patients who meet the criteria laid out by recent defibrillator trials [5,83,84], which might be expected to reduce waiting list mortality substantially. Extending this argument for the use of adjunctive device therapy, the use of CRT too could be argued, in order to provide at least symptomatic benefit for a select group of waiting list patients. The impact of device therapy upon the morbidity and mortality of these ambulant patients should be monitored with great interest.

The risk of death or deterioration within the first year for ambulant patients is increased by 50% if patients have one or more of the following criteria: inotrope dependence or NYHA class IV status at listing, PCWP>25mmHg, raised serum creatinine or an ischaemic aetiology of heart failure [82]. For these reasons, ambulant patients are reviewed at least every six months at a "tracking visit" where several prognostic indices are reassessed eg. right heart catheterisation, CPET, metabolic screen, echocardiography, etc. In general, males tend to wait longer than females (due to the need for weight matching) and those with blood group O longer than groups A or B, who in turn wait longer than group AB. With an increasing demand for organs as waiting lists grow, waiting times have inevitably increased [38].

Cardiac re-transplantation

Although rarely undertaken, the most common conditions for which retransplantation [85] is undertaken are allograft vasculopathy and early graft failure (including rejection). Results are inferior to primo-transplantation and hence, there is considerable debate regarding its appropriateness.

Conclusions

There is overwhelming evidence that cardiac transplantation is a viable and better alternative (both prognostically and in terms of quality of life) to the many current therapies available to patients with very severe heart failure. In less severe heart failure, in ambulant patients, the evidence is less certain and each patient requires careful detailed assessment to weigh the relative merits of transplantation over alternative treatments.

Recommendations	Evidence level
◆ Transplantation for heart failure NYHA class IV.	III/B
◆ Transplantation for heart failure NYHA class II and III.	IV/C
◆ Cardiac retransplantation.	IV/C

References

1. Ganesh S. UK Transplant activity. (personal communication) www.uktransplant.org.uk.
2. Costanzo M, Augustine S, Bourge R, *et al.* Selection and Treatment of Candidates for Heart Transplantation: A Statement for Health Professionals From the Committee on Heart Failure and Cardiac Transplantation of the Council on Clinical Cardiology. *Circulation* 1995; 92: 3593-3612.
3. Edwards LB, Keck BM. Thoracic organ transplantation in the US. *Clin Transpl* 2002; 29-40.
4. Caine N, Sharples LD, English TA, *et al.* Prospective study comparing quality of life before and after heart transplantation. *Transplant Proc* 1990; 22: 1437-1439.
5. Salukhe TV, Francis DP, Sutton R. Comparison of medical therapy, pacing and defibrillation in heart failure (COMPANION) trial terminated early; combined biventricular pacemaker-defibrillators reduce all-cause mortality and hospitalization. *Int J Cardiol* 2003; 87(2-3): 119-20.
6. Drummond MF. Economic evaluation and the rational diffusion and use of health technology. *Health Policy* 1987; 7: 309-324.
7. Deng MC, De Meester JM, Smits JM, *et al.* Effect of receiving a heart transplant: analysis of a national cohort entered on to a waiting list, stratified by heart failure severity. Comparative Outcome and Clinical Profiles in Transplantation (COCPIT) Study Group. *BMJ* 2000; 321: 540-545.
8. Kirsch M, Baufreton C, Naftel DC, *et al.* Pretransplantation risk factors for death after transplantation: the Henry Mondor experience. *J Heart Lung Transplant* 1999; 17: 268-277.
9. Hosenpud JD, Bennett LE, Keck BM, *et al.* The Registry of the International Society for Heart and Lung Transplantation: sixteenth official report 1999. *J Heart Lung Transplant* 1999; 18: 611-626.
10. 1995 Annual Report of the US Scientific Registry for Transplant Recipients and the Organ Procurement and Transportation Network. Data 1988-1994. UNOS, Richmond, Va, and the Division of Transplantation, Bureau of Health Resources Development, Health Resources, and Services Administration. US Department of Health and Human Services, Rockville, Md.
11. Satchithananda DK, Stoica SC, Parameshwar J, *et al.* Effect of receiving a heart transplant *BMJ* 2001; 322: 1179a.
12. Franciosa JA, Wilen M, Ziesche S, *et al.* Survival in men with severe chronic left ventricular failure due to either coronary heart disease or idiopathic dilated cardiomyopathy. *Am J Cardiol* 1983; 51: 831.
13. Kaul TK, Agnihotri TK, Fields BL, *et al.* Coronary artery bypass grafting in patients with an ejection fraction of twenty per cent or less. *J Thorac Cardiovasc Surg* 1996; 111: 1001.
14. Louie HW, Laks H, Milgalter E, *et al.* Ischaemic cardiomyopathy: criteria for coronary revascularisation and cardiac transplantation. *Circulation* 1991; 84(suppl III): III-290.
15. Kron IL, Flanagan TL, Blackbourne LH, *et al.* Coronary revascularisation rather than cardiac transplantation for chronic ischaemic cardiomyopathy. *Ann Surg* 1989; 210: 348.
16. Rahimtoola SH. Chronic myocardial hibernation. *Circulation* 1994; 89(4): 1907-8.
17. Tubau JF, Rahimtoola SH. Hibernating myocardium: a historical perspective. *Cardiovasc Drugs Ther* 1992; 6(3): 267-71.
18. Lewis ME, Pitt MP, Bonser RS, *et al.* Coronary artery surgery for ischaemic heart failure: the surgeon's view. *Heart Fail Rev* 2003 (2): 175-9.
19. Pagano D, Camici PG, Bonser RS. Revascularisation for chronic heart failure: a valid option? *Eur J Heart Fail* 1999; 1(3): 269-73.
20. Pagano D, Bonser RS, Camici PG. Myocardial revascularization for the treatment of post-ischemic heart failure. *Curr Opin Cardiol* 1999; 14(6): 506-9.
21. Joyce D, Loebe M, Noon GP, *et al.* Revascularization and ventricular restoration in patients with ischemic heart failure: the STICH trial. *Curr Opin Cardiol* 2003(6): 454-7.
22. Cleland JG, Freemantle N, Ball SG, *et al.* The heart failure revascularisation trial (HEART): rationale, design and methodology. *Eur J Heart Fail* 2003; 5(3): 295-303.
23. Faxon DP, Myers WO, McCabe CH, *et al.* The influence of surgery on the natural history of angiographically documented left ventricular aneurysm. The Coronary Artery Surgery Study. *Circulation* 1986: 74; 110-118.
24. Dor V, Sabatier M, Di Donato M, *et al.* Late haemodynamic results after left ventricular patch repair associated with coronary grafting in patients with postinfarction akinetic or dyskinetic aneurysm of the left ventricle. *J Thorac Cardiovasc Surg* 1995: 110; 1291-1299; discussion 1300-1301.
25. Carrier M, Perrault LP, Bouchard D *et al.* Effect of left ventricular assist device bridging to transplantation on donor waiting time and outcomes in Canada. *Can J Cardiol* 2004; 20(5): 501-504.
26. Birks EJ, Yacoub MH, Banner NR, *et al.* The role of bridge to transplantation: should LVAD patients be transplanted? *Curr Opin Cardiol* 2004; 19(2): 148-53.

27. Batista RJV, Santos LJV, Takeshita N, *et al.* Partial left ventriculectomy to improve left ventricular function in end-stage heart disease. *J Card Surg* 1996; 11: 96.
28. Dowling RD, Koeni S, Laureano MS, *et al.* Results of parital left ventriculectomy in patients with end-stage idiopathic dilated cardiomyopathy. *J Heart Lung Transpl* 1998; 17: 1208.
29. Dor V, Sabatier M, Donato M, *et al.* Efficacy of endoventricular patch plasty in postinfarction akinetic scar and severe left ventricular dysfunction: comparison with a series of large dyskinetic scars. *J Thorac Cardiovasc Surg* 1998; 116: 50-59.
30. Lange R, Sack FU Voss B, *et al.* Treatment of dilated cardiomyopathy with dynamic cardiomyoplasty: the Heidelberg experience. *Ann Thoracic Surg* 1995; 60: 1219.
31. Kirklin JK, Young JB, McGiffin DC. In: *Heart Transplantation.* Churchill Livingstone, 2002.
32. Salukhe TV, Dimopoulos K, Francis D. Cardiac resynchronisation may reduce all-cause mortality: meta-analysis of preliminary COMPANION data with CONTAK-CD, InSync ICD, MIRACLE and MUSTIC. *Int J Cardiol* 2004; 93(2-3): 101-3.
33. Coletta AP, Clark AL, Seymour AM, Cleland JG. Clinical trials update from the European Society of Cardiology Heart Failure meeting: COMET, COMPANION, Tezosentan and SHAPE. *Eur J Heart Fail* 2003; 5(4): 545-8.
34. Cleland JG, Ghosh J, Khan N, Hurren S, Kaye G. Ongoing trials of cardiac resynchronisation. *Minerva Cardioangiol* 2003; 51(2): 197-207.
35. Thackray S, Coletta A, Jones P, *et al.* Clinical trials update: Highlights of the Scientific Sessions of Heart Failure 2001, a meeting of the Working Group on Heart Failure of the European Society of Cardiology. CONTAK-CD, CHRISTMAS, OPTIME-CHF. *Eur J Heart Fail* 2001; 3(4): 491-4.
36. Paisey JR, Morgan JM. Advanced pacing techniques in congestive heart failure. *Br J Cardiol* (Acute Interv Cardiol) 2004; 11: AIC 17- AIC 23.
37. Hosenpud JD, Bennett LE, Keck BM, *et al.* The registry of the International Society for Heart and Lung Transplantation: 15th Official Report. / *J Heart and Lung Transplant* 1998; 17: 656-668.
38. UNOS United Network for Organ Sharing - Annual Report. Annual Report 2000.
39. Bourge RC, Naftel DC, Hill JA, *et al.* The emergence of co-morbid diseases impacting upon survival after cardiac transplantation; a ten year multi-institutional experience (Abstr). *J Heart Lung Tranpl* 2001; 20: 167.
40. Miller LW, Kubo SH, Young JB, *et al.* Report of the consensus conference on candidate selection for heart transplantation - 1993. *J Heart and Lung Transplant* 1995; 14: 562-571.
41. Rickenbacher PR, Haywood G, Fowler MB. Selecting candidates for cardiac transplantation. How to assess exclusion criteria and predict who will benefit. *J Crit Illn* 1995; 10(3): 199-206.
42. Anguita M, Torres F, Gimenez D, *et al.* For whom and when is a heart transplant indicated. *Rev Esp Cardio* 1995; 48 Suppl 7: 13-8.
43. Reichenspurner H, Hildebrandt A, Boehm D, *et al.*: Heterotopic heart transplantation in 1988 - recent selective indications and outcome. *J Heart Transplant* 1989; 8(5): 381-6.
44. Glogar D, Pacher R, Stefenelli T, *et al.* Heart transplantation: indication, selection criteria and patient management *Wien Med Wochenschr* 1990 15; 140(10-11): 287-9.
45. Stevenson L, Couper G, Natterson B, *et al.* Target heart failure populations for newer therapies. *Circulation* 1995; 92 Suppl II: 174-181.
46. Ho K, Anderson K, Grossman WK, *et al.* Survival after the onset of congestive heart failure in Framingham Heart Study subjects. *Circulation* 1993; 20: 301-3060.
47. Hochberg MS, Parsonet V, Gielchinsky I, *et al.* Coronary artery bypass grafting in patients with ejection fractions below forty per cent: early and late results in 466 patients. *J Thorac Cardiovasc Surg* 1983; 86: 519-527.
48. Wechsler AS. Coronary artery bypass grafting in patients with an ejection fraction of twenty per cent or less. *J Thorac Cardiovasc Surg* 1996; 111: 998-1000.
49. Livi U, Milano A, Bortolotti U, *et al.* Results of heart transplantation by extending recipient selection criteria. *J Cardiovasc Surg (Torino)* 1994; 35(5): 377-82.
50. Stevenson LW, Fowler MB, Schroeder JS, *et al.* Poor survival of patients with idiopathic cardiomyopathy considered too well for transplantation. *Am J Med* 1987; 83: 871-876.
51. Stevenson LW, Fowler MB, Schroeder JS *et al.*: Poor survival of patients with idiopathic cardiomyopathy considered too well for transplantation. *Am J Med* 1991; 18: 919-925.
52. Costanzo MR, Augustine S,Bourge RD, *et al.* Selection and treatment of candidates for heart transplantation. *Circulation* 1995; 92: 3953-3612.
53. Likoff MJ,Chandler SL, Kay HR. Clinical determinants of mortality in chronic congestive heart failure secondary to idiopathic dilated or to ischaemic cardiomyopathy. *Am J Cardiol* 1987; 59: 634-638.
54. Cohn J, Johnson G, Shebetai R, *et al.* Ejection fraction, peak exercise oxygen consumption, cardiothoracic ratio, ventricular arrhythmias and plasma norepinephrine as determinants of prognosis in heart failure. *Circulation* 1993; 87(Suppl VI): VI-5-VI-16.
55. Behrendt DM. Use and misuse of the ejection fraction. *Ann Thoacic Surg* 1995; 60: 1166-1168.
56. Cintron G, Johnson G, Francis G. Prognostic significance of serial changes in left ventricular ejection fraction in patients with congestive heart failure. *Circulation* 1993; 87: 17-22.
57. Stiemle AE, Stevenson LW, Fonarow GC, *et al.* Prediction of improvement in recent onset cardiomyopathy after referral for heart transplantation: *J AM Coll Cardiol* 1994; 23: 553-559.
58. DiSalvo DG, Mathier M, Semigran MJ, *et al.* Preserved right ventricular ejection fraction predicts exercise capacity and survival in advanced heart failure. *J Am Coll Cardiol* 1995; 25: 1143-1151.
59. Rickenbacher PR, Trindade PT, Haywood JA. Transplant candidates with severe left ventricular dysfunction managed with medical treatment: characteristics and survival. *J Am Coll Cardiol* 1996; 27: 1192-1197.

60. Weber K, Kinasewitz G, Janicki J, *et al.* Oxygen utilization and ventilation during exercise in patients with congestive heart failure. *Circulation* 1982; 65: 1213-1223.
61. Mancini D, LeJemtel T and Aaronson K. Peak VO_2: a simple yet enduring standard. *Circulation* 2000; 101: 1080-1082.
62. Fletcher GF, Balady GJ, Amsterdam EA, *et al.* Exercise Standards for Testing and Training: A Statement for Healthcare Professionals From the American Heart Association. *Circulation* 2001; 104: 1694-1740.
63. Mancini D, Eisen H, Kussmaul W, *et al.* Value of peak exercise oxygen consumption for optimal timing of cardiac transplantation in ambulatory patients with heart failure. *Circulation* 1991; 83: 778-786.
64. Bussieres LM, Cardella CJ, Daly PA, *et al.* Relationship between preoperative pulmonary status and outcome after heart transplantation. *J Heart Lung Transplant* 1990; 9: 124-128.
65. Weber KT, Janicki JS, McElroy PA, *et al.* Concepts and applications of cardiopulmonary exercise testing. *Chest* 1988; 93: 843-847.
66. Lee WH, Packer M. Prognostic importance of serum sodium concentration and its modification by converting enzyme inhibition in patients with severe chronic heart failure. *Circulation* 1986; 73: 257-267.
67. Francis GS, Cohn J, Johnson G, *et al.* Plasma norepinephrine, plasma renin activity, and congestive heart failure: relations to survival and the effects of therapy in V-HeFT II: the V-HeFt va cooperative Studies Group. *Circulation* 1993; 87(Suppl 6): VI-40-VI-48.
68. Troughton RW, Prior DL, Pereira JJ, *et al.* Plasma B-type natriuretic peptide levels in systolic heart failure: importance of left ventricular diastolic function and right ventricular systolic function. *J Am Coll Cardiol* 2004 Feb 4; 43(3): 416-22.
69. Park MH, Uber PA, Scott RL, *et al.* B-type natriuretic peptide in heart transplantation: an important marker of allograft performance. *Heart Fail Rev* 2003; 8(4): 359-63.
70. Grady KL, White Williams C, Naftel D, *et al*, and the Cardiac Transplant Research Database (CTRD). Are preoperative obesity and cachexia risk factors for post heart transplant morbidity and mortality: a multi-institutional study of preoperative weight-height indices (abstract). *J Heart Lung Transplant* 1999; 18: 750-763.
71. Young JB. Redevelopment of disease in cardiac allografts. *Graft* 1999; 2: S54-S59.
72. Aberegg SK. Cardiac transplantation in an HIV-1-infected patient. *N Engl J Med* 2003; 349(14): 1388-9.
73. Hosenpud JD, DeMarco T, Frazier OH, *et al.* Progression of systemic disease and reduced long-term survival in patients with cardiac amyloidosis undergoing heart transplantation: follow-up results of a multicenter study. *Circulation* 1991; 84: 338.
74. O' Connell JB, Dec W, Goldenberg IF, *et al.* Results of heart transplantation for acute lymphocytic myocarditis. *J Heart Lung Transplant* 1990; 9: 351.
75. Crespo MG, Pulpon LA, Pradas G, *et al.* Heart transplantation for cardiac angiosarcoma: should its indication be questioned? *J Heart Lung Transplant* 1993; 12(3): 527-30.
76. Fritz S, Stegmann T. Pericarditis as unusual indication for orthotopic heart transplantation. *Clin Transpl* 1989: 320-1.
77. Koerner MM, Tenderich G, Minami K, *et al.* Heart transplantation for end-stage heart failure caused by iron overload. *Br J Haematol* 1997; 97(2): 293-6.
78. Conraads V, Paelinck B, Vorlat A, *et al.* Isolated non-compaction of the left ventricle: a rare indication for transplantation. *J Heart Lung Transplant.* 2001; 20(8): 904-7.
79. Koelling TM, Joseph S, Aaronson KD. Heart failure survival score continues to predict death or UNOS 1 transplant in heart failure patients receiving beta-blockers. *J Am Coll Cardiol* 2003; 4: 517.
80. De Marco T, Goldman L. Predicting Outcomes in Severe Heart Failure. *Circulation* 1997; 95: 2597-2599).
81. Aaronson KD, Schwartz JS, Chen T, *et al.* Development and prospective validation of a clinical index to predict survival in ambulatory patients referred for cardiac transplantation. *Circulation* 1997; 95: 2660-2667.
82. Kubo S, Stevenson L, Miller L, *et al.* Outcomes in non-urgent patients (status II) awaiting transplantation: risk factors for death or deterioration to status I (urgent status) (abstract). *J Heart Lung Transplant* 1997; 16: 42.
83. Bourge RC, Stevenson L, Naftel, *et al.* Death awaiting cardiac transplantation: impact of the implantable cardioverter defibrillator (abstract). *J Heart Lung Transplant* 1998; 17: 61.
84. Greenberg H, Case RB, Moss AJ, *et al.* MADIT-II Investigators. Analysis of mortality events in the Multicenter Automatic Defibrillator Implantation Trial (MADIT-II). *J Am Coll Cardiol* 2004; 43(8): 1459-65.
85. Michler RE, Edwards NM, Hsu D, *et al.* Pediatric retransplantation. *J Heart Lung Transplant* 1993; 12(6 Pt 2): S319-27.

Chapter 28

Prophylaxis for postoperative atrial tachyarrhythmia in cardiac and general thoracic surgery

Artyom Sedrakyan MD ScC
Honorary Lecturer and Research Scholar

The Royal College of Surgeons of England and
The London School of Hygiene and Tropical Medicine, London, UK

Introduction

Atrial tachyarrhythmia (AT) remains a common complication after cardiac surgery with a reported incidence ranging from 20% to 45%[1-3]. AT typically occurs in the early postoperative period and has the potential to result in embolic stroke, haemodynamic instability[4], a prolonged hospital stay that is estimated to be 2-5 additional days and increased costs of up to $10,000 per incidence[1,2,5].

There are a number of studies and systematic reviews addressing prophylaxis of arrhythmias with anti-arrhythmic medications after cardiac surgery. However, the effectiveness of anti-arrhythmics in general thoracic surgery (GTS) is not known. As in cardiac surgery, atrial tachyarrhythmia (AT), predominantly atrial fibrillation (AF), is the most common complication after GTS and is associated with stroke, a longer hospital stay, higher health care costs[6-9] and mortality[8]. The reported incidence of AT ranges from 13% to 46%[8-10], which is comparable to AT incidence after coronary artery bypass grafting (CABG). An important consideration in the general thoracic setting is that most patients have a long-term history of chronic obstructive pulmonary disease and undergo surgery for lung cancer. Beta-blockers and medications with a similar action may potentially worsen pulmonary dysfunction that is associated with their use[11,12].

Topics of the review

Anti-arrhythmic prophylaxis in cardiac surgery

- Calcium channel blockers.
- Beta-blockers.
- Amiodarone.
- Sotalol.
- Atrial pacing.

Anti-arrhythmic prophylaxis in general thoracic surgery

- Calcium channel blockers.
- Beta-blockers.
- Digitalis.
- Others.

Methodology

Systematic reviews and RCTs were identified by searching the MEDLINE, EMBASE and the Cochrane Controlled Trials Register from 1980 to 2003. Only studies in humans were considered and no language restriction was applied. In addition, we searched the reference lists of RCTs and reviews to look for further studies. A standard RCT filter was used for MEDLINE and EMBASE (available at http://www.sign.ac.uk/methodology/filters.html). There were a number of systematic reviews with meta-analyses found for AT prophylaxis in cardiac surgery. However, no meta-analyses were found in general thoracic surgery addressing AT prophylaxis. We performed fixed effect model based meta-analyses of RCTs in general thoracic surgery. The risk estimates in the medication and placebo groups were assessed separately for each medication. Relative risk and 95% confidence intervals (CI) were calculated. Numbers needed to treat (NNT) and their confidence intervals (CIs) were also calculated using risk difference (RD) analysis. RevMan 4.2 developed by the Cochrane Collaboration was used in all analyses.

Assessing the evidence

Cardiac surgery

Calcium channel blockers

The most recent systematic review[13] has shown that non-dihydropyridines (diltiazem, verapamil) are associated with significant reduction in supraventricular tachyarrhythmia. There was a 34% reduction (95% CI 7%-59%) in the odds of these events in 41 trials including 3,327 patients. The review also reported that overall, there was a relative reduction of the odds of postoperative myocardial infarction (OR, 0.58; 95% CI 0.37-0.91) and myocardial ischaemia (OR, 0.53; 95% CI 0.39-0.72) in the trials of calcium channel blockers.

Beta-blockers

Crystal *et al* [14] performed a systematic review and meta-analysis based on 42 trials that randomised 3,840 patients into beta-blocker and placebo or no treatment groups. Almost all trials reported substantial reduction in the risk of AF. The incidence of AF was reduced from 33% to 19% and there was a 61% reduction in the risk of atrial fibrillation in these trials (95% CI 48%-72%). The study also reported a tendency toward 0.66 days reduction in the length of stay (LOS) (95% CI -2.04-0.72). There was no stroke reduction observed in the trials of beta-blockers. No other outcomes were reported.

Amiodarone

The effect of this medication was assessed in the meta-analytic study by Crystal *et al* [14] who assessed the effectiveness of this medication in nine trials including 1,384 patients. Wurdeman *et al* [15] reported the effectiveness and safety of amiodarone in five trials. Overall, there was a 52% reduction in the rate of atrial fibrillation (95% CI 39%-63%) [14]. The difference between amiodarone and placebo groups with regard to adverse drug reaction (ADR) was not substantial (ADR, 2%; 95% CI -2.5-11%) [15]. In the five trials reporting LOS, amiodarone was associated with a 0.91 days reduction in LOS (95% CI -1.59 to -0.24) [14]. As in the case of beta-blockers, no stroke reduction was observed in these trials [14].

One recent randomised clinical trial [16,17] has shown that oral amiodarone is effective even in patients who received pre-operative beta-blocker prophylaxis as a standard of care (22.5% vs 38%, p=0.01). The study also reported reduction of cerebrovascular accidents (1.7% vs 7.0%, p=0.04). However, the rates of atrial fibrillation (38%) and cerebrovascular accidents (7%) in the control group was much higher than it would have been expected in the beta-blocker treated population [14].

Sotalol

There were eight trials combined in the review by Crystal *et al* [14]. Trials enrolled 1,294 patients and there was a 65% reduction in the odds of AF (95% CI 51%-74%). AF incidence was reduced from 37% to 17%. There were four trials enrolling 900 patients that directly compared sotalol with other beta-blockers. AF incidence was reduced from 22% to 12% as compared to other beta-blockers (OR, 0.50; 95% CI 0.34-0.74). However, in five trials combined by Wurdeman [15], sotalol was associated with significant ADRs, that resulted in discontinuation of the medication (difference between drug and placebo 9.7%, p=0.048). Additionally, there was only a tendency toward reduction in LOS (-0.4 days; 95%CI -0.87-0.08) and no stroke reduction was observed [14]. Finally, although sotalol might be cheaper than amiodarone, it can be associated with renal problems and decreased cardiac output as compared to amiodarone. Thus, it should be reserved for healthier patients if ever considered [15].

Pacing

The issue of atrial pacing was highlighted by the prospective cohort study report that found a higher risk of atrial fibrillation in patients who have had an experience of atrial pacing [2]. However, these results might have been biased by the use of atrial pacing in patients who already had atrial fibrillation and non-consideration of timing. There were ten randomised clinical trials conducted after this report and the combined effect of these trials has shown a decrease in the odds of atrial fibrillation ranging from 32% to 54%, conditional on the mode of pacing employed [14]. Daoud *et al* [18] combined the results of eight trials and reported a 2.6 fold reduction in the odds of atrial fibrillation (95% CI 1.4-4.8) associated with overdrive bi-atrial pacing and a 2.5 fold reduction associated with fixed high-rate bi-atrial pacing. Right atrial pacing seemed to be a little less effective (OR, 1.8; 95% CI 1.1-2.7). As most of these trials were published less than five years ago, they are not yet widely applicable and further studies comparing or combining this strategy with pharmacologic prophylaxis are warranted.

General thoracic surgery

Calcium channel blockers

Atrial tachyarrhythmia

Four trials on calcium channel blockers [7,19-21] (three studies of verapamil and one study of diltiazem) assessed AT and enrolled 618 patients. The overall incidence was 10.6% in the medication group and 21.5% in the placebo group (RR, 0.50; 95% CI 0.34-0.73). There was evidence of 11 ATs averted per 100 patients treated (95% CI -17 to -5) (Figure 1).

Hypotension and bradycardia

All four trials reported the incidence of hypotension and three trials (total n=290) reported the incidence of bradycardia. The overall incidence of hypotension was 7.4% in the medication group and 0.6% in the placebo group.

Severe pulmonary complications

All four trials (total n=618) reported ARDS incidence. Overall incidence was 2.6% in the medication group and 2.0% in the placebo group (RR, 1.31; with a tendency of one additional event per 100 patients treated).

Beta-blockers

Atrial tachyarrhythmia

Two trials of beta-blockers [22,23] (one trial of metoprolol and one of propranolol) reported AT and enrolled 129 patients. The overall incidence was 9.4% in the medication group and 23.1% in the placebo group (RR, 0.40; 95% CI 0.17-0.95). There was evidence of 14 ATs averted per 100 patients treated (95% CI -26 to -2).

Hypotension and bradycardia

One trial [22] (n=99) reported this information. Hypotension incidence was 49.0% in the medication group and 26.0% in the placebo group.

Severe pulmonary complications

The overall incidence of pulmonary oedema was reported to be 14.1% in the medication group and 6.2% in the placebo group (RR, 2.15; with a tendency toward eight additional events per 100 patients treated). These findings were in line with the Cochrane review that reported a tendency toward a higher risk of pulmonary dysfunction associated with beta-blocker use in the COPD population [11,12].

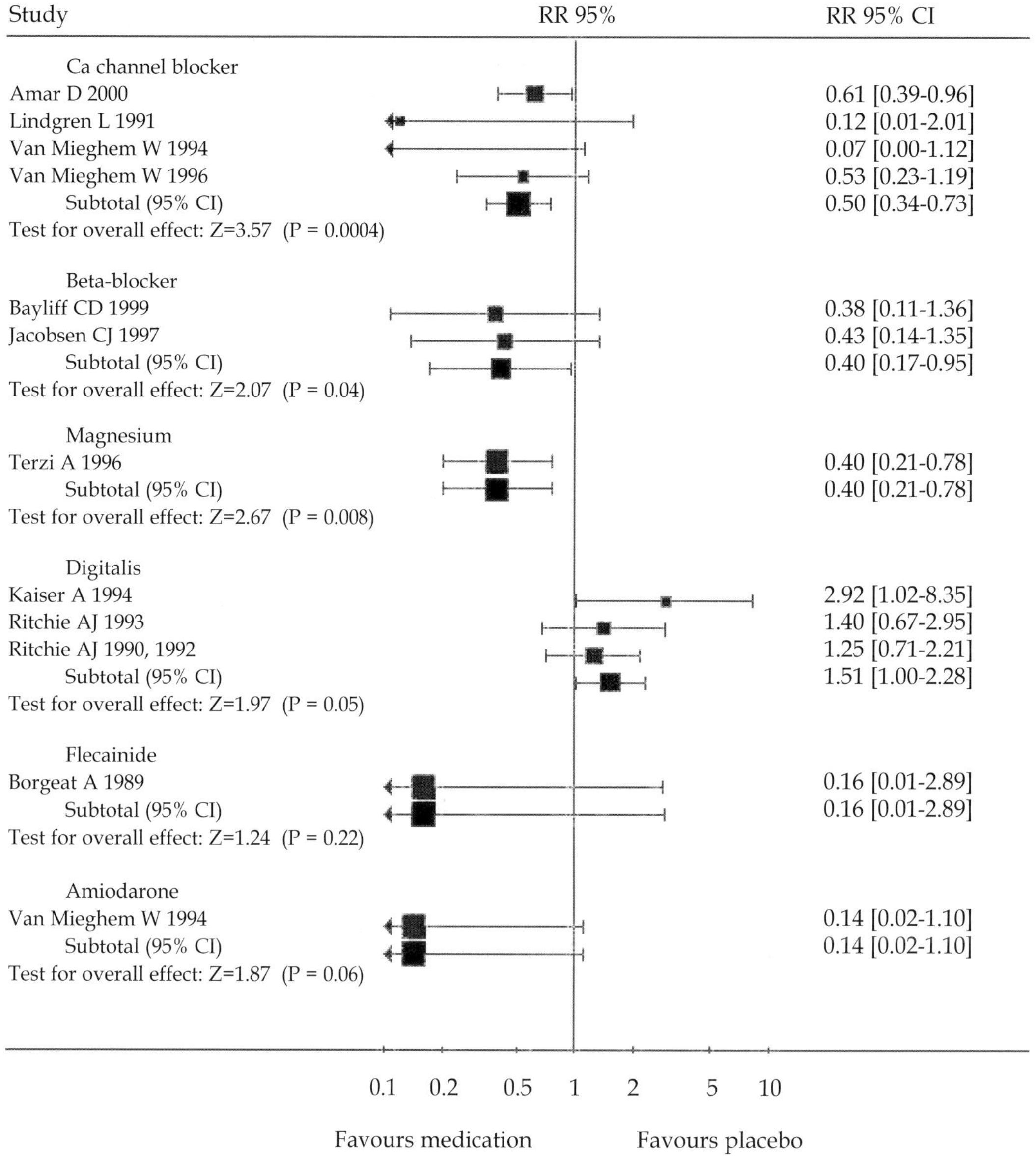

Figure 1. **Forest plot of relative risks (95% confidence intervals) of atrial tachyarrhythmia stratified by class of anti-arrhythmic medication in general thoracic surgery.**

Digitalis

Atrial tachyarrhythmia

There were three trials investigating the efficacy and safety of digitalis [24-26]. AT was assessed in all three trials of digitalis including 285 patients (Figure 1). In two of the trials "dysrhythmia" incidence was reported [24,25] while in the third trial, atrial tachyarrhythmia was determined. The overall incidence was 30.2% in the digitalis group and 19.9% in the placebo group (RR, 1.51; 95% CI 1.00-2.28).

Hypotension and bradycardia

No information on hypotension was available in the studies. Bradycardia was assessed in two trials including 209 patients. The overall incidence was 9.8% in the digitalis group and 1.9% in the placebo group.

Severe pulmonary complications

No information on the incidence of this outcome was available in the studies.

Others

Magnesium

Atrial tachyarrhythmia

There was one trial enrolling 194 patients [27]. The overall incidence was 10.7% in the medication group and 26.7% in the placebo group (RR, 0.40; 95% CI 0.21-0.78).

Hypotension and bradycardia

There were no events of hypotension and bradycardia reported in the trial.

Severe pulmonary complications

There was no information on the incidence of this outcome in the study.

Amiodarone

Atrial tachyarrhythmia

There was one trial enrolling 62 patients [20]. The overall incidence of AT was 3.1% in the medication group and 21.9% in the placebo group (RR, 0.14; 95% CI 0.02-1.10).

Hypotension and bradycardia

The incidence of hypotension was 3.1% in the medication group and 3.1% in the placebo group. Bradycardia occurred in 3.1% of the medication group and 0% of the placebo group.

Severe pulmonary complications

The overall incidence reported was ARDS and it occurred in 9.4% of the medication group and 0% of the placebo group with a tendency toward nine additional events per 100 patients treated.

Flecainide

Atrial tachyarrhythmia

There was one trial enrolling 30 patients [28]. The overall incidence was 0% in the medication group and 18.7% in the placebo group (RR, 0.16; 95% CI 0.01-2.89).

Hypotension and bradycardia

The overall incidence of hypotension was 57.1% in the medication group and 0% in the placebo group. There were no events of bradycardia reported in 30 enrolled patients.

Severe pulmonary complications

There were no events reported in the trial (n=30).

Recommendations - Cardiac surgery	Evidence level
◆ Further trials comparing anti-arrhythmic medications with placebo are not necessary.	I/A
◆ Beta-blockers should be considered a first choice as they seem to be effective, relatively safe and less costly.	I/A
◆ A rigorous cost-effectiveness analysis of amiodarone as a combination therapy with beta-blockers should be performed.	I/A
◆ Sotalol seems to be the least safe alternative and although it might be more effective than beta-blockers, it should be reserved for the healthiest population of patients.	I/A
◆ Calcium channel blockers and atrial pacing are associated with a reduced risk of atrial tachyarrhythmia after surgery. Further studies should clarify their indications.	I/A
Recommendations - General thoracic surgery	
◆ Calcium channel blockers and beta-blockers are associated with a reduction in AT to less than half of the incidence in the controls.	I/A & I/B
◆ There is a theoretical possibility that beta-blockers may interact with operative stress in the general thoracic surgical setting and worsen pre-existing pulmonary dysfunction in lung cancer patients. Calcium channel blockers on the other hand are known to reduce pulmonary vascular resistance and right ventricular pressure in addition to their anti-arrhythmic effect [19,29]. Thus, calcium channel blockers should be considered a first choice, as they seem to be a relatively safer alternative.	I/A & I/B
◆ RCTs do not support the use of digitalis for antiarrythmia prophylaxis in general thoracic surgery. Magnesium, amiodarone and flecainide were each tested in one trial and their effects are associated with uncertainty. The value of magnesium as a supplement to the main anti-arrhythmia regimen warrants further investigation [30].	I/A & I/B

References

1. Aranki SF, Shaw DP, Adams DH, *et al.* Predictors of atrial fibrillation after coronary artery bypass surgery. Current trends and impact on hospital resources. *Circulation* 1996; 94(3): 390-7.
2. Mathew JP, Parks R, Savino JS, *et al.* Atrial fibrillation following coronary artery bypass graft surgery: predictors, outcomes, and resource utilization. Multicenter study of perioperative ischemia research group. *JAMA* 1996; 276(4): 300-6.
3. Almassi GH, Schowalter T, Nicolosi AC, Aggarval A, Moritz TE, Henderson WG. Atrial fibrillation after cardiac surgery: a major morbid event? *Ann Surg* 1997; 226(4): 501-11; discussion 511-3.
4. Creswell LL, Schuessler RB, Rosenbloom M, Cox JL. Hazards of postoperative atrial arrhythmias. *Ann Thorac Surg* 1993; 56: 539-49.
5. Nickerson NJ, Murphy SF, Davila-Roman VG, Schechtman KB, Kouchoukos NT. Obstacles to early discharge after cardiac surgery. *Am J Manag Car*e 1999; 5(1): 29-34.
6. De Decker K, Jorens PG, Van Schil P. Cardiac complications after noncardiac thoracic surgery: an evidence-based current review. *Ann Thorac Surg* 2003; 75(4): 1340-8.
7. Amar D, Roistacher N, Rusch VW, *et al.* Effects of diltiazem prophylaxis on the incidence and clinical outcome of atrial arrhythmias after thoracic surgery. *J Thorac Cardiovasc Surg* 2000; 120(4): 790-8.
8. Amar D, Burt M, Reinsel RA, Leung DH. Relationship of early postoperative dysrhythmias and long-term outcome after resection of non-small cell lung cancer. *Chest* 1996; 110(2): 437-9.
9. Curtis JJ, Parker BM, McKenney CA, *et al.* Incidence and predictors of supraventricular dysrhythmias after pulmonary resection. *Ann Thorac Surg* 1998; 66(5): 1766-71.
10. Lanza LA, Visbal AI, DeValeria PA, Zinsmeister AR, Diehl NN, Trastek VF. Low-dose oral amiodarone prophylaxis reduces atrial fibrillation after pulmonary resection. *Ann Thorac Surg* 2003; 75(1): 223-30; discussion 230.
11. Salpeter S, Ormiston T, Salpeter E, Wood-Baker R. Cardioselective beta-blockers for reversible airway disease (Cochrane Review). In: *The Cochrane Library*, Issue 2, 2003, Oxford.
12. Salpeter SS, Ormiston T, Salpeter E, Poole P, Cates C. In: *The Cochrane Library*, Issue 2, 2003, Oxford.
13. Wijeysundera DN, Beatie WS, Rao V, Karski J. Calcium antagonists reduce cardiovascular complications after cardiac surgery: a meta-analysis. *J Am Coll Cardiol* 2003; 41(9): 1506-9.
14. Crystal E, Connoly SJ, Sleik K, Ginger TJ, Yusuf S. Interventions on prevention of postoperative atrial fibrillation in patients undergoing heart surgery. *Circulation* 2002; 106: 75-80.
15. Wurdeman RJ, Moss AN, Mohiuddin SM, Lenz TL. Amiodarone vs Sotalol as prophylaxis against atrial fibrillation/flutter after heart surgery. *Chest* 2002; 121: 1203-1210.
16. Giri S, White CM, Dunn AB, *et al.* Oral amiodarone for prevention of atrial fibrillation after open heart surgery, the Atrial Fibrillation Supression Trial (AFIST): a randomised placebo-controlled trial. *Lancet* 2001; 357(9259): 830-6.
17. Kluger J, White CM. Amiodarone prevents symptomatic atrial fibrillation and reduces the risk of cerebrovascular accidents and ventricular tachyarrhythmia after open heart surgery: results of the Atrial Fibrillation Supression trial (AFIST). *Card Electrophysiol Rev* 2003; 7(2): 165-7.
18. Daoud EG, Snow R, Hummel JD, Kalbfleisch SJ, Weiss R, Augostini R. Temporary atrial epicardial pacing as prophylaxis against atrial fibrillation after heart surgery: a meta analysis. *J Cardiovasc Electrophysiol* 2003; 14(2): 127-32.
19. Lindgren L, Lepantalo M, von Knorring J, Rosenberg P, Orko R, Scheinin B. Effect of verapamil on right ventricular pressure and atrial tachyarrhythmia after thoracotomy. *Br J Anaesth* 1991; 66(2): 205-11.
20. Van Mieghem W, Coolen L, Malysse I, Lacquet LM, Deneffe GJ, Demedts MG. Amiodarone and the development of ARDS after lung surgery. *Chest* 1994; 105(6): 1642-5.
21. Van Mieghem W, Tits G, Demuynck K, *et al.* Verapamil as prophylactic treatment for atrial fibrillation after lung operations. *Ann Thorac Surg* 1996; 61(4): 1083-5; discussion 1086.
22. Bayliff CD, Massel DR, Inculet RI, *et al.* Propranolol for the prevention of postoperative arrhythmias in general thoracic surgery. *Ann Thorac Surg* 1999; 67(1): 182-6.
23. Jakobsen CJ, Bille S, Ahlburg P, Rybro L, Hjortholm K, Andresen EB. Perioperative metoprolol reduces the frequency of atrial fibrillation after thoracotomy for lung resection. *J Cardiothorac Vasc Anesth* 1997; 11(6): 746-51.
24. Ritchie AJ, Bowe P, Gibbons JR. Prophylactic digitalization for thoracotomy: a reassessment. *Ann Thorac Surg* 1990; 50(1): 86-8.
25. Ritchie AJ, Tolan M, Whiteside M, McGuigan JA, Gibbons JR. Prophylactic digitalization fails to control dysrhythmia in thoracic esophageal operations. *Ann Thorac Surg* 1993; 55(1): 86-8.
26. Kaiser A, Zund G, Weder W, Largiader F. [Preventive digitalis therapy in open thoracotomy]. *Helv Chir Acta* 1994; 60(6): 913-7.
27. Terzi A, Furlan G, Chiavacci P, Dal Corso B, Luzzani A, Dalla Volta S. Prevention of atrial tachyarrhythmias after non-cardiac thoracic surgery by infusion of magnesium sulfate. *Thorac Cardiovasc Surg* 1996; 44(6): 300-3.
28. Borgeat A, Biollaz J, Bayer-Berger M, Kappenberger L, Chapuis G, Chiolero R. Prevention of arrhythmias by flecainide after noncardiac thoracic surgery. *Ann Thorac Surg* 1989; 48(2): 232-4.
29. Amar D, Roistacher N, Burt M, Reinsel RA, Ginsberg RJ, Wilson RS. Clinical and echocardiographic correlates of symptomatic tachydysrhythmias after noncardiac thoracic surgery. *Chest* 1995; 108(2): 349-54.
30. Wilkes NJ, Mallett SV, Peachey T, Di Salvo C, Walesby R. Correction of ionized plasma magnesium during cardiopulmonary bypass reduces the risk of postoperative cardiac arrhythmia. *Anesth Analg* 2002; 95(4): 828-34.